Antimicrobial Prescribing and Stewardship, 1st Volume

Antimicrobial Prescribing and Stewardship, 1st Volume

Editor

Diane Ashiru-Oredope

MDPI • Basel • Beijing • Wuhan • Barcelona • Belgrade • Manchester • Tokyo • Cluj • Tianjin

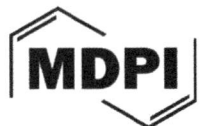

Editor
Diane Ashiru-Oredope
HCAI and AMR Division
UK Health Security
London
United Kingdom

Editorial Office
MDPI
St. Alban-Anlage 66
4052 Basel, Switzerland

This is a reprint of articles from the Special Issue published online in the open access journal *Antibiotics* (ISSN 2079-6382) (available at: www.mdpi.com/journal/antibiotics/special_issues/prescribing_antibiotic).

For citation purposes, cite each article independently as indicated on the article page online and as indicated below:

LastName, A.A.; LastName, B.B.; LastName, C.C. Article Title. *Journal Name* **Year**, *Volume Number*, Page Range.

ISBN 978-3-0365-7255-0 (Hbk)
ISBN 978-3-0365-7254-3 (PDF)

© 2023 by the authors. Articles in this book are Open Access and distributed under the Creative Commons Attribution (CC BY) license, which allows users to download, copy and build upon published articles, as long as the author and publisher are properly credited, which ensures maximum dissemination and a wider impact of our publications.

The book as a whole is distributed by MDPI under the terms and conditions of the Creative Commons license CC BY-NC-ND.

Contents

About the Editor ix

Preface to "Antimicrobial Prescribing and Stewardship, 1st Volume" xi

Gina Maki, Ingrid Smith, Sarah Paulin, Linda Kaljee, Watipaso Kasambara and Jessie Mlotha et al.
Feasibility Study of the World Health Organization Health Care Facility-Based Antimicrobial Stewardship Toolkit for Low- and Middle-Income Countries
Reprinted from: *Antibiotics* **2020**, *9*, 556, doi:10.3390/antibiotics9090556 1

Nasser M. Kaplan, Yousef S. Khader, Mahmoud A. Alfaqih, Rami Saadeh and Lora Al Sawalha
Implementation of the WHO Approved "Tailoring Antimicrobial Resistance Programs (TAP)" Reduces Patients' Request for Antibiotics
Reprinted from: *Antibiotics* **2020**, *9*, 507, doi:10.3390/antibiotics9080507 17

Wei Ping Khor, Omotayo Olaoye, Nikki D'Arcy, Eva M. Krockow, Rasha Abdelsalam Elshenawy and Victoria Rutter et al.
The Need for Ongoing Antimicrobial Stewardship during the COVID-19 Pandemic and Actionable Recommendations
Reprinted from: *Antibiotics* **2020**, *9*, 904, doi:10.3390/antibiotics9120904 29

Diane Ashiru-Oredope, Frances Kerr, Stephen Hughes, Jonathan Urch, Marisa Lanzman and Ting Yau et al.
Assessing the Impact of COVID-19 on Antimicrobial Stewardship Activities/Programs in the United Kingdom
Reprinted from: *Antibiotics* **2021**, *10*, 110, doi:10.3390/antibiotics10020110 41

David Musoke, Freddy Eric Kitutu, Lawrence Mugisha, Saba Amir, Claire Brandish and Deborah Ikhile et al.
A One Health Approach to Strengthening Antimicrobial Stewardship in Wakiso District, Uganda
Reprinted from: *Antibiotics* **2020**, *9*, 764, doi:10.3390/antibiotics9110764 55

Gwen M. Rees, Alison Bard and Kristen K. Reyher
Designing a National Veterinary Prescribing Champion Programme for Welsh Veterinary Practices: The Arwain Vet Cymru Project
Reprinted from: *Antibiotics* **2021**, *10*, 253, doi:10.3390/antibiotics10030253 71

Usman O. Adekanye, Abel B. Ekiri, Erika Galipó, Abubakar Bala Muhammad, Ana Mateus and Roberto M. La Ragione et al.
Knowledge, Attitudes and Practices of Veterinarians Towards Antimicrobial Resistance and Stewardship in Nigeria
Reprinted from: *Antibiotics* **2020**, *9*, 453, doi:10.3390/antibiotics9080453 89

Ana Belén Guisado-Gil, Manuela Aguilar-Guisado, Germán Peñalva, José Antonio Lepe, Ildefonso Espigado and Eduardo Rodríguez-Arbolí et al.
Long-Term Impact of an Educational Antimicrobial Stewardship Program on Management of Patients with Hematological Diseases
Reprinted from: *Antibiotics* **2021**, *10*, 136, doi:10.3390/antibiotics10020136 105

Leah F. Jones, Heidi Williamson, Petronella Downing, Donna M. Lecky, Diana Harcourt and Cliodna McNulty
A Qualitative Investigation of the Acceptability and Feasibility of a Urinary Tract Infection Patient Information Leaflet for Older Adults and Their Carers
Reprinted from: *Antibiotics* 2021, 10, 83, doi:10.3390/antibiotics10010083 119

Atsushi Uda, Katsumi Shigemura, Koichi Kitagawa, Kayo Osawa, Kenichiro Onuma and Yonmin Yan et al.
Risk Factors for the Acquisition of *Enterococcus faecium* Infection and Mortality in Patients with Enterococcal Bacteremia: A 5-Year Retrospective Analysis in a Tertiary Care University Hospital
Reprinted from: *Antibiotics* 2021, 10, 64, doi:10.3390/antibiotics10010064 135

Olaolu Oloyede, Emma Cramp and Diane Ashiru-Oredope
Antimicrobial Stewardship: Development and Pilot of an Organisational Peer-to-Peer Review Tool to Improve Service Provision in Line with National Guidance
Reprinted from: *Antibiotics* 2021, 10, 44, doi:10.3390/antibiotics10010044 147

Varidhi Nauriyal, Shankar Man Rai, Rajesh Dhoj Joshi, Buddhi Bahadur Thapa, Linda Kaljee and Tyler Prentiss et al.
Evaluation of an Antimicrobial Stewardship Program for Wound and Burn Care in Three Hospitals in Nepal
Reprinted from: *Antibiotics* 2020, 9, 914, doi:10.3390/antibiotics9120914 155

Lesley A. Hawes, Jaclyn Bishop, Kirsty Buising and Danielle Mazza
Feasibility and Validity of a Framework for Antimicrobial Stewardship in General Practice: Key Stakeholder Interviews
Reprinted from: *Antibiotics* 2020, 9, 900, doi:10.3390/antibiotics9120900 167

Francesco Cogliati Dezza, Ambrogio Curtolo, Lorenzo Volpicelli, Giancarlo Ceccarelli, Alessandra Oliva and Mario Venditti
Are Follow-Up Blood Cultures Useful in the Antimicrobial Management of Gram Negative Bacteremia? A Reappraisal of Their Role Based on Current Knowledge
Reprinted from: *Antibiotics* 2020, 9, 895, doi:10.3390/antibiotics9120895 179

Elisa Barbieri, Maia De Luca, Marta Minute, Carmen D'Amore, Marta Luisa Ciofi Degli Atti and Stefano Martelossi et al.
Impact and Sustainability of Antibiotic Stewardship in Pediatric Emergency Departments: Why Persistence Is the Key to Success
Reprinted from: *Antibiotics* 2020, 9, 867, doi:10.3390/antibiotics9120867 195

Flavien Bouchet, Vincent Le Moing, Delphine Dirand, François Cros, Alexi Lienard and Jacques Reynes et al.
Effectiveness and Acceptance of Multimodal Antibiotic Stewardship Program: Considering Progressive Implementation and Complementary Strategies
Reprinted from: *Antibiotics* 2020, 9, 848, doi:10.3390/antibiotics9120848 211

Danielle McDonald, Christina Gagliardo, Stephanie Chiu and M. Cecilia Di Pentima
Impact of a Rapid Diagnostic Meningitis/Encephalitis Panel on Antimicrobial Use and Clinical Outcomes in Children
Reprinted from: *Antibiotics* 2020, 9, 822, doi:10.3390/antibiotics9110822 225

Sam Ghebrehewet, Wendi Shepherd, Edwin Panford-Quainoo, Saran Shantikumar, Valerie Decraene and Rajesh Rajendran et al.
Implementation of a Delayed Prescribing Model to Reduce Antibiotic Prescribing for Suspected Upper Respiratory Tract Infections in a Hospital Outpatient Department, Ghana
Reprinted from: *Antibiotics* 2020, 9, 773, doi:10.3390/antibiotics9110773 235

Stéphanie Sirard, Claire Nour Abou Chakra, Marie-France Langlois, Julie Perron, Alex Carignan and Louis Valiquette
Is Antimicrobial Dosing Adjustment Associated with Better Outcomes in Patients with Severe Obesity and Bloodstream Infections? An Exploratory Study
Reprinted from: *Antibiotics* **2020**, *9*, 707, doi:10.3390/antibiotics9100707 247

Miroslav Fajfr, Michal Balik, Eva Cermakova and Pavel Bostik
Effective Treatment for Uncomplicated Urinary Tract Infections with Oral Fosfomycin, Single Center Four Year Retrospective Study
Reprinted from: *Antibiotics* **2020**, *9*, 511, doi:10.3390/antibiotics9080511 259

David Y. Graham
Transitioning of *Helicobacter pylori* Therapy from Trial and Error to Antimicrobial Stewardship
Reprinted from: *Antibiotics* **2020**, *9*, 671, doi:10.3390/antibiotics9100671 269

Giovanni Autore, Luca Bernardi and Susanna Esposito
Update on Acute Bone and Joint Infections in Paediatrics: A Narrative Review on the Most Recent Evidence-Based Recommendations and Appropriate Antinfective Therapy
Reprinted from: *Antibiotics* **2020**, *9*, 486, doi:10.3390/antibiotics9080486 287

Louise Ackers, Gavin Ackers-Johnson, Maaike Seekles, Joe Odur and Samuel Opio
Opportunities and Challenges for Improving Anti-Microbial Stewardship in Low- and Middle-Income Countries; Lessons Learnt from the Maternal Sepsis Intervention in Western Uganda
Reprinted from: *Antibiotics* **2020**, *9*, 315, doi:10.3390/antibiotics9060315 301

Jacqueline Sneddon, Daniel Afriyie, Israel Sefah, Alison Cockburn, Frances Kerr and Lucie Byrne-Davis et al.
Developing a Sustainable Antimicrobial Stewardship (AMS) Programme in Ghana: Replicating the Scottish Triad Model of Information, Education and Quality Improvement
Reprinted from: *Antibiotics* **2020**, *9*, 636, doi:10.3390/antibiotics9100636 319

Panagiotis Efthymiou, Despoina Gkentzi and Gabriel Dimitriou
Knowledge, Attitudes and Perceptions of Medical Students on Antimicrobial Stewardship
Reprinted from: *Antibiotics* **2020**, *9*, 821, doi:10.3390/antibiotics9110821 331

Omotayo Olaoye, Chloe Tuck, Wei Ping Khor, Roisin McMenamin, Luke Hudson and Mike Northall et al.
Improving Access to Antimicrobial Prescribing Guidelines in 4 African Countries: Development and Pilot Implementation of an App and Cross-Sectional Assessment of Attitudes and Behaviour Survey of Healthcare Workers and Patients
Reprinted from: *Antibiotics* **2020**, *9*, 555, doi:10.3390/antibiotics9090555 345

About the Editor

Diane Ashiru-Oredope

Professor Diane Ashiru-Oredope PhD FFRPS, FRPharmS is the Lead Pharmacist for healthcare-associated infections (HCAI) and antimicrobial resistance (AMR) at the UK Health Security Agency, and she is the chair of the English Surveillance Programme for Antimicrobial Utilisation and Resistance (ESPAUR). She is the Honorary Chair and Professor of Pharmaceutical Public Health at the University of Nottingham.

An antimicrobial pharmacist by background, Diane has led several projects that have shaped national and international policy in tackling antimicrobial resistance, including creating the global Antibiotic Guardian campaign in 2014. From 2016 to March 2022, she was an advisor and Global AMR leader for the Commonwealth Pharmacists Association. Diane remains active in research areas, with more than 70 peer-reviewed publications, and she is one of the editors for the BMC Public Health journal. She recently led a UK-wide evidence review on Pharmaceutical Public Health, commissioned by the four UK Chief Pharmaceutical Officers. In 2022, she was credentialed as a consultant pharmacist through the Royal Pharmaceutical Society's national credentialing and assessment processes. She has been recognised nationally, including through awards, nominations to deliver two TEDx talks, and fellowships with the Royal Pharmaceutical Society (FRPharmS and FFRPS).

Preface to "Antimicrobial Prescribing and Stewardship, 1st Volume"

Antimicrobial stewardship as coherent set of actions which promote using antimicrobials in ways that ensure sustainable access to effective therapy for all who need them"(Dyar, O.J.; 2017) is critical (alongside, e.g., infection prevention and control strategies) for tackling antimicrobial resistance/drug-resistant infections.

This Antimicrobial Prescribing and Stewardship Issue (Volume 1) consist of manuscripts, including original research, review articles, case series, and opinion papers for topics related to antimicrobial (antibiotic, antifungal) stewardship, including:

Disease-based/organism-based antimicrobial stewardship;

Diagnostic stewardship;

Influence of antimicrobial utilisation changes in antimicrobial resistance;

Impact of antimicrobial stewardship on quality performance measures and patient outcomes;

Novel antimicrobial stewardship education and training approaches or interventions aimed at the public and/or healthcare workers;

Behavioural change approaches to antimicrobial stewardship;

Collaborative practice agreements in antimicrobial stewardship;

Antimicrobial stewardship in special populations (e.g., paediatrics, geriatrics, emergency medicine, hematology/oncology);

Tackling AMR through antimicrobial stewardship in low- and middle-income countries;

Antimicrobial stewardship for animal health;

Antimicrobial stewardship in alternative settings (e.g., community practice, long-term care, and resource-limited small and rural hospitals);

Antimicrobial use and stewardship in the context of the COVID-19 pandemic;

Global collaborations to tackle AMR through antimicrobial stewardship.

This edition also aimed to include articles that recognize the theme for World Antimicrobial Awareness Week 2020, "United to preserve antimicrobials", with papers which consider the impact of global collaborations and health partnerships being invited to contribute.

World Antimicrobial Awareness Week (WAAW), led globally by the WHO, aims to increase awareness of global antimicrobial resistance (AMR) and to encourage best practices among the public, health workers, and policy makers to avoid the further emergence and spread of drug-resistant infections.

We also built on the success of this edition and there is a second volume on "Antimicrobial Prescribing and Stewardship, 2nd Volume".

Diane Ashiru-Oredope
Editor

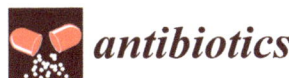

Article

Feasibility Study of the World Health Organization Health Care Facility-Based Antimicrobial Stewardship Toolkit for Low- and Middle-Income Countries

Gina Maki [1,*], Ingrid Smith [2], Sarah Paulin [2], Linda Kaljee [3], Watipaso Kasambara [4], Jessie Mlotha [4], Pem Chuki [5], Priscilla Rupali [6], Dipendra R. Singh [7], Deepak C. Bajracharya [8], Lisa Barrow [9], Eliaser Johnson [9], Tyler Prentiss [3] and Marcus Zervos [1,10]

1. Division of Infectious Disease, Henry Ford Health System, Detroit, MI 48202, USA; mzervos1@hfhs.org
2. World Health Organization, 1202 Geneva, Switzerland; ismith@who.int (I.S.); paulins@who.int (S.P.)
3. Global Health Initiative, Henry Ford Health System, Detroit, MI 48202, USA; LKaljee1@hfhs.org (L.K.); TPRENTI1@hfhs.org (T.P.)
4. Ministry of Health, 207218 Lilongwe, Malawi; watipasokasa@yahoo.com (W.K.); rhodamgb@gmail.com (J.M.)
5. Jigme Dorji Wangchuck National Referral Hospital, 11001 Thimpu, Bhutan; pchuki@jdwnrh.gov.bt
6. Department of Infectious Diseases, Christian Medical College, Vellore 632004, India; priscillarupali@yahoo.com
7. Ministry of Health and Population, 44600 Kathmandu, Nepal; dipendra2028@gmail.com
8. Group for Technical Assistance, 44600 Kathmandu, Nepal; bajra.deepak@gmail.com
9. Department of Health & Social Affairs, 96941 Pohnpei, Federated States of Micronesia; lbarrow@fsmhealth.fm (L.B.); ejohnson@fsmhealth.fm (E.J.)
10. School of Medicine, Wayne State University, Detroit, MI 48202, USA
* Correspondence: gmaki1@hfhs.org; Tel.: +1-313-829-5751

Received: 20 July 2020; Accepted: 28 August 2020; Published: 29 August 2020

Abstract: Antimicrobial stewardship (AMS) has emerged as a systematic approach to optimize antimicrobial use and reduce antimicrobial resistance. To support the implementation of AMS programs, the World Health Organization developed a draft toolkit for health care facility AMS programs in low- and middle-income countries. A feasibility study was conducted in Bhutan, the Federated States of Micronesia, Malawi, and Nepal to obtain local input on toolkit content and implementation of AMS programs. This descriptive qualitative study included semi-structured interviews with national- and facility-level stakeholders. Respondents identified AMS as a priority and perceived the draft toolkit as a much-needed document to further AMS program implementation. Facilitators for implementing AMS included strong national and facility leadership and clinical staff engagement. Barriers included lack of human and financial resources, inadequate regulations for prescription antibiotic sales, and insufficient AMS training. Action items for AMS implementation included improved laboratory surveillance, establishment of a stepwise approach for implementation, and mechanisms for reporting and feedback. Recommendations to improve the AMS toolkit's content included additional guidance on defining the responsibilities of the committees and how to prioritize AMS programming based on local context. The AMS toolkit was perceived to be an important asset as countries and health care facilities move forward to implement AMS programs.

Keywords: antimicrobial resistance; antimicrobial stewardship; low- and middle-income countries; barriers and enablers

1. Introduction

The misuse of antimicrobials is one of the main drivers for the development of antimicrobial resistance (AMR) [1,2]. Antimicrobial stewardship (AMS) programs have been shown to be effective in reducing unneeded antimicrobial use and slowing AMR in high-income countries; however, there are limited data on the feasibility of AMS programs in low- and middle-income countries (LMIC) [3–6]. As a response, the World Health Organization (WHO) has developed a practical toolkit for health care facility-based AMS programs in LMIC (hereafter referred to as the "AMS toolkit") [7].

In 2015, at the 68th World Health Assembly, AMR was recognized as a threat to public health. A global action plan, including an objective to optimize the use of antimicrobials, was endorsed during the Assembly. AMS programs aim not only to optimize antimicrobial use, but also to improve patient outcomes, decrease rates of AMR, and reduce health care costs [8–11]. With few new antimicrobials being produced and the decreased effectiveness of existing antimicrobials, AMS programs are an essential component of a One Health approach to address AMR [12]. Many LMIC have inadequate AMS policies and treatment guidelines at both the national and health care facility levels, resulting in a disproportionate impact of AMR in these countries [1,2,11,13–15]. Intraregional, interdisciplinary collaborations and partnerships are needed at the national and facility level to adapt, implement, and disseminate AMS programs that are locally salient [16–18].

The AMS toolkit is divided into six sections: (1) Structural Core Elements for AMS Implementation at the National Level; (2) Structural Core Elements for AMS Implementation at the Facility Level; (3) Planning AMS programs; (4) Performing AMS interventions; (5) Assessing AMS programs; (6) Education and Training. As part of the AMS toolkit's development, a feasibility study was undertaken in Bhutan, the Federated States of Micronesia (FSM), Malawi, and Nepal. The study objectives were to (1) assess local knowledge and perceptions regarding AMR, AMS, and key concepts of the AMS toolkit; (2) identify barriers and facilitators for the implementation of AMS programs and policies; (3) identify recommendations to revise the AMS toolkit draft to ensure it meets the needs of a broad range of LMIC settings; (4) to provide recommendations to the countries on initiating and strengthening AMS programs. The study countries were selected based on geographic regions where AMR is a significant issue and where, to date, there are limited resources and AMS programs. These countries also represent different regions and varying healthcare systems (Table 1).

Table 1. Information on Health Care Systems, AMR Stewardship, and Pharmaceutical Sales by Country.

Country/Population	Country-Specific Details
Bhutan 727,000	**Health Care System:** Majority public funded health system with some private providers. The National Health System provides free health care, including pharmaceuticals. **AMR Stewardship:** The Bhutan NAP on AMR was launched by the Bhutan cabinet in May 2017. AMS is prioritized in the NAP; a hospital-based AMS program has been initiated and the National Referral Hospital will function as the National AMS Coordination Center. **Pharmaceutical Sales:** Sales of antimicrobials by prescription-only is regulated by the Drug Regulatory Authority and the ban of irrational fixed-dose combinations (FDCs) is consistent with the WHO restricted list of FDCs.
Federated States of Micronesia (FSM) 100,000	**Health Care System:** There is one public hospital within each of the four island states and a fifth private hospital on the island of Pohnpei. The Department of Health Services in each state provides medical and public health services through a hospital, community health centers, and dispensaries. Each state system is autonomous. Health services are highly subsidized by the state governments, except in private clinics. There are six private health clinics in the country and one private hospital. Transportation difficulties between islands often prevent outer island residents from accessing hospital services.[1]

Table 1. Cont.

Country/Population	Country-Specific Details
	AMR Stewardship: The NAP on AMR in FSM has been drafted, but not yet implemented country-wide. A technical working group (TWG) comprised of national-level policymakers has worked on the implementation of the NAP, but it has not yet been endorsed by Congress. An AMS program across hospitals and other community health facilities has been identified as a priority in the NAP. Representatives from each of the four states have also worked on the revising and editing of the NAP to make it applicable across the entirety of FSM. **Pharmaceutical Sales:** A bill on prescription-only regulation of all antibiotic sales is currently under advisement in the National Congress. Many patients within FSM are served by community dispensaries, particularly in the outer islands of the region where few qualified healthcare professionals are practicing. These dispensaries are undergoing a review of standards. Antibiotic purchasing is handled at the state level, guided by the National Essential Medicines List. When antibiotic inefficacy is suspected, quality control testing is undertaken in connection with the Therapeutic Goods Administration in Australia.
Malawi 18.6 million	**Health Care Services:** Health services in Malawi are provided by public, private for profit (PFP), and private not for profit (PNFP) sectors. Health services in the public sector are free-of-charge at the point of use. The PFP sector consists of private hospitals, clinics, laboratories, and pharmacies. Traditional healers are also prominent and would be classified as PFP. The PNFP sector comprises of religious institutions, nongovernmental organizations (NGOs), statutory corporations and companies.[2] **AMR Stewardship:** In 2015, a situational analysis of AMR was undertaken by the Ministry of Health. In 2017–2018, a NAP on AMR based on a One Health approach was developed and approved. **Pharmaceutical Sales:** Regulations to restrict nonprescription sale of antibiotics are limited and antibiotics are readily available in communities throughout Malawi. There are national-level guidelines, which were implemented in 2014; however, there is a need for revision to reflect the specific patterns of resistance throughout Malawi. A majority of antibiotics are prescribed without any definitive laboratory data on pathogen or resistance. Hospitals are dependent on donations for many pharmaceuticals, including antibiotics, and certain antibiotics may be overprescribed because of limited options.
Nepal 26 million	**Health Care System:** Nepal's health system includes public, private, and not-for-profit facilities. As part of the new federalist government system's restructuring, the public health system is being decentralized, with 16 tertiary hospitals being managed by the federal government and primary and secondary hospitals being managed at the provincial level. At the same time, the Ministry of Health and Population (MOHP) is expanding access to Universal Health Care throughout the country. **AMR Stewardship:** The MOHP has also established a multisector AMR Steering Committee inclusive of a TWG, which has been approved by the Deputy Prime Minister. As of 2019, a NAP on AMR has been drafted and includes AMS as a priority. **Pharmaceutical Sales:** Regulations to restrict nonprescription sale of antibiotics are limited, with little monitoring and enforcement of existing policies. Many remote areas do not have access to trained physicians, so other health providers must dispense antibiotics in public health centers.

[1] World Health Organization Western Pacific Region. 2017. Federated States of Micronesia: WHO Country Cooperation Strategy, 2018-2022. [2] Ministry of Health and Population, Republic of Malawi. The Health Care System. Available at: https://www.health.gov.mw/index.php/2016-01-06-19-58-23/national-aids.

2. Results

The following results are organized by national and health care facility core elements and health care facility-based interventions as described within the AMS toolkit. In addition, we have included data on actionable items and recommendations for the draft toolkit. A summary of demographic information is found in Table 2.

Table 2. Clinical Staff Demographics.

Demographic Description		Bhutan	Federated States of Micronesia	Malawi	Nepal
Total staff interviewed	-	16	21	16	12
Members of IPC committee	Yes	10	5	9	6
	No	6	12	2	5
	No IPC at institution	-	3	3	1
	No response	-	1	2	-
Average years at institution	-	8.0 (range 2–19)	14.2 (range 0.33–30)	7.2 years (range 0.75–14)	15.4 (range 1–35)
Average years working on AMR	-	6.9 (range 1–28)	9.8 (range 1–26)	5.1 years (range 0.33–21)	6.4 (range 1.5–20)
Facility classification	Public	16	20	16	5
	Private	0	1	0	4
	Non-profit	-	-	-	3

AMR—antimicrobial resistance; IPC—infection prevention and control.

Key findings from this study are shown in Table 3.

Table 3. Key findings for Implementation of AMS in LMIC.

Implementation Category	Key Findings
AMS implementation facilitators	• Strong national and health care facility leadership. • Clinical staff engagement in AMS committees.
AMS implementation barriers	• Inadequate human and financial resources. • Limited supplies of antibiotics, particularly in remote regions. • Lack of enforcement of regulations for prescription-only sales of antibiotics. • AMS competencies among health care workers and limited training and education in AMR, AMS, and IPC.
Recommendations to strengthen health care facility-based AMS	• Dedicated financial resources and AMS leaders and champions. • Use of stepwise approaches for AMS implementation based on country and health care facility contexts. • Mechanisms for reporting and feedback. • Implementation of interdisciplinary AMS training workshops and AMS curricula.

AMR—antimicrobial resistance; AMS—antimicrobial stewardship; IPC—infection prevention and control.

2.1. National Core Elements

The national core elements include (1) National Plan and Strategies; (2) Regulations and Guidelines; (3) Education and Training; (4) Supporting Technologies and Data.

2.1.1. National Plan and Strategies

All study countries identified AMR as a growing threat and have drafted an AMR National Action Plan (NAP); however, the countries were at various levels in terms of NAP implementation. Relatively few respondents outside of the national government were aware of the NAP content.

Remark 1. *"I have heard of the National Plan, but it is not being implemented in our medical college . . . ."* (Hospital Administrator, Nepal)

Study participants aware of the NAP reported dedicated high-level national leadership in support of the NAP. In addition, some countries have obtained outside funding to support portions of the NAP. However, across the four countries, numerous barriers were identified that affected the implementation of NAP policies and programs. These barriers included the need for additional financial support and technical assistance, limited laboratory capacity, including infrastructure and expertise, and lack of technical expertise on AMR-specific issues.

Remark 2. *" . . . again, it involves a lot of resources. You need to see the sensitivity and (do) surveillance . . . to review sensitivities . . . A lot of budget is involved in that. So, funding is another part (in terms of) feasibility or not. And of course, the human side and human resources are also important...."* (National Level, Nepal)

2.1.2. Regulations and Guidelines

Facilitators for AMR regulations and guidelines included the existence of drafted standard antibiotic prescribing guidelines, which have been developed in Bhutan, Malawi, and Nepal. In FSM, there is an antibiotic prescribing guideline that has been reviewed with national stakeholders and external technical expertise. FSM, Malawi, and Nepal are in the process of developing and implementing policies for prescription-only antibiotic sales. In Bhutan, prescription-only regulations are implemented and enforced. The key barriers identified included inadequate monitoring and evaluation at the national and regional levels for infection prevention and control (IPC) and AMS including adherence to guidelines, inadequate laboratory facilities to provide empiric diagnostic data and support, implementation of the AWaRe (Access, Watch, Reserve) classification of antibiotics, challenges with the supply chain of medications in hospital pharmacies, and lack of prescribers (physicians) in remote areas.

Remark 3. *" . . . .I'm not claiming that just writing in law will be sufficient to really restrict prescriptions for selling . . . we have so many pharmacies which have been already selling without prescriptions . . . we need to really go and then take action against those who are selling the antibiotics . . . at the same time in the public sector we are promoting some antibiotics to be used by [non-physicians] . . . because neonatal mortality [is] very high . . . "* (National Level, Nepal)

Remark 4. *" . . . If we don't have the drugs [in the hospital], the doctor will prescribe and then the patient is obligated to buy in a pharmacy . . . ."* (National Level, Malawi)

2.1.3. Awareness, Training, and Education

At the national level, there was strong support to enhance education and training in AMR/AMS for physicians, nurses, pharmacists, and laboratory staff. At the broader community level, AMS awareness, training, and education included public antibiotic information campaigns. Barriers included lack of dedicated financial support and limited training and technical expertise. Respondents also reported the need for more community advocacy and awareness of AMR.

Remark 5. *"... and we are also thinking to develop some sort of dramatizing ... learning materials and publishing to the media (for the community). So that type of materials we're planning to do. That requires a little bit budget so we are constrained with budget so we're planning anyway ... and also planning to do some training for health professionals ... primary, community levels–upper-level health professionals also need to have training ...." (National Level, Nepal)*

2.1.4. Supporting Technologies and Data

Bhutan, Malawi, and Nepal are recipients of Fleming Fund grants to expand microbiology laboratory capacity and strengthen surveillance systems [16]. Respondents perceived this support as a starting point to significantly enhance NAP implementation. However, respondents also recognized the need for more sustained funding and training in diagnostic testing, laboratory surveillance, and information technologies, and the struggle with inadequate local expertise in monitoring antimicrobial use and consumption.

Remark 6. *"So, we are so glad that at least one of our key priorities for the NAP–AMR surveillance—we have a country grant to support improving lab capacity and surveillance. So, that's a very good plus for us ...." (National Level, Malawi)*

2.2. Health Care Facility Core Elements

Health care facility core elements include (1) Leadership Commitment; (2) Accountability and Responsibilities; (3) Education and Training; (4) Monitoring and Surveillance; (5) Reporting and Feedback.

2.2.1. Leadership Commitment

A key component of facility-based AMS is dedicated support from facility leadership to encourage the development of AMS and IPC committees and implement programs. Facility leaders stated that the recommended AMS activities in the toolkit are feasible and necessary to decrease AMR. Barriers to leadership commitment included inadequate dedicated human and financial resources for AMS programs, and inadequate internal communication between administrators, management, and staff.

Remark 7. *"A successful stewardship program can only work when there is good collaboration between top management and middle-level management. Because middle-level management, they are the ones that are in touch with the staff on the ground there." (Hospital Administrator, Malawi)*

Remark 8. *"Stressing the importance of leadership commitment is really important. Because nothing really happens without leadership commitment." (National Level, FSM)*

2.2.2. Accountability and Responsibilities

Respondents described active IPC committees, quality improvement teams, and drug and therapeutic committees. These committees are engaged in routine activities and provide important feedback and training to clinical personnel. Building on these committees, leaders and clinical staff were enthusiastic about future implementation of AMS committees and antibiotic prescribing guidelines.

Remark 9. *"... we don't have an AMS team but the infection control committee they have nurse staff. They do regular monitoring of cultures of different areas of the theatre ... they take a routine culture on a regular basis ...." (Hospital Administrator, Nepal)*

Barriers included physicians' reluctance to change their prescribing practices, even with the available evidence-based guidelines, and provider-heavy workloads, which decreased interest in devoting time to an AMS committee.

Remark 10. *"We have an issue of shortages of staff ... we also have issues of people wearing too many hats, so that is part of, I guess, it's kind of like we're not sure who's going to take care of it, and wonder who which program is." (Clinical Staff, FSM)*

2.2.3. Education and Training

There was a high level of enthusiasm for expanding AMS education and training within health care facilities. Currently, some study facilities have an established education infrastructure (e.g., continuing medical education) that can support additional AMR/AMS training. However, despite enthusiasm, time and resources were barriers. Many facilities lack space and available expertise to support trainings. At some sites, even IPC trainings are limited due to inadequate resources. In addition, some respondents emphasized the need for a 'hands-on' approach to support sustained knowledge.

Remark 11. *"Major barriers as of right now is lack of knowledge mainly. We have high staff turnover, so in the last three years there have been no new trainings. Almost 75% of the staff may not be aware of the IP (infection prevention) practices ... ." (Clinical Staff, Malawi)*

Remark 12. *"So hands-on is a very, very important part of it. As compared to just reading and looking at the modules. But you have to apply, the application of that knowledge needs to be implemented as well. With the hands-on skills I think it will stick and will stay there longer, and be more useful to the people. In my opinion, I think two or more models of education is probably the best suitable for us in this setting."*

2.2.4. Monitoring and Surveillance

Among microbiologists and laboratory staff, there was a strong desire for capacity building and international support for up-to-date equipment and supplies and development of AMR surveillance systems. However, in most health care facility sites, there was inadequate capacity to conduct point prevalence surveys and routine surveillance of susceptibility patterns, including health care facility-specific antibiogram data.

Remark 13. *"For the lab, our major challenges are both human and material resources ... we have a very big challenge procuring laboratory microbiology supplies. Either maybe because of the budget or our major supplier—the central medical stores—they don't have them in stock ... ... we have the knowledge, but resources are not there ... ." (Clinical Staff, Malawi)*

2.2.5. Reporting and Feedback

In health care facilities with developed IPC committees, there are existing reporting and feedback structures in place that can be expanded to include AMS. However, in most facilities, there are inadequate structures for reporting these data to facility management and clinical staff. Study participants noted there was little communication between laboratory and clinical personnel, decreasing opportunities for information exchange about AMR patterns and impact of the use of specific antibiotics.

Remark 14. *" ... We are very much lacking in reporting and feedback. We can do something but this is one area we really have to really have to think and discuss with regards to core elements ... there are so many challenges, which we have to sit together and discuss and see how to move things forward." (Clinical Staff, Bhutan)*

2.3. Action Items at the National and Health Care Facility Level

Multiple action items were identified at both the national and facility level to move forward with implementation of the NAP and the WHO toolkit and development and implementation of AMS committees and other supporting programs and policies. Identification of sustainable funding and technical expertise in human, animal, and environmental health was essential across each of the core elements. Action items at the national and facility level are found in Boxes 1 and 2.

Box 1. National-level action items to support AMS and toolkit implementation.

- Establish terms of reference for National AMR technical working groups.
- Perform needs assessments of local laboratory capacity at the national and local levels.
- Update National Essential Medicine Lists or equivalent documents, including integration of the WHO AWaRe categories.
- Sensitize health care providers about AwaRE categories.
- Review, update, and implement national and district/state/regional antibiotic prescribing guidelines informed by available AMR surveillance data.
- Develop needed resources for health care facility leadership to ensure antibiotic prescribing guidelines are followed consistently across the country.
- Increase national antibiotic awareness campaigns.
- Develop or expand age-relevant education AMR/AMS programs in public school systems.
- Strengthen microbiology laboratory capacity and expand training to facility-based laboratory staff to support and encourage engagement in AMS and national surveillance.

AMR—antimicrobial resistance; AMS—antimicrobial stewardship.

Box 2. Health care facility-level action items to support AMS and toolkit implementation.

- Identify funding sources to support facility-level AMS.
- Sensitize facility leaders about the urgency of AMR as a health risk.
- Increase facility leaders' awareness of National Action Plan (NAP) content, government roll out plans, and potential funding and resources to support facility-based AMS.
- Develop stepwise approaches to implement AMS considering facility capacities throughout the country.
- Standardize IPC committee roles and responsibilities.
- Identify dedicated leaders and champions within facilities who will take responsibility for establishing AMS committees and implement AMS programs. In many instances, individuals involved in IPC, QIT, and DTC committees can serve as key stakeholders in this process.
- Develop/adapt standard antibiotic prescribing guidelines informed by local AMR surveillance data patterns.
- Strengthen laboratory capacity to ensure annual output of aggregate antibiograms and support regular reporting to national laboratories for AMR surveillance.
- Establish mechanisms for reporting and feedback on the implementation of AMS interventions and adherence to antibiotic prescribing guidelines based on international consensus and local input.
- Integrate AMS training into existing CME programs and IPC training initiatives across all health disciplines.
- Develop interdisciplinary training programs to support increased understanding and communication between wards and departments.
- Develop training-of-trainer workshops on AMS and cascade training to other health care providers in the health care facilities.

AMR—antimicrobial resistance; AMS—antimicrobial stewardship; CME—continuing medical education; DTC—drug and therapeutic committees; IPC—infection prevention and control; QIT—quality improvement teams.

2.4. Health Care Facility-Based AMS Interventions

The WHO toolkit provides a detailed overview of evidence-based health care facility AMS interventions including (1) persuasive, educational, and feedback; (2) restrictive; (3) structural interventions. The toolkit also includes information on planning, implementing, and assessing AMS programs. Identified enablers to support AMS interventions included strong leadership support at the health care facility administration level, overall strong interest in education and training in IPC, AMR, and AMS among clinical staff, and perceptions among staff that AMS interventions decrease unnecessary antibiotic use. Barriers included inadequate local infectious disease, AMR and AMS expertise, and limited financial and human resources to implement interventions and conduct program monitoring and evaluation.

Remark 15. *"When it comes to interventions I think they are very much appropriate because many of these problems do exist in our ... day-to-day practices. But we are not really assessing them ... to the fullest extent about the interventions." (Clinical Staff, Bhutan)*

2.5. Summary of Recommendations for the Draft WHO Toolkit

Study participants suggested recommendations on the improvement of content, organization, and presentation of materials, which were incorporated into the final version of the WHO AMS toolkit (Table 4). Participants also noted that the review of the AMS toolkit needs to be an iterative process as implementation of the toolkit and AMS programs and policies progress in each country.

Table 4. Key recommendations and implemented changes in the WHO AMS toolkit

Study Participants' Recommendations	Specific Changes to Toolkit	Toolkit Reference
Easy-to-follow directions in terms of which chapters were most relevant for specific audiences	Key target audience was added	Top of first page of all chapters
Additional information on how to prioritize AMS activities (short-, medium-, and long-term) and guidance on stratification of interventions and assessment procedures based on local resources. Guidance in prioritizing AMS activities based on available resources, establishing stronger linkages between existing programs, e.g., IPC and AMS, and instituting the roles and responsibilities of members of AMS committees.	• Key steps in establishing a national AMS program to enable facility AMS; • Key steps to establishing a health care facility AMS program; • Indicators from the Tripartite M&E framework for the Global Action Plan on AMR relevant to AMS programs; • Preparation for developing and implementing an AMS program in a health care facility; • Sample AMS review form.	Ch. 1, Page 3, Box 1 Ch. 1 Page 4, Box 2 Ch. 2, Page 10, Table 3 Ch. 4, Page 18, Table 5 Page 67, Annex IV
Definition of the role and function of an AMS champion. Definition of roles within AMS interventions for various types of health providers (e.g., physician, nurse, and microbiologist).	• Sample terms of reference national AMS technical working group; • Sample terms of reference health care facility AMS committee; • Sample terms of reference health care facility AMS team.	Page 63, Annex I Page 64, Annex II Page 66, Annex III
Information or resource links that can guide countries in the development of AMS and AMR antibiotic prescribing guidelines in regions without hospitals and physicians.	• Snapshot of GLASS; • Sample pre-authorization/restricted prescribing form; • Sample medical chart; • Sample bug–drug chart; • Sample cumulative antibiogram for Gram-negative bacteria;	Ch. 4, Page 29, Box 7 Page 68, Annex V Page 69, Annex VI Page 70, Annex VII Page 71, Annex VIII

Table 4. *Cont.*

Study Participants' Recommendations	Specific Changes to Toolkit	Toolkit Reference
Training information to support effective AMS and IPC committees in terms of leadership skills, division of staff roles and responsibilities, reporting and feedback systems, and interdisciplinary communication.	• Core components of IPC and the link to AMS;	Ch. 4, Page 23, Box 4
	• Step-by-step guide for setting up an AMC surveillance program at the facility level;	Ch. 4, Page 25, Box 5
	• Step-by-step guide for setting up a health care facility PPS;	Ch. 4, Page 26, Box 6
	• The quality improvement model in more detail;	Ch. 5, Page 34, Figure 15
	• Core steps for implementing an educational program.	Ch. 7, Page 60, Box 9

Remark 16. *"I think it's a good start. It has more stuff, areas that need to be stringent, if we kind of have an impact on this issue. And I think it's pretty comprehensive in a sense ... But I think it should be an organic process, as we move along and identify issues, we address them and continue to make improvements." (Clinical Staff, FSM)*

3. Discussion

The toolkit was universally well-received by policy makers, facility management, and clinical staff levels throughout the four study countries. Data were obtained from a diverse multinational and interdisciplinary group of stakeholders. Identification of possible enablers and barriers for toolkit implementation at the national and facility level supported revisions to ensure that the toolkit meets the needs of a broad range of LMIC settings. Each study country presented different contextual factors to consider regarding AMS implementation and use of the AMS toolkit. Varying factors included different health priorities at both the national and facility level, current status of nationalized universal health care plans, variances in public health funding, availability and use of antibiotics, and development and enforcement of prescription-only regulations. These factors must be considered on a country-by-country basis for stakeholder engagement and evaluating pathways to toolkit implementation.

Key facilitators and enablers included strong leadership commitment at the national, local, and facility levels, increases in funding mechanisms to support development of surveillance systems within countries, and increased awareness of AMR. Key barriers to AMS implementation included limited human and financial resources, inadequate supporting technologies (e.g., monitoring and surveillance), and communication challenges between facility administration and staff, and between staff members. These barriers can be mitigated using a clear step-by-step approach, as indicated in the WHO AMS toolkit, tailored to specific country and facility contexts and needs. In addition, a multidisciplinary training and education approach can potentially strengthen AMS commitment and communication within health care facilities.

Prior studies have described the core elements of AMS programs in LMIC settings, including the need to build laboratory capacity, enhance IPC, and establish surveillance systems of both infections and antibiotic use [15,19–25]. Feasibility study data support these needs, as well as other essential elements of AMS. Overall, respondents stated that leadership support at the national and senior facility management levels was needed for successful implementation. In addition, stepwise implementation strategies were universally considered to be useful. At the national level, respondents supported the urgent need for the development and implementation of antibiotic treatment guidelines. AMS must be identified as a national priority and included in facility key performance indicators, requiring dedicated support, accountability, and assigned roles and responsibilities. Within health care facilities, AMS must include written strategies, implementation of a formal multidisciplinary structure including laboratory surveillance and IPC, and identification of dedicated staff with clearly defined roles. These strategies must include support and expertise on infection management, access to timely laboratory/imaging/information technology services and available trained and experienced professionals in AMR and infectious disease.

Respondents reported the need for increased and consistent education and training. A first step towards strengthening educational initiatives includes understanding current clinical staff competencies and building tailored projects and programs that emphasize and develop knowledge and skills. Education must be ongoing, hands on, and practical, and include incentives and a broad range of resources (e.g., face-to-face and web-based).

Respondents felt the toolkit provided important information on appropriate antibiotic use and consumption and the means to utilize less expensive and technologically based approaches appropriate to LMIC contexts. AMS committees were considered at the heart of effective facility-based stewardship. Therefore, these committees must be formed and members must receive regular training in antimicrobial prescribing practices and stewardship. The committee should be responsible for reviewing and auditing courses of therapy for specified antimicrobial agents and clinical conditions. There is also the need for an established and effective communication strategy between the AMS committee, leadership, and clinical staff.

In terms of health care facility-based AMS, evidence-based antibiotic treatment guidelines were identified as a key component of AMS. Where possible, guidelines should be based on local antibiotic resistance patterns and availability and cost-effectiveness of agents. Day-to-day guidelines should be kept simple and include empiric antibiotic selection, definitive antibiotic selection, organism and disease states, intravenous to oral conversion, renal dosing, and duration of therapy. In conjunction with those guidelines, AMS programs are needed to reduce the overuse and overprescribing of antibiotics, the use of broad-spectrum antibiotics and dose combinations, and delayed prescribing.

Health care facilities in LMIC need capacity building both in terms of human and technological resources to develop a formulary and auditing process, antibiotic prescribing documentation policies and procedures, and regulations regarding drug restrictions including use of the WHO AWaRe (Access, Watch, Reserve) classifications. Health care facility monitoring and surveillance capabilities need to be developed to support AMS initiatives including measures to monitor quality/quantity of antimicrobial use at the unit and facility-wide level, compliance with specific interventions, and identification of antibiotic susceptibility rates for locally significant pathogens.

Limitations

The feasibility study was conducted in only four countries with a sample size of 12 national leaders, 21 facility administrators, and 65 clinical staff. Only one country was selected from Africa and there were no LMIC from Latin America, the Caribbean, the Middle East, or Europe included. Despite the small sample size, purposeful sampling was undertaken to ensure that different regions of the study countries were included with a diverse group of national- and facility-based stakeholders. These data provide a general overview of barriers and facilitators for implementation of AMS programs and the AMS toolkit. As implementation of the toolkit moves forward, additional data from other countries will continue to contribute to future versions. In addition, the feasibility study was focused on health facilities which provide inpatient care. Respondents discussed the need for AMS within community health facilities and education for patients. Future research and development of community-based AMS training and interventions are needed to address the high consumption of antibiotics outside of inpatient facilities.

4. Materials and Methods

4.1. Overview

The feasibility study was conducted from February 2019 to May 2019. The project was a partnership inclusive of a multinational and interdisciplinary team with expertise in AMR and AMS, infectious diseases, IPC, public health, nursing sciences, pharmacy, and social sciences. The study countries were selected by both WHO staff and the HFHS feasibility study team, based on geographic regions where AMR is a significant issue and where, to date, there are limited resources and AMS programs. These countries represent diverse contexts and challenges associated with the implementation of health care facility-based AMS programs. In addition, WHO and/or HFHS had worked with AMS leaders in the four selected countries, which facilitated rapid implementation of the feasibility study.

The study population included national- and local-level policymakers, facility administrators, and clinical staff. Study health care facilities were identified by in-country investigators and coordinators, and represented various facilities (e.g., public, private, and non-profit) and diverse geographic regions within each country. All facilities included inpatient care and ranged in size from 36 to 850 beds. Participating clinical staff included physicians, nurses, pharmacists, microbiologists, and laboratory technicians.

The study used a qualitative design based on key domains for program feasibility studies [26,27]. These included (1) acceptability of the toolkit; (2) demand and anticipated use; (3) practicality of the toolkit for use in LMIC; (4) integration of the toolkit within existing infrastructures; (5) adaptability of the toolkit within local contexts; (6) implementation and dissemination enablers and barriers to toolkit sustainability and scale-up within LMIC. The qualitative approach provided opportunity to engage with multiple partners from the selected sites throughout the development, implementation, and dissemination of the study. Through this engagement, conversations about AMR during meetings, workshops, and interviews provided visibility to local, national, and international issues related to AMR, the role of stewardship in the contexts of LMIC, and the potential for adaptation of the WHO toolkit to support AMR stewardship at the policy and programmatic levels in multiple settings.

In each country, the project was undertaken after an initial meeting with in-country study investigators and local governmental, nongovernmental, and health care facility stakeholders. After completion of the study, dissemination stakeholder workshops were convened within each country. These workshops provided opportunity for local input on (1) the interpretation of the feasibility study data; (2) ways to address facilitators and barriers to implementation of the AMS toolkit and AMS programs and policies; (3) identification of actionable items to promote implementation. This input from each country is reflected in the final reports and subsequently, in this paper.

4.2. Sample Size and Recruitment

Overall, 12 policy makers were recruited and interviewed, and 15 health care facilities were selected between the four countries. With the facilities, a total of 21 administrators, 20 physicians, 21 nurses, 11 pharmacists, and 13 laboratory personnel were interviewed (Table 5). When the study started, the research team estimated the sample size with the stipulation that it could be smaller or larger depending on data saturation. In each site, the team felt confident that the data collected reached saturation and no significant additional information was being recorded to justify additional interviews.

National-level respondents were identified by in-country principal investigators and coordinators as well as recommendations from the WHO Country Offices and included individuals involved in the development of AMS NAP and other experts in AMR and AMS. At the facility level, administrators or managers were invited to participate in the study. Clinical staff selection criteria included individuals engaged in current or past IPC programs and/or those engaged in existing AMS committees. A range of staff were interviewed, including ward physicians and nurses, laboratory staff, and pharmacists. In each country, the international and local partners worked closely together to approach potential respondents to explain the purpose of the study and request their participation. At the policy and hospital administration level, all of those approached made themselves available for the interviews. At the clinical level, the study team requested interviews with representatives from nursing, medicine, pharmacy, and microbiology/laboratory staff (Table 5). Potential participants were provided with an abbreviated version of the toolkit with sections specific to their position (e.g., policy maker, administrator, and staff) and a list of key topics to be covered in the interview [28].

Table 5. Study sites, health care facility types, and sample sizes for policy makers, facility administrators, and clinical staff.

Country	Location	Facility	Policy Makers	Administrators	Staff
Bhutan	Central	Public	3	5	6 physicians 4 nurses 3 pharmacists 3 laboratory
	Western	Public			
	Eastern	Public			
FSM	Chuuk State	Public	3	7	8 physicians 6 nurses 2 pharmacists 4 laboratory
	Kosrae State	Public			
	Pohnpei State	Public			
	Yap State	Public			
Malawi	Lilongwe	Public	3	5	3 physicians 6 nurses 4 pharmacists 4 laboratory
	Lilongwe	Public			
	Mzuzu	Public			
	Blantyre	Public			
Nepal	Kathmandu	Non-profit	3	4	3 physicians 5 nurses 2 pharmacists 2 laboratory
	Kathmandu	Public			
	Nepalgunj	Private			
	Dharan	Private			
TOTAL	-	-	12	21	20 physicians 21 nurses 11 pharmacists

4.3. Research Instruments

Three interview guides and demographic forms were developed specific to the population groups (policymakers, health care facility administrators, and clinical staff). Draft interview guides and demographic forms were provided to in-country investigators to review and revise to ensure they reflected local contexts. Interview guide items and probes focused on the research objectives, the toolkit core elements for health care facility-based AMS in LMIC, and the 6 program feasibility key domains. Demographic forms included items on current institutional affiliation (e.g., city/district, type of institution, and number of beds), respondents' education and employment (e.g., current position and years in current position), and engagement in AMR, AMS, and IPC programs at the health care facility or national levels (see Table S1).

4.4. Data Collection and Management

Data collection was led by team members from the Henry Ford Health System in partnership with local staff. In Bhutan, additional data collection support was provided by investigators/infectious disease specialists from Christian Medical College, Vellore, India. Interviews were conducted in English, with interpretation to local language verbally as required. Interviews were audiotaped and transcribed. Transcribed data were entered into Ethnograph, version 6, a qualitative data management software. A data coding dictionary was developed based on the interview guides and emergent themes from team members' field experiences and the transcribed text.

4.5. Data Analysis

After initial coding was completed, groups of code words were organized under common topics including the AMS core elements, the key domains for the feasibility study, and emergent themes. Searches were conducted within common themes, study country, and population (policymakers, administrators, and staff). Search documents were saved and reviewed to identify key findings and recommendations within and across countries in terms of barriers and facilitators for health care facility-based AMS policies and programs, action items to strengthen AMS policies and programs including implementation of the AMS toolkit, and specific recommendations for the AMS toolkit's content and organization. Illustrative text within the transcripts were identified to support the summary conclusions. Country-specific draft reports were sent to in-country investigators and other stakeholders for their review and input.

4.6. Ethical Approval

The project was approved by ethical review boards in each country, the Henry Ford Health System Institutional Review Board (Detroit, MI, USA), and the WHO Ethical Review Committee (Geneva) (Approval February 2019, #ppp3131/004479)]. All participants provided written informed consent.

5. Conclusions

There was clear consensus that optimal implementation and use of the toolkit requires recognition of country-specific contexts. These include diagnostic challenges, laboratory capacity, and high burdens of infectious diseases. Health care workers responsible for prescribing antibiotics have a broad range of education, training, and experience. Development of antibiotic prescribing guidelines may often be limited by inadequate local data on disease burden and susceptibility patterns. Many LMIC have poorly regulated prescription-only policies or limited access to essential antibiotics

Despite these challenges, the consensus among study respondents was that the toolkit will be an important asset as countries and health care facilities move forward to combat AMR and implement AMS programs. More information will be needed to address implementation strategies and many barriers need to be addressed to increase likelihood of successful implementation within the study countries and other LMIC. The road ahead must include commitment at the national and facility levels to prioritize AMR and develop sustainable national and local initiatives. The WHO toolkit provides a comprehensive review of core elements of AMS, strategies for intervention adaptation and implementation, and expansion of training and educational platforms. With growing global concerns regarding AMR, the WHO toolkit can provide practical guidance and support to LMIC worldwide [1].

Supplementary Materials: The following are available online at http://www.mdpi.com/2079-6382/9/9/556/s1, Table S1. Interview guides.

Author Contributions: Conceptualization, G.M., I.S., S.P., L.K., T.P., M.Z.; methodology, I.S., S.P., L.K.; formal analysis, G.M., I.S., S.P., L.K., P.C., T.P.; investigation, G.M., L.K., W.K., J.M., P.C., P.R., D.R.S., D.C.B., L.B., E.J., T.P., M.Z.; writing—original draft preparation, G.M., L.K., T.P., M.Z.; writing—review and editing, G.M., L.K., T.P., M.Z.; project administration, I.S., S.P., M.Z.; funding acquisition, M.Z. All authors have read and agreed to the published version of the manuscript. The authors S.P. and I.S. are staff members of the World Health Organization. The author alone is responsible for the views expressed in this publication and they do not necessarily represent the views, decisions or policies of the World Health Organization.

Funding: This research was funded by the World Health Organization, grant number D30521.

Acknowledgments: We would like to thank the following national experts and WHO country office staff involved in the feasibility studies: Sonam Yangchen and Pema Yangzom (Bhutan); Kelias Msyamboza (Malawi); Eunyoung Ko (Federated States of Micronesia); and Rajan Rayamajhi and Reuben Samuel (Nepal). We would also like to thank the many individuals who participated in the study in the four study countries.

Conflicts of Interest: The authors declare no conflict of interest.

References

1. Review on Antimicrobial Resistance. In *Tackling Drug-Resistant Infections Globally: Final Report and Recommendations*; Review on Antimicrobial Resistance: London, UK, 2016.
2. Planta, M.B. The role of poverty in antimicrobial resistance. *J. Am. Board Fam. Med.* **2007**, *20*, 533–539. [CrossRef]
3. Van Dijck, C.; Vlieghe, E.; Arnoldine Cox, J. Antibiotic stewardship interventions in hospitals in low- and middle-income countries: A systematic review. *Bull. World Health Organ.* **2018**, *96*, 266–280. [CrossRef] [PubMed]

4. Wilkinson, A.; Ebata, A.; MacGregor, H. Interventions to reduce antibiotic prescribing in LMICs: A scoping review of evidence from human and animal health systems. *Antibiotics* **2018**, *8*, 2. [CrossRef] [PubMed]
5. National Center for Emerging and Zoonotic Infectious Diseases; Centers for Disease Control and Prevention. *Core Elements of Hospital Antibiotic Stewardship Programs*; US Department of Health and Human Services: Atlanta, GA, USA, 2014.
6. National Center for Emerging and Zoonotic Infectious Diseases; Centers for Disease Control and Prevention. *The Core Elements of Antibiotic Stewardship Programs in Resource-Limited Settings: National and Hospital Settings*; US Department of Health and Human Services: Atlanta, GA, USA, 2018.
7. World Health Organization. *Antimicrobial Stewardship Programmes in Health-Care Facilities in Low- and Middle-Income Countries: A WHO Practical Toolkit*; World Health Organization: Geneva, Switzerland, 2019.
8. Davey, P.; Marwick, C.A.; Scott, C.L.; Charani, E.; McNeil, K.; Brown, E.; Gould, I.M.; Ramsay, C.R.; Michie, S. Interventions to improve antibiotic prescribing practices for hospital inpatients. *Cochrane Database Syst. Rev.* **2017**, *2*, CD003543. [CrossRef] [PubMed]
9. Schuts, E.C.; Hulscher, M.E.J.L.; Mouton, J.W.; Verduin, C.M.; Cohen Stuart, J.W.T.; Overdiek, H.W.P.M.; van der Linden, P.D.; Natsch, S.; Hertogh, C.M.P.M.; Wolfs, T.F.W.; et al. Current evidence on hospital antimicrobial stewardship objectives: A systematic review and meta-analysis. *Lancet Infect. Dis.* **2016**, *16*, 847–856. [CrossRef]
10. Dellit, T.H.; Owens, R.C.; McGowan, J.E., Jr.; Gerding, D.N.; Weinstein, R.A.; Burke, J.P.; Huskins, W.C.; Paterson, D.L.; Fishman, N.O.; Carpenter, C.F.; et al. Infectious Diseases Society of America and the Society for Healthcare Epidemiology of America guidelines for developing an institutional program to enhance antimicrobial stewardship. *Clin. Infect. Dis.* **2007**, *44*, 159–177. [CrossRef] [PubMed]
11. World Health Organization. *Global Action Plan on Antimicrobial Resistance*; World Health Organization: Geneva, Switzerland, 2015.
12. McEwen, S.A.; Collignon, P.J. Antimicrobial resistance: A one Health perspective. *Microbiol. Spectr.* **2018**, *6*, 521–547.
13. Prentiss, T.; Weisberg, K.; Zervos, J. Building capacity in infection prevention and antimicrobial stewardship in low- and middle-income countries: The role of partnerships inter-countries. *Curr. Treat. Options Infect. Dis.* **2018**, *10*, 7–16. [CrossRef]
14. Travis, P.; Egger, D.; Davies, P.; Mechbal, A. *Towards Better Stewardship: Concepts and Critical Issues*; World Health Organization: Geneva, Switzerland, 2002.
15. Cox, J.A.; Vlieghe, E.; Mendelson, M.; Wertheim, H.; Ndegwa, L.; Villegas, M.V.; Gould, I.; Levy Hara, G. Antibiotic stewardship in low-and middle-income countries: The same but different? *Clin. Microbiol. Infect.* **2017**, *23*, 812–818. [CrossRef] [PubMed]
16. Saha, S.K.; Hawes, L.; Mazza, D. Effectiveness of interventions involving pharmacists on antibiotic prescribing by general practitioners: A systematic review and meta-analysis. *J. Antimicrob. Chemother.* **2019**, *74*, 1173–1181. [CrossRef] [PubMed]
17. Flowers, P. Antimicrobial resistance: A biopsychosocial problem requiring innovative interdisciplinary and imaginative interventions. *J. Infect. Prev.* **2018**, *19*, 195–199. [CrossRef] [PubMed]
18. Shallcross, L.; Lorencatto, F.; Fuller, C.; Tarrant, C.; West, J.; Traina, R.; Smith, C.; Forbes, G.; Crayton, E.; Rockenschaub, P.; et al. PASS Research Group. An interdisciplinary mixed-methods approach to developing antimicrobial stewardship interventions: Protocol for the Preserving Antibiotics through Safe Stewardship (PASS) Research Programme. *Wellcome Open Res.* **2020**, *14*, 8. [CrossRef] [PubMed]
19. Fleming Fund. Grants. Available online: https://www.flemingfund.org/grants/?type=country-grant (accessed on 12 January 2020).
20. World Health Organization; Food and Agriculture Organization of the United Nations; World Organization for Animal Health. *Antimicrobial Resistance: A Manual for Developing National Action Plans*; World Health Organization, Food and Agriculture Organization of the United Nations, World Organization for Animal Health: Geneva, Switzerland, 2016.

21. Pulcini, C.; Binda, F.; Lamkang, A.S.; Trett, A.; Charani, E.; Goff, D.A.; Harbarth, S.; Hinrichsen, S.L.; Levy-Hara, G.; Mendelson, M.; et al. Developing core elements and checklist items for global hospital antimicrobial stewardship programmes: A consensus approach. *Clin. Microbiol. Infect.* **2019**, *25*, 20–25. [CrossRef] [PubMed]
22. Regional Office for South-East Asia; World Health Organization. *Step-By-Step Approach for Development and Implementation of Hospital Antibiotic Policy and Standard Treatment Guidelines*; Regional Office for South-East Asia, World Health Organization: New Delhi, India, 2011.
23. World Health Organization. Promoting rational use of medicines: Core components. *WHO Policy Perspect. Med.* **2002**, *5*, 1–6.
24. World Health Organization. Guidelines on Core Components of Infection Prevention and Control. In *Programmes at the National and Acute Health Care Facility Level*; World Health Organization: Geneva, Switzerland, 2016.
25. Mendelson, M.; Morris, A.M.; Thursky, K.; Pulcini, C. How to start an antimicrobial stewardship programme in a hospital. *Clin. Microbiol. Infect.* **2020**, *26*, 447–453. [CrossRef] [PubMed]
26. Bowen, D.J.; Kreuter, M.; Spring, B.; Cofta-Woerpel, L.; Linnan, L.; Weiner, D.; Bakken, S.; Kaplan, C.P.; Squiers, L.; Fabrizio, C.; et al. How we design feasibility studies. *Am. J. Prev. Med.* **2009**, *36*, 452–457. [CrossRef] [PubMed]
27. Keith, R.E.; Crosson, J.C.; O'Malley, A.S.; Cromp, D.; Taylor, E.F. Using the Consolidated Framework for Implementation Research (CFIR) to produce actionable findings: A rapid-cycle evaluation approach to improving implementation. *Implement. Sci.* **2017**, *12*, 15. [CrossRef] [PubMed]
28. Antimicrobial stewardship programmes in health-care facilities in low- and middle-income countries. In *A Practical Toolkit*; Licence CC BY-NC-SA 3.0 IGO; World Health Organization: Geneva, Switzerland, 2019.

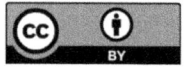

© 2020 World Health Organization; Licensee MDPI, Basel, Switzerland. This is an open access article distributed under the terms of the Creative Commons Attribution IGO License (CC BY) license (http://creativecommons.org/licenses/by/3.0/igo/legalcode), which permits unrestricted use, distribution, and reproduction in any medium, provided the original work is properly cited. In any reproduction of this article there should not be any suggestion that WHO or this article endorse any specific organisation or products. The use of the WHO logo is not permitted.

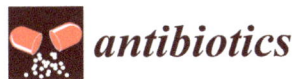 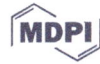

Article

Implementation of the WHO Approved "Tailoring Antimicrobial Resistance Programs (TAP)" Reduces Patients' Request for Antibiotics

Nasser M. Kaplan [1], Yousef S. Khader [2], Mahmoud A. Alfaqih [3,*], Rami Saadeh [2] and Lora Al Sawalha [4]

1. Department of Pathology and Microbiology, Faculty of Medicine, Jordan University of Science and Technology, 22110 Irbid, Jordan; nmkaplan@just.edu.jo
2. Department of Community Medicine and Public Health, Faculty of Medicine, Jordan University of Science and Technology, 22110 Irbid, Jordan; yskhader@just.edu.jo (Y.S.K.); rasaadeh@just.edu.jo (R.S.)
3. Department of Physiology and Biochemistry, Faculty of Medicine, Jordan University of Science and Technology, 22110 Irbid, Jordan
4. Anti-Microbial-Resistance Officer, World Health Organization, Jordan Country Office, 11181 Amman, Jordan; alsawalhal@who.int
* Correspondence: maalfaqih@just.edu.jo; Tel.: +962-2-7201000

Received: 7 June 2020; Accepted: 4 August 2020; Published: 12 August 2020

Abstract: The misuse of antibiotics is a worldwide public health concern. Behavioral Intervention programs that aim to reduce patients' own request for antibiotics during their visit to primary care clinics is an attractive strategy to combat this problem. We tested the effectiveness of a behavioral modification method known as the Tailoring Antimicrobial resistance Programs (TAP) in reducing the request for antibiotics by patients visiting primary care clinics for mild upper respiratory tract infections (URTIs). A stratified cluster randomized design with two groups pre-post, comparing intervention with the control, was conducted in six health centers. TAP was implemented for eight weeks. Request for antibiotics was assessed before (period 1) and after introducing TAP (period 2). The percentage of patients or their escorts who requested antibiotics in period 1 was 59.7% in the control group and 60.2% in the intervention group. The percentage of patients who requested antibiotics did not significantly change between period 1 and 2 in the control group, who continued to receive the standard of care. The above percentage significantly decreased in the intervention group from 60.2% to 38.5% ($p < 0.05$). We conclude that behavioral change programs including TAP are a viable alternative strategy to address antibiotic misuse in Jordan.

Keywords: antibiotics; microbial resistance; upper respiratory tract infections

1. Introduction

Antimicrobial resistance is a threat to the public health sector worldwide [1]. Many factors contribute to this problem; however, the misuse and/or overuse of antibiotics are established as the major driving forces [2,3]. Indeed, it was estimated that up to 50% of all antimicrobials globally prescribed to patients are not even necessary [4,5]. It is interesting to note that most of the unnecessary antibiotic prescription takes place in the primary care setting [6], with the biggest percentage of unnecessary antibiotics being prescribed for patients with upper respiratory tract infections (URTIs) [6].

Jordan is a developing country in the Middle East and North Africa (MENA) region. The misuse of antibiotics by consumers, including the use of antibiotics without prescriptions, was widely documented in Jordan and in the region [7–12]. Other forms of antibiotic misuse in the MENA region include the use of antibiotics for improper indications, including to fight viral infections [13–16].

Despite the magnitude of the antibiotic misuse problem, most of the countries in the MENA region have no laws and/or legislations that prohibit dispensing antibiotics without a proper prescription [8,17]. Moreover, countries that have relevant legislation in place do not have proper surveillance systems and/or do not adequately enforce relevant laws [18]. Interestingly, knowledge about antibiotic misuse and antimicrobial resistance by itself, without being coupled with behavioral change interventions, does not seem to be an efficient strategy to enforce better antibiotic stewardship [19–21]. This observation might be explained by the complexity of the factors that affect antibiotic misuse which appears to be influenced by a plethora of cultural and social factors [19,21]. For example, several reports demonstrated that the specialty of the health care provider, patient education and other patient socio-economic factors guide the antibiotic prescription patterns of physicians [22–25].

Tailoring Antimicrobial Resistance Programs (TAP) is a behavioral change methodology developed by the World Health Organization (WHO) Eastern Mediterranean Regional Office (EMRO) to modify the behaviors that drive antimicrobial resistance (AMR). TAP methodology not only aims to identify barriers against proper behavior but also identifies the incentives that drive such a behavior. TAP proposes guidelines for (a) the design of proper behavioral change strategies, (b) implementation of such strategies and (c) evaluation of the results of any behavioral intervention. The Ministry of Health in Jordan joined the WHO TAP in November 2018 to pilot a behavioral change intervention that aims to reduce the prescription of antibiotics for viral URTIs in a primary healthcare setting. This study presents and discusses the findings of the TAP intervention, specifically its effect in reducing the percentage of patients that request antibiotics. Additionally, the study investigated the association of several socioeconomic factors with changes in antibiotic request by the patients following TAP intervention.

2. Results

2.1. The Characteristics of the Study Subjects

A total of 855 subjects (506 in the control group and 349 in the intervention group) participated in the study in period 1 before the implementation of the intervention. In period 2, following the intervention, a total of 1025 subjects (576 in the control group and 449 in the intervention group) were enrolled in the study (Figure 1).

A stratified cluster randomized trial with two groups pre-post design, comparing intervention with the control (standard care), was used in the study. The study was performed in six health centers in Amman. The centers were randomized into two groups (three centers each). In period 1, there was a pre-assessment of antibiotic request. In period 2, following application of the intervention or maintenance of standard treatment care, there was a re-evaluation of antibiotic request among enrolled patients.

The socio-demographic characteristics of the subjects of the control and intervention groups in periods 1 and 2 are shown in Table 1. In period 1, 17.8% of the subjects in the control group and 7.2% of the subjects in the intervention group were children ($p < 0.001$). In period 2, almost one quarter of the subjects in both groups were children ($p = 0.320$). In period 1, subjects of the intervention group were significantly younger. Moreover, a significantly higher number of the above subjects did not hold a university degree. More than half of the subjects (55.9%) in the control group and 33% of the subjects in the intervention group were new patients. In period 2, a significantly lower number of subjects in the intervention group received college/university education than subjects in the intervention group ($p < 0.001$). The characteristics of the subjects significantly differed between period 1 and period 2 in both control and intervention groups.

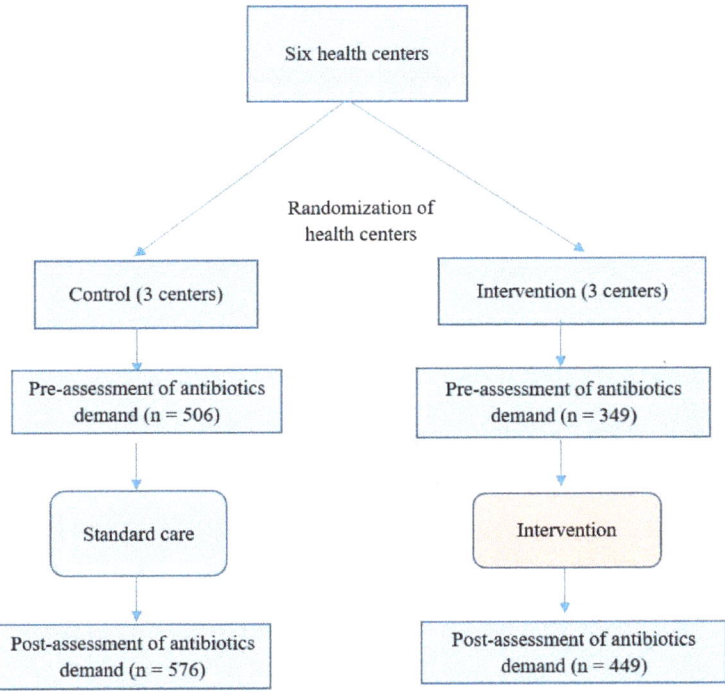

Figure 1. A flow chart that explains the design of the study.

Table 1. The socio-demographic characteristics of patients in the control and intervention groups during period 1 and period 2.

	Period 1 (Pretest)					Period 2 (Posttest)				
Variable	Control Group		Intervention Group		p-Value	Control Group		Intervention Group		p-Value
	n	%	n	%		n	%	n	%	
Gender					0.666					0.488
Male	297	58.7	210	60.2		369	64.1	297	66.1	
Female	209	41.3	139	39.8		207	35.9	152	33.9	
Age					<0.001					0.320
Children (<18 year)	90	17.8	25	7.2		142	24.7	123	27.4	
Adults (≥18 year)	416	82.2	324	92.8		434	75.3	326	72.6	
Nationality										
Jordanian	475	93.9	332	95.1		558	96.9	427	95.1	
Non-Jordanian	31	6.1	17	4.9		18	3.1	22	4.9	
Education					<0.001					<0.001
No formal education	72	14.2	43	12.3		68	11.8	60	13.4	
Primary education	84	16.6	98	28.1		106	18.4	141	31.4	
Secondary education	155	30.6	114	32.7		161	28	151	33.6	
Professional training	35	6.9	16	4.6		20	3.5	3	0.7	
College/University education	160	31.6	78	22.3		221	38.4	94	20.9	
Marital status					<0.001					0.158
Married	332	65.6	265	75.9		359	62.3	284	63.3	
Single	60	11.9	30	8.6		43	7.5	29	6.5	
Divorced/Widow	24	4.7	29	8.3		32	5.6	13	2.9	
Children	90	17.8	25	7.2		142	24.7	123	27.4	
Patient's type					<0.001					0.606
New	283	55.9	115	33		298	51.7	225	50.1	
Regular	223	44.1	234	67		278	48.3	224	49.9	

2.2. Effect of TAP Intervention on Antibiotics Request among Study Subjects

The percentage of patients or their escorts who requested antibiotics in period 1, before the implementation of the intervention, was 59.7% in the control group and 60.2% in the intervention group ($p = 0.886$) (Figure 2). While the percentage of requesting antibiotics did not change significantly between period 1 and 2 in the control group ($p = 0.393$), this percentage decreased significantly in the intervention group from 60.2% to 38.5% ($p < 0.05$) (expressed as no request in Figure 2). The relative percent of reduction in the percentage of subjects who requested antibiotics between the two periods in the intervention group was 36% (absolute difference of 21.7%).

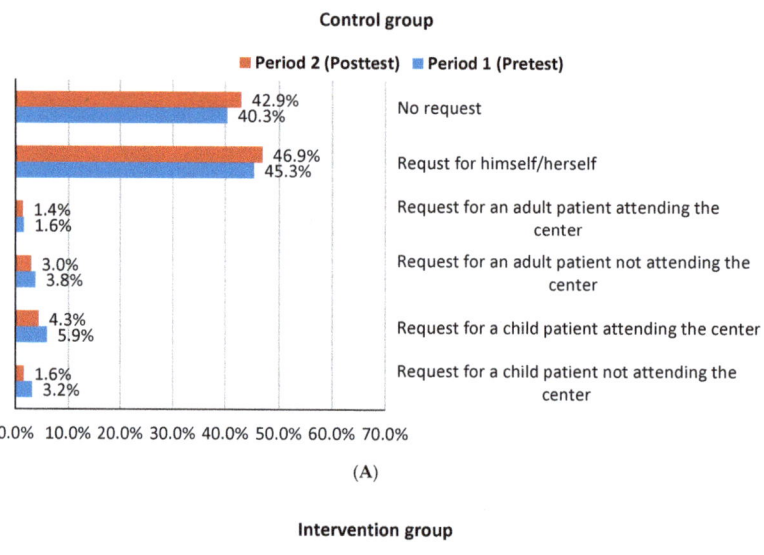

(A)

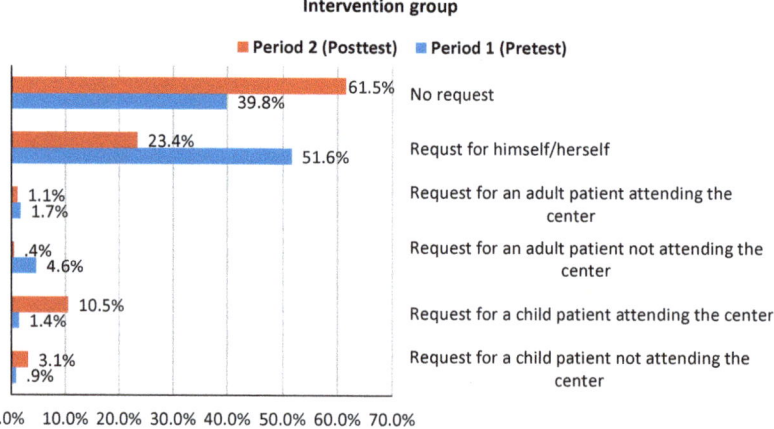

(B)

Figure 2. The pattern of antibiotics requests in the control or intervention groups. A horizontal bar graph displaying the pattern of antibiotics request in period 1 (**blue**) and period 2 (**red**) in (**A**) Control or (**B**) Intervention groups. Each bar represents the percentage of individuals that either did not request the antibiotics, requested the antibiotics from themselves, requested the antibiotics for an adult patient attending the center, requested the antibiotics for an adult patient not attending the center, requested the antibiotics for a child patient attending the center or requested the antibiotics for a child patient not attending the center.

2.3. Pattern of Antibiotics Request

In the intervention group, the percentage of patients or their escorts who requested antibiotics for themselves decreased from 51.6% before the intervention to 23.4% following the intervention, with a relative percent of reduction of 45.7% (Figure 2). In the control group, the above described percentage did not change significantly between period 1 and period 2 ($p = 0.359$). About 45.3% and 46.9% of participants requested antibiotics for themselves in period 1 and period 2, respectively.

2.4. Reasons for Requesting Antibiotics

Overall, among those who requested antibiotics in both the control and intervention groups (n = 1014), the most common reasons were sore throat (36.7%) followed by cough (27.5%). The health-related complaints that motivated subjects of this study to request antibiotics differed between the control and intervention groups (Table 2). In the control group, the most common reasons for requesting antibiotics were sore throat, followed by flu, and then cough (Table 2). In the intervention group, the main complaints were sore throat, followed by pain upon swallowing, fever, and then cough (Table 2).

Table 2. The most frequent patient complaints associated with requesting antibiotics in the control and intervention groups in period 1 or 2.

Complaint	Control				Intervention			
	Period 1 (Pretest)		Period 2 (Posttest)		Period 1 (Pretest)		Period 2 (Posttest)	
	n	%	n	%	n	%	n	%
Sore Throat	104	34.4	118	35.9	103	49.0	56	32.4
Flu	67	22.2	64	19.5	33	15.7	32	18.5
Cough	84	27.8	119	36.2	34	16.2	42	24.3
Pain on swallowing	39	12.9	50	15.3	40	19.0	42	24.3
Cold	31	10.3	21	6.4	8	3.8	27	15.6
Influenza	61	20.2	62	18.8	27	12.9	40	23.1
Fever	58	19.2	50	15.2	16	7.6	49	28.3
Nasal Congestion	42	13.9	30	9.1	18	8.6	14	8.1
Breathing Difficulties	33	10.9	59	17.9	11	5.2	12	6.9
Nasal secretion	34	11.3	24	7.3	11	5.3	9	5.2
Sneezing	27	8.9	22	6.7	5	2.4	7	4.0
Weakness	16	5.3	14	4.3	14	6.7	8	4.6

2.5. Type of Antibiotics Requested

Of those who requested antibiotics, 961 (94.8%) requested a specific type of antibiotics (data not shown). It is interesting to note that more than three quarters (78.1%) requested amoxicillin/clavulanic acid (Amoclan) (data not shown).

2.6. Factors That Influence Antibiotics Request

Table 3 shows a multivariate analysis of the effect of multiple factors on the decision of the study subjects to request antibiotics from the prescriber (i.e., physician). In the control group, the variables that were significantly associated with requesting antibiotics by the patients were age of the patient, type of patient (regular vs. first appointment), level of education of the patient and the specialty of the health care provider. Antibiotics were more likely to be requested by, or for, adult patients compared to patients who were children (Odds Ratio (OR) = 1.7) (Table 3). Regular patients were more likely to request antibiotics compared to patients visiting that specific physician for the first time (OR = 2.5) (Table 3). Patients with no formal education, primary education, secondary education or with professional training were more likely to request antibiotics than patients with college/university education. Patients who were visiting a family doctor were less likely to request antibiotics than patients visiting general practitioners (OR = 0.5). On the other hand, in the intervention group, our analysis showed that antibiotic request by subjects was significantly lower following the implementation of the intervention (OR = 0.4). The only other variable in the intervention group to significantly affect antibiotic request was primary or secondary education compared to having no formal education. Our results showed that having primary or secondary education significantly increased the odds of requesting antibiotics.

Table 3. Multivariate analysis of factors associated with antibiotics demand in the control and intervention groups.

Variable	Control Group			Intervention Group			
	OR	95% Confidence Interval		p-Value	OR	95% Confidence Interval		p-Value
Time (post vs. pre)	1.0	0.8	1.4	0.713	0.4	0.3	0.6	<0.001
Specialty of health care provider								
General practitioner	1				1			
Family Medicine	0.5	0.4	0.7	<0.001	1.2	0.8	1.6	0.366
Pediatrics	1.1	0.8	1.7	0.519	1.0	0.6	1.6	0.927
Internal Medicine	0.9	0.5	1.7	0.792				
Education								
No formal education	2.9	1.9	4.5	<0.001	1.0	0.6	1.7	0.968
Primary education	2.3	1.6	3.3	<0.001	1.8	1.1	2.7	0.010
Secondary education	1.7	1.3	2.4	0.001	1.9	1.3	2.8	0.002
Professional training	5.7	2.8	11.6	<0.001	0.8	0.3	2.3	0.74
College/university education	1							
Age of patient (adults vs. children)	1.7	1.1	2.5	0.006	1.3	0.8	2.1	0.229
Type of patient (regular vs. new)	2.5	1.9	3.3	<0.001	1.2	0.9	1.7	0.153

3. Discussion

The misuse of antibiotics in primary care is a major contributor to antibiotic resistance [5]. URTIs are common presentations seen in the general practice [26]. URTI without complications is most often caused by a virus [27]. Antibiotics have no efficacy in the treatment of viral infections, but are nevertheless often prescribed for their treatment [28,29].

In this study, using a stratified cluster randomized trial with two groups pre-post design, we evaluated the effect of the TAP intervention in reducing the percentage of patients that request antibiotics. The above design allowed for a comparison of the intervention group receiving TAP with a control group in which standard care was maintained. In addition to collecting information on the percentage of patients who requested antibiotics, the research team collected data of several factors previously reported to affect antibiotic vigilance such as gender, age, level of education of the patient and the specialty of the health care provider. The study design also differentiated between patients visiting the physician for the first time and returning patients. Recruitment to the study was restricted to patients complaining from URTIs.

In this pilot study conducted on patients visiting six health centers in the capital city of Jordan, Amman, we were the first group to demonstrate the efficacy of the TAP program in reducing the percentage of patients that request antibiotics from their health care provider in a primary care setting. Notably, our findings also indicated that the TAP program achieved its goal independent of all the other variables that might influence antibiotic requests by the patients.

In the absence of any intervention (in our case the TAP program) our findings indicated that more than half of the patients diagnosed with mild URTIs would request antibiotics for the treatment of their illness. This result is analogous with other reports which suggested that patient pressure or "perceived pressure" is a major driver of the lack of antibiotic vigilance [30,31]. The above figure, showing that most patients request antibiotics from their primary health care provider as a result of illnesses that do not normally require antibiotics, may reflect the lack of public awareness programs on the harmful effects of the unnecessary use of antibiotics. Although this observation is alarming from a public health standpoint, the fact that the TAP method successfully reduced the number of patients that request antibiotics shows that positive behavioral change could be achieved in the patient population and invites the application of the TAP method on a larger scale.

An interesting finding of this investigation was the difference observed in the percentage of patients that request antibiotics based on the specialty of the health care provider. For example, in the control group, it was observed that patients were more likely to request antibiotics from general practitioners vs. family medicine specialists. In Jordan, general practitioners start their appointment following one year of vocational training only (internship), without enrollment in any residency program. On the other hand, to become a family medicine specialist in Jordan, candidates must finish their vocational training, enroll in a structured residency program and pass a national board exam. The exact reason behind the above disparity in antibiotic request between patients seen by different specialists is unknown but could be related to family medicine specialists building better communication and assertive skills during their residency programs [32]. If the above explanation turns out to be partially responsible for this disparity, a solution for this problem would be to offer general practitioners Continuing Medical Education (CME) courses in communication skills and antibiotic stewardship. These courses would help mend the gap created by a longer study path to become a family medicine specialist.

This investigation has a few limitations. First, this study was conducted in Amman, the capital city of Jordan. Although the findings of this study are very promising, the adoption of the TAP program as a method to achieve better antibiotic vigilance requires testing the program across different geographic regions. For example, the level of education, a variable shown in this study to affect antibiotic stewardship, might be different in Amman from other geographic regions in the country. Second, the research team failed to collect information on the volume of patients examined by physicians on a single day in the clinic. This variable was shown in several reports to affect consultation time with the patient, and was significantly associated with an excess, often unnecessary, antibiotic prescription [33,34]. Indeed, it would be interesting to evaluate if implementation of the TAP actually increased the consultation time with the patients and how that affected the overall revenue of the medical practice/clinic. Despite these limitations, this study is the first in Jordan and should be informative to public health policy makers and health care workers interested in antibiotic stewardship with regards to the size of the antibiotic misuse problem and the feasibility of reducing this problem with a simple behavioral approach.

4. Materials and Methods

4.1. Study Design, Site Selection and Randomization

A stratified cluster randomized trial with two groups pre-post design, comparing intervention with the control (standard care), was conducted in the period between August and November of 2019. The standardized behavior change intervention was implemented for eight weeks in the intervention group. The demand for antibiotics was assessed among patients with mild URTIs attending the intervention and control centers before and after introducing the behavior change intervention. Written consent was requested from all patients before the interviews. No identifiers were collected. Approval from the Jordan Ministry of Health Ethical Review Board was obtained prior to conducting the study. All interviews were conducted in a closed room to ensure privacy and confidentiality.

Six health centers in Amman, Jordan were selected using a stratified cluster randomized sampling strategy. The centers were classified into three strata—small, medium and large—based on the number of physicians and monthly patient visits obtained from statistics of the year 2018. Out of each stratum, one center was randomized to the intervention group and another center to the control group, resulting in three centers in each group.

4.2. Patient Recruitment

General practitioners, family medicine specialists, pediatricians and internal medicine specialists were trained to interview patients attending the clinic for mild URTIs or to obtain medications for relatives with mild URTIs. The practitioners used a semi-structured questionnaire before and after the intervention to assess the demand for antibiotics. The questionnaire was pilot tested on 30 patients and revised accordingly. All consecutive patients of all ages diagnosed with URTIs who visited the selected health centers during the working hours for the duration of the study period were included. Only patients visiting general practitioners, family medicine specialists, pediatricians, and internal medicine specialists were included. Patients diagnosed with infections other than URTIs were excluded.

4.3. Intervention

A strategic behavior change intervention package was designed and implemented in the three intervention centers. As part of the intervention, physicians were trained, by a WHO expert in the area of antimicrobial resistance and a consultant in communication, to adopt a more proper behavior relevant to antibiotic prescription and to communicate with patients who insist on receiving antibiotics for viral URTIs. A 1-day training workshop was held in the premises of the Ministry of Health (MoH). During the training, physicians were trained on the current national guidelines for prescribing antibiotics to patients with URTIs and were trained on the best approaches to manage discussions with difficult patients. The physicians in the intervention centers received a copy of the clinical guidelines for the diagnosis and treatment of URTIs and were instructed to adopt the guidelines in their practices. A commitment was obtained from prescribers to become advocates for the proper use of antibiotics for URTIs and to join the intervention by signing a commitment board.

Posters were placed in the waiting areas to advise patients not to request antibiotics from their doctors and to always consult a doctor before antibiotics' administration, and leaflets about the proper use of antibiotics were distributed to patients. During the routine patient consultation in the intervention centers, physicians requested each patient to answer a quiz about the indication and proper use of antibiotics. Then, the physician held a short discussion (2–3 min) about the answers to the questions, encouraged patients to reduce their requests for antibiotics, and provided patients with information about the antibiotics and the consequences of improper prescription. Peer-to-peer weekly coffee sessions were held and moderated by the MoH staff to strengthen the bonds between colleagues and managers as a single entity that reduced the unnecessary use of antibiotics. Moreover, the strategies used to implement the behavior change, including the roles of the prescribers and patients, are shown in Table 4.

Table 4. Behavioral change strategies for prescribers or patients.

	Behavioral Barrier	Behavioral Domain	Intervention Function	Intervention	Activities
	Behavioral change strategies and activities for prescribers				
1	Limited communication skills to manage patient pressure of antibiotics for viral infections	Skills	Physical capability	To improve counselling and negotiation skills of doctor to better manage patient demand for antibiotics for viral infections	A training workshop for communication skills
2	Limited knowledge of guidelines and alternative treatments for viral infections	Knowledge	Psychological capability	To increase doctors' knowledge of guidelines and alternatives to antibiotics	A prescriber reference booklet including national guidelines for viral Upper Respiratory Tract Infections (URTIs)
3	Social norms: patient culture of demanding antibiotics and expecting to best know the suitable treatment for self and family.	Social	Social opportunity	To emphasize the professional role of doctors as the best one to diagnose illness and prescribe antibiotics	A conversation/quiz with patients Commitment board
4	Peer pressure to prescribe antibiotics for viral infections	Professional role	Reflective motivation	To strengthen the bonds between colleagues and managers as one entity that reduced unnecessary use of antibiotics	Peer to peer weekly coffee session
	Behavioral change strategies and activities for patients				
1	Limited knowledge of proper use of antibiotics and Antimicrobial Resistance (AMR)	Knowledge	Psychological capability	To raise knowledge about antibiotics and AMR	A quiz during patient consultation
2	Limited knowledge that antibiotics are not a solution for viral infections	Knowledge		To raise awareness about alternative therapies	A quiz during patient consultation
3	Limited understanding of the consequences of improper use of antibiotics	Belief in consequences	Reflective motivation	To label families who do not consume antibiotics for viral infections as healthy and wealthy families	A quiz during patient consultation **Poster**
4	Social norms linked with beliefs that people know which antibiotics work best for them	Social	Social environment	To emphasize doctors' role as the best to diagnose patients following the Arabic proverb "give the bread to the baker".	A quiz during patient consultation **Poster:** Never demand antibiotics from your doctor. Always consult your doctor before taking antibiotics
5	No plans to change behavior	Intentions/goals		To encourage change in social norms by using people who do not use antibiotics as a reference group	Commitment board

The MoH staff coordinating the project regularly visited the clinics during the intervention, observed the physicians' practices, and filled out the monitoring forms. The monitoring form included information on the physicians' adherence to the study protocol and the number of patients treated.

4.4. Sample Size

A minimum sample size needed to assess the effect of the intervention on the change in the percentage of patients who request antibiotics for URTIs in a pretest-posttest nonequivalent control group design was calculated using G*Power. Assuming that the percentage of patients who request antibiotics for URTIs in the selected health centers is 50%, the sample size needed to detect a change of 12% in this percentage following the intervention (at a level of significance of 0.05 and a power of 80%) is 370 patients in the intervention group (370 at pretest and 370 at posttest) and 370 patients in the control group (370 at pretest and 370 at posttest). This is the minimum sample size with enough power to determine the impact of the intervention, taking into consideration that the analysis will be stratified by demographic and clinical characteristics.

4.5. Statistical Analysis

Data were analyzed using IBM SPSS, version 20 (IBM Corp., Armonk, NY, USA). Data were described using means, standard deviations, and percentages. Chi-square test was used to compare the percentage of patients who requested antibiotics for URTIs between intervention and control groups and between the two periods within each group. The same test was used to compare demographic and other categorical variables between intervention and control groups and between the two periods within each group. Binary logistic regression was used to test for the change in request for antibiotics over time, after adjusting for patients' characteristics. The interaction term between period (pretest (period 1)/ posttest (period 2)) and group (intervention/control) was tested. A p-value of less than 0.05 was considered statistically significant.

5. Conclusions

In conclusion, in this pilot study evaluating the TAP program as a measure to achieve proper antibiotic stewardship in Jordan, we provide evidence on its efficacy, simplicity and feasibility. Given the small scale of this investigation, we recommend testing the program on a larger scale and across multiple health sectors in the country. We anticipate that the interventional program described in this investigation might be adopted as a public health method to address the misuse of antibiotics in Jordan.

Author Contributions: Conceptualization, N.M.K.; Formal analysis, Y.S.K. and R.S.; Funding acquisition, L.A.S.; Methodology, Y.S.K.; Project administration, N.M.K., Y.S.K., M.A.A. and L.A.S.; Validation, R.S.; Writing—original draft, M.A.A.; Writing—review and editing, M.A.A. All authors have read and agreed to the published version of the manuscript.

Funding: This work was supported by the World Health Organization (WHO) office in Amman.

Acknowledgments: The authors would like to thank officials at the Ministry of Health in Jordan for facilitating completion of the study. BMJ 1998, 317, 609–610.

Conflicts of Interest: The authors would like to report no conflict of interest.

Abbreviations

Abbreviation	Full Term
TAP	Tailoring Antimicrobial resistance Program
URTIs	Upper Respiratory Tract Infections
MENA	Middle East and North Africa
WHO	World Health Organization
EMRO	Eastern Mediterranean Regional Office
AMR	Antimicrobial resistance

SPSS	Statistical Package for the Social Sciences
OR	Odds Ratio
CME	Continuing Medical Education

References

1. Wise, R.; Hart, T.; Cars, O.; Streulens, M.; Helmuth, R.; Huovinen, P.; Sprenger, M. Antimicrobial Resistance: Is a major threat to public health. *BMJ* **1998**, *317*, 609–610. [CrossRef] [PubMed]
2. Holmes, A.H.; Moore, L.S.; Sundsfjord, A.; Steinbakk, M.; Regmi, S.; Karkey, A.; Guerin, P.J.; Piddock, L.J. Understanding the mechanisms and drivers of antimicrobial resistance. *Lancet* **2016**, *387*, 176–187. [CrossRef]
3. Laxminarayan, R.; Duse, A.; Wattal, C.; Zaidi, A.K.; Wertheim, H.F.; Sumpradit, N.; Vlieghe, E.; Hara, G.L.; Gould, I.M.; Goossens, H. Antibiotic resistance—the need for global solutions. *Lancet Infect. Dis.* **2013**, *13*, 1057–1098. [CrossRef]
4. Levy, S.B.; Marshall, B. Antibacterial resistance worldwide: Causes, challenges and responses. *Nat. Med.* **2004**, *10*, S122–S129. [CrossRef] [PubMed]
5. Atlanta, G. *Antibiotic Resistance Threats in the United States*; Centers for Disease Control and Prevention: Atlanta, GA, USA, 2013.
6. Harris, A.M.; Hicks, L.A.; Qaseem, A. Appropriate antibiotic use for acute respiratory tract infection in adults. *Ann. Intern. Med.* **2016**, *164*, 425–434. [CrossRef]
7. Abasaeed, A.; Vlcek, J.; Abuelkhair, M.; Kubena, A. Self-medication with antibiotics by the community of Abu Dhabi Emirate, United Arab Emirates. *J. Infect. Dev. Ctries.* **2009**, *3*, 491–497. [CrossRef]
8. Al-Azzam, S.; Al-Husein, B.; Alzoubi, F.; Masadeh, M.; Ali, M. Self-medication with antibiotics in Jordanian population. *Int. J. Occup. Med. Environ. Health* **2007**, *20*, 373–380. [CrossRef]
9. Awad, A.I.; Aboud, E.A. Knowledge, attitude and practice towards antibiotic use among the public in Kuwait. *PLoS ONE* **2015**, *10*, e0117910. [CrossRef]
10. Sabry, N.A.; Farid, S.F.; Dawoud, D.M. Antibiotic dispensing in Egyptian community pharmacies: An observational study. *Res. Soc. Adm. Pharm.* **2014**, *10*, 168–184. [CrossRef]
11. Jamhour, A.; El-Kheir, A.; Salameh, P.; Hanna, P.A.; Mansour, H. Antibiotic knowledge and self-medication practices in a developing country: A cross-sectional study. *Am. J. Infect. Control* **2017**, *45*, 384–388. [CrossRef]
12. Barah, F.; Gonçalves, V. Antibiotic use and knowledge in the community in Kalamoon, Syrian Arab Republic: A cross-sectional study. *EMHJ-East. Mediterr. Health J.* **2010**, *16*, 516–521. [CrossRef]
13. Mouhieddine, T.H.; Olleik, Z.; Itani, M.M.; Kawtharani, S.; Nassar, H.; Hassoun, R.; Houmani, Z.; El Zein, Z.; Fakih, R.; Mortada, I.K. Assessing the Lebanese population for their knowledge, attitudes and practices of antibiotic usage. *J. Infect. Public Health* **2015**, *8*, 20–31. [CrossRef] [PubMed]
14. Darwish, D.A.; Abdelmalek, S.; Dayyih, W.A.; Hamadi, S. Awareness of antibiotic use and antimicrobial resistance in the Iraqi community in Jordan. *J. Infect. Dev. Ctries.* **2014**, *8*, 616–623. [CrossRef] [PubMed]
15. El Zowalaty, M.E.; Belkina, T.; Bahashwan, S.A.; El Zowalaty, A.E.; Tebbens, J.D.; Abdel-Salam, H.A.; Khalil, A.I.; Daghriry, S.I.; Gahtani, M.A.; Madkhaly, F.M. Knowledge, awareness, and attitudes toward antibiotic use and antimicrobial resistance among Saudi population. *Int. J. Clin. Pharm.* **2016**, *38*, 1261–1268. [CrossRef] [PubMed]
16. Taufiq, M.; Zuberi, R.W. Overuse of antibiotics in children for upper respiratory infections (URIs): A Dilemma. *J. Coll. Physicians Surg. Pak.* **2011**, *21*, 59–60.
17. Albsoul-Younes, A.; Wazaify, M.; Yousef, A.-M.; Tahaineh, L. Abuse and misuse of prescription and nonprescription drugs sold in community pharmacies in Jordan. *Subst. Use Misuse* **2010**, *45*, 1319–1329. [CrossRef]
18. Wazaify, M.; Abood, E.; Tahaineh, L.; Albsoul-Younes, A. Jordanian community pharmacists' experience regarding prescription and nonprescription drug abuse and misuse in Jordan–An update. *J. Subst. Use* **2017**, *22*, 463–468. [CrossRef]
19. Charani, E.; Edwards, R.; Sevdalis, N.; Alexandrou, B.; Sibley, E.; Mullett, D.; Franklin, B.D.; Holmes, A. Behavior change strategies to influence antimicrobial prescribing in acute care: A systematic review. *Clin. Infect. Dis.* **2011**, *53*, 651–662. [CrossRef]

20. Charani, E.; Castro-Sanchez, E.; Sevdalis, N.; Kyratsis, Y.; Drumright, L.; Shah, N.; Holmes, A. Understanding the determinants of antimicrobial prescribing within hospitals: The role of "prescribing etiquette". *Clin. Infect. Dis.* **2013**, *57*, 188–196. [CrossRef]
21. Rawson, T.M.; Charani, E.; Moore, L.S.P.; Hernandez, B.; Castro-Sánchez, E.; Herrero, P.; Georgiou, P.; Holmes, A.H. Mapping the decision pathways of acute infection management in secondary care among UK medical physicians: A qualitative study. *BMC Med.* **2016**, *14*, 208. [CrossRef]
22. Kandeel, A.; El-Shoubary, W.; Hicks, L.A.; Fattah, M.A.; Dooling, K.L.; Lohiniva, A.L.; Ragab, O.; Galal, R.; Talaat, M. Patient attitudes and beliefs and provider practices regarding antibiotic use for acute respiratory tract infections in Minya, Egypt. *Antibiotics* **2014**, *3*, 632–644. [CrossRef] [PubMed]
23. Dooling, K.L.; Kandeel, A.; Hicks, L.A.; El-Shoubary, W.; Fawzi, K.; Kandeel, Y.; Etman, A.; Lohiniva, A.L.; Talaat, M. Understanding antibiotic use in Minya District, Egypt: Physician and pharmacist prescribing and the factors influencing their practices. *Antibiotics* **2014**, *3*, 233–243. [CrossRef] [PubMed]
24. Joseph, H.A.; Agboatwalla, M.; Hurd, J.; Jacobs-Slifka, K.; Pitz, A.; Bowen, A. What Happens When "Germs Don't Get Killed and They Attack Again and Again": Perceptions of Antimicrobial Resistance in the Context of Diarrheal Disease Treatment Among Laypersons and Health-Care Providers in Karachi, Pakistan. *Am. J. Trop. Med. Hyg.* **2016**, *95*, 221–228. [CrossRef] [PubMed]
25. Shahid, A.; Iftikhar, F.; Arshad, M.K.; Javed, Z.; Sufyan, M.; Ghuman, R.S.; Tarar, Z. Knowledge and attitude of physicians about antimicrobial resistance and their prescribing practices in Services Hospital, Lahore, Pakistan. *JPMA J. Pak. Med Assoc.* **2017**, *67*, 968. [PubMed]
26. Bush, K.; Courvalin, P.; Dantas, G.; Davies, J.; Eisenstein, B.; Huovinen, P.; Jacoby, G.A.; Kishony, R.; Kreiswirth, B.N.; Kutter, E. Tackling antibiotic resistance. *Nat. Rev. Microbiol.* **2011**, *9*, 894–896. [CrossRef] [PubMed]
27. Monto, A.S. Epidemiology of viral respiratory infections. *Am. J. Med.* **2002**, *112*, 4–12. [CrossRef]
28. Nyquist, A.-C.; Gonzales, R.; Steiner, J.F.; Sande, M.A. Antibiotic prescribing for children with colds, upper respiratory tract infections, and bronchitis. *JAMA* **1998**, *279*, 875–877. [CrossRef]
29. Gonzales, R.; Steiner, J.F.; Sande, M.A. Antibiotic prescribing for adults with colds, upper respiratory tract infections, and bronchitis by ambulatory care physicians. *JAMA* **1997**, *278*, 901–904. [CrossRef]
30. Fletcher-Lartey, S.; Yee, M.; Gaarslev, C.; Khan, R. Why do general practitioners prescribe antibiotics for upper respiratory tract infections to meet patient expectations: A mixed methods study. *BMJ Open* **2016**, *6*, e012244. [CrossRef]
31. Hamm, R.M.; Hicks, R.J.; Bemben, D. Antibiotics and respiratory infections: Are patients more satisfied when expectations are met? *J. Fam. Pract.* **1996**, *43*, 56–62.
32. Morgan, E.R.; Winter, R.J. Teaching communication skills: An essential part of residency training. *Arch. Pediatrics Adolesc. Med.* **1996**, *150*, 638–642. [CrossRef] [PubMed]
33. Kumar, S.; Little, P.; Britten, N. Why do general practitioners prescribe antibiotics for sore throat? Grounded theory interview study. *BMJ* **2003**, *326*, 138. [PubMed]
34. Biezen, R.; Brijnath, B.; Grando, D.; Mazza, D. Management of respiratory tract infections in young children—A qualitative study of primary care providers' perspectives. *NPJ Prim. Care Respir. Med.* **2017**, *27*, 1–7. [CrossRef] [PubMed]

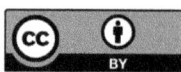

© 2020 by the authors. Licensee MDPI, Basel, Switzerland. This article is an open access article distributed under the terms and conditions of the Creative Commons Attribution (CC BY) license (http://creativecommons.org/licenses/by/4.0/).

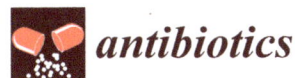

Perspective

The Need for Ongoing Antimicrobial Stewardship during the COVID-19 Pandemic and Actionable Recommendations

Wei Ping Khor [1], Omotayo Olaoye [1], Nikki D'Arcy [1], Eva M. Krockow [2], Rasha Abdelsalam Elshenawy [3], Victoria Rutter [1] and Diane Ashiru-Oredope [1,*]

1. Commonwealth Pharmacists Association, London E1W 1AW, UK; weiping.khor@commonwealthpharmacy.org (W.P.K.); omotayo.olaoye@commonwealthpharmacy.org (O.O.); nikki.darcy@commonwealthpharmacy.org (N.D.); victoria.rutter@commonwealthpharmacy.org (V.R.)
2. Department of Neuroscience, Psychology and Behaviour, University of Leicester, Leicester LE1 7RH, UK; emk12@leicester.ac.uk
3. FADIC School of Antimicrobial Stewardship, Muirfield Road, Watford WD19 6LN, UK; Rasha.Abdelsalam@fadic.net
* Correspondence: diane.ashiru-oredope@commonwealthpharmacy.org

Received: 14 November 2020; Accepted: 9 December 2020; Published: 14 December 2020

Abstract: The coronavirus disease (COVID-19) pandemic, which has significant impact on global health care delivery, occurs amid the ongoing global health crisis of antimicrobial resistance. Early data demonstrated that bacterial and fungal co-infection with COVID-19 remain low and indiscriminate use of antimicrobials during the pandemic may worsen antimicrobial resistance It is, therefore, essential to maintain the ongoing effort of antimicrobial stewardship activities in all sectors globally.

Keywords: antimicrobial stewardship; COVID-19; pharmacy

1. Introduction

Coronavirus disease (COVID-19), caused by the novel severe acute respiratory syndrome coronavirus 2 (SARS-CoV-2), has been exerting a significant impact on global health care delivery across both primary and secondary care, since it was first reported in December 2019 [1]. As of 20 September 2020, 30 million people globally have tested positive for COVID-19, of which 3.1% have died [2]. It is critical that normal acute infection management is maintained, and potential COVID-19 complications are anticipated. For the majority of patients, COVID-19 will run an uncomplicated course, hospital admission will not be required, and secondary infection will be uncommon [3].

The current SARS-CoV-2 pandemic occurs amid the already ongoing global health crisis of antimicrobial resistance (AMR). Infections caused by antimicrobial-resistant pathogens are estimated to cause 700,000 deaths each year globally and may complicate the care of COVID-19 patients, potentially leading to increased mortality [4], and result in significant economic burden. Resistant infections have previously been highlighted (pre-pandemic era) as causing economic burden and estimated to cost more than 100 trillion US dollars by 2050 if left unaddressed [4]; these are likely to be even more significant in the current pandemic and the post-pandemic era. At time of writing, it is reported that approximately 5% of COVID-19 patients require admission to intensive care units (ICU) and those with significant co-morbidity may require ventilatory support [5]. ICU admission and mechanical ventilation significantly increase the risk of patients acquiring secondary viral, bacterial and fungal infections [6,7].

One risk during a pandemic is that all resources may be diverted to treating patients infected with the pandemic agent, and other key health care priorities may be overlooked or deprioritised. However, antimicrobial stewardship (AMS) programmes remain essential and are likely more important at a time when needs for healthcare resources may exceed capacity [8]. Inappropriate access to and use of antimicrobials during the current SARS-CoV-2 pandemic may worsen AMR globally. This paper aims to contribute to highlighting the need for ongoing action to tackle the global AMR crisis during the COVID-19 pandemic and the need to uphold and continue the principal of AMS programmes among pharmacy teams. First, it focuses on reviewing the key challenges of optimising infection management and minimising AMR during the pandemic. For this, a literature search was performed by extracting published articles from PubMed with the search terms of "antibiotic stewardship", "antimicrobial stewardship", "antimicrobial resistance" and "COVID-19". Subsequently, the article makes actionable recommendations for clinical practice in the context of COVID-19.

2. Key Challenges of Optimising Infection Management and Minimising AMR

2.1. Continued Occurrence of Common Infections

Amid the current SARS-CoV-2 pandemic, common infections including e.g., seasonal influenza, bacterial infections, tropical infections or malaria will continue to be present [9]. There is no evidence that these common infections should be managed differently during the pandemic [9]. Local, and/or national primary and secondary care infection management guidelines and AMS principles should continue to be followed. Inappropriate use of antibiotics to treat viral infections and indiscriminate use of broad-spectrum antibiotics may reduce availability and lead to resistance and/or increased *Clostridiodes difficile* infections. Chronic infections such as human immunodeficiency virus (HIV) and tuberculosis remain global health issues and may be heavily impacted by the ongoing pandemic, in which diagnosis and treatment may be delayed, inappropriate or interrupted [10].

As governments across the world are closing down cities and restricting movements to flatten the curve of the pandemic, a large proportion of healthcare resources as well as staff are being diverted to halt the spread of COVID-19 [11]. In addition, there is emerging evidence that healthcare staff that lead on AMS have been asked to prioritise COVID-19 response and management, leading to reduced AMS activities.

2.2. Empiric Use of Antimicrobials in Patients with Suspected or Proven COVID-19

Testing for SARS-CoV-2 is currently not widely available globally, and the reverse transcription polymerase chain reaction (RT-PCR) test that is currently the gold-standard diagnostic test has a high false negative rate [12]. In the absence of diagnostic confirmation of SARS-CoV-2 infection, it is important that clinical features are carefully assessed to determine the likely source of infection. However, clinical features of SARS-CoV-2 infection are non-specific and can be indistinguishable from bacterial or influenza pneumonia. Some published initial recommendations were to consider empirical broad-spectrum antibiotics and neuraminidase inhibitors when patients presenting with COVID-19 symptoms are admitted to intensive care units [13]. However, it is important to note that the use of broad-spectrum antibiotics can lead to *Clostridiodes difficile* infection and a rise in AMR.

WHO guidance on the clinical management of COVID-19 suggests that antibiotics should not be prescribed for the prevention or treatment of mild COVID-19; while for suspected or confirmed moderate COVID-19 cases, antibiotic therapy should only be offered if there is clinical suspicion of bacterial infection [14]. However, for patients who have suspected or confirmed severe COVID-19, early empirical antimicrobials can be administered to treat all likely pathogens based on clinical judgement, patient host factors and local epidemiology [14].

Other international guidance, for example, The National Institute for Health and Care Excellence (NICE, London, UK) guidelines from the UK, suggest that antibiotics for the treatment or prevention of pneumonia in community settings should not be offered if SARS-CoV-2 is likely to be the cause or if the symptoms are mild [15]. Similarly, in Africa, the Uganda Ministry of Health guidelines do not advocate the use of antibiotics if the patient only suffers from mild COVID-19 symptoms [16].

In spite of this guidance, the empirical use of antibiotics in hospital settings is likely to increase globally because of the ongoing pandemic. In published case studies from China, it has been shown that 100% of severe and moderate cases were treated empirically with antimicrobials such as moxifloxacin and/or cephalosporin [17]. Indeed, this appears to have been standard practice in many hospitals in China [18].

In one hospital in Wuhan, 95% of admitted patients with suspected SARS-CoV-2 infection received antibiotics [19]. Of 191 patients included in the study, 181 patients received antibiotics, but this was shown to have no effect on survival ($p = 0.15$) while 41 patients received antiviral agents, which also had no effect on survival ($p = 0.87$) [19]. Similarly, in a review paper assessing 9 studies conducted in China and the United States including 806 SARS-CoV-2 positive patients, while some patients were found to develop bacterial or fungal co-infection, the comparatively low proportion (8%) did not justify the reported antimicrobial prescribing rates, which included 72% of patients receiving empirical broad-spectrum antimicrobial therapy [20]. A study conducted in the United Kingdom by Hughes et al. showed that the number of bacterial coinfections is low, occurring in 3.2% (27/836) of cases [21]. No evidence of fungal co-infection during early COVID-19 hospital presentation (0–5 days post-admission) was observed [21]. These findings demonstrate that there are currently limited data to support widespread usage of antimicrobial therapy on COVID-19 patients, and there is a need to develop global and regional antimicrobial policies and strengthen AMS interventions to prevent inappropriate use of antimicrobial therapy during the pandemic.

2.3. Falsified and Substandard Antimicrobial Medicines

Another challenge during the pandemic response in many countries is combating falsified and substandard medicines and pharmaceutical supplies. Falsified medicines are medicines which have no or little active ingredients and have not undergone any quality control evaluation, while substandard medicines are authorised medical products that fail to meet either their quality standards or specifications or both [22]. Past studies have shown that falsified or substandard antimicrobials are highly likely to promote the emergence and spread of AMR [23]. Recent studies have also shown that the resistance of *Escherichia coli* and *Mycobacterium smegmatis* to rifampin occurred as a result of exposure to substandard medicines; this presents a potential threat to tuberculosis treatment [24,25]. Over the years, it has been recognised that addressing the problem of substandard or falsified medicines will require the united action of all relevant stakeholders including government bodies, policy makers, regulatory and law enforcement agencies, public health professionals, patients and the general public. Pharmacists play a pivotal role in combating falsified and substandard medicines by working on strengthening supply chain procurement processes to ensure uninterrupted access to safe and effective medicines during the pandemic [26–29].

2.4. Stock Management and Supply Chain of Antimicrobials

Global antimicrobial supply chains are likely to be affected by the pandemic, and the cost may be increased due to travel restrictions or cancellations, therefore risking patients' lives and potentially contributing to drug resistance [11]. This is particularly challenging in countries that are highly dependent on imported medicines and pharmaceuticals [30]. Hence, there is a need to apply new innovative supply chain management strategies and diverse supply chains to ensure and protect the supply of essential medicines during the COVID-19 pandemic and beyond [31,32].

2.5. Healthcare Associated Infections

Whilst data are currently scant and there is no evidence to suggest that patients with COVID-19 are more likely to be infected by multidrug resistant bacteria and fungi, there is increased possibility that healthcare-associated infections will occur in COVID-19 patients with prolonged hospitalisation [33]. A large proportion of patients admitted to hospital due to severe symptoms required mechanical ventilation (75%), in a Seattle study [34]. Patients may be at increased risk of developing hospital-acquired pneumonia (HAP) and ventilator-associated pneumonia (VAP), which are often associated with drug-resistant bacterial strains. In the first documented outbreak of SARS-CoV-2 in Wuhan, China, VAP occurred in 31% of patients requiring mechanical ventilation and was associated with increased mortality [19]. There is evidence to suggest that a large proportion of deaths during the 1918 Influenza pandemic were due to secondary bacterial infection [35]. Secondary fungal infections must also be considered; putative invasive pulmonary aspergillosis was found in almost one third of critically ill COVID-19 patients at a Parisian hospital [6].

3. Recommendations for Adaptations of Clinical Practice in the Context of COVID-19

3.1. Consider Existing AMS Principles

Adherence to the local, national and international guideline recommendations is vital to prevent over- and inappropriate prescribing of antimicrobials during the pandemic. To support ease of access to antimicrobial prescribing and COVID-19 management guidelines, the Commonwealth Pharmacists Association (London, UK) developed a new repository of resources on COVID-19 prevention and management via the Commonwealth Partnerships for Antimicrobial Stewardship (CwPAMS) app, which is a smartphone app that consists of national antimicrobial prescribing guidelines from Ghana, Tanzania, Uganda and Zambia as well as international guidelines from the World Health Organization and International Pharmaceutical Federation (FIP) (The Hague, The Netherlands) [36]. A repository of useful resources on COVID-19 may be found in the Supplementary Materials File S1.

Despite limited evidence for the effectiveness of AMS interventions in low- and middle-income countries, AMS alongside infection prevention and control (IPC) remain the cornerstone to tackle AMR [37,38]. Appropriate use of antimicrobials may also reduce the economic burden and ensure availability of antimicrobials given the economic crises during the pandemic [38]. National and/or local levels should continue to develop action plans and policies to promote and perform AMS programmes [38,39]. In recent development, the Commonwealth Pharmacists Association published a CwPAMS toolkit, which outlines strategies and projects that a healthcare facility can implement as part of an AMS workplan. This may serve as a guidance especially for resource-limited countries to initiate AMS programmes [40].

Patient education on the appropriate use of antimicrobials is important as there is no evidence that antibiotics can be used for the treatment of viruses, and research/clinical trials on the use of certain antimicrobials in the management of COVID-19 is still ongoing. On 23 April 2020, the Africa Centres for Disease Control released a statement on medications to treat COVID-19. In the statement, the Africa CDC made the following recommendation:

> "Physicians should not prescribe, and individuals should not take, chloroquine or hydroxychloroquine to prevent or treat COVID-19 except under clinical trial or monitored emergency use of unregistered and investigational interventions (MEURI) as these drugs can cause neurologic, ophthalmic, cardiac, and other forms of toxicity and Physicians should not prescribe, and individuals should not take, Lopinavir/Ritonavir, Remdesivir or other medications to prevent or treat COVID-19 except under clinical trial or MEURI" [41].

The WHO's interim guidance on the clinical management of COVID-19 released on 27 May 2020 also makes the same recommendation stating that:

> "Chloroquine and hydroxychloroquine (+/− azithromycin); antivirals including but not limited to Lopinavir/ritonavir, remdesivir, umifenovir, favipiravir; Immunomodulators, including but not limited to tocilizumab and Interferon-β-1a, and plasma therapy should not be administered as treatment or prophylaxis for COVID-19, outside of the context of clinical trials" [14].

Key AMS components that can be promoted and practiced amid the current ongoing COVID-19 pandemic are described below. Actionable recommendations are sub-divided into different sectors of care.

3.1.1. Hospital Care

To improve infection management and reduce AMR in hospital patients, the following principles are likely to be vital [14,39]:

- Appropriate microbiological tests by culture or serological tests based on availability should be obtained before the initiation of empirical antibiotic therapy.
- Local infection management guidelines should be promoted. An initial choice of empirical antibiotic treatment should be selected based on local antibiograms, and institutional antimicrobial guidelines should be based upon local antibiogram results.
- Antibiotic treatment should be evaluated daily, and be deescalated or discontinued if clinical markers are not suggestive of bacterial infection.
- If antibiotic treatment is continued, the choice of antibiotic should be guided by microbiological test results.
- Conversion from an intravenous route to an oral route should be performed as soon as possible, as long as the oral route is not compromised, and the patient has shown clinical improvement.
- The duration of antibiotic treatment can be limited to five days for the majority of respiratory indications.
- Careful patient monitoring is necessary for potential drug interactions or toxicity, e.g., QTc prolongation (macrolides and quinolones), cation drug interactions (doxycycline and quinolones) and other drug interactions (macrolides and quinolones).
- Prophylactic use of antibiotics to prevent bacterial pneumonia should not occur.

3.1.2. Community Care/Primary Care

Primary care providers have the responsibility to support and guide patients through managing COVID-19 symptoms, explaining [42]:

- The common symptoms, which are mostly pyrexia, cough and loss of the ability to smell or taste as well as breathlessness and/or delirium, weakness, headache, muscle pain and sore throat in certain individuals.
- Guidelines to be followed by people caring for them in line with their country's guidance on self-isolation and protection for vulnerable people.
- The possible outcomes of the disease depending on the severity. If the symptoms are mild, they are likely to feel much better within a week.
- The appropriate health authorities to contact in their country/region if their symptoms get worse, for example NHS 111 online in the UK.

3.2. Harness the AMS Role of Pharmacists and Their Teams

Pharmacy teams in the community especially, also play a strategic role in ensuring the rational use of medicines and, as a result, are critically placed to help address AMR [43]. Pharmacists, along with other healthcare professionals, are crucial to ensuring that knowledge and evidence are effectively gathered and provided to members of the public. This ensures the judicious use of medications and prevention of stockpiling of medicines, especially the precious commodities of anti-infective drugs. Individual countries should devise and strengthen prescription-monitoring schemes to monitor the safety and efficacy of any off-label drugs being used for COVID-19 management [44].

Community pharmacists' dual roles as healthcare providers and retailers has also become very apparent during the pandemic [45], emphasizing their indispensable place as providers of safe and effective medicines and medicines information. Pharmacists and pharmacy associations have a vital role in engaging the public and providing education in communities to ensure timely delivery of scientifically proven and reliable information on COVID-19 prevention and management. In line with this, the CPA alongside other pharmacy bodies such as FIP (The Hague, The Netherlands) and the Royal Pharmaceutical Society (London, UK) organised webinars aimed at ensuring that pharmacists across the Commonwealth, worldwide and UK respectively were equipped with knowledge and the right resources to support the COVID-19 response during the peak of the pandemic. The webinars were designed strategically to prevent common occurrences of misinformation and rumours during the pandemic, which can lead to misuse of medicines and a negative impact on public health [46]. This has been highlighted in the cases of chloroquine, a drug which has a long history of being used for malaria treatment, and hydroxychloroquine, which is commonly used for autoimmune disease treatment. These drugs have come into the limelight through the media as potential COVID-19 treatments. There is currently no randomised controlled trial that suggests their efficacy in preventing or treating COVID-19, and indiscriminate promotion and widespread use of chloroquine and hydroxychloroquine have led to drug shortages, self-treatment, fatal overdoses and potential drug resistance [44]. This is of considerable health concern especially in countries, which are endemic with malaria or have poor assess to reliable and accurate health information.

Community pharmacists are well placed to promote AMS and often have the right knowledge, adequate opportunity and inherent dedication required. Despite this, there is limited information on AMS interventions at a community level with the community pharmacist role being less established and harnessed [47]. Similarly, there is a paucity of data on how community pharmacists have applied the principles of AMS to combat AMR in low- and middle-income countries during the COVID-19 pandemic. Community pharmacists can promote AMS in the context of COVID-19 through [47]:

- Promoting the appropriate use of prescribed antimicrobials for treating infections by advising patients on compliance to the dosage regimen, possible adverse effects and any risk of drug interactions.
- Serving as an interface between prescribers and patients; discussing and consulting with prescribers on antibiotic prescriptions to promote adherence to prescribing guidelines and optimal treatment regimens.
- Advocating for an adequate and effective supply chain to ensure continuous medicines supply and prevent drug shortages.
- Providing advice, counseling and support as well as educating patients on Infection Prevention and Control (IPC) practices, AMR and basic hygiene, including hand washing and COVID-19 transmission, nutritional tips during self-quarantine and the best use of over the counter (non-prescription) medications such as pain relief/symptom control medicines, vitamin C, D and zinc, among other vital medications, especially with special populations such as pregnant and elderly patients [48,49].
- Effectively addressing the increased demand for antimicrobials by providing adequate drug information and a literature review on the treatment options for self-limiting illnesses and guidance on when to see a doctor.
- Utilising the media to organise health education and promotion campaigns on the correct use of antimicrobials during the pandemic, including the provision of guidelines for the proper disposal of old/unused antibiotics or expired medicines to maintain safe antibiotic disposal to reduce medicines in the environment.
- Providing prescribers with updates on the use of antibiotics in bacterial co-infections in COVID-19 patients. This is highly important during the current pandemic, as the WHO reports that the use of azithromycin with hydroxychloroquine is highly prevalent although its use is not yet approved outside of COVID-19 clinical trials [14].

Pharmacy teams across all sectors are at the forefront of contributing to the COVID-19 crisis emergency preparedness. A recent study on global contributions by pharmacists during the COVID-19 pandemic in nine countries discussed how pharmacists worked at the frontline of the pandemic to provide care spanning across a broad range of areas including community pharmacies, hospitals, clinics, public health and care homes among other vital areas [50]. It is, therefore, important for pharmacy teams to be equipped with emergency preparedness skills as well as knowledge on prevention measures for COVID-19 whilst carrying out their duties. This includes [51]:

- Insistence on the adherence to IPC guidelines on hand hygiene, respiratory hygiene and the use of medical masks by patients exhibiting respiratory symptoms.
- The right application of contact and droplet precautions when dealing with suspected cases.
- The provision of health education on the early identification of symptoms, necessary precautions to take and right health facilities patients and families should utilise.
- The application of medication therapy management to ensure patients are receiving right medications properly with regards to their clinical conditions, as well as comprehensive medication management.

3.3. Address Issues of Falsified and Substandard Antimicrobial Medicines

As professionals charged with the final custody of medicines, pharmacists have a vital role to play in ensuring that the quality and efficacy of medicines is maintained in these settings, especially with impending challenges in drug supply and access to quality medicines as a result of the pandemic. Substandard and falsified medicines pose significant safety, quality and efficacy risks to patients [52]. In the context of falsified medicines, community pharmacists as frontline healthcare workers have specific duties including:

- Educating patients about the risk of obtaining medicines from unknown and unsafe sources such as unlicensed medicine shops online and medicine hawkers.
- Providing proper documentation and creating a feedback system to identify and track adverse drug events associated with the use of falsified or substandard antimicrobials, coupled with advising patients and providers to report on changes in the efficacy of all medicines.
- Advising governments, healthcare organisations and policymakers to design and implement policies to control the production and importation of falsified and substandard medicines, as well as to improve the detection of the same.

3.4. Manage Access to Effective Antimicrobials

Preparedness to ensure hospitals do not run out of antibiotics and other critical drugs is key, and guidance for which medicines stocks to increase should be provided. The WHO has recently published a COVID-19 Essential Supplies Forecasting Tool, which provides guidance on essential drugs including antimicrobials and consumables required to treat severe or critically ill patients [53]. Individual countries will need to conduct active surveillance and establish early warning mechanisms to receive alerts whenever a drug shortage is anticipated by evaluating a drug utilisation review especially for antibiotics. This is particularly important for antibiotics, which are commonly used for community-associated bacterial to lower respiratory tract infections, as shortages are expected to increase urgent care consultations and potentially increase hospital admissions. There has been increasing demand and evidence for the incorporation of digital technology as a tool to monitor stock levels, which provides feedback mechanisms that would ensure the continuity of medication supply.

3.5. Ensure Effective Infection Prevention and Control (IPC) Practices

IPC and appropriate use of personal protective equipment (PPE) have been well recognised as ways to control AMR [54]. During a pandemic, these measures are critical and should be expanded to contain the spread of the infections (both the spread of SARS-CoV-2 as well as other hospital-acquired infections [54]. Dedicated, trained IPC teams should be in place where possible. In countries where IPC is limited or non-existent, minimum requirements for IPC must be implemented as soon as possible, both at the national and facility level.

The WHO has issued five strategies to prevent or limit the transmission of SARS-CoV-2 in health care settings. It specifies:

- Ensuring triage, early recognition and source control (isolating patients with suspected COVID-19).
- Applying standard IPC precautions for all patients.
- Implementing empiric additional precautions (droplet and contact and, whenever applicable, airborne precautions) for suspected cases of COVID-19.
- Implementing administrative controls.
- Using environmental and engineering controls.

Hand hygiene and respiratory measures are essential, and all health care workers should be aware of and apply the WHO's 5 Moments for Hand Hygiene approach [54]. Appropriate selection of hand rub is equally important to ensure optimal antimicrobial efficacy [54]. In accordance with the WHO guidance on local production of hand rub formulation, the Commonwealth Pharmacists Association responded to the COVID-19 pandemic by launching a training video to support pharmacy teams in the production of WHO-formula alcohol-based hand sanitisers to further support IPC in hospitals and prevent the spread of infections, including COVID-19 [55,56].

Whilst access to PPE may be limited, IPC teams should, at the earliest opportunity, assess and quantify demand for masks and hand sanitisers. Local manufacturers of PPE should be identified and engaged to ensure supply where possible. Teams should be trained in appropriate use of gloves and masks—how to use, remove and dispose of them. Interventions to minimise the need for PPE include the use of telemedicine to identify COVID-19 cases, physical barriers such as windows at points of patient contact, restriction in access to patients by visitors and non-essential healthcare workers [57]. PPE should only be used where appropriate to minimise shortages. Environmental cleaning and disinfection procedures should be adhered to.

The use of IPC measures must be supported by administrative controls, including the availability of resources, appropriate infrastructure to allow the segregation of infected patients from the uninfected and distancing of healthcare workers and patients, the development of clear IPC policies and the access to laboratory testing.

3.6. Advocate for AMS at the Governmental Level (State or Federal)

The harm of AMR has a widespread effect on not only human health but also other critical priorities including the achievement of universal health coverage and sustainable development goals (SDGs). For example, combatting AMR is important for achieving SDG 3 of "good health and well-being", because the availability of effective antimicrobials is essential for restoring health where an infection is present. Effective antimicrobials also support the prevention of maternal, neonatal and childhood deaths as well as epidemics of communicable diseases such as tuberculosis, HIV and gonorrhea [58]. Other related SDG goals which AMR can impact include SDG 2 "zero hunger", SDG 8 "decent work and economic growth", SDG 6 "clean water and sanitation", SDG 12 "responsible consumption and production" and SDG 17 "partnerships for the goals" [58]. Considering that AMS is the key action to combat AMR, advocacy at the government level is therefore, an important determinant of its success. Identifying gaps is an important initial step for advocacy; for this, assessing the current level of AMS activities using the WHO checklist of essential national/regional and facility core elements for AMS programmes is recommended [59].

National and international advocacy as well as advocacy through civil societies is particularly important in resource-limited areas [60]. Through the effort of governmental and international collaborations to share established strategies, policies and skills; resource-limited countries may benefit from the experience of countries with existing AMS programmes. This can provide a framework to kickstart and expand AMS programmes without unnecessary delays [60].

4. Conclusions

The COVID-19 pandemic is a significant and new public health threat, putting tremendous pressure on all healthcare professionals. However, the ongoing global crisis of AMR must not be neglected. We highlight key challenges of infection management including continued occurrence of common infections, empiric use of antibiotics to treat COVID-19 patients, problematic access to effective antimicrobials and hospital-acquired infections. Given these challenges, we advocate that urgent actions are required to continue AMS practices during the pandemic. Specifically, we highlight the need for the reliance on existing principles of AMS across the hospital sector, primary care and community pharmacy. Other recommendations include ensuring access to effective antimicrobials as well as upholding the principles of IPC. Finally, advocacy for AMS must continue at all levels during the current pandemic and in the post-pandemic era.

Supplementary Materials: The following are available online at http://www.mdpi.com/2079-6382/9/12/904/s1. Supplementary Materials File S1: A repository of useful resources on COVID-19.

Author Contributions: Conceptualisation, D.A.-O., V.R. and N.D.; funding acquisition, D.A.-O. and V.R.; methodology, D.A.-O., N.D., O.O. and W.P.K.; data Curation, O.O., W.P.K. and D.A.-O.; project administration, W.P.K.; supervision, D.A.-O. and N.D.; writing of the original draft, W.P.K. and O.O.; writing of review and editing, W.P.K., O.O., E.M.K., R.A.E., N.D. and D.A.-O. All authors have read and agreed to the published version of the manuscript.

Funding: This project was funded as part of the CwPAMS supported by the Tropical Health and Education Trust (THET) and the CPA using official development assistance (ODA) funding, through the Department of Health and Social Care's Fleming Fund. The Fleming Fund is a £265 million UK aid investment to tackle antimicrobial resistance by supporting low- and middle-income countries to generate, use and share data on AMR. The programme is managed by the UK Department of Health and Social Care. The views expressed in this publication are those of the author(s) and not necessarily those of the NHS, the Fleming Fund, the Department of Health and Social Care, THET or CPA.

Conflicts of Interest: The authors declare no conflict of interest.

References

1. COVID-19 Significantly Impacts Health Services for Noncommunicable Diseases. Available online: https://www.who.int/news-room/detail/01-06-2020-covid-19-significantly-impacts-health-services-for-noncommunicable-diseases (accessed on 2 July 2020).
2. Coronavirus Disease (COVID-19). Available online: https://www.who.int/docs/default-source/coronaviruse/situation-reports/20200921-weekly-epi-update-6.pdf?sfvrsn=d9cf9496_6 (accessed on 25 September 2020).
3. Langford, B.J.; So, M.; Raybardhan, S.; Leung, V.; Westwood, D.; MacFadden, D.R.; Soucy, J.-P.R.; Daneman, N. Bacterial co-infection and secondary infection in patients with COVID-19: A living rapid review and meta-analysis. *Clin. Microbiol. Infect.* **2020**, *26*, 1622–1629. [CrossRef] [PubMed]
4. Review on Antimicrobial Resistance, Antimicrobial Resistance: Tackling a Crisis for the Health and Wealth of Nations; Review on Antimicrobial Resistance. 2014. Available online: https://amr-review.org/Publications.html (accessed on 29 November 2020).
5. Alanio, A.; Dellière, S.; Fodil, S.; Bretagne, S.; Mégarbane, B. Prevalence of putative invasive pulmonary aspergillosis in critically ill patients with COVID-19. *Lancet. Respir. Med.* **2020**, *8*, e48–e49. [CrossRef]
6. Lescure, F.-X.; Bouadma, L.; Nguyen, D.; Parisey, M.; Wicky, P.-H.; Behillil, S.; Gaymard, A.; Bouscambert-Duchamp, M.; Donati, F.; Le Hingrat, Q.; et al. Clinical and virological data of the first cases of COVID-19 in Europe: A case series. *Lancet Infect. Dis.* **2020**, *20*, 697–706. [CrossRef]
7. Kim, D.; Quinn, J.; Pinsky, B.; Shah, N.H.; Brown, I. Rates of co-infection between SARS-CoV-2 and other respiratory pathogens. *JAMA* **2020**, *323*, 2085–2086. [CrossRef]
8. Getahun, H.; Smith, I.; Trivedi, K.; Paulin, S.; Balkhy, H.H. Tackling antimicrobial resistance in the COVID-19 pandemic. *Bull. WHO* **2020**, *98*, 442. [CrossRef]

9. World Health Organization. *Clinical Care for Severe Acute Respiratory Infection Toolkit*; World Health Organization: Geneva, Switzerland, 2020.
10. Jiang, H.; Zhou, Y.; Tang, W. Maintaining HIV care during the COVID-19 pandemic. *Lancet HIV* **2020**, *7*, e308–e309. [CrossRef]
11. Adepoju, P. Tuberculosis and HIV responses threatened by COVID-19. *Lancet HIV* **2020**, *7*, e319–e320. [CrossRef]
12. Xiao, A.T.; Tong, Y.X.; Zhang, S. False-negative of RT-PCR and prolonged nucleic acid conversion in COVID-19: Rather than recurrence. *J. Med. Virol.* **2020**, *92*, 1755–1756. [CrossRef]
13. Phua, J.; Weng, L.; Ling, L.; Egi, M.; Lim, C.M.; Divatia, J.V.; Shrestha, B.R.; Arabi, Y.M.; Ng, J.; Gomersall, C.D.; et al. Intensive care management of coronavirus disease 2019 (COVID-19): Challenges and recommendations. *Lancet Respir. Med.* **2020**, *8*, 506–517. [CrossRef]
14. World Health Organization. *Clinical Management of COVID-19 Interim Guid.—May 2020*; World Health Organization: Geneva, Switzerland, 2020.
15. National Institue for Health and Care Excellence. *COVID-19 Rapid Guideline: Managing Suspected or Confirmed Pneumonia in Adults in the Community*; National Institue for Health and Care Excellence: London, UK, 2020.
16. Ministry of Health. *National Guidelines for Management of COVID-19*; Ministry of Health: Kampala, Uganda, 2020.
17. Chen, G.; Wu, D.; Guo, W.; Cao, Y.; Huang, D.; Wang, H.; Wang, T.; Zhang, X.; Chen, H.; Yu, H.; et al. Clinical and immunological features of severe and moderate coronavirus disease 2019. *J. Clin. Investig.* **2020**, *130*, 2620–2629. [CrossRef]
18. Wang, D.; Hu, B.; Hu, C.; Zhu, F.; Liu, X.; Zhang, J.; Wang, B.; Xiang, H.; Cheng, Z.; Xiong, Y.; et al. Clinical characteristics of 138 hospitalized patients with 2019 novel coronavirus–infected pneumonia in Wuhan, China. *JAMA* **2020**, *323*, 1061–1069. [CrossRef] [PubMed]
19. Zhou, F.; Yu, T.; Du, R.; Fan, G.; Liu, Y.; Liu, Z.; Xiang, J.; Wang, Y.; Song, B.; Gu, X.; et al. Clinical course and risk factors for mortality of adult inpatients with COVID-19 in Wuhan, China: A retrospective cohort study. *Lancet* **2020**, *395*, 1054–1062. [CrossRef]
20. Rawson, T.M.; Moore, L.S.; Zhu, N.; Ranganathan, N.; Skolimowska, K.; Gilchrist, M.; Satta, G.; Cooke, G.; Holmes, A. Bacterial and fungal co-infection in individuals with coronavirus: A rapid review to support COVID-19 antimicrobial prescribing. *Clin. Infect. Dis.* **2020**, ciaa530. [CrossRef] [PubMed]
21. Hughes, S.; Troise, O.; Donaldson, H.; Mughal, N.; Moore, L.S. Bacterial and fungal coinfection among hospitalized patients with COVID-19: A retrospective cohort study in a UK secondary-care setting. *Clin. Microbiol. Infect.* **2020**, *26*, 1395–1399. [CrossRef] [PubMed]
22. Fight the Fakes. A Fight the Fakes Factsheet. Available online: http://fightthefakes.org/resources/a-fight-the-fakes-factsheet/ (accessed on 23 November 2020).
23. Newton, P.N.; Fernandez, F.M.; Green, M.D.; Primo-Carpenter, J.; White, N.J. Counterfeit and substandard anti-infectives in developing countries. In *Antimicrobial Resistance in Developing Countries*; Sosa, A., Byarugaba, D., Amábile-Cuevas, C., Hsueh, P.R., Kariuki, S., Okeke, I., Eds.; Springer: New York, NY, USA, 2010; pp. 413–443.
24. Weinstein, Z.B.; Zaman, M.H. Evolution of Rifampin resistance in Escherichia coli and Mycobacterium smegmatis due to substandard drugs. *Antimicrob. Agents Chemother.* **2019**, *63*, e01243-18. [CrossRef] [PubMed]
25. Davies, J.; Davies, D. Origins and evolution of antibiotic resistance. *Microbiol. Mol. Biol. Rev.* **2010**, *74*, 417–433. [CrossRef]
26. Zaman, M.H. *Bitter Pills: The Global War on Counterfeit Drugs*; Oxford University Press: New York, NY, USA, 2018.
27. Hamilton, W.L.; Doyle, C.; Halliwell-Ewen, M.; Lambert, G. Public health interventions to protect against falsified medicines: A systematic review of international, national and local policies. *Health Policy Plan.* **2016**, *31*, 1448–1466. [CrossRef]
28. Member State Mechanism on Substandard/Spurious/Falsely-Labelled/Falsified/Counterfeit Medical Products. Available online: https://apps.who.int/gb/ebwha/pdf_files/WHA70/A70_23-en.pdf (accessed on 20 August 2020).

29. Ravinetto, R.; Vandenbergh, D.; Macé, C.; Pouget, C.; Renchon, B.; Rigal, J.; Schiavetti, B.; Caudron, J.M. Fighting poor-quality medicines in low-and middle-income countries: The importance of advocacy and pedagogy. *J. Pharm. Policy Pract.* **2016**, *9*, 1–4. [CrossRef]
30. Adebisi, Y.A.; Jumoke, A.A.; Carolyn, O.O. Coronavirus disease-19 and access to medicines in Africa. *Int. J. Health Allied Sci.* **2020**, *9*, 120. [CrossRef]
31. British Society for Antimicrobial Therapy. How Can We Ensure the Pharma Industry Protects the Supply of Essential Medicines during the COVID-19 Pandemic and Beyond? Available online: http://www.bsac.org.uk/how-can-we-ensure-the-pharma-industry-protects-the-supply-of-essential-medicines-during-the-covid-19-pandemic-and-beyond/ (accessed on 6 November 2020).
32. Asia Analysis. Highlighting Key Areas Across Asia. EU Pharma Strategy: COVID-19 Shows the Need for Diverse Supply Chains. Available online: https://www.openaccessgovernment.org/eu-pharma-strategy-covid-19-shows-the-need-for-diverse-supply-chains/96896/ (accessed on 6 November 2020).
33. Hassan, M.; Tuckman, H.; Patrick, R.; Kountz, D.; Kohn, J.L. Hospital length of stay and probability of acquiring infection. *Int. J. Pharm. Healthc. Mark.* **2010**, *4*, 324–338. [CrossRef]
34. Bhatraju, P.K.; Ghassemieh, B.J.; Nichols, M.; Kim, R.; Jerome, K.R.; Nalla, A.K.; Greninger, A.L.; Pipavath, S.; Wurfel, M.M.; Evans, L.; et al. Covid-19 in Critically Ill Patients in the Seattle Region—Case Series. *New Engl. J. Med.* **2020**, *382*, 2012–2022. [CrossRef] [PubMed]
35. Brundage, J.F. Interactions between influenza and bacterial respiratory pathogens: Implications for pandemic preparedness. *Lancet Infect. Dis.* **2006**, *6*, 303–312. [CrossRef]
36. Olaoye, O.; Tuck, C.; Khor, W.P.; McMenamin, R.; Hudson, L.; Northall, M.; Panford-Quainoo, E.; Asima, D.M.; Ashiru-Oredope, D. Improving access to antimicrobial prescribing guidelines in 4 African countries: Development and pilot implementation of an App and cross-sectional assessment of attitudes and behaviour survey of healthcare workers and patients. *Antibiotics* **2020**, *9*, 555. [CrossRef] [PubMed]
37. Cox, J.A.; Vlieghe, E.; Mendelson, M.; Wertheim, H.; Ndegwa, L.; Villegas, M.V.; Gould, I.; Hara, G.L. Antibiotic stewardship in low-and middle-income countries: The same but different? *Clin. Microbiol. Infect.* **2017**, *23*, 812–818. [CrossRef] [PubMed]
38. Huebner, C.; Flessa, S.; Huebner, N.O. The economic impact of antimicrobial stewardship programmes in hospitals: A systematic literature review. *J. Hosp. Infect.* **2019**, *102*, 369–376. [CrossRef] [PubMed]
39. Huttner, B.; Catho, G.; Pano-Pardo, J.R.; Pulcini, C.; Schouten, J. COVID-19: Don't neglect antimicrobial stewardship principles! *Clin. Microbiol. Infect.* **2020**, *26*, 808–810. [CrossRef] [PubMed]
40. Commonwealth Pharmacists Association. Commonwealth Partnership for Antimicrobial Stewardship (CwPAMS) Toolikit. Available online: https://commonwealthpharmacy.org/launch-of-the-commonwealth-partnerships-for-antimicrobial-stewardship-cwpams-toolkit/ (accessed on 28 November 2020).
41. Africa CDC. Statement on Medications to Treat Novel Coronavirus Disease (COVID-19). Available online: https://africacdc.org/download/statement-on-medications-to-treat-novel-coronavirus-disease-covid-19/ (accessed on 22 August 2020).
42. National Institute of Health and Care Excellence (NICE). *COVID-19 Rapid Guideline: Managing Symptoms (Including at the End of Life) in the Community*; NICE: London, UK, 2020.
43. Howard, P.; Ashiru-Oredope, D.; Gilchrist, M. Time for pharmacy to unite in the fight against antimicrobial resistance. *Pharm. J.* **2013**, *291*, 537.
44. Abena, P.M.; Decloedt, E.H.; Bottieau, E.; Suleman, F.; Adejumo, P.; Sam-Agudu, N.A.; TamFum, J.J.M.; Seydi, M.; Eholie, S.P.; Mills, E.J.; et al. Chloroquine and Hydroxychloroquine for the Prevention or Treatment of COVID-19 in Africa: Caution for Inappropriate Off-label Use in Healthcare Settings. *Am. J. Trop. Med. Hyg.* **2020**, *102*, 1184–1188. [CrossRef]
45. Chan, A.H.Y.; Rutter, V.; Ashiru-Oredope, D.; Tuck, C.; Babar, Z.U.D. Together we unite: The role of the Commonwealth in achieving universal health coverage through pharmaceutical care amidst the COVID-19 pandemic. *J. Pharm. Policy Pract.* **2020**, *13*, 1–7. [CrossRef]
46. O'Connor, C.; Murphy, M. Going viral: Doctors must tackle fake news in the covid-19 pandemic. *BMJ* **2020**, *24*, 1587. [CrossRef]
47. Essack, S.; Bell, J.; Shephard, A. Community pharmacists–Leaders for antibiotic stewardship in respiratory tract infection. *J. Clin. Pharm.* **2018**, *43*, 302–307. [CrossRef] [PubMed]

48. WHO Regional Office for Europe. Food and Nutrition Tips during Self-Quarantine. Available online: https://www.euro.who.int/en/health-topics/health-emergencies/coronavirus-covid-19/publications-and-technical-guidance/food-and-nutrition-tips-during-self-quarantine (accessed on 6 November 2020).
49. Pharmacy Times. Evaluating the Efficacy of Adjunctive Therapies Used to Treat COVID-19: The Role of Vitamin C and Zinc. Available online: https://www.pharmacytimes.com/news/evaluating-the-efficacy-of-adjunctive-therapies-used-to-treat-covid-19-the-role-of--vitamin-c-and-zinc (accessed on 6 November 2020).
50. Goff, D.A.; Ashiru-Oredope, D.; Cairns, K.A.; Eljaaly, K.; Gauthier, T.P.; Langford, B.J.; Mahmoud, S.F.; Messina, A.P.; Michael, U.C.; Saad, T.; et al. Global contributions of pharmacists during the COVID-19 pandemic. *J. Am. Coll Clin. Pharm.* **2020**, *3*, 1480–1492. [CrossRef]
51. World Health Organization. Infection Prevention and Control during Health Care When Coronavirus Disease (COVID-19) Is Suspected or Confirmed. Available online: https://www.who.int/publications/i/item/WHO-2019-nCoV-IPC-2020.4 (accessed on 1 July 2020).
52. Ferrario, A.; Orubu, E.S.F.; Adeyeye, M.C.; Zaman, M.H.; Wirtz, V.J. The need for comprehensive and multidisciplinary training in substandard and falsified medicines for pharmacists. *BMJ Glob. Health* **2019**, *4*, e001681. [CrossRef] [PubMed]
53. COVID-19 Essential Supplies Forecasting Tool. Available online: https://www.who.int/publications/m/item/covid-19-essential-supplies-forecasting-tool (accessed on 1 July 2020).
54. World Health Organization. *WHO Guidelines on Hand Hygiene in Health Care—First Global Patient Safety Challenge Clean Care is Safer Care*; World Health Organization: Geneva, Switzerland, 2009.
55. World Health Organization. *Guide to Local Production: WHO-Recommended Handrub Formulations*; World Health Organization: Geneva, Switzerland, 2010.
56. How to Manufacture Alcohol Hand Rub: Training Video Launched to Support COVID-19 Response. Available online: https://commonwealthpharmacy.org/press-release-how-to-manufacture-alcohol-hand-rub-training-video-launched-to-support-covid-19-response/ (accessed on 1 September 2020).
57. World Health Organization. *Rational Use of Personal Protective Equipment (PPE) for Coronavirus Disease (COVID-19) Interim Guidance-19 March 2020*; World Health Organization: Geneva, Switzerland, 2020.
58. World Health Organization, Regional Office for Europe. *The Fight against Antimicrobial Resistance Is Closely Linked to the Sustainable Development Goals*; World Health Organization: Copenhagen, Denmark, 2019; Available online: https://www.euro.who.int/en/health-topics/disease-prevention/antimicrobial-resistance/publications/2019/antimicrobial-resistance-advocacy-briefs-2019 (accessed on 5 December 2020).
59. World Health Organization Practical Toolkit: Antimicrobial Stewardship Programmes in Health-Care Facilities in LMICs. Available online: https://apps.who.int/iris/bitstream/handle/10665/329404/9789241515481-eng.pdf (accessed on 7 December 2020).
60. Tattevin, P.; Hara, G.L.; Toumi, A.; Enani, M.; Coombs, G.; Voss, A.; Wertheim, H.; Poda, A.; Daoud, Z.; Laxminarayan, R.; et al. Advocacy for increased international efforts for antimicrobial stewardship actions in low-and middle-Income countries on behalf of alliance for the Prudent Use of Antimicrobials (APUA), under the auspices of the International Society of Antimicrobial Chemotherapy (ISAC). *Front. Med.* **2020**, *7*, 503. [CrossRef]

Publisher's Note: MDPI stays neutral with regard to jurisdictional claims in published maps and institutional affiliations.

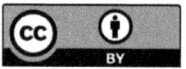

© 2020 by the authors. Licensee MDPI, Basel, Switzerland. This article is an open access article distributed under the terms and conditions of the Creative Commons Attribution (CC BY) license (http://creativecommons.org/licenses/by/4.0/).

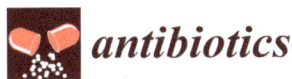

Article

Assessing the Impact of COVID-19 on Antimicrobial Stewardship Activities/Programs in the United Kingdom

Diane Ashiru-Oredope [1,*], Frances Kerr [2], Stephen Hughes [1], Jonathan Urch [1], Marisa Lanzman [1], Ting Yau [1], Alison Cockburn [2], Rakhee Patel [1], Adel Sheikh [1], Cairine Gormley [3], Aneeka Chavda [1], Tejal Vaghela [1], Ceri Phillips [4], Nicholas Reid [4] and Aaron Brady [3]

1. The Pharmacy Infection Network (PIN), United Kingdom Clinical Pharmacy Association (UKCPA), Leicester LE2 5BB, UK; Stephen.Hughes2@chelwest.nhs.uk (S.H.); jonathan.urch@nhs.net (J.U.); marisa.lanzman@nhs.net (M.L.); ting.yau@nhs.net (T.Y.); rakhee.patel1@nhs.net (R.P.); adel.sheikh@porthosp.nhs.uk (A.S.); aneeka.chavda1@nhs.net (A.C.); t.vaghela@nhs.net (T.V.)
2. Association of Scottish Antimicrobial Pharmacists (ASAP), Room 48, Ward 41, Regional Infectious Diseases Unit, Western General Hospital, Crewe Road, Edinburgh EH4 2XU, UK; frances.kerr@nhs.scot (F.K.); alison.cockburn@nhslothian.scot.nhs.uk (A.C.)
3. Northern Ireland Regional Antimicrobial Pharmacists Network, Medicines Optimisation Innovation Centre (MOIC), Bretten Hall, Antrim Area Hospital Site, Bush Road, Antrim BT41 2RL, UK; Cairine.Gormley@westerntrust.hscni.net (C.G.); Aaron.brady@qub.ac.uk (A.B.)
4. All Wales Antimicrobial Pharmacists Group, Cardiff CF10 4BZ, UK; ceri.phillips@wales.nhs.uk (C.P.); Nicholas.Reid@wales.nhs.uk (N.R.)
* Correspondence: diane.ashiru-oredope@phe.gov.uk

Abstract: Since first identified in late 2019, the acute respiratory syndrome coronavirus (SARS-CoV2) and the resulting coronavirus disease (COVID-19) pandemic has overwhelmed healthcare systems worldwide, often diverting key resources in a bid to meet unprecedented challenges. To measure its impact on national antimicrobial stewardship (AMS) activities, a questionnaire was designed and disseminated to antimicrobialstewardship leads in the United Kingdom (UK). Most respondents reported a reduction in AMS activity with 64% (61/95) reporting that COVID-19 had a negative impact on routine AMS activities. Activities reported to have been negatively affected by the pandemic include audit, quality improvement initiatives, education, AMS meetings, and multidisciplinary working including ward rounds. However, positive outcomes were also identified, with technology being increasingly used as a tool to facilitate stewardship, e.g., virtual meetings and ward rounds and increased acceptance of using procalcitonin tests to distinguish between viral and bacterial infections. The COVID-19 pandemic has had a significant impact on the AMS activities undertaken across the UK. The long-term impact of the reduced AMS activities on incidence of AMR are not yet known. The legacy of innovation, use of technology, and increased collaboration from the pandemic could strengthen AMS in the post-pandemic era and presents opportunities for further development of AMS.

Keywords: COVID-19; antimicrobial stewardship (AMS); antimicrobial resistance (AMR); coronavirus; SARS-CoV-2

1. Introduction

The novel coronavirus, SARS-CoV-2, has dominated all aspects of healthcare since it was first identified at the end of 2019 [1,2]. The coronavirus disease (COVID-19) has overwhelmed healthcare systems in those countries affected and diverted resources away from established services, as clinical teams look to manage this pandemic [3]. The antimicrobial stewardship (AMS) services, established to optimize anti-infectives and minimize the spread and impact of antimicrobial resistance (AMR), have been severely impacted by COVID-19 [4]. Whilst we battle against this pandemic, it is essential that we do not lose sight of the long-term AMR priorities.

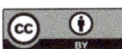

The long-term impact of COVID-19 on AMR has been much debated in the recent literature [5,6]. The highlighted importance of infectious disease and microbiology teams in managing this emerging pandemic, the increased awareness of and use of personal protective equipment and greater focus on hand hygiene are all expected to support existing AMR strategies. Limiting patient contact and social distancing may lead to reductions in healthcare-associated transmission of disease. These benefits are likely offset by prioritized allocation of isolation rooms to COVID-19 patients over those with multi-drug resistant organisms and the reallocation of resource to fight this pandemic. Many infectious disease and microbiology teams have been repurposed to manage complex COVID-19 patients and thus established AMS services have suffered. High antibacterial prescribing in patients presenting with COVID-19 is expected to propagate AMR and presents an immediate challenge for AMR [7]. Reports of low prevalence of confirmed bacterial and fungal co-infections with COVID-19 are emerging yet high rates of empiric antibacterial prescribing are evident [8,9]. Challenges differentiating COVID-19 presentations with classical bacterial pneumonia, the established concerns with bacterial co-infection with other viral infections (e.g., influenza), and often reduced diagnostic resources all contribute to difficulties when differentiating COVID-19 from potential concurrent bacterial infection [10–15]. Understandably, in the absence of robust evidence and clear guidance, antibacterials are often added as a precaution. This is complicated further by early conflicting evidence purporting the potential antiviral role of azithromycin, subsequently leading to increased use of macrolides for non-bacterial indications [16–19].

The infection pharmacist has been central to the delivery of care on the frontline and supporting the traditional AMS role. With the increased pressure on the health system during the pandemic, infection pharmacists have been called upon as key members of the healthcare team to support and alleviate the burden on over-stretched emergency departments, intensive care units, and to support medical staff with the management of high acuity patients. In addition, AMS roles have developed in response to local needs and resource availability. Availability of new technologies and reduced patient contact have also transformed traditional services and provide unique challenges and opportunities for antimicrobial teams [20]. The expected impact of COVID-19 on existing AMS services and on antimicrobial prescribing; thus, AMR remains unknown [6].

The challenge for pharmacists to balance the demands of daily clinical duties with those of maintaining an oversight of the rapidly emerging evidence base is great. Frequent reviews of the literature, drafting local guidelines, managing the effects of fragile medication supply chains, and introducing novel anti-infective therapies within trial or compassionate use settings as well as effectively communicating these changes have become an essential role for infection pharmacists. The Pharmacy Infection Network (PIN) of the United Kingdom Clinical Pharmacy Association (UKCPAPIN) during the first wave of the pandemic in the UK sought to support pharmacists, providing peer support, and creating the opportunities for shared learning to help reduce the burden for individual pharmacists. To better understand what was being done, what the barriers were, and the potential impact of COVID-19 on existing AMS services the UKCPAPIN developed a survey for distribution to all UKCPAPIN members within the United Kingdom. The survey was purposed to explore the intended and unintended changes of AMS services, to quantify (where possible) these changes at a national level, to guide future interventions by the UKCPA to better support colleagues and advocate for relevant actions based on recommendations from the survey results.

This manuscript provides an overview of this survey, conducted in June 2020, describing the challenges and opportunities that exist in the AMS teams across the UK and Ireland and identifies how the UKCPA can better support antimicrobial pharmacists in their goals to optimize patient care in these unprecedented times.

2. Results and Discussion

2.1. Demographics of Respondents

Overall, there were responses on behalf of 95 of 169 acute trusts or health boards (56%) in the UK: 79/143 acute trusts in England, 5/14 health boards (Scotland), 7/7 health boards (Wales), and 4/5 health and social care trusts (Northern Ireland) (Table 1). This is the widest survey to date that authors can locate on the effects of the COVID-19 pandemic on AMS activities, covering almost a hundred healthcare providers (56%) across the four nations of the UK. Majority of the responding organizations were hospital trusts consisting of district/general hospitals (41%) followed by teaching hospitals (26%) (Table 1).

Table 1. Country distribution of responses (n = 95).

Country	Number of Trusts/Health Boards with Responses	% of Respondents
England	79	83.2
Scotland	5	5.3
Wales	7	7.4
Northern Ireland	4	4.2
Type of hospital/organization	Number	% of respondents
Teaching	25	26.3
District/General	39	41.1
Acute Trust with multiple types of hospitals	13	13.7
Specialist	7	7.4
Others	11	11.6
Community Trust, Mental Health Trust, or Clinical Commissioning Groups (CCG)/Primary care/Primary Care Network	0	0
Reported estimated number of COVID-19 cases by respondents	Number of respondents	% of respondents
0–50	4	4.2
51–200	10	10.5
201–500	16	16.8
501–1000	21	22.1
1000–2000	12	12.6
>2000	4	4.2
Unsure	25	26.3
Do not wish to answer	3	3.2

The approximate number of hospitalized COVID-19 cases as estimated by the respondents in the organizations (up until 31 May 2020) ranged from 0 to >2000; the majority reported having more than 500 hospitalized cases of COVID-19 at the time of the survey and four organizations reported having more than 200 hospitalized cases.

The majority of the respondents were lead antimicrobial or infection pharmacists (90%; 85/95), members of the infection/AMS pharmacy team (7%; 7/95) or microbiologist (1%; 1/95) who would have good insight into the AMS challenges and changes within their organizations. Two (2%) of the respondents were clinical pharmacists. There were no AMS nurse respondents.

2.2. Impact of COVID-19 on Antimicrobial Stewardship (AMS) Activities/Initiatives

When asked how much of an impact COVID-19 had had on their routine AMS activities (i.e., "In your opinion, how much impact would you say COVID-19 has had on your routine AMS activities?), 65% (61/95) felt that COVID-19 had a negative impact on routine AMS activities, with 31% (29/95) stating it had a very negative impact and 34% (32/95) describing some negative impact. While no one felt it had a very positive effect, 7% (7/95) did feel that the overall effect of COVID-19 was positive, whereas 25% (25/95) respondents thought that overall there were both positive and negative effects on AMS with the COVID-19 pandemic. Only 2 (2%) participants felt that COVID-19 had no impact on AMS activity within their hospital and one respondent stated they were unsure/unable to assess.

Most of the activities listed in Figure 1 were considered to have been negatively affected by the pandemic. The greatest impact was on audit, quality improvement initiatives, education, training, AMS meetings, and multidisciplinary workings including ward rounds. Qualitative data collected through open questions also supported this, with respondents highlighting core AMS work such as reviewing and writing non-COVID-19 guidelines as being the most affected. Respondents were concerned about increased antibiotic use, including increased use of broad-spectrum antibiotics, delayed IV to oral switches (IVOST), and prolonged antibiotic durations. However, they were not able to accurately quantify increases due to the impact on routine AMS surveillance activities. In addition, there were concerns of inappropriate prescribing of antimicrobials in patients with COVID-19 infection. Although these concerns cannot be accurately quantified at present due to the UK-wide decrease in audit activities undertaken by antimicrobial pharmacists, the suspicion of increased 'just in case' prescribing of antimicrobials is supported by PHE Fingertips data. Analysis of this national surveillance database indicates a substantial increase in antibiotic prescribing (DDD/1000 admissions) for the current COVID-19 period in comparison to all previous quarters going back to 2017 [21]. Notably, this trend was also seen across all NHS Acute Trusts in England.

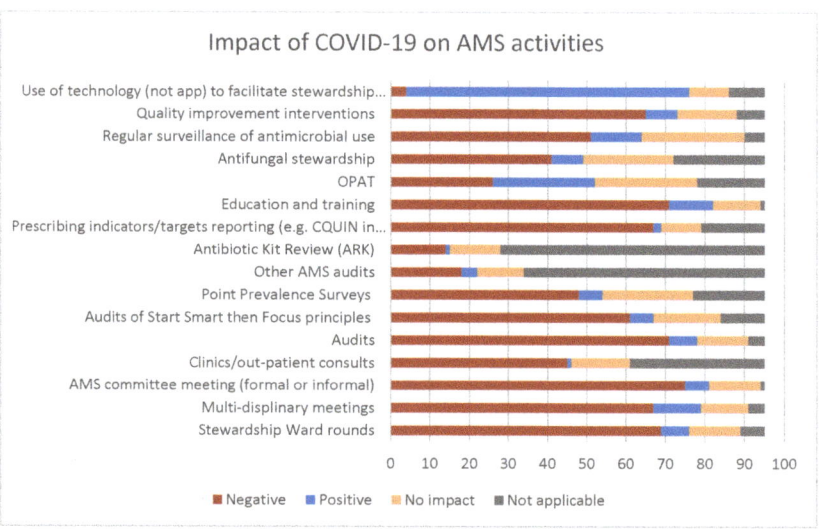

Figure 1. Impact of coronavirus 2019 (COVID-19) on antimicrobial stewardship (AMS) activities (n = 95 survey respondents).

Furthermore, PHE Fingertips data also reported a reduction in the WHO-classified 'Access' group of antibiotics which are typically narrow-spectrum and indicated as first-line treatment agents. Conversely, an increase in both the WHO-classified 'Watch' and Reserve' groups of antibiotics (typically more broad-spectrum and/or last resort antibiotics) were recorded nationally [21].

This suggests that nationwide use of antibiotics is not only increasing in overall volume but, more concerningly, in the number and volume of broad-spectrum agents prescribed. It is beyond the scope of this paper, but this trend has obvious implications for antimicrobial resistance in the months and years to

Open questions within the survey indicated that respondents were concerned that cases of *Clostridioides difficile* infection (CDI) were rising in some hospitals. It is however difficult to attribute increasing CDI rates with reduced AMS activities as there are multiple confounding factors involved. National surveillance of CDI also shows that cases were already rising pre-COVID-19 pandemic [21]. Moreover, when inquiring into what causes the increased concern for pharmacists, we found that physical limitations on conducting ward rounds, the inability to conduct regular antimicrobial audits, and the inability to see patients in person to confirm patient medication histories were most commonly cited. Stock shortages were also identified as time consuming and difficult to manage due to overwhelmed supply chains for antibiotics, antivirals and in some cases personal protective equipment (PPE). Some stock shortages for some antimicrobials such as levofloxacin appear to have commenced worldwide before the pandemic [22]. Due to the lack of routine AMS activity, it was felt that the full picture was not yet available to fully quantify the impact of COVID-19 on AMS and AMR.

Positive outcomes were also identified, with technology being increasingly used as a tool to facilitate stewardship, e.g., virtual meetings and ward rounds. The COVID-19 pandemic was also seen to break down barriers, resulting in increased collaboration. Other outcomes which respondents considered as positive were the increased introduction of novel biomarkers (e.g., procalcitonin) for differentiating viral and bacterial infections and better use of technology including virtual platforms and remote working. In addition, the use of hospital electronic prescribing systems facilitated AMS activities by antimicrobial pharmacists; allowing them to target their activities, for example identification of patients receiving excessive durations of antibiotics. There has also been a positive increase in multidisciplinary working where pharmacist contributions have been welcomed in an ever-changing evidence-based environment and pharmacists feeling valued for their contribution. Increased awareness of antimicrobial guidelines and improvements seen in infection prevention control have also been highlighted as likely to have a positive impact on AMS and resistance in the longer term. Innovation has also been key with some adapting services such as outpatient clinics and outpatient parenteral antibiotic therapy (OPAT) and changing current inpatient processes such as COVID-19 patients receiving a senior review more quickly. A virtual hospital model has been suggested as helpful to tackle the COVID-19 pandemic [23].

The majority of the respondents (73%) did not consider that there were non-COVID-19 related confounding factors that might have impacted AMS activities since the declaration of the pandemic in the UK (March 2020). For those that highlighted that there were confounding factors, these included staffing challenges within the infection team (i.e., lack of a stewardship lead microbiologist, antimicrobial pharmacists either not being in post or pharmacist AMS leads being redeployed, or needing to focus on clinical trials), drug shortages, increased post infection reviews for MRSA bacteremia and *Clostridioides difficile* cases. Positive confounding factors were also highlighted for example suspension of local meetings and national quality improvement schemes which allowed more time to review patients or target patients on high risk antibiotics.

Recently, Lynch et al. suggested that "AMS has become a casualty of the COVID-19 pandemic" [24]. In this survey we highlighted that while routine AMS activities were indeed a casualty of the COVID-19 pandemic, there were some opportunities presented and some positive outcomes. A recent review by Monnet and Harbarth reviewed the various determinants that may result in either an increase or, inversely, a decrease in AMR. They found that these determinants to be balanced [25]. However, the true impact of the

COVID-19 pandemic on AMR will not become clear for months, possibly years, when full surveillance data on antimicrobial use and resistance become available. In addition, the changes in AMR will vary depending on the settings, e.g., hospital types/units (ICU vs. other units) and facilities available in these settings; the reduction in usual hospital activities (such as routine surgery), availability of electronic prescribing and stock management systems; community vs. hospital settings, the number of COVID-19 cases as well as AMS activities that continue to be implemented through the pandemic.

2.3. COVID-19 Specific Changes to the Management of Pneumonia

Figure 2 illustrates the identified changes in AMS activity in the management of patients with community acquired pneumonia (CAP) during the COVID-19 surge in April 2020 against a baseline of 31 January 2020. It highlights for example that the pandemic led to increased use of procalcitonin in the management of respiratory tract infection both within and outside of the ICU, guiding antibiotic de-escalation and initiation. 53% (50/95) of respondents had updated guidelines on CAP before the release of the COVID-19 rapid guideline: managing suspected or confirmed pneumonia in adults in hospital by the National Institute for Health and Care Excellence (NICE) on 1 May 2020 [26]. There was also decreased AMS monitoring through audits such as the Start Smart then Focus (SSTF) studies, and the use of the CURB65 scoring system decreased slightly. The NICE guideline for CAP highlighted that CURB65 tool for CAP had not been validated for people with COVID-19. NICE guidance for the management of pneumonia in adults in hospital specified that there is insufficient evidence to recommend routine procalcitonin testing to guide decisions about antibiotics and encouraged centers already using procalcitonin tests to participate in research and data collection [27]. However, many organizations incorporated adherence to the CURB 65 scoring and advocated use of procalcitonin within their guidelines for management of COVD-19 patients.

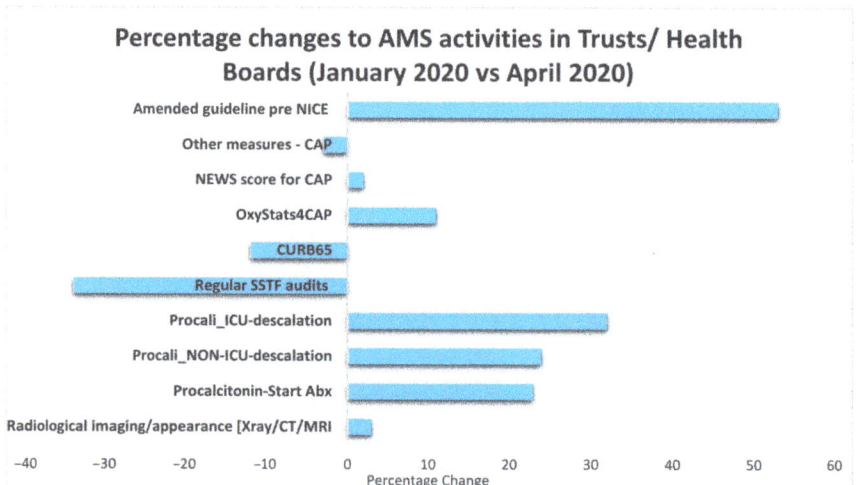

Figure 2. Changes to AMS initiatives as a result of the COVID-19 surge (*n* = 95). Key for the Y-axis: **Procalcitonin-Start Abx:** procalcitonin use to inform starting antibiotics. **Procali_NON-ICU-de-escalation:** Procalcitonin use in non-intensive care unit (ICU) settings to inform de-escalation and stopping antimicrobial stewardship activity. **Procalcitonin_ICU-de-escalation:** Procalcitonin use in ICU settings only to inform de-escalation and stopping antimicrobial stewardship activity. **Regular SSTF audits:** Regular (weekly or monthly) audit of review of antimicrobial prescriptions (Start Smart then Focus principles). **CURB65:** CURB 65 is specified in the guideline for assessing severity of Community Acquired Pneumonia **OxyStats4CAP**: Oxygen Saturations is specified in the guideline for assessing severity of Community Acquired Pneumonia. **NEWS score for CAP:** NEWS2 score is specified in the guideline for assessing severity of Community Acquired Pneumonia. **Other measures, CAP:** Other measures specified in the guideline for assessing severity of Community Acquired Pneumonia. **Radiological imaging/appearance (X-ray/CT/MRI):** Radiological imaging/appearance (X-ray/CT/MRI) to facilitate antibiotic review (de-escalating or stopping antibiotic) **Amended guideline pre NICE:** Amended antimicrobial prescribing guidance for COVID19 (pre NICE Guidance publications).

2.4. Participation in COVID-19 Clinical Trials*

At the time of the survey, almost all responding organizations (n = 95) were participating in the Randomised Evaluation of COVID-19 Therapy (RECOVERY) clinical trial (98%) with 75% and 58% participating in the Easy Access to Medicine Scheme (EAMS)–Remdesivir and Randomised, Embedded, Multi-factorial, Adaptive Platform Trial for Community-Acquired Pneumonia (REMAP-CAP) clinical trials respectively. Other trials and schemes taking place within responding Trusts included the since-discontinued expanded access program (EAP) for remdesivir (9%), Accelerating COVID-19 Research & Development (ACCORD-2) (8%), Safety and Efficacy of Tocilizumab in Patients With Severe COVID-19 Pneumonia (COVACTA) (6%), Platform Randomised trial of INterventions against COVID-19 In older peoPLE (PRINCIPLE) (4%), Adaptive COVID-19 Treatment Trial (ACTT) (4%), and Azithromycin versus usual care In Ambulatory COVID-19 (ATOMIC2) (2%). Two respondents reported that none of these trials were taking place in their organization. More than half of respondents also stated that their organization were part of the Early Access to Medicines Scheme (EAMS) for remdesivir.

As of 30 June 2020, there were 1142 clinical trials recruiting patients for COVID-19 management in hospitals or ICU settings globally with 62 of these registered for patients in the UK [28,29]. As perhaps expected, all organizations except two participated in the RECOVERY trial (RECOVERY; ISRCTN50189673), which was one of the two clinical trials globally that received the greatest media and scientific attention at the time. The other trial was the WHO "Solidarity" trial (ISRCTN83971151), which did not include sites in the UK. The lead role that many AMS teams had in management of these clinical trials may have contributed to the impact noted on routine AMS activities. Lack of resources for AMS because of re-allocation to COVID-19 planning and management, such as multiple trials, has also been highlighted by others [30]

2.5. Update of Local Guidelines and Implementation of National Guidelines

A third of responding organizations (UK-wide) had updated their local guidelines based on the NICE national guidelines for CAP and hospital-acquired pneumonia (HAP) published in April 2020; with just over 40% stating they were already aligned with the published guidelines whilst 12% of organizations stated they did not plan to update their guidelines based on national guidelines (Table 2).

Table 2. Organizations updating guidance in line with NICE recommendations (n = 95 respondents).

National Guidelines	Yes (%)	Already Aligned (%)	Still Discussing (%)	Don't Plan to (%)	NA (%)
Update CAP guidelines following publication of NICE NG 165 (n = 95)	29.5	42.1	9.5	11.6	7.4
Update HAP guidelines following publication of NICE NG173 (n = 95)	29.5	41.1	10.5	11.6	7.4
NICE criteria on when to stop antibiotics been implemented/promoted (n = 95)	36.8	27.4	24.2	5.3	6.3

A high proportion of organizations reviewed or updated their CAP, HAP, or healthcare associated infections (HCAI) guidelines as part of COVID-19 planning or during the COVID-19 surge. Three quarters of organizations (77%) also developed dedicated COVID-19 infection management guidelines (Figure 3). Other activities which had been affected during the COVID-19 first wave are highlighted in Table 3.

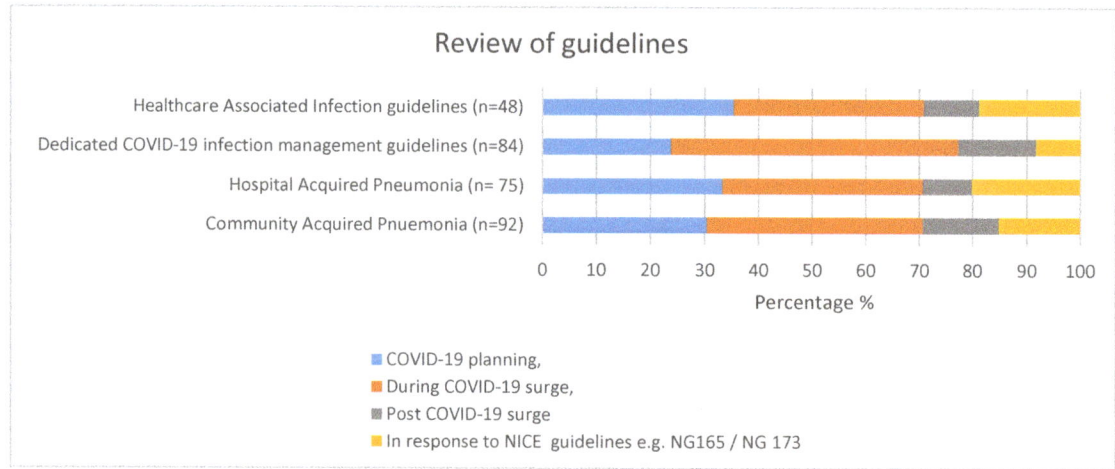

Figure 3. Percentage of organizations that reviewed their guidelines (*n* = 95 respondents).

Table 3. Other activities undertaken in organizations during the COVID-19 pandemic (*n* = 95).

Other Activities–Yes Responses	Number	%
Does your Trust have electronic prescribing for inpatients?	43	45.3
Has face to face clinical pharmacy time per patient reduced?	72	75.8
Has your organization published a specific antibiotic guideline for COVID-19?	62	65.3
Have you collected data on antibiotic use in COVID-19 patients since March 2020?	45	47.4
Is there formal recommendation/guidance/communication to stop antibiotics if patient is COVID + ve and no evidence of bacterial infection?	69	72.6
Have you collected data on bacterial co-infections since March 2020?	22	23.2

2.6. Communication Methods within Secondary Care Settings (*n* = 95)

Digital methods were the most common methods of communication within organizations during the COVID-19 first surge (Table 4). A variety of methods were employed to keep staff up to date with current best practice in an ever changing evidence base including the local intranet, an antibiotic app, and an increase in virtual meetings and teleconferences.

Table 4. Communication methods by organizations during the COVID-19 Pandemic.

Method of Communication within Organizations	Number	%
Intranet	54	56.8
Antibiotic App	50	52.6
Virtual meetings/teleconference	34	35.8
No specific cascade of messages on antibiotic use	16	16.8
Emails to staff	13	13.7
Grand rounds	13	13.7
Specific guidelines	10	10.5
Online learning, e.g., internal webinars	7	7.4

2.7. Staff Changes during COVID-19 Epidemic

COVID-19 has had a considerable impact on the roles and responsibilities of antimicrobial pharmacists (Table 5). More than half (57%) of antimicrobial pharmacists were seconded to other clinical roles within the pharmacy team and wider hospital with many having to undertake more than one role (Table 5). The main roles pharmacists were seconded to were ICU and general medicine. A small proportion of pharmacists also were seconded to roles outside pharmacy.

Table 5. New responsibilities for infection management pharmacy teams.

New Responsibilities during COVID-19 Response	Number	%
Secondment to other clinical specialties at any point for more than 0.5WTE of usual AMS activities time	54	56.8
Secondment to ICU	42	44.2
Secondment to general medicine	44	46.3
Secondment to technical services	6	6.3
Secondment to other roles within pharmacy	29	30.5
Secondment to other roles outside pharmacy	5	5.3

Antimicrobial pharmacists and antimicrobial pharmacy teams also undertook additional responsibilities as demonstrated in Table 6, with the highest number reporting additional responsibility for managing drug shortages, for both antimicrobial and non-antimicrobial medication. Managing supply of medication to patients with COVID-19 and providing PPE advice was also an additional role undertaken by many pharmacists during the initial COVID-19 pandemic. It is also evident that antimicrobial pharmacists had considerable involvement in the provision of infection prevention and control advice which may well have been part of the multidisciplinary ward round activities. The extension of antimicrobial pharmacists' roles beyond traditional duties/activities has also been highlighted by Goff et al. (2020) [31]. In addition, a recent review proposed recommendation for harnessing the AMS role of pharmacists and their teams in the context of COVID-19 and importance of continuing to advocate for AMS [32].

Table 6. Additional activities undertaken by AMS (n = 95) pharmacy teams.

Additional Organization-Wide (External to Pharmacy) Roles AMS Pharmacy Teams Were Involved in as Part of the COVID-19 Response	Number	%
Communications	67	70.5
Development of treatment guidelines linked to COVID	16	16.8
Development of other guidelines	48	50.5
Managing drug shortages (excluding antimicrobials)	29	30.5
Managing antimicrobial drug shortages	77	81.1
Monitor compliance with antimicrobial treatment guidelines	54	56.8
Management of patient's own drugs for COVID-19 patients	53	55.8
Providing infection prevention and control advice	57	60.0
Providing personal protective equipment (PPE) advice	33	34.7
Others (wider pharmacy management responsibilities)	5	5.3

More than half of respondents (56%) (Table 7) had to undertake additional training on their own time with only 37% being able to complete additional training and learning needs around COVID-19 within work. There was no training available for COVID-19 during the first surge as it was new to all. More than three months after the start of the pandemic, no hospital was able to provide formalized mandated training on COVID-19; this is likely to change as understanding of COVID-19 progresses and when a vaccine becomes available, which will require large scale training before administration. Learning on the job, reading papers being published from China and joining various webinars were the typical opportunities available during the surge. Our survey results showed that 92% of the respondents undertook this learning in their own time or as on the job training. This is further emphasized by the respondents in the increase in multidisciplinary team (MDT) working as the teams were learning as a team.

Table 7. Opportunity for additional learning undertaken during the COVID-19 Pandemic (n = 95).

Source of Significant Proportion of Learning/Training on COVID-19	Number	%
I learned on my own time	53	55.8
I have learnt on the job	35	36.8
I have not been able to dedicate time to learn about COVID-19 specifically	5	5.3
I received formal training which my hospital mandated	0	0

3. Materials and Methods

A quantitative survey-based approach was adopted using a 20-item questionnaire developed from the literature on AMS in the context of COVID-19 and consensus from infection/antimicrobial pharmacists (Supplementary Materials 1). Demographic data on the organization of each respondent included: which UK country, type of hospital (teaching, district/general, larger organization with multiple hospital sites, specialist), number of COVID-19 cases up until 31 May 2020, and the role of respondents. The survey was reviewed and refined by discussion with a working group comprised of members from the UKCPA Pharmacy Infection Network (UKCPAPIN), Association of Scottish Antimicrobial Pharmacists, All Wales Antimicrobial Pharmacists Group, and Northern Ireland Regional Antimicrobial Pharmacists Network. The survey was then hosted on Google Forms, a web-based survey platform, then pilot tested with five individuals across the UK. Following this initial testing, the final survey was disseminated by UKCPAPIN, Association of Scottish Antimicrobial Pharmacists, All Wales Antimicrobial Pharmacists Group, and Northern Ireland Regional Antimicrobial Pharmacists Network. The survey was also promoted via UKCPAPIN social media channels, and antimicrobial pharmacists/local network WhatsApp groups.

3.1. Respondent Eligibility

Pharmacy infection professionals (pharmacists, pharmacy technicians, and dispensers) across all UK secondary care and acute institutions/hospitals were the intended audience for the completion of the survey. Participation was voluntary, with the questionnaire being open for responses over a 2-week period (4 to 10 June2020).

3.2. Data Management

All data were held securely and in line with the General Data Protection Regulation 2016/679 (17). Study approval was also obtained from the UKCPAPIN

3.3. Data Analysis

Descriptive statistics on the frequency distributions and percentages were used to analyze the responses. Data were analyzed using Microsoft® Excel (2010). The survey tool is provided as Supplementary Information 1.

4. Conclusions

The findings of our survey provides, for the first time, quantitative and qualitative data on the impact of the COVID-19 pandemic on AMS activities undertaken across the UK.

Key stewardship activities that were negatively impacted include AMS ward rounds, MDT AMS meetings, quality improvement, audits, and education/training. The long-term impact of COVID-19 and the full extent of reduced AMS activities, as well as the impact of this on AMR, is unlikely to become clear for months and possibly years. We will know more when surveillance data on antimicrobial use and resistance become available, which will likely vary depending on setting and incidence of COVID-19 within each health system. Monitoring the impact of any harm caused by reduced AMS activities such as *C. difficile*, increased multidrug resistant organisms, and increased hospital admission or length of stay and mortality further reinforced the need to preserve this vital activity in future pandemic or COVID-19 surges. An additional survey to compare the impact of AMS activity during the first wave and subsequent waves or overall would add to the evidence.

Positive impacts identified within participating organizations highlighted through the survey (linked to measures to control the pandemic) included the increased acceptance of using procalcitonin to discriminate between viral and bacterial pneumonia-reducing inappropriate antimicrobial use in viral pneumonia patients in the post pandemic era. Technology was embraced to bring some of the historic AMS activities into the digital age and should be further harnessed and promoted. Using virtual platforms for education and training, multidisciplinary team meetings, AMS meetings, AMS rounds, and virtual clinics could also continue to be encouraged for AMS activities.

While the impact of the COVID-19 pandemic on AMS activity has been quantified, the psychological impact of additional roles, secondment to other specialties, and additional responsibilities that antimicrobial pharmacists have undertaken has yet to be evaluated and may form the basis of further studies. It is important that those who lead on AMS continue to have protected time to focus on AMS during current or future pandemics.

As expected wide scale participation in clinical trials for treatments of COVID-19 have been observed across the whole of the UK. The large number of participants has contributed to and will continue to progress the understanding of treatment options for COVID-19 for the benefit of future patients.

The legacy of innovation, use of technology, and increased collaboration/links with non-infection specialists, which the pandemic made necessary, could in fact strengthen AMS in the post-pandemic era and presents further opportunities for development of the antimicrobial stewardship roles. In addition, the networking and support network that has been developed will continue to support pharmacists in this role in future.

Supplementary Materials: The following are available online at https://www.mdpi.com/2079-6382/10/2/110/s1. Survey Form UKCPAPIN COVID-19 Survey.

Author Contributions: Conceptualization, D.A.-O.; data curation, D.A.-O.; formal analysis, D.A.-O. and F.K.; methodology, D.A.-O., J.U., M.L., T.Y., A.C. (Aneeka Chavda), R.P., A.S., C.G., A.C. (Alison Cockburn), T.V., C.P., N.R., and A.B.; project administration, D.A.-O.; writing–original draft, D.A.-O., F.K., and S.H.; writing–review and editing, D.A.-O., F.K., J.U., M.L., T.Y., A.C. (Aneeka Chavda), R.P., A.S., C.G., A.C. (Alison Cockburn), T.V., C.P., and A.B. All authors have read and agreed to the published version of the manuscript.

Funding: This project received no external funding.

Institutional Review Board Statement: The survey was conducted as part of service improvement of the Pharmacy Infection Network; no ethical approval was required

Informed Consent Statement: The following statement was included on the survey form and needed to be completed before completion of the survey "The survey is completely voluntary and part of UKCPA Pharmacy Infection Network support provision. You have the right to refuse to answer questions or withdraw at any time. By proceeding to the next page: I consent to UKCPAPIN collecting and using the information about me that I voluntarily provide for the purposes of the survey I have read, understand and agree to the information provided above".

Data Availability Statement: The data presented in this study are available on request from the corresponding author. The data are not publicly available due to organisation privacy.

Acknowledgments: We are grateful to all infection colleagues across the NHS in England, Scotland, Wales and Northern Ireland who replied to the survey. The views expressed are not those of the NHS or their respective organizations. We also acknowledge Elizabeth Beech who made important contributions to the design of the survey.

Conflicts of Interest: The authors declare no conflict of interest. The organizations the authors of this manuscript have their substantive infection lead roles in are listed: D.A.-O. (Public Health England); F.K. (NHS Lanarkshire, Scotland); S.H. (Chelsea and Westminster Hospital NHS Trust); J.U.(Great Western Hospitals NHS Foundation Trust); M.L. (Royal Free London NHS Foundation Trust); T.Y. (St George's University Hospitals NHS Foundation Trust); A.C. (Alison Cockburn) (NHS Lothian, Scotland); A.S. (Portsmouth Hospitals University NHS Trust); R.P. (Dartford And Gravesham NHS Trust); C.G. (Western Trust, Northern Ireland); A.C. (Aneeka Chavda) (Imperial College Healthcare NHS Trust); T.V. (West Hertfordshire Hospitals NHS Trust); C.P. (Aneurin Bevan University Health Board, Wales); N.R. (Public Health Wales); A.B. (Queens University, Belfast).

References

1. Phelan, A.L.; Katz, R.; Gostin, L.O. The Novel Coronavirus Originating in Wuhan, China: Challenges for Global Health Governance. *JAMA J. Am. Med. Assoc.* **2020**, *323*, 709–710. [CrossRef]
2. Zhu, N.; Zhang, D.; Wang, W.; Li, X.; Yang, B.; Song, J.; Zhao, X.; Huang, B.; Shi, W.; Lu, R.; et al. A novel coronavirus from patients with pneumonia in China, 2019. *N. Engl. J. Med.* **2020**, *382*, 727–733. [CrossRef]
3. Zhou, F.; Yu, T.; Du, R.; Fan, G.; Liu, Y.; Liu, Z.; Xiang, J.; Wang, Y.; Song, B.; Gu, X.; et al. Clinical course and risk factors for mortality of adult inpatients with COVID-19 in Wuhan, China: A retrospective cohort study. *Lancet* **2020**, *395*, 1054–1062. [CrossRef]
4. Huttner, B.D.; Catho, G.; Pano-Pardo, J.R.; Pulcini, C.; Schouten, J. COVID-19: Don't neglect antimicrobial stewardship principles! *Clin. Microbiol. Infect.* **2020**, *26*, 808–810. [CrossRef]
5. Mazdeyasna, H.; Nori, P.; Patel, P.; Doll, M.; Godbout, E.; Lee, K.; Noda, A.J.; Bearman, G.; Stevens, M.P. Antimicrobial Stewardship at the Core of COVID-19 Response Efforts: Implications for Sustaining and Building Programs. *Curr. Infect. Dis. Rep.* **2020**, *22*, 1–6. [CrossRef]
6. Rawson, T.M.; Moore, L.S.P.; Castro-Sanchez, E.; Charani, E.; Davies, F.; Satta, G.; Ellington, M.J.; Holmes, A.H. COVID-19 and the potential long-term impact on antimicrobial resistance. *J. Antimicrob. Chemother.* **2020**, *75*, 1681–1684. [CrossRef]
7. Rawson, T.M.; Moore, L.S.P.; Zhu, N.; Ranganathan, N.; Skolimowska, K.; Gilchrist, M.; Satta, G.; Cooke, G.; Holmes, A. Bacterial and fungal co-infection in individuals with coronavirus: A rapid review to support COVID-19 antimicrobial prescribing. *Clin. Infect. Dis.* **2020**. [CrossRef]
8. Hughes, S.; Troise, O.; Donaldson, H.; Mughal, N.; Moore, L.S. Bacterial and fungal coinfection among hospitalised patients with COVID-19: A retrospective cohort study in a UK secondary care setting. *Clin. Microbiol. Infect.* **2020**, *26*. [CrossRef]
9. Langford, B.J.; So, M.; Raybardhan, S.; Leung, V.; Westwood, D.; MacFadden, D.R.; Soucy, J.-P.R.; Daneman, N. Bacterial co-infection and secondary infection in patients with COVID-19: A living rapid review and meta-analysis. *Clin. Microbiol. Infect.* **2020**, *26*. [CrossRef]
10. Klein, E.Y.; Monteforte, B.; Gupta, A.; Jiang, W.; May, L.; Hsieh, Y.H.; Dugas, A. The frequency of influenza and bacterial coinfection: A systematic review and meta-analysis. *Influenza Other Respir. Viruses* **2016**, *10*, 394–403. [CrossRef]
11. Rodriguez-Morales, A.J.; Cardona-Ospina, J.A.; Gutiérrez-Ocampo, E.; Villamizar-Peña, R.; Holguin-Rivera, Y.; Escalera-Antezana, J.P.; Alvarado-Arnez, L.E.; Bonilla-Aldana, D.K.; Franco-Paredes, C.; Henao-Martinez, A.F.; et al. Clinical, laboratory and imaging features of COVID-19: A systematic review and meta-analysis. *Travel Med. Infect. Dis.* **2020**, *34*, 101623. [CrossRef]
12. Xiong, Y.; Sun, D.; Liu, Y.; Fan, Y.; Zhao, L.; Li, X.; Zhu, W. Clinical and High-Resolution CT Features of the COVID-19 Infection: Comparison of the Initial and Follow-up Changes. *Investig. Radiol.* **2020**, *55*, 332–339. [CrossRef]
13. Cox, M.J.; Loman, N.; Bogaert, D.; O'Grady, J. Co-infections: Potentially lethal and unexplored in COVID-19. *Lancet Microbe* **2020**, *1*, e11. [CrossRef]
14. Morris, D.E.; Cleary, D.W.; Clarke, S.C. Secondary Bacterial Infections Associated with Influenza Pandemics. *Front. Microbiol.* **2017**, *8*, 1041. [CrossRef]
15. Schauwvlieghe, A.F.A.D.; Rijnders, B.J.A.; Philips, N.; Verwijs, R.; Vanderbeke, L.; Van Tienen, C.; Lagrou, K.; Verweij, P.E.; Van de Veerdonk, F.L.; Gommers, D.; et al. Invasive aspergillosis in patients admitted to the intensive care unit with severe influenza: A retrospective cohort study. *Lancet. Respir. Med.* **2018**, *6*, 782–792. [CrossRef]
16. Arabi, Y.M.; Deeb, A.M.; Al-Hameed, F.; Mandourah, Y.; Almekhlafi, G.A.; Sindi, A.A.; Al-Omari, A.; Shalhoub, S.; Mady, A.; Alraddadi, B.; et al. Macrolides in critically ill patients with Middle East Respiratory Syndrome. *Int. J. Infect. Dis.* **2019**, *81*, 184–190. [CrossRef]
17. Gautret, P.; Lagier, J.C.; Parola, P.; Hoang, V.T.; Meddeb, L.; Sevestre, J.; Mailhe, M.; Doudier, B.; Aubry, C.; Amrane, S.; et al. Clinical and microbiological effect of a combination of hydroxychloroquine and azithromycin in 80 COVID-19 patients with at least a six-day follow up: A pilot observational study. *Travel Med. Infect. Dis.* **2020**, *34*. [CrossRef]

18. Cavalcanti, A.B.; Zampieri, F.G.; Rosa, R.G.; Azevedo, L.C.P.; Veiga, V.C.; Avezum, A.; Damiani, L.P.; Marcadenti, A.; Kawano-Dourado, L.; Lisboa, T.; et al. Hydroxychloroquine with or without Azithromycin in Mild-to-Moderate Covid-19. *N. Engl. J. Med.* **2020**. [CrossRef]
19. Arshad, S.; Kilgore, P.; Chaudhry, Z.S.; Jacobsen, G.; Wang, D.D.; Huitsing, K.; Brar, I.; Alangaden, G.J.; Ramesh, M.S.; McKinnon, J.E.; et al. Treatment with hydroxychloroquine, azithromycin, and combination in patients hospitalized with COVID-19. *Int. J. Infect. Dis.* **2020**, *97*, 396–403. [CrossRef]
20. Stevens, R.W.; Estes, L.; Rivera, C. Practical Implementation of COVID-19 Patient Flags into an Antimicrobial Stewardship Program's Prospective Review. *Infect. Control Hosp. Epidemiol.* **2020**, *41*, 1–2. [CrossRef]
21. PHE Fingertips. AMR Local Indicators. Available online: https://fingertips.phe.org.uk/profile/amr-local-indicators (accessed on 30 November 2020).
22. Department of Health and Social Care. Drug Shortages Update. Supply Issues Update for Primary and Secondary Care: March/April 2020. Available online: https://www.lmc.org.uk/visageimages/Covid-19/Supply%20issues%20update%20for%20primary%20and%20secondary%20care%20March%20April%202020.pdf21 (accessed on 30 November 2020).
23. Knight, M.; Evans, D.; Vancheeswaran, R.; van der Watt, M.; Smith, A.N.; Oliver, C.; Kelso, P.; Spencer, C.; Barlow, A. A Virtual Hospital Model Can Help Tackle the Covid-19 Pandemic. Available online: https://www.hsj.co.uk/technology-and-innovation/a-virtual-hospital-model-can-help-tackle-the-covid-19-pandemic/7027340.article (accessed on 30 November 2020).
24. Lynch, C.; Mahida, N.; Gray, J. Antimicrobial stewardship: A COVID casualty? *J. Hosp. Infect.* **2020**, *106*, 401–403. [CrossRef]
25. Monnet, D.L.; Harbarth, S. Will coronavirus disease (COVID-19) have an impact on antimicrobial resistance? *Eurosurveillance* **2020**, *25*, 2001886. [CrossRef]
26. National Institute for Health and Care Excellence (NICE). COVID-19 Rapid Guideline: Managing Suspected or Confirmed Pneumonia in Adults in the Community (NG 165). Available online: https://www.nice.org.uk/guidance/ng165/ (accessed on 28 November 2020).
27. National Institute for Health and Care Excellence (NICE). COVID-19 Rapid Guideline: Antibiotics for Pneumonia in Adults in Hospital (NG 173). Available online: https://www.nice.org.uk/guidance/ng173/ (accessed on 28 November 2020).
28. Thorlund, K.; Dron, L.; Park, J.; Hsu, G.; Forrest, J.I.; Mills, E.J. A real-time dashboard of clinical trials for COVID-19. *Lancet Digit. Health* **2020**, *2*, e286–e287. [CrossRef]
29. Cytlel. Global Coronavirus COVID-19 Clinical Trial Tracker. Available online: https://www.covid-trials.org/ (accessed on 28 November 2020).
30. Martin, E.; Philbin, M.; Hughes, G.; Bergin, C.; Talento, A.F. Antimicrobial stewardship challenges and innovative initiatives in the acute hospital setting during the COVID-19 pandemic. *J. Antimicrob. Chemother.* **2021**. [CrossRef]
31. Goff, D.A.; Ashiru-Oredope, D.; Cairns, K.A.; Eljaaly, K.; Gauthier, T.P.; Langford, B.J.; Mahmoud, S.F.; Messina, A.P.; Michael, U.C.; Saad, T.; et al. Global contributions of pharmacists during the COVID-19 pandemic. *J. Am. Coll. Clin. Pharm.* **2020**, 1–13. [CrossRef]
32. Khor, W.P.; Olaoye, O.; D'Arcy, N.; Krockow, E.M.; Elshenawy, R.A.; Rutter, V.; Ashiru-Oredope, D. The Need for Ongoing Antimicrobial Stewardship during the COVID-19 Pandemic and Actionable Recommendations. *Antibiotics* **2020**, *9*, 904. [CrossRef]

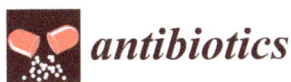 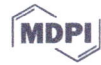

Article

A One Health Approach to Strengthening Antimicrobial Stewardship in Wakiso District, Uganda

David Musoke [1,*], Freddy Eric Kitutu [2], Lawrence Mugisha [3], Saba Amir [4], Claire Brandish [5], Deborah Ikhile [6], Henry Kajumbula [7], Ismail Musoke Kizito [8], Grace Biyinzika Lubega [1], Filimin Niyongabo [1], Bee Yean Ng [5], Jean O'Driscoll [5], Kate Russell-Hobbs [5], Jody Winter [9] and Linda Gibson [6]

[1] Department of Disease Control and Environmental Health, School of Public Health, College of Health Sciences, Makerere University, Kampala P.O. Box 7072, Uganda; gracelubega45@gmail.com (G.B.L.); filiminniyongabo@gmail.com (F.N.)
[2] Department of Pharmacy, School of Health Sciences, College of Health Sciences, Makerere University, Kampala P.O. Box 7072, Uganda; kitutufred@gmail.com
[3] College of Veterinary Medicine, Animal Resources and Biosecurity (COVAB), Makerere University, Kampala P.O. Box 7062, Uganda; mugishalaw@gmail.com
[4] School of Animal, Rural and Environmental Sciences, Nottingham Trent University, Nottingham NG25 0QF, UK; saba.amir@ntu.ac.uk
[5] Buckinghamshire Healthcare NHS Trust, Aylesbury HP21 8AL, UK; claire.brandish@nhs.net (C.B.); beeyean.ng@nhs.net (B.Y.N.); jean.odriscoll1@nhs.net (J.O.); kate.russellhobbs@nhs.net (K.R.-H.)
[6] Institute of Health and Allied Professions, School of Social Sciences, Nottingham Trent University, Nottingham NG1 4FQ, UK; deborah.ikhile@ntu.ac.uk (D.I.); linda.gibson@ntu.ac.uk (L.G.)
[7] Department of Medical Microbiology, School of Biomedical Sciences, College of Health Sciences, Makerere University, Kampala P.O. Box 7072, Uganda; henrykajumbula427@gmail.com
[8] Entebbe Regional Referral Hospital, Entebbe P.O. Box 29, Uganda; ismailkizito11@gmail.com
[9] Department of Biosciences, School of Science and Technology, Nottingham Trent University, Nottingham NG11 8NS, UK; jody.winter@ntu.ac.uk
* Correspondence: dmusoke@musph.ac.ug; Tel.: +25-67-1298-7736

Received: 29 August 2020; Accepted: 19 October 2020; Published: 31 October 2020

Abstract: Antimicrobial stewardship (AMS), as one of the global strategies to promote responsible use of antimicrobials to prevent antimicrobial resistance (AMR), remains poor in many low-and middle-income countries (LMICs). We implemented a project aimed at strengthening AMS in Wakiso district, Uganda using a One Health approach. A total of 86 health practitioners (HPs), including animal health workers, and 227 community health workers (CHWs) participated in training workshops, and over 300 pupils from primary schools were sensitized on AMR, AMS, and infection prevention and control (IPC). We further established two multidisciplinary online communities of practice (CoPs) for health professionals and students, with a current membership of 321 and 162, respectively. In addition, a Medicine and Therapeutics Committee (MTC) was set up at Entebbe Regional Referral Hospital. The project evaluation, conducted three months after training, revealed that the majority of the HPs (92.2%) and CHWs (90.3%) reported enhanced practices, including improved hand washing (57.3% and 81.0%, respectively). In addition, 51.5% of the HPs reported a reduction in the quantity of unnecessary antibiotics given per patient. This project demonstrates that AMS interventions using a One Health approach can promote understanding of the prudent use of antimicrobials and improve practices at health facilities and in communities.

Keywords: antimicrobial resistance; antimicrobial stewardship; community health workers; health practitioners; infection prevention and control; multidisciplinary; one health; Uganda; UK

1. Introduction

Antimicrobial resistance (AMR) poses a global public health concern that relates to humans, animals, and the environment. Several factors contribute to the escalation of AMR, including inappropriate prescription, misuse and overuse of, and lack of effective stewardship of antimicrobials [1]. In 2015, the World Health Assembly endorsed a global action plan to tackle the worldwide problem of AMR [1]. This plan has at its core the use of a One Health multi-sectoral approach, and calls for collaboration and co-ordination globally and locally. In response, Uganda developed and released its 5-year AMR National Action Plan (NAP) in 2018, which sets out a framework of actions to address the undertakings across the country [2]. The NAP acknowledges limited awareness of AMR and data pertaining to antimicrobial use, rising rates of AMR in the country, and the comprehensive steps that need to be taken to contain and control this threat to global health [2–4].

One Health refers to a collaborative, co-ordinated, and multidisciplinary approach to ensure the health and wellbeing of humans, animals, and the environment across different spatial levels [5]. A One Health approach is necessary as AMR is an ecological challenge that is affected by the interrelations between humans, animals and the environment [5]. The implementation of interventions and actions of multiple actors towards the optimization of antimicrobial use is known as antimicrobial stewardship (AMS) [6]. Despite increasing evidence for the need for a multidisciplinary approach to tackle AMR, the use of One Health in addressing AMS challenges has been minimal. A recent systematic review showed that there is a dearth in the practice and implementation of AMS programs across Africa [7]. Whereas there is increasing evidence on challenges affecting AMS in Uganda, there is little literature on antimicrobial use in animals and its relationship to human health and the environment [8–10]. This therefore calls for more interventions to use a multidisciplinary approach to improve AMS across the country as stipulated in the NAP [2].

With support from the Commonwealth Partnership for Antimicrobial Stewardship (CwPAMS) scheme [11], an initiative of Commonwealth Pharmacists Association (CPA) and Tropical Health and Education Trust (THET) under the Fleming Fund of the UK Department of Health and Social Care (DHSC), our health partnership aimed to strengthen AMS in Wakiso district, Uganda. The focus of the project was on capacity building, multidisciplinary stakeholder engagement, and knowledge exchange using a One Health approach. The project drew on a multidisciplinary partnership and expertise from: the Schools of Social Sciences, Animal, Rural and Environmental, and Science and Technology at Nottingham Trent University (NTU); Buckinghamshire Healthcare NHS Trust (BHT); Colleges of Health Sciences, and Veterinary Medicine, Animal Resources and Biosecurity at Makerere University (Mak); and Entebbe Regional Referral Hospital (ERRH) in Uganda.

It is acknowledged that antimicrobials are used widely in both humans and animals, and are commonly present in the environment [12], hence the need for a broader One Health approach in addressing AMR. Although most AMS interventions have been health facility based, a large proportion of antimicrobials are used in the community, both as part of outpatient care [13] and integrated community case management (iCCM) for the treatment of childhood illnesses. In iCCM, community health workers (CHWs) are involved in the diagnosis of malaria, diarrhea, and pneumonia among children under five years of age. CHWs are the frontline health cadre at the community level in many low- and middle-income countries (LMICs), including Uganda, and so, they have a key role in ensuring proper use of antimicrobials in their communities. Therefore, this project was designed with interventions at both health facility and community levels to ensure wide reach and impact. It was also planned for knowledge to cascade from healthcare professionals into the wider communities through the CHWs. Specifically, the project aimed to: strengthen AMR awareness and upskill human and animal health practitioners (HPs) in AMS and infection prevention and control (IPC); utilize a training of trainers approach with the HPs and CHWs to improve community-wide awareness of AMR; establish communities of practices (CoPs) for sustainable engagement and resource sharing to support AMS; and facilitate knowledge exchange and sharing of best practice between Uganda and

UK. In this paper, we describe the main activities and achievements of the project, including results from the evaluation of the HPs and CHWs who were involved in the training workshops.

2. Materials and Methods

2.1. Project Site and Setting

The 15-month project, as part of the CwPAMS scheme, was implemented in Wakiso district, central Uganda. Wakiso district has a total surface area of 2807.75 square kilometers, and a population of 2,007,700 people at an estimated growth rate of 4.1% [14]. ERRH, located in Entebbe municipality, Wakiso district, is the health facility where the main project interventions were implemented. ERRH has a 200-bed capacity, serving approximately 300 to 400 out-patients per day. Services offered at the hospital include but are not limited to: dental, pharmacy, peadiatrics, radiology, laboratory, maternity, maternal and child health, general surgery, internal medicine, and orthopedics. The hospital is led by a medical director, and approximately 10% of its staff are prescribers, including medical officers, dental surgeons, and clinical officers. ERRH serves a population of over 300,000, including the community in Entebbe municipality and neighboring areas, some being islands on Lake Victoria [14]. The community component of the project was implemented in Busiro South Health Sub District (HSD) in Wakiso district, which is comprised of three town councils (Kajjansi, Kasanje, and Katabi) and one sub county (Bussi). The HSD has a population of approximately 243,420 people. With a high number of households in Busiro South and the wider Wakiso district engaged in poultry and livestock farming, antimicrobials are used extensively [15,16]. The animal health workers involved in the project worked in Entebbe municipality either with the local government or as private practitioners. These health workers carry out diagnosis and treatment of animals mainly in the community. The CHWs in Busiro South HSD involved in the project not only treat childhood illnesses of diarrhoea, pneumonia, and malaria but also participate in educating the community on key public health issues, including AMR.

2.2. Project Team and Reciprocal Visits

This project was delivered as part of a 10-year international partnership between NTU, UK, and School of Public Health at Mak, Uganda. The partnership co-opted a multidisciplinary team for delivery of the project. This was essential due to the nature of the multifactorial challenges of AMR in humans, animals, and the environment. From the UK, specialist antimicrobial pharmacists and a medical microbiologist from BHT, a microbiology lecturer from School of Science and Technology, and an animal specialist from the School of Animal, Rural and Environmental Studies (ARES) at NTU took part in the interventions. In Uganda, project partners included: public health specialists, pharmacists including a clinical pharmacist, a veterinary doctor, and a microbiologist from Mak with support from health professionals from the Ministry of Health (MOH), ERRH, Wakiso district local government, and Entebbe Municipal Council. As part of the project, reciprocal visits between members from the UK and Uganda for planning, scoping, implementation, knowledge exchange, and sharing of best practices were held.

2.3. Project Planning and Stakeholder Engagement

The multidisciplinary project team conducted several meetings both physically and virtually before, during, and after implementation. The virtual meetings were held monthly using Skype and were attended by partners from both the UK and Uganda. The meetings facilitated project planning, implementation, monitoring, and evaluation as well as keeping track of the achievement of set goals. Other day-to-day communication to support implementation and timely completion of project tasks was achieved using a WhatsApp group. A google drive account was also set up for the team to access project documentation, such as previous meeting minutes, photos, and training materials. These communication avenues were invaluable for tracking progress of ongoing project activities and enhancing team work. Before and during project implementation, the project team held several meetings and engagements with various stakeholders in Uganda to ensure ownership, buy-in, and participation in planned activities. These stakeholders included government ministries (MOH and Ministry of Agriculture, Animal Industry and Fisheries—MAAIF), governmental parastatals (such as the National Drug Authority), professional associations (the Pharmaceutical Society of Uganda), training institutions (Mak), local governments (Wakiso district), health facilities (ERRH and lower level health facilities, such as health centre IIs, IIIs and IVs), local leaders (such as local council chairpersons), and the general community. The project team specifically engaged the MOH Technical Working Committee (TWC) on AMS, optimal access, and use, which is mandated to provide technical oversight of all AMS activities in the country. This engagement involved collaborative planning as well as regularly providing project updates in the TWC meetings and getting feedback that informed ongoing activities.

2.4. Enhancing Capacity of Health Practitioners, Community Health Workers, and School Pupils

The project held training workshops for HPs from both human and animal health to create awareness on AMR/AMS/IPC using a One Health approach. The workshops targeted selected HPs from government health facilities, including ERRH, as well as animal health workers in Wakiso district. The selection of HPs involved in the workshops was done in consultation with contacts at ERRH, Entebbe Municipal Council, and Wakiso District Health Office. Using the 'training of trainers' model, selected trained HPs were involved in training workshops for CHWs in AMR/AMS/IPC also using a One Health approach. The CHWs were from Kajjansi town council in Wakiso district where earlier NTU–Mak partnership interventions had been implemented [17]. All CHWs in the town council available at the time were involved in the workshops. In addition to the training of HPs and CHWs, the project also sensitised pupils in two primary schools in Wakiso district (St. Theresa and Kawotto Saviours Primary Schools) on AMR/AMS/IPC. St. Theresa's is a government school in Entebbe municipality while Kawotto Saviours is a private school in Kajjansi town council, both in Wakiso district. These schools were selected in consultation with key stakeholders in Wakiso district.

2.5. Establishment of One Health Communities of Practice and University Student Engagement

The project set up two online CoPs involving individuals from human health, animal health, and the environment. The first CoP was for health professionals, including HPs, researchers, policy makers, and academics, while the second targeted undergraduate students of Mak from various disciplines, including environmental health, veterinary medicine, pharmacy, biomedical sciences, social sciences, and computer sciences. In addition to the CoPs, multidisciplinary students at Mak and microbiology students at NTU were involved in various activities to promote AMR/AMS/IPC, including seminars, webinars, and competitions. The competitions, which were to design AMS messages using innovative approaches, were held to commemorate WAAW 2019. The winners of the competition were recognized as a form of motivation to continue being antibiotic guardians in their respective settings.

2.6. Establishment of a Medicine and Therapeutics Committee

Working closely with the hospital pharmacist, the project supported the establishment of a MTC at ERRH. This included appointing a multi-disciplinary team, in accordance with the MOH MTC manual [18]. The aim of the MTC is to support the safe and effective use of medicines through evaluation of usage, and to develop guidelines and protocols for medicine prescription and administration, as well as other health commodity related activities at the hospital. The MTC at ERRH has 12 members and three sub-committees reflecting the main functions: supply chain; pharmacovigilance, and AMS. During the course of the project, the MTC held three meetings to elect members, establish roles and responsibilities, develop work plans including a procurement plan for the 2020/21 financial year, and define standard IPC practices at the hospital. The MTC was specifically involved in: selection of medicines to be used; monitoring and ensuring rational use of medicines as per the standard treatment guidelines; development of draft treatment protocols; as well as developing Standard Operating Procedures (SOPs) during the management of COVID-19 patients.

2.7. Project Evaluation

The final project evaluation involved assessment of practices of the beneficiary HPs and CHWs, which was carried out three months after their respective training workshop. Specifically, the evaluation was aimed at establishing any changes in practices of the HPs and CHWs related to AMR/AMS/IPC following the workshops conducted as part of the project. The practices assessed among the HPs included: increased use of the Uganda Clinical Guidelines (UCG) when prescribing antimicrobials; increased diagnosis based on laboratory results; improved handwashing; and more patient guidance and counselling when they do not require antimicrobials. For the CHWs, practices, such as improved hand washing with soap as well as increased community sensitization on avoiding self-medication, consulting animal health professionals whenever animals were ill, and avoiding the use of human prescribed medicines in animals including poultry, were assessed. The evaluation among the HPs used a self-administered questionnaire while for the CHWs, a researcher-administered questionnaire was used. In addition, key informant interviews using telephone were held with selected key individuals from the various stakeholders involved in the project. The interviews included HPs and CHWs who participated in the workshops, particularly those with leadership roles, CoP members, Wakiso district health office staff, and facilitators of the training. In this paper, we present a summary of the key findings from the evaluation. The diagrammatic summary of the project implementation is shown in Figure 1.

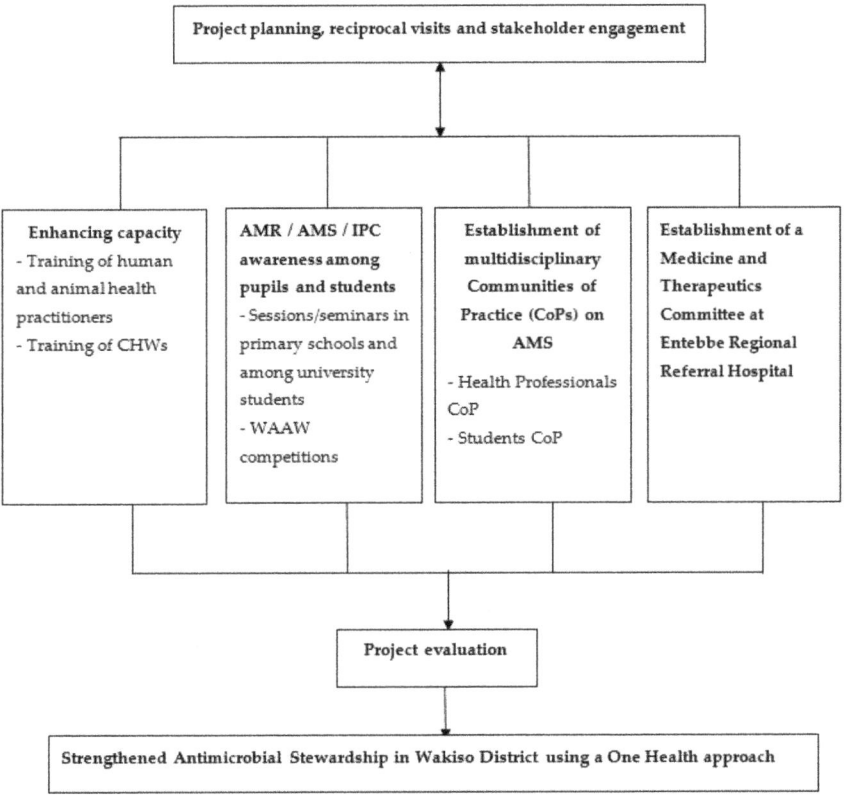

Figure 1. Summary of the project implementation.

3. Results

3.1. Reciprocal Visits

The project exchange visits lasted between one and two weeks depending on the timing of activities as well as the availability of the team members. The timing of these visits was crucial for the different teams to appreciate the level of, and approaches to AMS in the host country. The first UK team visit to Uganda in April 2019 was organised as a scoping visit. This was necessary to appreciate AMS activity in the country, including challenges, knowledge gaps, areas of sub-optimal antibiotic use, development needs at ERRH, and animal health AMS concerns to inform the project activities, including training of HPs and capacity support to ERRH. During this visit, several meetings were held with the ERRH administration, Wakiso district health and veterinary staff, MOH Department of Pharmaceuticals and Natural Medicines, and College of Veterinary Medicine, Animal Resources and Biosecurity at Mak. The second exchange visit was that of the ERRH pharmacist to the UK in June 2019. The pharmacist was involved in AMS discussions involving multi-disciplinary teams from BHT and NTU (City, Brackenhurst, and Clifton campuses). While at the Brackenhurst campus, which houses the School of Animal, Rural and Environment Sciences at NTU, the pharmacist learnt about the various animal projects there, including research on AMS. The pharmacist also spent some time in the microbiology department at the Clifton campus where he made a presentation to share experiences of AMS at ERRH and generally in Uganda among faculty. At BHT, the pharmacist spent time seeing AMS in practice on clinical ward rounds and in the pathology laboratory, and visited the medical microbiology laboratory where he gave a presentation to scientists. The pharmacist met with the medical director to discuss a potential memorandum of understanding with ERRH and how future work may be undertaken to support other collaborative activities. In the UK, the pharmacist was also involved in further project planning and work shadowing to learn more about AMS practices. The third exchange visit was of the UK team in September 2019 that involved a series of activities including: facilitation of three two-day AMS trainings among human and animal HPs; AMS seminars at Mak; and visits to primary schools to sensitize them on AMR and to launch an awareness competition. The final visit was by a Ugandan clinical pharmacist and lecturer at Mak in September 2020. This visit focused on AMS / AMR knowledge exchange, potential expansion of partnership work, discussions on final project activities including evaluation and dissemination, as well as exploring avenues for future collaboration between Uganda and the UK. In total, six UK members, including antimicrobial pharmacists, microbiologists, and an animal health specialist from NTU and BHT, travelled to Uganda over the two visits, while two Uganda pharmacists visited the UK as part of the project.

3.2. Training of Health Practitioners

In September 2019, the project team held training workshops for a multidisciplinary group of 86 health professionals from human and animal health on AMR/AMS/IPC. Among the trained HPs, 56 were from ERRH, 20 were from lower level health facilities in Wakiso district (Nsaggu HC II, Nakawuka HC III, Kajjansi HC IV, Zzinga HC II, Kitala HC II, Bussi HC II, and Kasanje HC III), and 10 were animal health professionals working within Entebbe municipality. Whereas all the human health HPs were selected from government health facilities, some of the animal health HPs were in private practice. The workshops for the HPs from both animal and human health were greatly appreciated by the participants as they shared experiences among themselves, and realised the similarities and close linkage between AMS among their professions. All HPs trained were involved in either prescription, administration, issuance of antimicrobials, or related clinical work. They included pharmacists, medical doctors, laboratory technicians, clinical officers, nurses, and veterinary practitioners. The two-day training workshops, held in Entebbe, were facilitated jointly by the UK and Uganda members of the project team. This ensured the local context of material and applicability was delivered during the training. The UK trainers included three antimicrobial pharmacists, two microbiologists, and an animal health specialist, while the Uganda team included three pharmacists, a veterinary doctor, and two environmental health scientists. The workshop sessions included: introduction to AMR/AMS/IPC; the World Health Organization (WHO) AMR competency framework for human health; prudent antibiotic use, actions, and barriers in human and animal health; use of UCG incuding how to use the Microguide app that hosts these guidelines provided by CwPAMS; the One Health approach; hand hygiene; and sharing of gained knowledge with others using the capability, opportunity, and motivation behaviour (COM-B) change model [19]. The workshop sessions were interactive and engaged participants in order to facilitate adult learning. Specifically, sessions included a pre- and post-assessment, group discussions, e-Bug AMR balloon experiment [20], hand washing demonstration using the Glow Germ Gel kit™ [21], case studies from both human and animal health, interactive games, sharing of past experiences, and a certificate awarding ceremony. From the pre- and post-training assessment, there was an improvement in the knowledge levels of the HPs after the trainings. Out of the 80 HPs who participated in the post assessment, 64 (80%) correctly defined AMR compared to 63.9% (53/83) who had done so during the pre-assessment. In the post-training evaluation, 73.8% (59/80) of the HPs stated that inadequate hand hygiene is one of the contributing factors of AMR compared to 21.7% (18/83) who did so during the pre-training assessment.

3.3. Training of Community Health Workers

A total of 227 CHWs from Kajjansi town council took part in training workshops conducted by a team of three HPs who were among those trained in the project as part of the 'training of trainers' model. The one-day workshop for CHWs, in groups of approximately 30, was conducted using interactive and engaging sessions similar to those used with HPs. Given that CHWs are involved in treatment of only three diseases (malaria, diarrhoea, and pneumonia) for infants less than five years under iCCM, and health promotion on key public health issues, their training was largely focused on creating awareness on AMR/AMS/IPC in their communities. The workshops included sessions on: introduction to antimicrobials and AMR; AMS at the community level; prevention of AMR in animals and humans; water, sanitation, and hygiene; food hygiene and safety; and IPC in communities. Similar to the workshops of HPs, a pre- and post-training assessment was undertaken for the CHWs. There was a notable improvement in knowledge of the CHWs in the post-training assessment in comparison with the pre-training survey. Out of the 212 CHWs who participated in the post-training assessment, 97.1% (206/212) reported that microorganisms can fail to respond to antimicrobials compared to 49.3% (111/225) in the pre-training assessment. In addition, 96.2% (204/212) of the CHWs reported in the post-training assessment that antimicrobials dumped in the environment can lead to AMR compared to 33.3% (75/225) in the pre-training assessment. Furthermore, 97.6% (204/212) of the CHWs agreed in the post-training assessment that inappropriate use of antimicrobials in livestock can lead to AMR compared to 36.4% (82/225) in the pre-training assessment. In the post-training assessment, all the CHWs (100%) felt that they were knowledgeable enough to educate their communities on preventing AMR through improved AMS and IPC following the training.

3.4. Increasing Awareness on AMS to Primary School Pupils and University Students

The project introduced and created awareness on AMR/AMS among over 300 pupils at St. Theresa and Kawotto Saviours primary schools in Wakiso district. These sessions were attended by pupils mainly in the upper classes of the schools (primary 5 to 7) as well as their teachers. These schools were twinned with two schools in the UK (Wingrave Church of England and Longwick Church of England primary schools). Pupils in both the Ugandan and UK schools also participated in a competition to develop AMR/AMS/IPC messages in commemoration of World Antibiotic Awareness Week (WAAW) 2019, and the winners received various awards. Winners in Uganda and the UK were selected for best poster / song / performance. Award ceremonies were held at the schools in Uganda and the UK to share the winning material among pupils, teachers, and parents to reinforce the messages and illustrate the importance of the global issue of AMR. Winners (four from Uganda and four from the UK) received an award of 25 GBP, a young antibiotic guardian t-shirt, and a certificate of appreciation for their participation. As part of the twinning of the Uganda and UK schools, ideas were shared on future collaboration, which will be explored in future. An initial activity carried out as part of the twinning was pupils from the Uganda schools writing pen pal letters to their UK counterparts and vice versa, which was well received by both groups and the administration of the schools. At Mak, the project organised three seminars and workshops on AMR / AMS /IPC, and interactions with NTU students. The seminars were attended by over 120 students from the UK and Uganda from different programs, including environmental health, pharmacy, microbiology, and environment. The project also launched an AMR awareness competition among Makerere University Environmental Health Students' Association (MUEHSA) and NTU students for them to design appropriate messages for community sensitization. During the World Antibiotic Awareness Week (WAAW) in November 2019, the project held an award giving ceremony in which the four winners of the competition from Mak and NTU each received a cash prize of 25 GBP as well as a certificate of appreciation.

3.5. Establishment of One Health AMS Communities of Practice

Through stakeholder engagement at initiation of the project, the need for two online CoPs, one for health professionals and the other for students (as opposed to the earlier planned one), was identified and established. The aim of the CoPs was to provide a platform for sharing resources, opportunities, and materials on AMR, AMS, and IPC targeting both human and animal health, as well as enhance sustainability as these would continue after the project duration. The *Antimicrobial Stewardship, Optimum Access and Use in Uganda* CoP for health professionals is hosted by the MOH TWC on AMS, optimum access, and use. The *Students for Antimicrobial Stewardship* CoP is a Facebook group that was formed after the realisation of the need for students to work together, in a multidisciplinary setting, at an early stage in their careers to tackle AMR. This platform is managed by five AMR champions from the following schools at Mak: veterinary medicine; biosecurity; biotechnical, and laboratory science; health sciences; and public health. Currently, the students' CoP has 162 members while the one for health professionals has 321 members, with membership of both groups steadily increasing. The health professionals' CoP has sent out over 50 emails with resources, opportunities, and other materials concerning AMR/AMS from Uganda, the UK, and globally. One example of how this has changed engagement with this work is that some members of the health professionals CoP have submitted abstracts to conferences, which they learnt about from the online platform. The students CoP has sent over 20 messages on opportunities for students to participate in. These opportunities have included attending webinars and conferences, such as the 4th National Conference on AMR held in Kampala, Uganda in 2019. In addition, students on their CoP have appreciated the importance of working in multi-disciplinary teams to tackle AMR, which they are likely to utilize during their future professional work.

3.6. Evaluation of the Trained HPs and CHWs

From the project evaluation, there was a positive change in practices among the HPs and CHWs following the training. Out of the 77 HPs who participated in the evaluation, 68 (88.3%) stated that they had adopted new practices from the project training. Out of the 68 HPs who adopted new practices, 39 (57.3%) reported improved handwashing, over half 36 (52.9%) reported an increase in use of the UCG when prescribing antimicrobials, and 35 (51.5%) reported a reduction in the quantity of unnecessary antibiotics given per patient. Among the 77 HPs, 48 (62.3%) reported having faced challenges when attempting to become an antimicrobial steward in their setting. These challenges included stock out of drugs, 29 (60.4%); lack of personal protective equipment (PPE), including gloves and masks, 19 (39.6%); and insufficient laboratory capacity, 17 (27.1%) (Table 1).

Table 1. Evaluation results of health practitioners.

	Frequency (N = 77)	Percentage (%)
Gender		
Male	29	37.7
Female	48	62.23
Nature of practitioner		
Human health worker	72	93.5
Animal health worker	5	6.5
Found the training helpful in their day-to-day activities		
Yes	71	92.2
No	6	7.8
Presence of new practices adopted after training		
Yes	68	88.3
No	6	7.8
Not sure	3	3.9
***Adopted new practices after training (n = 68)**		
Increased use of UCG when prescribing antimicrobials	36	52.9
Diagnosis based on laboratory results	30	44.1
Sending more samples to the laboratory	24	35.3
Improved handwashing	39	57.3
Monitoring of my prescribing patterns	26	38.2
Patient guidance and counselling when they do not need antibiotics	31	45.6
Reduction of the number of antibiotics given per patient	35	51.5
Reduction of the use of injectables at out-patient department	19	27.9
** Others	32	47.1
Were using the CwPAMS microguide app		
Yes	33	43.4
No	39	50.0
Not applicable because they are Veterinary officers	5	6.6
Faced challenges when attempting to become antimicrobial stewards		
Yes	48	62.3
No	29	37.7
Challenges faced (n = 48)		
Drug stock outs	29	60.4
Lack of prescribing materials/guidelines	11	22.9
Lack of hand washing facilities and/or supplies	11	22.9
Lack of gloves, masks and/or other PPE	19	39.6
Insufficient laboratory capacity	17	27.1
Lack of first line antibiotics	13	16.9
Supervisors not very supportive in AMS matters	5	10.4
*** Others	22	45.8

* Multiple response question; ** Other practices included advising against self-medication, encouraging use of organic feeds for poultry and livestock, health education on adherence to drugs, waste segregation, and training other HPs who did not attend the training; *** Other challenges included poor attitude of fellow HPs, patients demanding for antibiotics, self-medication by patients, and lack of flexibility among some prescribers.

From the qualitative evaluation of the project, the HPs reported that they were using the UCG more during the prescribing of antimicrobials, and they had also reduced the quantities of antibiotics given per patient when appropriate to do so. Improved prescription practices among the HPs also led to improved availability of antimicrobials at the various health facilities as demonstrated in the quotation below.

"At the facility nowadays, I only give out amoxicillin where necessary as per the guidelines. I do not just give out antibiotics anymore. For this reason, I am now able to save amoxicillin tablets for patients who really need them, and I also give out the medication in the right dose. This has helped me reduce on the number of times I go to look for medicines from other facilities due to reduced stock-outs at my facility." Health worker, Bussi health centre II

Among the 226 CHWs who participated in the evaluation, 204 (90.3%) reported improved practices attributable to the training. The majority, 183 (81%), of the CHWs reported increased handwashing with soap, 175 (77.4%) had encouraged community members to improve personal hygiene and general sanitation, 151 (66.8%) had encouraged community members to take the full dose of their prescribed medication, while 130 (57.2%) had encouraged farmers to always consult veterinary professionals whenever their animals were ill. Following the training, 69 CHWs (30.5%) reported having reached between 50 to 100 community members and health educated them on AMR, while 27 (12%) reached over 100 community members (Table 2).

Table 2. Evaluation results of community health workers.

Gender	Frequency (N = 226)	Percentage (%)
Male	47	20.8
Female	179	79.2
Nature of CHW		
Involved in iCCM	111	49.1
Not involved in iCCM	115	50.9
Change in practice after the training		
Yes	204	90.3
No	22	9.7
* New practices adopted individually after the training (n = 204)		
Increased use of treatment guidelines for childhood illness	90	39.8
Patient guidance/counselling when they do not need antibiotics	74	32.7
Proper disposal of medical waste and medicine	111	49.1
Encouraged community members to take full dose of medication	151	66.8
Encouraged community members to stop self-medication	159	70.4
Encouraged community members to follow doctors' prescriptions	144	63.7
Increased hand washing with soap	183	81.0
Encouraged community members to improve personal hygiene and general sanitation	175	77.4
Encouraged food hygiene and safety	135	59.7
Promoted the safe water chain	172	76.1
Encouraged farmers to consult veterinary doctors whenever animals were ill	130	57.2
Encouraged farmers not to use human medicines in poultry and animals	112	49.6
** Others	69	30.5
Number of people sensitized about AMR in the community		
<50	130	57.5
50–100	69	30.5
>100	27	12.0

Table 2. *Cont.*

Gender	Frequency (N = 226)	Percentage (%)
Faced challenges when attempting to become antimicrobial guardians in the community		
Yes	208	92.0
No	18	8.0
Challenges faced when attempting to become antimicrobial guardians (n = 208)		
People do not understand AMR	132	62.9
Needed more training	136	64.8
AMR is complicated	44	21.0
*** Others	61	29.1

* Multiple response question. ** Others included advising against sharing of drugs, proper drug storage, advising against eating of dead animals, and burying dead animals. *** Other challenges included poor attitude of community members, poverty, and disrespect for CHWs.

Qualitative evaluation among the CHWs confirmed improved practices amongst them regarding the prevention of AMR in the community, particularly regarding animal husbandry, such as observing antibiotic withdrawal periods among animals before consuming their products, not eating deceased animals that were recently on treatment, reduction of self-prescription for animals, and reduction in use of human-prescribed antimicrobials among animals as mentioned in the quotations below.

"Before the training, I was among the people who used to slaughter sick chicken which were under treatment or those that had died while receiving medication. During the training, I learnt that we should never slaughter sick animals undergoing treatment. I now also know that to slaughter a chicken recently on treatment for consumption, you must wait for 7 or more days so that the medication is no longer present in its body hence not consuming small doses of the drug from the chicken which can contribute to AMR." Female CHW, Kajjansi Town Council

"For us, we thought that medicine that has been prescribed for humans could be used the way we wanted to treat animals especially antiretroviral drugs which we used to give pigs, and amoxicillin capsules to chicken. However, at the training I learnt that it is very dangerous to give human medicine to animals, and we should always call the veterinary doctor to treat our animals and prescribe the medicine for them, other than treating the animals ourselves." Male CHW, Kajjansi Town Council

4. Discussion

Improper use of antimicrobials including non-compliance with guidelines is a contributing factor to AMR [4], hence the need for interventions targeting improvement of access to and appropriate use of antimicrobials. There is limited data on AMS programs in Africa, including Uganda [7,22], hence our project provides an important contribution to the existing body of knowledge on how to address the growing burden of AMR. The need for a One Health approach to promote AMS is well established internationally [5], and is translated into the local Ugandan context through the NAP [2]. The One Health approach used in the project was made possible through the multidisciplinary nature of our team with expertise in human and animal health, and environmental health. The strength of this team was fostered through reciprocal relationships and engagement with a variety of in-country stakeholders, including policy makers, such as the MOH and MAAIF. The project was delivered through multiple parallel interventions, including the training of HPs and CHWs, the creation of AMS awareness among university students and school pupils, as well as the establishment of CoPs and a hospital MTC. Our project is one of the few that have delivered multiple interventions at both health facility and community levels using a One Health approach in Uganda so provides a good contribution to the NAP in the fight against AMR.

In line with WHO recommendations, our training approach focused on both human and animal HPs [9]. In addition, the training of HPs on AMR/AMS/IPC took a One Health approach where an emphasis was given to the use of antimicrobials in humans and animals, and their link to the environment. This was necessary to truly embed the principles of One Health into the training component of our project. Indeed, with a multidisciplinary team from Uganda and the UK facilitating the training, the goal of ensuring One Health was achieved. The project was able to translate AMS principles across various primary health care levels in Uganda as the training involved HPs from ERRH and lower level health facilities. Whereas these lower level health facilities in Uganda (health centre IIs, IIIs and IVs) are often ignored for AMS and other interventions, they provide health care to a good portion of the population, particularly in rural areas that have limited access to hospitals [23]. The use of UK trainers in addition to those from Uganda was of benefit for both countries. These trainers brought their unique expertise around infection prevention and the UK's principles of AMR and AMS practice. On the other hand, the UK trainers were exposed to the issues of AMS and AMR in a developing country context, and community-based approaches of tackling global health challenges, particularly AMR. The project also facilitated bi-directional learning between the two countries, which can inform other health partnerships. The use of participatory training techniques, such as demonstrating handwashing using the Glow Germ Gel Kits, facilitated learning and knowledge retention as opposed to traditional didactic methods.

In addition to the training of HPs, our project trained CHWs on AMR/AMS/IPC using the 'training of trainers' model. AMS programs are largely hospital based and have predominantly focused on HPs, such as laboratory scientists, nurses, clinicians, pharmacists, and microbiologists [24]. Our study went beyond this and involved CHWs as they are key to health service delivery at the community level in Uganda as well as other developing countries. The CHWs trained in our project have a primary responsibility of health education and promotion in their communities while some had an extra role on iCCM. From the evaluation results, it was evident that training of the CHWs enhanced their capacity to contribute to AMR through sensitization of the general population on the appropriate use of antibiotics, particularly in humans, but also in animals among other related issues. Miscommunication at the community level has been identified as a major challenge to addressing AMR in Africa [25], hence CHWs are a critical part of the health workforce to contribute to the NAP in the local setting. Given the training of CHWs had a component of IPC, they were subsequently invaluable in the promotion of sanitation and hygiene during the emergency public health measures undertaken in response to the COVID-19 pandemic in the communities. The use of the 'training of trainers' model, where the trained HPs later trained CHWs, is an indication of the health partnership's commitment towards building local capabilities in primary health care delivery. In addition, using trained practitioners to train another health cadre enhances health promotion and ensures cultural appropriateness [26].

Awareness of basic hygiene principles and infection control are at the core of AMR education [5]. The AMS activities we implemented in schools will help to promote intergenerational awareness on AMR, as well as facilitate pupils becoming antimicrobial guardians in the future. Such pupils are also likely to promote proper AMS and IPC practices, such as handwashing with soap, at critical times among peers and family members. Our project also involved undergraduate students from various disciplines concerning human and animal health from Uganda and the UK in AMR awareness-raising activities, including seminars, webinars, and competitions. Although these students may have earlier been exposed to AMR as part of their studies, it cannot be guaranteed that they had adequate knowledge and skills on AMS, which would be reflected in their practice. At the undergraduate level, many prescribers and students of other professions may not be confident in their preparedness to deal with AMS. For instance, a survey among fourth-year medical students in the United States revealed that only one-third of those surveyed considered themselves as being adequately prepared in basic antimicrobial use [27]. Similarly, a study among paramedical students in Ethiopia revealed that less than half of the students surveyed had adequate knowledge of AMR [28]. These gaps in knowledge among university students reflect the need for AMS awareness initiatives to be incorporated into educational training curricula. Involving pupils and students in AMS / IPC interventions is therefore important as they are the future generation, and it also contributes to ensuring the sustainability of project activities.

Our project facilitated the establishment of an MTC at ERRH to support appropriate prescribing of antimicrobials and related activities. Having an MTC at a hospital is one of the recommended steps in setting up an AMS program [29], hence it is an important contribution to the NAP. During the COVID-19 pandemic, ERRH was the first facility to handle cases with disease in the country, and the rapid and comprehensive support from the MTC to guide the hospital response was timely. The current existence and operation of the MTC at the hospital is a key achievement of our project given that it continues to support day-to-day operations at the facility, hence contributing to the sustainability of our project interventions. Establishment of the CoPs on AMS was also instrumental in ensuring sustainability as they continue to enhance knowledge exchange among human and animal health professionals and students. The CoPs continue to be integral to building awareness and sharing best practices on AMR/AMS/IPC. Given the COPs are online, the UK project team are able to stay engaged and be involved when not in Uganda. Indeed, online CoPs have been demonstrated to have a wider reach and keep participants engaged in comparison with physical ones, particularly in this digital age [30,31]. Having set-up the health professionals' CoP as part of the MOH TWC on AMS, optimum access and use will also contribute towards its sustainability beyond the project duration.

The pre- and post-training assessment and project evaluation revealed an improvement in HPs' and CHWs' knowledge of AMR and their practices to promote AMS and IPC. Specifically, the evaluation results showed that the training of HPs substantially improved the organizational culture for the majority, with 88.3% adopting new practices around AMR/AMS/IPC in line with the national requirement as prescribed in the UCG. Studies in different parts of Africa, such as South Africa [32], have also recorded change in organizational culture following the implementation of an AMS program. This change in practice among HPs involved in our study resulted in improved availability of antimicrobials as prescriptions and use were optimized. However, the evaluation revealed that health systems challenges, such as stock out of medicine, inadequate human resources, and lack of PPE for hospital staff, could impede AMS promotion if not equally tackled. In the case of CHWs, the evaluation results demonstrated how training them has a wider impact on improving positive health outcomes across communities, with many CHWs having sensitized between 50 and 100 community members on AMR/AMS within three months following the training. In addition, training the CHWs was instrumental in promoting the One Health approach, which was evident through encouraging livestock farmers to consult with a veterinary specialist regarding the health of their animals in the community. Animal husbandry is an important practice in the project community [15] and the East African region in general [25] so it is critical it is considered while implementing AMS interventions. This practice is reported to bring with it a high burden of what Ampaire et al. [25] referred to as "community-acquired infections". There is a high rate of antibiotics misuse and poor engagement with veterinary professionals among livestock farmers at the community level in Africa [33]. Therefore, the ability of CHWs to support improved practices regarding management of animal conditions should be integrated in future AMS activities to contribute to the fight against AMR in Uganda and beyond.

One of the strengths of our project is that it was implemented as part of a 10-year established health partnership between NTU and Mak with existing structures, intellectual capital, as well as local and global resources and networks that will contribute to strengthening the primary health care system in Uganda. In addition, our project embraced the One Health approach and targeted AMS interventions at both the health facility and community levels as well as including primary schools and university students, which is worth mentioning. A limitation of our project was its limited scope given it involved one hospital, a few lower level health facilities, two primary schools, and selected university students. The involvement of animal health workers in project activities was also low compared to those from human health, which can be improved in the future. Nevertheless, being a small pilot project, the achievements and lessons learnt will be instrumental in informing our future partnership activities to strengthen AMS in Uganda and further contribute to the NAP.

5. Conclusions

Adoption of a One Health approach in our project facilitated multidisciplinary efforts, including training human and animal HPs, to increase awareness and contribute towards improving AMS at health facilities and in the community. Reciprocal visits and establishment of CoPs fostered bi-directional learning and knowledge transfer on AMS between the UK and Uganda. The achievements of this project can inform the design of large-scale AMS interventions in support of implementation of the Uganda AMR National Action Plan.

Author Contributions: D.M. and L.G. are the Uganda and UK health partnership leads respectively and initiated the project idea. F.E.K., L.M., C.B., H.K., I.M.K., B.Y.N., J.O., K.R.-H. and J.W. contributed to conceptualization of the project. All authors including S.A., D.I., G.B.L. and F.N. participated in project implementation and writing the manuscript. All authors have read and agreed to the published version of the manuscript.

Funding: This project was funded as part of the Commonwealth Partnerships on Antimicrobial Stewardship (CwPAMS) supported by Tropical Health and Education Trust (THET) and Commonwealth Pharmacists Association (CPA) using Official Development Assistance (ODA) funding, through the Department of Health and Social Care's Fleming Fund. The views expressed in this publication are those of the author(s) and not necessarily those of the NHS, the Fleming Fund, the Department of Health and Social Care, THET or CPA.

Acknowledgments: We thank all stakeholders who supported the implementation of the project including from the: Ministry of Health; Ministry of Agriculture, Animal Industry and Fisheries; Entebbe Regional Referral Hospital; Makerere University College of Health Sciences; Makerere University College of Veterinary Medicine, Animal Resources and Biosecurity; Entebbe Municipal Council; Wakiso District Health Office; Kajjansi Health Centre (HC) IV; Nakawuka HC III; Kasanje HC III; Nsaggu HC II; Zzinga HC II; Kitala HC II; and Bussi HC II.

Conflicts of Interest: The authors declare no conflict of interest. The funders had no role in the design of the project; in the collection, analyses, or interpretation of data; in the writing of the manuscript, or in the decision to publish the results.

References

1. Global Action Plan on Antimicrobial Resistance. Available online: https://apps.who.int/iris/bitstream/handle/10665/193736/9789241509763_eng.pdf?sequence=1 (accessed on 31 July 2020).
2. Government of Uganda. *Antimicrobial Resistance National Action Plan 2018–2023*; Government of Uganda: Kampala, Uganda, 2018.
3. Fujita, A.W.; Mbabazi, O.; Akampurira, A.; Najjuka, C.F.; Izale, C.; Meya, D.; Boulware, D.; Manabe, Y.; Kajumbula, H. Antimicrobial Resistance in Uganda and the Urgent Need for Standardized Reporting and a National Surveillance Program. *Open Forum Infect. Dis.* **2015**, *2*, 1472. [CrossRef]
4. Tadesse, B.T.; Ashley, E.A.; Ongarello, S.; Havumaki, J.; Wijegoonewardena, M.; González, I.J.; Dittrich, S. Antimicrobial resistance in Africa: A systematic review. *BMC Infect. Dis.* **2017**, *17*, 616. [CrossRef] [PubMed]
5. McEwen, S.A.; Collignon, P.J. Antimicrobial resistance: A one health perspective. In *Antimicrobial Resistance in Bacteria from Livestock and Companion Animals*; ASM Press: Washington, DC, USA, 2018; pp. 521–547.
6. Dyar, O.J.; Huttner, B.; Schouten, J.; Pulcini, C. What is antimicrobial stewardship? *Clin. Microbiol. Infect.* **2017**, *23*, 793–798. [CrossRef] [PubMed]
7. Akpan, M.R.; Isemin, N.U.; Udoh, A.E.; Ashiru-Oredope, D. Implementation of antimicrobial stewardship programmes in African countries: A systematic literature review. *J. Glob. Antimicrob. Resist.* **2020**, *22*, 317–324. [CrossRef]
8. Ackers, L.; Ackers-Johnson, G.; Seekles, M.; Odur, J.; Opio, S. Opportunities and Challenges for Improving Anti-Microbial Stewardship in Low-and Middle-Income Countries; Lessons Learnt from the Maternal Sepsis Intervention in Western Uganda. *Antibiotics* **2020**, *9*, 315. [CrossRef]
9. Dyar, O.J.; Obua, C.; Chandy, S.; Xiao, Y.; Stålsby Lundborg, C.; Pulcini, C. Using antibiotics responsibly: Are we there yet? *Future Microbiol.* **2016**, *11*, 1057–1071. [CrossRef]
10. Yantzi, R.; van de Walle, G.; Lin, J. 'The disease isn't listening to the drug': The socio-cultural context of antibiotic use for viral respiratory infections in rural Uganda. *Glob. Public Health* **2019**, *14*, 750–763. [CrossRef]

11. Commonwealth Partnerships for Antimicrobial Stewardship. Available online: https://www.flemingfund.org/grants/commonwealth-partnerships-for-antimicrobial-stewardship-2/ (accessed on 31 July 2020).
12. World Health Organization. *WHO Competency Framework for Health Workers' Education and Training on Antimicrobial Resistance*; WHO: Geneva, Switzerland, 2018.
13. Dobson, E.L.; Klepser, M.E.; Pogue, J.M.; Labreche, M.J.; Adams, A.J.; Gauthier, T.P.; Turner, R.B.; Su, C.P.; Jacobs, D.M.; Suda, K.J. Outpatient antibiotic stewardship: Interventions and opportunities. *J. Am. Pharm. Assoc.* **2017**, *57*, 464–473. [CrossRef]
14. Wakiso District Local Government. Development Profile/Investment Plan FY 2015/16-2019/20. Investment opportunities and Doing Business. Wakiso District. 2016. Available online: http://www.wakiso.go.ug/sites/default/files/Wakiso%20District%20Profile_0.pdf (accessed on 20 August 2020).
15. Uganda Bureau of Statistics. The National Population and Housing Census 2014—Area Specific Profile Series—Wakiso District. 2017. Available online: https://www.ubos.org/wp-content/uploads/publications/2014CensusProfiles/WAKISO.pdf (accessed on 20 August 2020).
16. Bashahun, D.; Odoch, T. Assessment of antibiotic usage in intensive poultry farms in Wakiso District, Uganda. *Livest. Res. Rural Dev.* **2015**, *27*, 12.
17. Musoke, D.; Gibson, L.; Mukama, T.; Khalil, Y.; Ssempebwa, J.C. Nottingham Trent University and Makerere University School of Public Health partnership: Experiences of co-learning and supporting the healthcare system in Uganda. *Glob. Health* **2016**, *12*, 11. [CrossRef]
18. Department of Pharmaceuticals and Natural Medicines, Ministry of Health. *Medicine and Therapeutics Committees Manual*; Ministry of Health: Kampala, Uganda, 2018.
19. Michie, S.; Van Stralen, M.M.; West, R. The behaviour change wheel: A new method for characterising and designing behaviour change interventions. *Implement. Sci.* **2011**, *6*, 42. [CrossRef]
20. Antibiotics: Peer Education. Available online: https://www.e-bug.eu/peereducation/download/english/Antibiotic%20Peer%20Education%20Lesson.pdf (accessed on 30 June 2019).
21. The Original Visual Tool for Teaching Proper Handwashing, Aseptic Techniques, and General Infection Control. Available online: https://www.glogerm.com (accessed on 20 August 2020).
22. Fadare, J.O.; Ogunleye, O.; Iliyasu, G.; Adeoti, A.; Schellack, N.; Engler, D.; Massele, A.; Godman, B. Status of antimicrobial stewardship programmes in Nigerian tertiary healthcare facilities: Findings and implications. *J. Glob. Antimicrob. Resist.* **2019**, *17*, 132–136. [CrossRef] [PubMed]
23. Ministry of Health. *Health Sector Development Plan 2015/16—2019/20*; Ministry of Health: Kampala, Uganda, 2015.
24. Chetty, S.; Reddy, M.; Ramsamy, Y.; Naidoo, A.; Essack, S. Antimicrobial stewardship in South Africa: A scoping review of the published literature. *JAC-Antimicrob. Resist.* **2019**, *1*, dlz060. [CrossRef]
25. Ampaire, L.; Muhindo, A.; Orikiriza, P.; Mwanga-Amumpaire, J.; Bebell, L.; Boum, Y. A review of antimicrobial resistance in East Africa. *Afr. J. Lab. Med.* **2016**, *5*, 1–6. [CrossRef] [PubMed]
26. Maruta, T.; Yao, K.; Ndlovu, N.; Moyo, S. Training-of-trainers: A strategy to build country capacity for SLMTA expansion and sustainability. *Afr. J. Lab. Med.* **2014**, *3*. [CrossRef]
27. Abbo, L.M.; Cosgrove, S.E.; Pottinger, P.S.; Pereyra, M.; Sinkowitz-Cochran, R.; Srinivasan, A.; Webb, D.J.; Hooton, T.M. Medical students' perceptions and knowledge about antimicrobial stewardship: How are we educating our future prescribers? *Clin. Infect. Dis.* **2013**, *57*, 631–638. [CrossRef]
28. Seid, M.A.; Hussen, M.S. Knowledge and attitude towards antimicrobial resistance among final year undergraduate paramedical students at University of Gondar, Ethiopia. *BMC Infect. Dis.* **2018**, *18*, 312. [CrossRef] [PubMed]
29. Mendelson, M.; Morris, A.M.; Thursky, K.; Pulcini, C. How to start an antimicrobial stewardship programme in a hospital. *Clin. Microbiol. Infect.* **2020**, *26*, 447–453. [CrossRef]
30. Gannon-Leary, P.; Fontainha, E. Communities of Practice and virtual learning communities: Benefits, barriers and success factors. *eLearning Pap.* **2007**, *5*, 1–13.
31. Zhang, W.; Watts, S. Online communities as communities of practice: A case study. *J. Knowl. Manag.* **2008**, *12*, 55–71. [CrossRef]

32. Junaid, E.; Jenkins, L.; Swanepoel, H.; North, Z.; Gould, T. Antimicrobial stewardship in a rural regional hospital–growing a positive culture. *S. Afr. Med. J.* **2018**, 108. [CrossRef] [PubMed]
33. Caudell, M.A.; Dorado-Garcia, A.; Eckford, S.; Creese, C.; Byarugaba, D.K.; Afakye, K.; Chansa-Kabali, T.; Fasina, F.O.; Kabali, E.; Kiambi, S. Towards a bottom-up understanding of antimicrobial use and resistance on the farm: A knowledge, attitudes, and practices survey across livestock systems in five African countries. *PLoS ONE* **2020**, *15*, e0220274. [CrossRef] [PubMed]

Publisher's Note: MDPI stays neutral with regard to jurisdictional claims in published maps and institutional affiliations.

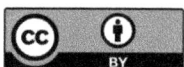

© 2020 by the authors. Licensee MDPI, Basel, Switzerland. This article is an open access article distributed under the terms and conditions of the Creative Commons Attribution (CC BY) license (http://creativecommons.org/licenses/by/4.0/).

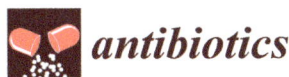

Article

Designing a National Veterinary Prescribing Champion Programme for Welsh Veterinary Practices: The Arwain Vet Cymru Project

Gwen M. Rees [1,2,*], Alison Bard [2] and Kristen K. Reyher [2]

1. Institute of Biological, Environmental and Rural Sciences (IBERS), Aberystwyth University, Penglais, Aberystwyth SY23 3DA, UK
2. Bristol Veterinary School, University of Bristol, Langford BS40 5DU, UK; alison.bard@bristol.ac.uk (A.B.); kristen.reyher@bristol.ac.uk (K.K.R.)
* Correspondence: gwr15@aber.ac.uk

Abstract: Antimicrobial use in agriculture has been identified as an area of focus for reducing overall antimicrobial use and improving stewardship. In this paper, we outline the design of a complex antimicrobial stewardship (AMS) intervention aimed at developing a national Veterinary Prescribing Champion programme for Welsh farm animal veterinary practices. We describe the process by which participants were encouraged to design and deliver bespoke individualised AMS activities at practice level by forging participant "champion" identities and communities of practice through participatory and educational online activities. We describe the key phases identified as important when designing this complex intervention, namely (i) involving key collaborators in government and industry to stimulate project engagement; (ii) grounding the design in the literature, the results of stakeholder engagement, expert panel input, and veterinary clinician feedback to promote contextual relevance and appropriateness; and (iii) taking a theoretical approach to implementing intervention design to foster critical psychological needs for participant motivation and scheme involvement. With recruitment of over 80% of all farm animal practices in Wales to the programme, we also describe demographic data of the participating Welsh Veterinary Prescribing Champions in order to inform recruitment and design of future AMS programmes.

Keywords: antimicrobial stewardship; veterinary; complex intervention

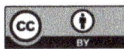

1. Introduction

Antimicrobial resistance (AMR) is a global One Health challenge of great significance [1]. The World Health Organisation describes AMR as a global health and development threat requiring urgent multisectoral action [2]. While the development and transmission of AMR is complex and not yet fully understood, antimicrobial use is known to be a major driver of resistance and there is broad consensus that antimicrobial stewardship (AMS) is a key component in addressing the issue [2–4]. Indeed, "the critical role of antimicrobial stewardship in tackling the problem of AMR is reflected in its inclusion as a key action in the UK five-year antibiotic resistance strategy" [5]. Extensive AMS programmes are commonly seen in human healthcare settings [4,6,7] and, although they form a part of many national and global AMR action plans [2,3,5], their implementation in veterinary practice remains sporadic and small scale [8].

Antimicrobial use in agriculture has been identified as an area of focus for reducing overall antimicrobial use and improving stewardship [3]. In the UK context, recent efforts have led to a decrease in overall antimicrobial use in food-producing animals of 45% since 2015 [9]. These reductions have been broadly industry-led, with industry bodies recognising a consumer demand for responsible antimicrobial use and an increasing political focus on the issue [10–12]. Responsible prescribing is defined by the UK AMR

5-Year National Action Plan as "The use of antimicrobials in the optimal way, for the right pathogen, at the right dose, for the right duration, for the treatment or prevention of infectious disease." [12].

In Wales, agriculture, animal health, and animal welfare are devolved policy areas over which the Welsh government has legislative powers [13]. AMR has been a policy focus in recent years, with the establishment of an Animals and the Environment AMR Delivery Group leading to the publication of the Welsh government's five-year AMR Implementation Plan [11]. This plan includes the key focus areas of improving standards of antimicrobial selection and prescribing, as well as improving standards of antimicrobial supply. AMS has been recognised as a vital component of national AMR strategies, although there is work to be done to improve implementation [5]. The agricultural industry represents a proportionally greater percentage of the national economy in Wales than it does for the UK as a whole, and the majority of Welsh farming is based on beef, sheep, and dairy production [14]. As such, the health and welfare—and related antimicrobial prescribing—of cattle and sheep, could be argued as being of relatively greater significance in Wales than the rest of the UK.

AMS programmes are complex interventions consisting of several interacting and inter-relational components, which present challenges to those designing, implementing, and analysing such programmes [15]. Successful design requires evaluation of the available evidence, engagement with theory and a good theoretical understanding of how an intervention may cause change [16]. A recent systematic review found the use of theory, engagement of end users, identifying barriers, and selecting appropriate intervention components to be key elements of the successful design of interventions for changing healthcare professionals' behaviour [17]. Additionally, involving stakeholders, understanding the intervention context and considering implementation in a "real world" setting have also been seen as essential principles for consideration [18].

The purpose of this paper is to outline the development and implementation of a national AMS scheme for farm animal veterinary practices through the establishment of a network of Veterinary Prescribing Champions (VPCs) as part of the wider Arwain Vet Cymru (AVC) programme in Wales. Arwain Vet Cymru is a collaborative initiative, which aims to train and support a national network of Veterinary Prescribing Champions across Wales to improve antibiotic prescribing in cattle and sheep. The project is participatory in approach, aiming to empower veterinary surgeons to develop and implement bespoke stewardship interventions, as well as share experiences and ideas. Both development and implementation of this scheme were informed by the self-determination theory (SDT), a broad theory of human motivation covering elements of interpersonal dynamics, goals and motives, individual differences, psychological needs, and psychological well-being [19]. SDT explicitly recognises that some behaviours are not intrinsically appealing and that the salient question when considering behaviour change is how to motivate individuals to value, self-regulate and (without external pressure) carry out and maintain, such behaviours. As such, SDT is particularly pertinent to the context of AMS, as it considers not just how and whether AMS behaviours are likely to be enacted, but the mechanisms by which these behaviours can become self-directed and, thus, maintained over time—elements critical to a national AMS scheme.

Aim and Objectives

As the Veterinary Prescribing Champion Network is a novel intervention—with similar programmes now being considered for England and Scotland—this paper aims to inform future national stewardship programmes about its design, methodology, and enactment, providing a much-needed evidence base for future complex interventions in the veterinary sphere. Specific objectives are to examine:

- The process through which this national AMS scheme was appropriately contextualised, involving the integration of complementary knowledge pathways in the development of intervention goals;

- How intervention goals were subsequently grounded within a theoretical framework, by identifying operational SDT conditions and associated guiding principles relevant and applicable to VPC participation; and
- How the individual components of the AVC programme can lead to improved prescribing practice.

2. Methods

The study obtained ethical approval from the University of Bristol Health Sciences Research Ethics Committee, Reference 99522.

2.1. Study Setting

Antimicrobial use in Wales is regulated by the Veterinary Medicines Directorate, an executive agency of the Department for the Environment, Food, and Rural Affairs. All antimicrobials used in food-producing animals are prescription-only medicines, which can only be prescribed by veterinary surgeons to animals "under their care" [20]. Farmers in Wales are in the relatively privileged position of being able to store antimicrobials on farm for use at a later date [21]. There is a requirement to maintain purchase and use records, although there is evidence that these records may not always be accurate [22]. Veterinary practices in Wales that provide farm animal services are members of one of two Veterinary Delivery Partnerships, established to allow the delivery of government tuberculosis testing across Wales. Practices are otherwise separate and private business entities, with farmers able to choose their veterinary practice freely. There are approximately 50 separate veterinary practices providing farm animal services in Wales, although some of these are located along the border in England.

2.2. Theoretical Basis

The AVC intervention aimed to facilitate a professional environment that would inspire VPCs to engage with and endorse the network and their new AMS behaviours. Given the disparate nature of current antimicrobial prescribing and stewardship in veterinary practice, it was recognised that each participant's context and behavioural opportunities would likely be different, and a one-size-fits-all approach to AMS was unlikely to be effective. This intervention was therefore founded on the selection, adoption, and implementation of AMS behaviour changes by AVC participants themselves, through participant involvement in the scheme cultivating a prescribing "champion" mindset to cement their intention to design and implement an AMS intervention within their own professional environments. In considering this target behaviour change through the lens of the widely used COM-B behaviour system (capability, opportunity and motivation) and the associated Behaviour Change Wheel [23], it was clear that achieving this goal necessitated a focus on delivering an intervention design that engaged core motivational drivers of individual AVC participants with regards to their engagement with AMS knowledge, principles, and activities. To this end, an evidence-based theoretical perspective was sought to inform the AVC process and activities with respect for—and targeted attention towards—fundamental VPC motivational needs. Few frameworks on motivation have spurred as much research as SDT, with a recent conceptual and empirical meta-analysis supporting key premises within the theory [24].

SDT identifies distinct types of motivation that are key to understanding how—and whether—behaviour becomes internalised by individuals and stimulates personal growth and change. The most fundamental distinction is between intrinsic motivation, which refers to carrying out a behaviour because it is inherently enjoyable or interesting, and extrinsic motivation, which refers to carrying out a behaviour because it leads to a separable outcome or instrumental value [25]. For example, a veterinary surgeon who spends her spare time reading a paper on responsible prescribing practices, purely because she is curious about the topic, does so because she is intrinsically motivated, whilst her colleague who carries out the same behaviour only because it has been mandated by their boss is extrinsically motivated.

Extrinsic motivation can be further classified by its underpinning reasons or goals, forming a continuum from internalised and agentic extrinsically motivated states to those that are more motivationally impoverished and externalised [25]. Those extrinsic behaviours that are more internalised (i.e., in line with an individual's closely held beliefs or values) are likely to be associated with better quality of engagement, more positive self-perception and greater persistence than those behaviours that are more externalised (i.e., those carried out due to external punishments and rewards or a focus on approval from others via, for example, pride, shame or guilt) [24,25]. As such, for the veterinary surgeon reading about responsible prescribing because his boss requires it, if he also views the activity as valuable in developing his professional knowledge and identity, he will be more effectively engaged than if he acts purely to avoid guilt or a reprimand.

Where the premise of this intervention was to encourage individuals to carry out behaviours that might not have been intrinsically motivated (otherwise, no intervention would arguably have been necessary), we believed promoting conditions that allowed VPCs to feel more in control—and to express internalised motivation in their AVC engagement and chosen AMS behaviours—to be critical to intervention success, given associated benefits in learning, engagement, creativity, and personal commitment [25]. SDT identifies three universal psychological conditions that—across cultures—are critical to promoting internalised forms of extrinsic motivation in individual behaviour: the needs to feel competence (perceived self-efficacy), autonomy (a sense of choice, being the origin of one's own behaviour), and relatedness (feeling understood and cared for by others) [26,27]. Significant consideration was therefore paid to fostering these conditions in all aspects of programme delivery to promote VPC self-direction in AVC activities and resulting AMS behaviour change goals (Table 1).

2.3. Engagement through Key Collaborators

The AVC project—which also includes quantitative antimicrobial use data collection and animal health planning schemes alongside the intervention—represents a collaboration between Bristol Vet School, Welsh government's Office of the Chief Veterinary Officer, the industry-controlled farmer cooperative Welsh Lamb and Beef Producers and the South Wales and North Wales Veterinary Delivery Partners, Iechyd da and Milfeddygon Gogledd Cymru, respectively. Development of a network of Veterinary Prescribing Champions is one part of the wider AVC project, which is aimed at addressing antimicrobial resistance in Welsh agriculture. This includes work to develop technology for improving the accuracy of medicine use recording by farmers, led by Welsh Lamb and Beef Producers, and benchmarking veterinary practice antimicrobial use, led by Iechyd Da. By engaging these key collaborators, the AVC intervention was supported by leading academic, governmental and industry representatives able to engage with potential participants and encourage active involvement in the programme. Each collaborator contributed to engagement in the following ways: The Office of the Chief Veterinary Officer was able to use established communication channels to encourage participation in an official capacity, with the Chief Veterinary Officer for Wales endorsing the programme and encouraging veterinary surgeons to take part. Welsh Lamb and Beef Producers are responsible for farm quality assurance schemes in Wales and, therefore, are a familiar industry body that Welsh farm animal veterinary surgeons understand to represent farmers' interests, which helped improve engagement. The Veterinary Delivery Partners were able to contribute to active recruitment by disseminating details of the project to their veterinary practice members through formal networks. The project lead (GR) had also worked as a farm animal veterinary surgeon in Wales and, therefore, was able to combine these formal recruitment pathways with informal networks to further promote engagement.

Participant demographic data were collected through an online questionnaire at the time of initial recruitment and registration.

Table 1. Operational conditions of self-determination theory posited by Silva, Marques, and Teixera [27] for consideration in intervention design and their adaptation to guiding principles for appropriate enactment within Arwain Vet Cymru.

SDT Construct	Operational Condition	Guiding Principle
Support for autonomy	Relevance	Provide a clear and meaningful rationale for both AVC and AMS activities throughout all inputs and training elements of the AVC programme (Figure 1), aiming to facilitate self-endorsement of activities by VPCs.
	Respect	Seek to actively acknowledge VPCs' perspectives, feelings, and agendas within network activities. Thoughtfully integrate opportunities within the programme for individuals to contribute to, shape, and offer reflection on the intervention process, foci, and goals as they unfold.
	Choice	Embed engagement with AVC activities with a sense of choice wherever possible, by providing varied options for process engagement (i.e., in educational training and network meeting participation) and encourage VPCs to follow their own interests, ideas, and goals in the selection, adoption, and implementation of AMS intervention activities.
	Avoidance of control	Commitment by those leading AVC to avoid directive, coercive, or authoritarian management of VPCs within the network; ensuring this ethos leads to the selection of collaborative partners who contribute to practical programme delivery (such as external facilitators).
Support for competence	Clarity of expectations	Ensuring that through recruitment, inputs and training activities within the AVC programme (Figure 1) discussion of what to expect and what not to expect from AVC participation is facilitated. Set up processes that encourage the setting of realistic and achievable behaviour change goals by VPCs in their adoption and integration of AMS options.
	Optimal challenge	Seek to encourage VPCs to select behaviour change goals where the challenge of the activity is highly balanced with their ability to successfully perform the behaviour (i.e., the change is a good fit for their practice and context, is something that they have the appropriate skill set to enact, and that is neither too easy nor too difficult for the VPC to implement).
	Feedback	Ensure VPCs have the opportunity to access relevant and non-judgmental feedback on their practice interventions throughout design and implementation processes, both individually (through accessibility of contact with G.R. as project lead) and in-group meetings where this is facilitated peer-to-peer within the network (i.e., workshops and discussion groups).
	Skills training	Commitment to providing education, training, guidance and support in key areas of AMS as identified through knowledge pathways in Phase One of intervention design, to ensure VPCs feel adequately equipped to identify and set their own AMS behaviour change goal(s).
Support for relatedness	Empathy	Ensuring group meetings (discussion groups, workshops) offer opportunities for VPCs to explore and reflect on their colleagues' perspectives at both peer-to-peer and group levels. Facilitate alternate perspective taking on any contentious issues if they arise within the group.
	Affection	Those coordinating the AVC scheme taking care to convey a sense of care and concern for participants prescribing and AMS challenges, in addition to genuine appreciation for VPC engagement.
	Attunement	Careful attention to, gathering knowledge about and responding to VPC perspectives both (i) by those coordinating the AVC scheme and (ii) facilitated peer-to-peer within the AVC network, to ensure VPCs needs to feel validated, accepted, affirmed, and significant within AVC are met [28], and to generate a felt sense of union with other VPCs in this process [29].
	Dedication of resources	Emphasising where and how AVC coordinators and wider project collaborators (industry, government) are investing time and energy into the scheme, in addition to creating project opportunities (workshops, discussion groups) where VPCs are connected by volunteering their time and energy to drive the momentum of AVC.
	Dependability	Ensuring VPCs feel that support is available to them via AVC in case of need on their AMS behaviour change journey, through guidance on how they can seek the input and advice of the project lead (GR) throughout.

Where SDT = self-determination theory, AMS = antimicrobial stewardship, AVC = Arwain Vet Cymru, VPC = veterinary prescribing champion, GR = Gwen Rees.

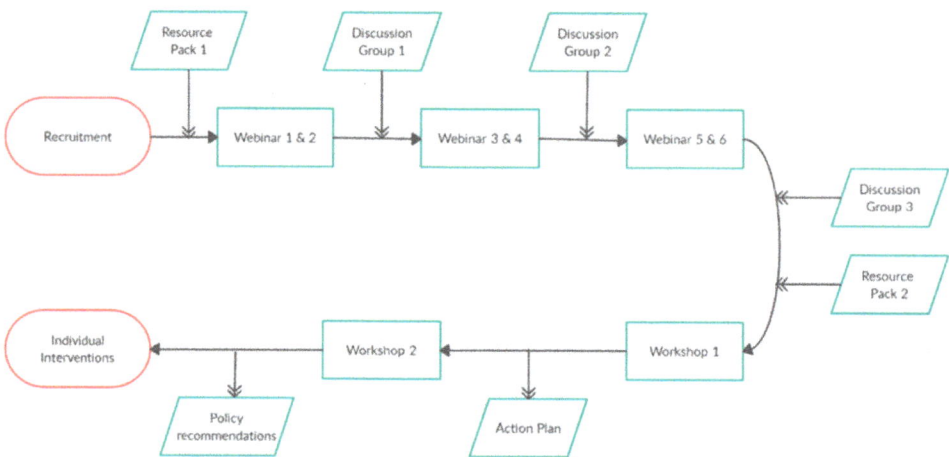

Figure 1. Flowchart showing the chronology of the inputs and outputs in the Arwain Vet Cymru programme.

2.4. Designing a National Stewardship Programme

The development of the AVC intervention model occurred in two phases (Figure 2). Firstly, identifying critical elements of the intervention—through the integration of the four knowledge pathways representing subject experts, relevant stakeholders, practicing veterinary surgeons, and the current evidence base for effective interventions targeting prescribing practice—enabled the design of a context-specific and appropriate intervention. Secondly, grounding the delivery of this intervention within the SDT theoretical framework—by identifying operational SDT conditions relevant and applicable to AVC participation—allowed for an understanding how the intervention was proposed to engage VPCs' internalised motivation.

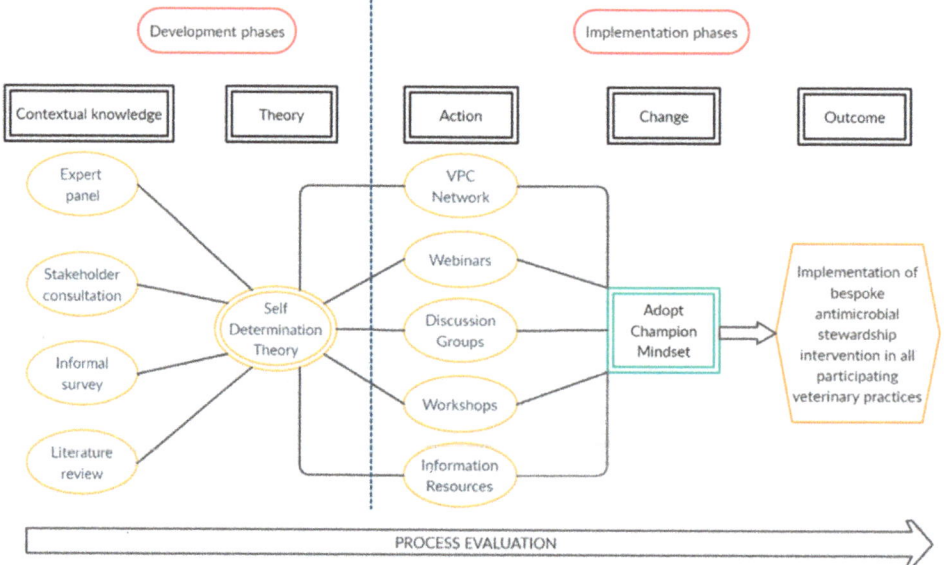

Figure 2. Design map of the Arwain Vet Cymru program, identifying the key phases of the design and implementation process.

2.4.1. Phase One: Contextual Knowledge

Four knowledge pathways were explored to appropriately contextualise the aims of the AMS program for VPCs in Wales.

Relevant stakeholders: key stakeholders were identified in the areas of veterinary professional regulation, specialist veterinary membership organisations, farming body representatives, government policy departments, and human public health. Stakeholders included the British Veterinary Association's Welsh Branch Council, Welsh government's AMR in Animals and the Environment Delivery Group, the Sheep Veterinary Society, the British Cattle Veterinary Association, Public Health Wales, and the National Farmers Union, among others. These stakeholders were contacted and invited to input into the design of the new national stewardship programme. Stakeholders involved in ongoing animal health projects in Wales were contacted in order to coordinate efforts and avoid duplication.

Practicing veterinary surgeons: practising farm animal veterinary surgeons in Wales were informally surveyed by the Veterinary Delivery Partners in order to identify key issues they felt important to be included in the design of the programme. This took the form of utilising existing communication networks between farm animal veterinary surgeons, including email and WhatsApp communications, to invite suggestions for stewardship intervention strategies and feedback on current policy.

Expert input: a broad range of expertise was available through the University of Bristol's "AMR Force" multidisciplinary research group, consisting of clinical veterinary practitioners, epidemiologists, veterinary academics, and social scientists. By drawing upon this expertise, intervention design was informed by the current research landscape and areas of clinical importance in order to focus on identified areas of key importance to research and clinical practice.

Literature review: an extensive literature review examining (i) complex intervention design theory; (ii) antimicrobial prescribing in agriculture; and (iii) AMS interventions was conducted. This review provided an evidence base for the intervention design, identified potential barriers, and enablers to stewardship in the veterinary context and highlighted known areas of high antimicrobial use for specific focus.

2.4.2. Phase Two: Integrating Theory

The second phase of AVC intervention design aimed to foster the motivational internalisation of AVC activities and AMS change for participating VPCs. To ensure VPCs' motivation was cultivated in this internalised, agentic form, active integration of the psychological needs highlighted within SDT was critical. Namely, the need for VPCs to feel AVC activities and selected AMS change(s) (i) enhanced their competence (perceived self-efficacy); (ii) supported their autonomy (a sense of choice, being the origin of one's own behaviour); and (iii) promoted their sense of relatedness (feeling understood and cared for by others) [26]. Operational conditions for these psychological needs have been detailed for consideration in the design of SDT-informed interventions of this kind [27]. These conditions were adapted to create guiding principles for the AVC intervention design (Table 1) informing the selection, content, and thoughtful delivery of activities within the AVC training schedule, as highlighted in Results.

3. Results

3.1. Participation of VPCs

A total of 43 farm animal veterinary surgeons were recruited to the AVC project from March 2020, representing 41 veterinary practices across Wales. Participants were offered no incentives for taking part in this study, although the training could be counted towards mandatory continuing professional development requirements of UK practicing veterinary surgeons. Out of the 50 Welsh practices involved in farm work (defined as practices with Official Veterinarians registered with the Veterinary Delivery Partners), nine did not take part in the programme. Of these, five stated that they did not do sufficient farm work within Wales to make participation worthwhile, one practice withdrew from the programme due to increased workload relating to the Coronavirus Disease (COVID-19) pandemic and no response was received from three practices. Demographics of participants can be seen in Table 2.

Table 2. Participant demographics of Veterinary Prescribing Champions (VPCs) enrolled on the Arwain Vet Cymru project in Wales.

Participant Characteristic	All VPCs		North Wales VPCs		South Wales VPCs	
All VPCs	43	100%	17	100%	26	100%
Gender						
Male	24	56%	11	65%	13	50%
Female	19	44%	6	35%	13	50%
Years qualified						
<5 years	2	5%	0	0%	2	8%
5–10 years	8	19%	4	24%	4	15%
10–20 years	11	25%	5	29%	6	23%
>20 years	22	51%	8	47%	14	54%
Position in practice						
Business Partner/Director	19	44%	7	41%	12	46%
Clinical Director	5	12%	2	12%	3	12%
Consultant	1	2%	1	6%	0	0%
Salaried Assistant	18	42%	7	41%	11	42%
Number of cattle herds served by the practice						
<100	7	16%	4	24%	3	12%
101–200	11	26%	4	24%	7	27%
201–300	12	28%	6	35%	6	23%
301–400	6	14%	1	6%	5	19%
>401	7	16%	2	11%	5	19%
Number of farm vets in the practice						
0-5	7	16%	3	18%	4	15%
6–10	23	54%	9	53%	14	55%
11–15	6	14%	2	11%	4	15%
>15	7	16%	3	18%	4	15%
Species cared for						
Farm only	7	16%	3	18%	4	15%
Mixed species	36	84%	14	82%	22	85%

Fifty-eight percent of the veterinary surgeons participating were either business partners or directors, consultants, or clinical directors, with the remaining 42% identifying as salaried assistants. Half of the participants had been graduated for >20 years, with only 5% having graduated fewer than five years prior to the programme beginning. Participants had a diverse range of interests across the spectrum of farm animal clinical work, with similar proportions interested in dairy, sheep, beef, mixed practice, and smallholder work. Twenty-six practices belonged to the South Wales Network, and 17 practices belonged to the North Wales Network. Eight practices were based over the Wales–England border, but served a significant number of Welsh farms. Nineteen participants (44%) were female and the remaining participants male.

The key barriers to implementation found so far in the AVC project can be best characterized as time constraints for participants and concern that restricting antimicrobial prescribing may lead to farming clients sourcing medicines elsewhere. However, despite a focus on these barriers during group discussions, they have not impacted significantly on participation in the programme to this point.

3.2. Defining the AVC Intervention Structure

Four knowledge pathways, as outlined in Methods, determined the structure, and focus of the overall intervention:

Stakeholder engagement: stakeholder response was positive, with all those contacted recognising the need for an AMS programme in Wales. Topics that emerged as important from the stakeholder engagement included a focus on responsible antimicrobial sales practices, the need for greater communication and collaboration between veterinary practices within a region, supporting veterinary surgeons to make responsible prescribing decisions and improving knowledge of relevant legislation and guidance.

Practicing veterinary surgeons: an informal survey of the needs and desires of farm animal veterinary surgeons in Wales indicated that they had similar areas of concern and focus as those identified by stakeholders. Of particular importance was the issue of responsible antimicrobial sales practices and improving communication between practices. Practising veterinary surgeons also outlined an interest in behaviour change principles, and how they could be applied when encouraging farmers to use medicines responsibly.

Expert input: interdisciplinary research group meetings outlined several key areas that were viewed as important in the design of this intervention. These included improving knowledge of the legal aspects, professional regulations, and industry guidelines surrounding prescribing, the principles of evidence-based veterinary medicine and the importance of participatory approaches to change.

Literature review: grounding the design in the theory of behaviour change and complex interventions in healthcare was identified as very important to the programme's success. Reviewing the literature indicated that the use of so-called "Champions" in health care interventions had been successful in other settings. The literature also highlighted the benefit of building sustainable communities of practice for complex healthcare interventions, and of combining education and training resources with reflective exercises and goal setting.

By combining the results of these four knowledge pathways, AVC's design was focussed around addressing the following key areas:

- Recruit and train one VPC from each farm animal veterinary practice in Wales.
- Improve VPCs' knowledge of AMS, the evidence base for prescribing decisions and the evidence base for legal and regulatory frameworks, human behaviour change, and species-specific considerations.
- Foster a sense of group identity as well as of community and collaboration between Champions.
- Encourage Champions to disseminate AMS messages within their practices.
- Facilitate the autonomous development, by each individual participant, of individual practical, fit-for-purpose stewardship interventions at each participating practice.

3.3. Enactment of the AVC Network: Combining Intervention Goals and Theoretical Drivers

The overall design of the implementation can be seen in Figure 2, and the training schedule can be seen in Table 3. Initially, implementation of the programme was designed to consist of several in-person meetings of all VPCs over the course of the first year. However, following the COVID-19 global pandemic and subsequent lockdown in the UK in March 2020, combined with the uncertain future of large gatherings, it was necessary to reimagine the AVC process in an entirely online format in early 2020. Each element of this online format within the AVC process will be discussed with reference to the operational conditions of SDT (Table 1) identified as critical guiding principles of the AVC intervention design.

Table 3. Arwain Vet Cymru Veterinary Prescribing Champion (VPC) training schedule developed as outlined in Figure 1.

Week	Activity	Topic
1	Webinar	Welcome and introduction to antimicrobial stewardship (AMS)
2	Webinar	Encouraging behaviour change for AMS
3	Discussion Group	Developing the "Champion mindset"
4	Webinar	Prescribing rules, regulations and guidelines in farm animals
5	Webinar	Sector-specific prescribing: dairy cattle, beef cattle and sheep
6	Discussion Group	Prescribing conduct and barriers to AMS
7	Webinar	Evidence-based prescribing and practical approaches to AMS
8	Webinar	Case studies and practical examples
9	Discussion Group	The future of the VPC Network
12	Workshop	Intervention design
13	Workshop	Policy recommendations

3.4. Webinars

In order to address the goal of improving VPCs' knowledge of the key areas of AMS identified in the knowledge pathways outlined above, an educational programme of six webinars was included in the overall design. Expert speakers were invited from a range of academic institutions, with content informed by the literature review and expert panel meetings along with veterinary and stakeholder engagement. Six one-hour webinars were co-designed with the speakers. These webinars were broadcast weekly on Wednesday afternoons, the day identified during recruitment as the best time for VPCs as routine tuberculosis testing does not usually occur on this day. Participants were given the opportunity to attend webinars during the live broadcast or to watch recordings asynchronously, at their convenience.

A brief description of the content of each webinar is outlined in Table 3. Briefly, webinars covered topics such as Welsh AMR policy, the concept of AMS, legislation and guidelines relevant to prescribing, behaviour change theory, evidence-based veterinary medicine, antimicrobial use benchmarking across the different species and a selection of case examples from practices that had successfully implemented various AMS schemes. These topics were selected based on the key areas identified in the literature review, stakeholder engagement, expert input, and informal survey of practicing veterinary surgeons, as outlined in Section 3.2.

The format and delivery of these webinars was chosen to actively promote operational conditions within SDT to enhance VPC engagement (Table 1). The provision of instrumental and practically relevant AMS training—in addition to clarifying VPCs' expectations of their involvement in the AVC Network—promoted support for VPC-perceived competence. Additionally, focusing on promoting VPC self-endorsement of AVC activities through provision of a variety of rationales from well-respected, expert speakers whilst providing choice in how webinars were accessed by participants (i.e., synchronous or asynchronous) embedded key attributes of autonomy support.

3.5. Discussion Groups

To develop a sense of community, collaboration, and group identity, informal online discussion sessions were held every third week of the nine-week training timeline (Table 3). VPCs were divided by region into North Wales and South Wales groups. Participants were given a choice of which group they wished to belong to, since those working in mid-Wales may have identified more strongly with a different region than might have been suggested geographically. Discussion sessions were hosted using online videoconferencing software and were facilitated by two researchers experienced in group facilitation (G.R. and A.B.).

Topics of discussion in each session were iterative and informed in part by the content of the previous webinars, in addition to topics raised during informal feedback and webinar question-and-answer sessions. These topics were guided by the facilitators, but were semi-structured in nature, allowing some freedom for participants to discuss issues they felt to be important at the time. Utilising interactive polling and small group breakout rooms, participants were asked to focus on and discuss specific areas related to veterinary prescribing before joining plenary discussion sessions where participants were able to share their views and discuss further with the whole group. Discussion group size varied from a minimum of five participants to a maximum of 17 participants between group meetings, and the facilitation of these groups was flexible in order to account for varying group size. Where discussion group size was greater than five, virtual "break-out rooms" were used, and participants were asked to discuss in small groups before returning to the main plenary discussion to report back on their discussions. This flexibility was important because the availability of participants to join discussion groups would vary depending on clinical veterinary duties on the day.

Discussion sessions enabled participants to outline the main challenges they perceived when considering implementing AMS programmes, along with exploring opportunities for change(s), and developing a sense of shared ownership over the outcomes of the project. Discussion sessions were also an opportunity to prepare Champions for the subsequent workshops. Promoting congruence with the tenets of SDT underpinned discussion session design. To cultivate a sense of autonomy for VPCs, attendance was made non-compulsory and VPCs chose their regional group allocation. The sessions were also opportunities for AVC facilitators to actively evoke and acknowledge VPCs' feelings and agendas with regards to the breadth of potential interventions covered in the webinar sessions. This, in turn, further promoted autonomy through respect for the VPCs' unique choices and intentions with regards to the AMS foci. To support VPCs' competence, the discussion groups offered facilitators the chance to provide relevant and non-judgemental feedback on VPC perspectives on AMS foci, whilst allowing facilitators to shape participatory activities to also encourage positive peer-to-peer feedback. Finally, enhanced relatedness was achieved through a focus on evoking, exploring and understanding VPC perspectives, both by the facilitators and through targeted peer-to-peer activities, creating opportunities for promoting group empathy and attunement (a felt sense of union) between AVC participants.

3.6. Workshops

Two three-hour facilitated workshops were included in the design of the programme and followed on from the webinars and discussion groups in order to enable goal setting and the creation of action plans by VPCs, as outlined below. The first workshop was intended to allow VPCs to develop the knowledge and ideas gained during the webinars and discussion groups and distil these into actionable goals designed specifically for their practice context. VPCs were responsible for designing their own context-specific AMS intervention, relevant to their veterinary practice's prescribing context. A second workshop, designed to inform policy, was included in order to allow VPCs the opportunity to contribute to the wider professional context with regards to matters of AMS.

3.6.1. Stewardship Intervention Design Workshop

The stewardship intervention design workshop aimed to enable each participating VPC to design and develop their own personal action plan, as well as a stewardship intervention for their practice. Examples of the kind of action plans discussed include:

- Reorganise the practice veterinary medicine dispensary to make certain antimicrobials more difficult to reach and/or more easily identified as second or third choice.
- Schedule training and improve communication with veterinary reception and dispensing staff at the practice to ensure all staff members are delivering a unified message around antimicrobial prescribing and dispensing.
- Begin to benchmark antimicrobial use among practice farms and include discussion of antimicrobial use in annual herd or flock health planning.
- Introduce on-farm medicine cupboard "health checks" into the annual herd or flock health planning.

This workshop was run by an experienced participatory action research facilitator and co-facilitated by two experienced facilitators familiar to the VPCs (G.R. and A.B.). Participants were asked to set goals and create action plans outlining how they would implement their stewardship intervention according to the SMART framework (Specific, Measurable, Attainable, Relevant, Timely) [30]. Structured discussions utilising online fora and breakout rooms allowed VPCs to consider their plans with their peers, helping to identify potential barriers to implementation and possible solutions by drawing on their collective experiences.

Central to the concept and design of this workshop was fostering VPCs' sense of autonomy in their AMS roles. Workshop activities consolidated VPCs' own ideas for an AMS intervention strategy depending on what they envisaged for their own practice context, whilst a primary facilitator experienced in non-directive, participant-led workshops emphasised the ethos of VPC choice and self-endorsement throughout. Workshop activities also aimed to encourage VPCs toward the choice of an optimal AMS challenge (i.e., not too easy nor too difficult) for their circumstances and skill set, to drive competence-infused practice change. Relatedness was embedded within workshop activities through, for example, informal and personal introductions in each workshop to foster rapport, by offering attending VPCs opportunities to vocalise fears, concerns, and thoughts on intervention interests for peer validation, and facilitating peer-to-peer exploration, reflection, and group feedback on personal perspectives of AMS activities and policy within Wales. Together, activities of this kind sought to foster empathy and union (attunement).

3.6.2. Policy Workshop

This workshop was designed to allow VPCs the opportunity to inform AMR policy at the national level. Participants were encouraged to identify important areas of focus, outline the policy support required to enable them to be responsible prescribers, and construct practical solutions to help address some of the barriers identified in the AVC project. This workshop was created with the support of Welsh government, who agreed that outcomes would be presented to the Welsh government's Animals and the Environment AMR Delivery Group.

This policy workshop offered VPCs the chance to develop a sense of personal influence over policy decisions impacting their profession; thus, engendering a feeling of self-endorsement critical to autonomous engagement. The premise of the workshop—highlighting the unique role of the AVC network as a valued voice in determining AMR strategy in Wales—emphasised the importance of this group influence of AVC Champions thus forging the relatedness of group members further. Providing another practical opportunity for VPCs to explore and construct solutions to AMS challenges, elevated to the national perspective within Wales, was a final training opportunity for VPC competence development.

3.7. Stewardship Intervention Implementation

The initial AVC programme outlined above required a time commitment of around 15 h by the VPCs. Following on from the workshops, VPCs are expected to disseminate the AMS messages to and implement their co-designed, individual AMS plans in their respective practices. This will lead to 41 different AMS schemes being implemented—one at each participating practice—beginning in January 2021. Participants will be asked to complete monthly reports outlining the implementation of their stewardship scheme as well as provide feedback on ease of implementation, relevant actors involved, scope of the changes, outcomes observed, and barriers encountered. Overall practice prescribing behaviours will be evaluated through a longitudinal prescribing audit.

Throughout implementation, AVC facilitators will manage VPCs through a continued ethos of avoiding directive, coercive, or authoritarian approaches, first and foremost emphasising VPC autonomy in the enactment of practice-based interventions and how VPCs choose to engage with the AVC Network, and support staff throughout this process.

Practices will be supported by the project as required, with AVC facilitators prioritising trust in VPC competencies in overseeing the implementation of these intervention choices, with a focus on responsive management determined by VPCs themselves. It is hoped that the attunement developed from peer-to-peer activities within the AVC Network (through discussion groups and workshops) will also be an avenue of relatedness support for participating veterinary surgeons during this implementation process.

4. Discussion

In a complex healthcare intervention such as this, multiple interconnected elements all inform and affect each other. The AVC design process included stakeholder engagement, reviewing current literature, drawing on theory and understanding context as laid out by O'Cathain et al. [18]. As such, it is difficult to appraise each individual element of such a programme, and the entire intervention must be considered as a whole. However, by examining some of the principal domains of the intervention design (Figure 2), it is possible to explore how they informed—and became intrinsic to—the programme structure. By attempting to understand the context, theoretical basis, and implementation of the intervention, we can examine how and why VPCs within the AVC network might promote change through their AMS interventions and lead to more responsible use of antimicrobials.

Considerable effort was spent throughout the intervention process in engaging and communicating with farm animal veterinary surgeons in Wales. By grounding the design in the available literature and accessing informal feedback, key barriers to implementation could be identified and attempts to overcome them could be incorporated into the design from the outset. A recent scoping review found that knowledge, responsibility (the influence of peer behaviour) and the veterinary surgeon–client relationship represented significant barriers to AMS for cattle veterinary surgeons [31]. The AVC implementation design sought to address these barriers through education and building communities of practice. In Golding et al.'s exploration of veterinary surgeons' beliefs about AMS, one perceived barrier to implementation was the concern that farming clients might simply change to a rival practice if denied the antimicrobial of their choice [32]. This was also identified by stakeholders and participants as a barrier to change. In response to this, the design of the AVC intervention included an emphasis on building a sense of common purpose between practices, encouraging open communication, and creating a community by incorporating informal discussion groups.

The demographic characteristics of the participants was hypothesised to play an important role in the likely success of the program. Experienced veterinary surgeons with a senior role in their practices were thought to have a greater degree of autonomy and authority with which to implement AMS interventions. The relatively few female participants (44%) compared with the 57% of females who make up the UK's veterinary workforce was statistically significant ($p = 0.0472$) using the N-1 Chi-Squared Test for two proportions and may be explained in part by the increasing "feminisation" of the profession and the under-representation of female veterinary surgeons in senior roles [33]; recruitment of older, senior veterinary surgeons meant they were more likely to be male. It would be interesting to understand whether the gender ratio of such a participant group—and its representativeness of the wider study population—influences the effectiveness of the intervention. Further research into the role of gender in complex intervention implementation through realist evaluation principles is required [34].

In identifying a theoretical driver for AVC, full consideration of the intervention context was essential. Following the recommendations within COM-B [23], AVC design considered (i) the target behaviour; (ii) intervention options; and (iii) content and implementation options. The target behaviour within AVC was complex, with the aim of participants cultivating a prescribing "Champion" mindset and cementing their intention to design and implement an AMS intervention within their own professional environments. Fundamentally, the AVC goal was therefore to create the facilitative conditions for this mindset and practice change to occur. Intervention options from the Behaviour Change

Wheel targeting training, environmental restructuring, and enablement appeared most appropriate for this purpose, influencing the multifaceted intervention design and the inclusion of webinars, discussion groups, and workshops informed by the four knowledge pathways [23]. Through consideration of how best to integrate these intervention foci effectively as drivers of capability, opportunity, and motivation with regards to a "Champion" mindset, a theoretical underpinning was sought to foster VPC engagement throughout.

Key to the aim of this intervention was the need for the "Champion" mindset to be sufficiently salient, psychologically, to drive VPC self-directed behaviour as VPCs are expected to implement their own AMS intervention in January 2021, following active engagement in the AVC scheme. Understanding the motivational factors that facilitate or undermine a sense of initiative and volition, in addition to the quality of performance, is central to SDT [19,23]. This theory therefore appeared uniquely adapted to the demands of the AVC scheme. The psychological conditions posited to encourage individuals to value, self-regulate and (without external pressure) carry out and maintain behaviour—competence, autonomy, and relatedness [26]—were adopted as guiding principles in the practical realisation of the intervention design. The strength of this intervention lies in having conducted a thorough assessment of: the behaviour change target in question, what might be needed to achieve this change, and where a theoretical underpinning resonating with the project aims might enrich implementation [35].

In the pursuit of forging individual identities within health interventions, the concept of using "Champions" as a means of motivating change in healthcare settings is not new. In Australia, Antibiotic Champions have been used to support an AMS campaign within Children's Health teams [36]. Medical, veterinary and dental students in the UK can register to become Antibiotic Guardian Champions [37], and the UK's National Health Service (NHS) has several Champion schemes, addressing such issues as social prescribing [38], diabetes [39], physical activity [40], perinatal metal health [41], and digital health [42]. In this programme, giving the participants an identity, as a VPC was a crucial part in developing a sense of community and leadership. Champions were representing the programme within their practices but were also representing their practice within the network.

Complementing this individual shift in perspective was the hypothesized creation of communities of practice, forging a group identity for AVC participants. The Situated Learning Theory [43], whereby professional learning occurs through interaction with peers and participation in practice, forms the basis for the concept of communities of practice. These are groups of people who interact on an ongoing basis in order to share expertise and deepen knowledge on an area of concern [44]. They have been utilised in healthcare settings as a means of improving performance and sharing knowledge "in response to the challenges of complex systems" [45,46]. By encouraging the development of a superordinate identity—in this case that of a national Prescribing Champion—alongside their professional identities as veterinary surgeons working in discrete private practice, it was intended that VPCs could overcome the professional barriers to AMS identified in the literature, as suggested by Bartunek et al. [47].

The inclusion of goal setting and action planning in this programme, through the intervention design workshop, allowed VPCs the opportunity to translate the knowledge and ideas gained during the initial training into defined, outcome-driven actions. By using the SMART framework [30], creating individual action plans based on overarching goals was expected to help narrow the intention–behaviour gap [48]. Literature establishes that planning within a particular context of who, when, where, and how is important when considering behaviour change [4]; indeed, it is at the heart of the theoretical underpinnings of the COM-B model [23]. Encouraging VPCs to consider these elements in their individual intervention designs will ideally facilitate AMS plans that appropriately echo tenets of the COM-B model, even in the absence of direct training on the intricacies of this model. A recent paper by Atkins et al. specifically called on National AMS intervention design to include goal setting and action planning, as they were areas identified as being underrepresented in current AMS programmes [49].

Educational interventions have been shown to improve knowledge of pharmacovigilance [50] and prescribing competency [51] as well as to strengthen AMS [52–54], although the effects may be short-lived. Online learning as part of AMS programmes has been playing an increasing role [55] and online training of GPs has been shown to reduce antimicrobial prescribing for respiratory disease [56]. An online process also enabled the inclusion of a diverse range of external expert speakers who may not have been able to attend in more traditional in person provision, potentially improving the overall content. Another unintended but positive effect of online provision was the distribution of training sessions over the course of several weeks, interspersed with other activities, thus potentially consolidating the VPCs' participation in the programme.

The Medical Research Council's new guidance for developing and analysing complex interventions [57] highlights the importance of practical effectiveness—that is, whether the intervention works "in the real world"—as a key measure when evaluating complex interventions. In order to answer this question, process evaluation can use ethnographic and qualitative methodology in order to explore the impact of the intervention, identify any unintended consequences and be able to describe the experience of the participants who take part in any intervention programme. Through an ongoing process evaluation combining ethnographic exploration of implementation and quantitative measures of prescribing, the implementation of the AVC programme will be under continuous appraisal until completion (September 2021). Results of this evaluation will be published separately.

It remains to be seen whether the Arwain Vet Cymru project produces workable AMS interventions in clinical veterinary prescribing practice as predicted. While it is hoped that this complex intervention is successful in improving responsible prescribing practices, further empirical evidence is currently being collected in order to enable full conclusions to be drawn. Any unforeseen negative consequences are of course also important, and all outcomes are meaningful when informing future development of similar programmes, both in Wales and further afield.

Limitations

While in an ideal world the design–evaluation–implementation process would occur in a relatively linear fashion and follow best-practice study design, practically this is not always possible. In this instance, the intervention took place in the context of political and industry-led pressure on the veterinary profession to improve prescribing, with an impact-led rather than research-led funding focus. As such, design, evaluation and implementation occurred in a more cyclical and iterative process in this study.

The establishment of this national Network of Prescribing Champions has been relatively labour-intensive, requiring high levels of ongoing engagement with key actors across many stakeholder groups. Participation in the project has involved around 15 h of time investment from participating VPCs, and the ongoing time commitment required to implement their action plans will be dependent on the complexity of the intervention each VPC has designed. The other stakeholders involved in the development of the AVC stewardship programme were not compensated for their time, and we believe their involvement to be motivated by a desire across the veterinary profession to improve antimicrobial prescribing both for the "greater good" and to improve the image of UK agriculture. Given the economic and political sensitivities of bringing individuals from separate, competing interests together to tackle a common concern, the very high level of recruitment to the programme is both surprising and encouraging. Establishing this pan-Wales network of highly motivated clinicians may make it possible to overcome some of the perceived barriers to change. The ongoing sustainability of the network—and its legacy after the end of the funded project—is an important area for development in the next stage of the programme. By moving to a self-sufficient model of participant-led network maintenance, it may be possible to continue the network beyond the lifespan of the project.

5. Conclusions

Designing a novel national AMS programme for farm animal veterinary surgeons requires several supporting factors. The applicability of this programme design to other parts of the UK and the rest of the world is difficult to predict; however, we believe that by focusing on a robust theoretical grounding and giving full consideration to the context of the intervention as evidenced in this paper, stewardship interventions can be improved worldwide. A favourable policy background, collaboration with key actors within the profession, stakeholder consultation, an emphasis on autonomy, and commitment to developing a sense of community have all helped to promote high levels of engagement in this voluntary national network of VPCs. Empirical data from both qualitative and quantitative process evaluations will help reveal the impact this type of complex intervention may have on AMS in rural veterinary medicine.

Author Contributions: Conceptualization, G.M.R.; methodology, G.M.R. and A.B.; investigation, G.M.R. and A.B.; writing—original draft preparation, G.M.R. and A.B.; writing—review and editing, K.K.R.; visualization, G.M.R.; supervision, K.K.R.; project administration, G.M.R.; funding acquisition, G.M.R. and K.K.R. All authors have read and agreed to the published version of the manuscript.

Funding: This research was funded by the Welsh government through the Rural Development Programme.

Institutional Review Board Statement: The study was conducted according to the guidelines of the Declaration of Helsinki, and approved by the Institutional Review Board (or Ethics Committee) of the University of Bristol Faculty of Health Sciences (protocol code 99522, 18 March 2020).

Informed Consent Statement: Informed consent was obtained from all subjects involved in the study.

Acknowledgments: The authors would like to thank the collaborative partners in this project, Iechyd Da and Welsh Lamb and Beef producers, along with all of the participants and stakeholders involved in development of this project.

Conflicts of Interest: The authors declare no conflict of interest.

References

1. World Health Organization. *Antimicrobial Resistance: A Manual for Developing National Action Plans*; Version 1; WHO: Geneve, Switzerland, 2016. Available online: https://apps.who.int/iris/handle/10665/2044702016 (accessed on 20 October 2020).
2. World Health Organisation. *Global Action Plan on Antimicrobial Resistance*; World Health Organization: Geneve, Switzerland, 2015. Available online: http://www.who.int/iris/handle/10665/193736 (accessed on 20 October 2020).
3. O'Neill, J. *Tackling Drug Resistant Infections Globally: Final Report and Recommendations. The Review on Antimicrobial Resistance*; Government of the United Kingdom: London, UK, 2016.
4. Davey, P.; Peden, C.; Charani, E.; Marwick, C.; Michie, S. Time for action-Improving the design and reporting of behaviour change interventions for antimicrobial stewardship in hospitals: Early findings from a systematic review. *Int. J. Antimicrob. Agents* **2015**, *45*, 203–212. [CrossRef]
5. Johnson, A.P.; Ashiru-Oredope, D.; Beech, E. Antibiotic Stewardship Initiatives as Part of the UK 5-Year Antimicrobial Resistance Strategy. *Antibiotics* **2015**, *4*, 467–479. [CrossRef] [PubMed]
6. Ashiru-Oredope, D.; Doble, A.; Akpan, M.R.; Hansraj, S.; Shebl, N.A.; Ahmad, R.; Hopkins, S. Antimicrobial Stewardship Programmes in Community Healthcare Organisations in England: A Cross-Sectional Survey to Assess Implementation of Programmes and National Toolkits. *Antibiotics* **2018**, *7*, 97. [CrossRef]
7. Howard, P.; Pulcini, C.; Levy Hara, G.; West, R.M.; Gould, I.M.; Harbarth, S.; Nathwani, D. An international cross-sectional survey of antimicrobial stewardship programmes in hospitals. *J. Antimicrob. Chemother.* **2015**, *70*, 1245–1255. [CrossRef] [PubMed]
8. Hardefeldt, L.Y.; Gilkerson, J.R.; Billman-Jacobe, H.; Stevenson, M.A.; Thursky, K.; Bailey, K.E.; Browning, G.F. Barriers to and enablers of implementing antimicrobial stewardship programs in veterinary practices. *J. Vet. Intern. Med.* **2018**, *32*, 1092–1099. [CrossRef] [PubMed]
9. UK-VARSS. *Veterinary Antibiotic Resistance and Sales Surveillance Report (UK-VARSS 2019)*; Addlestone Veterinary Medicines Directorate: Addlestone, UK, 2020.
10. RUMA. Targets Task Force Report 2020 Responsible Use of Antibiotics in UK Farming Progress against 2020 Targets New Targets 2021–2024. Available online: https://www.ruma.org.uk/wp-content/uploads/2020/11/RUMA-Targets-Task-Force-Report-2020_download.pdf (accessed on 20 October 2020).
11. Welsh Government. *Antimicrobial Resistance in Animals and the Environment: Five Year Implementation Plan for Wales 2019–2024*; Welsh Government: Cardiff, UK, 2019.
12. HM Government. *Tackling antimicrobial resistance 2019–2024: The UK's 5-Year National Action Plan*; HM Government: London, UK, 2019.

13. Government of Wales Act 2006, Schedule 7. Available online: https://www.legislation.gov.uk/ukpga/2006/32/contents (accessed on 20 October 2020).
14. Welsh Government. *Agriculture in Wales*; Welsh Government: Cardiff, UK, 2019.
15. Schweitzer, V.A.; van Werkhoven, C.H.; Rodriguez Bano, J.; Bielicki, J.; Harbarth, S.; Hulscher, M.; Huttner, B.; Islam, J.; Little, P.; Pulcini, C.; et al. Optimizing design of research to evaluate antibiotic stewardship interventions: Consensus recommendations of a multinational working group. *Clin. Microbiol. Infect.* **2020**, *26*, 41–50. [CrossRef]
16. MRC. *Developing and Evaluating Complex Interventions: New Guidance*; Medical Research Council: London, UK, 2019.
17. Colquhoun, H.L.; Squires, J.E.; Kolehmainen, N.; Fraser, C.; Grimshaw, J.M. Methods for designing interventions to change healthcare professionals' behaviour: A systematic review. *Implement. Sci.* **2017**, *12*, 30. [CrossRef] [PubMed]
18. O'Cathain, A.; Croot, L.; Duncan, E.; Rousseau, N.; Sworn, K.; Turner, K.M.; Yardley, L.; Hoddinott, P. Guidance on how to develop complex interventions to improve health and healthcare. *BMJ Open* **2019**, *9*, e029954. [CrossRef]
19. Deci, E.L.; Ryan, R.M. The "What" and "Why" of Goal Pursuits: Human Needs and the Self-Determination of Behavior. *Psychol. Inq.* **2000**, *11*, 227–268. [CrossRef]
20. Royal College of Veterinary Surgeons (2020) Code of Professional Conduct for Veterinary Surgeons. Available online: https://www.rcvs.org.uk/setting-standards/advice-and-guidance/code-of-professional-conduct-for-veterinary-surgeons/ (accessed on 20 October 2020).
21. Rees, G.M.; Barrett, D.C.; Buller, H.; Mills, H.L.; Reyher, K.K. Storage of prescription veterinary medicines on UK dairy farms: A cross-sectional study. *Vet. Rec.* **2018**, *184*, 153. [CrossRef] [PubMed]
22. Rees, G.M.; Barrett, D.C.; Sánchez-Vizcaíno, F.; Reyher, K.K. Measuring antimicrobial use on dairy farms: A method comparison cohort study. *J. Dairy Sci.* **2021**, in press. [CrossRef] [PubMed]
23. Michie, S.; van Stralen, M.M.; West, R. The behaviour change wheel: A new method for characterising and designing behaviour change interventions. *Implement. Sci.* **2011**, *6*, 1–12. [CrossRef] [PubMed]
24. Van den Broeck, A.; Ferris, D.L.; Chang, C.-H.; Rosen, C.C. A Review of Self-Determination Theory's Basic Psychological Needs at Work. *J. Manag.* **2016**, *42*, 1195–1229. [CrossRef]
25. Ryan, R.M.; Deci, E.L. Intrinsic and Extrinsic Motivations: Classic Definitions and New Directions. *Contemp. Educ. Psychol.* **2000**, *25*, 54–67. [CrossRef] [PubMed]
26. Ryan, R.M.; Deci, E.L. Self-determination theory and the facilitation of intrinsic motivation, social development, and wellbeing. *Am. Psychol.* **2000**, *55*, 68–78. [CrossRef]
27. Silva, M.N.; Marques, M.M.; Teixeira, P.J. Testing theory in practice: The example of self-determination theory-based interventions. *Eur. Health Psychol.* **2014**, *16*, 171–180.
28. Erskine, R.G. Attunement and involvement: Therapeutic responses to relational needs. In *Relational Patterns, Therapeutic Presence Concepts and Practice of Integrative Psychotherapy*; Routledge: London, UK, 2015; Chapter 3.
29. Kossak, M.S. Therapeutic attunement: A transpersonal view of expressive arts therapy. *Arts Psychother.* **2009**, *36*, 13–18. [CrossRef]
30. Doran, G.T. There's a S.M.A.R.T. way to write management's goals and objectives. *Manag. Rev.* **1981**, *70*, 35–36.
31. Gozdzielewska, L.; King, C.; Flowers, P.; Mellor, D.; Dunlop, P.; Price, L. Scoping review of approaches for improving antimicrobial stewardship in livestock farmers and veterinarians. *Prev. Vet. Med.* **2020**, *180*, 105025. [CrossRef]
32. Golding, S.E.; Ogden, J.; Higgins, H.M. Shared Goals, Different Barriers: A Qualitative Study of UK Veterinarians' and Farmers' Beliefs About Antimicrobial Resistance and Stewardship. *Front. Vet. Sci.* **2019**, *6*, 132. [CrossRef]
33. Gender Statistics about Veterinary Surgeons in the UK. Available online: https://www.vetfutures.org.uk/download/gender-statistics-about-veterinary-surgeons-in-the-uk/ (accessed on 20 October 2020).
34. Fletcher, A.; Jamal, F.; Moore, G.; Evans, R.E.; Murphy, S.; Bonell, C. Realist complex intervention science: Applying realist principles across all phases of the Medical Research Council framework for developing and evaluating complex interventions. *Evaluation* **2016**, *22*, 286–303. [CrossRef]
35. Michie, S.; Atkins, L.; Gainforth, H.L. Changing Behaviour to Improve Clinical Practice and Policy. In *Novos Desafios, Novas Competências: Contributos Atuais da Psicologia*; Axiom: Stepney, Australia, 2016; pp. 41–60.
36. Children's Health Queensland. Antibiotic Champion Network. Available online: https://www.childrens.health.qld.gov.au/chq/health-professionals/antimicrobial-stewardship/antibiotic-champion-network/2020 (accessed on 20 October 2020).
37. BSAC. Healthcare Students—Antibiotic Guardian Champion Badge. Available online: https://antibioticguardian.com/Resources/healthcare-students-ag-champion-badge/2020 (accessed on 20 October 2020).
38. College of Medicine and Integrated Health. National Social Prescribing Student Champion Scheme the Social Prescribing Network, the College of Medicine, and NHS England. Available online: https://collegeofmedicine.org.uk/national-social-prescribing-student-champion-scheme-the-social-prescribing-network-the-college-of-medicine-and-nhs-england/ (accessed on 20 October 2020).
39. Diabetes UK. The Clinical Champions Programme. Available online: https://www.diabetes.org.uk/professionals/resources/clinical-champions-and-networks (accessed on 20 October 2020).
40. Carlin, L.; Musson, H.; Adams, E. Evaluation of the Clinical Champions' Physical Activity Training programme. *OSF Prepr.* **2020**. preprint.
41. Institute of Health Visiting. Perinatal Mental Health Champions Training. Available online: https://ihv.org.uk/training-and-events/training-programme/courses/perinatal-depression-champions-training/ (accessed on 20 October 2020).

42. NHS Digital. Digital Champions for Health: A Blueprint for Success. Available online: https://digital.nhs.uk/about-nhs-digital/our-work/transforming-health-and-care-through-technology/empower-the-person-formerly-domain-a/widening-digital-participation/digital-champions-for-health2020 (accessed on 20 October 2020).
43. Lave, J.; Wenger, E. *Situated Learning: Legitimate Peripheral Participation*; Cambridge University Press: Cambridge, UK, 1990.
44. Wenger, E. *Communities of Practice: Learning, Meaning, and Identity*; Cambridge University Press: New York, NY, USA, 1998.
45. McKellar, K.A.; Pitzul, K.B.; Yi, J.Y.; Cole, D.C. Evaluating communities of practice and knowledge networks: A systematic scoping review of evaluation frameworks. *Ecohealth* **2014**, *11*, 383–399. [CrossRef] [PubMed]
46. Ranmuthugala, G.; Plumb, J.J.; Cunningham, F.C.; Georgiou, A.; Westbrook, J.I.; Braithwaite, J. How and why are communities of practice established in the healthcare sector? A systematic review of the literature. *BMC Health Serv. Res.* **2011**, *11*, 273. [CrossRef] [PubMed]
47. Bartunek, J.M. Intergroup relationships and quality improvement in healthcare. *BMJ Qual. Saf.* **2011**, *20* (Suppl. S1), i62–i66. [CrossRef]
48. Mann, T.; de Ridder, D.; Fujita, K. Self-regulation of health behavior: Social psychological approaches to goal setting and goal striving. *Health Psychol.* **2013**, *32*, 487–498. [CrossRef] [PubMed]
49. Atkins, L.; Chadborn, T.; Bondaronek, P.; Ashiru-Oredope, D.; Beech, E.; Herd, N.; de la Morinière, V.; González-Iraizoz, M.; Hopkins, S.; McNulty, C. Content and Mechanism of Action of National Antimicrobial Stewardship Interventions on Management of Respiratory Tract Infections in Primary and Community Care. *Antibiotics* **2020**, *9*, 512. [CrossRef] [PubMed]
50. Opadeyi, A.O.; Fourrier-Reglat, A.; Isah, A.O. Educational intervention to improve the knowledge, attitude and practice of healthcare professionals regarding pharmacovigilance in South-South Nigeria. *Ther. Adv. Drug Saf.* **2019**, *10*, 2042098618816279. [CrossRef] [PubMed]
51. Kamarudin, G.; Penm, J.; Chaar, B.; Moles, R. Educational interventions to improve prescribing competency: A systematic review. *BMJ Open* **2013**, *3*, e003291. [CrossRef] [PubMed]
52. Magrini, N.; Formoso, G.; Capelli, O.; Maestri, E.; Nonino, F.; Paltrinieri, B.; del Giovane, C.; Voci, C.; Magnano, L.; Daya, L.; et al. Long term effectiveness on prescribing of two multifaceted educational interventions: Results of two large scale randomized cluster trials. *PLoS ONE* **2014**, *9*, e109915. [CrossRef] [PubMed]
53. Wei, X.; Zhang, Z.; Walley, J.D.; Hicks, J.P.; Zeng, J.; Deng, S.; Zhou, Y.; Yin, J.; Newell, J.N.; Sun, Q.; et al. Effect of a training and educational intervention for physicians and caregivers on antibiotic prescribing for upper respiratory tract infections in children at primary care facilities in rural China: A cluster-randomised controlled trial. *Lancet Glob. Health* **2017**, *5*, e1258–e1267. [CrossRef]
54. Maki, G.; Smith, I.; Paulin, S.; Kaljee, L.; Kasambara, W.; Mlotha, J.; Chuki, P.; Rupali, P.; Singh, D.R.; Bajracharya, D.C.; et al. Feasibility Study of the World Health Organization Health Care Facility-Based Antimicrobial Stewardship Toolkit for Low- and Middle-Income Countries. *Antibiotics* **2020**, *9*, 556. [CrossRef] [PubMed]
55. Rocha-Pereira, N.; Lafferty, N.; Nathwani, D. Educating healthcare professionals in antimicrobial stewardship: Can online-learning solutions help? *J. Antimicrob. Chemother.* **2015**, *70*, 3175–3177. [CrossRef] [PubMed]
56. Little, P.; Stuart, B.; Francis, N.; Douglas, E.; Tonkin-Crine, S.; Anthierens, S.; Cals, J.W.L.; Melbye, H.; Santer, M.; Moore, M.; et al. Effects of internet-based training on antibiotic prescribing rates for acute respiratory-tract infections: A multinational, cluster, randomised, factorial, controlled trial. *Lancet* **2013**, *382*, 1175–1182. [CrossRef]
57. Skivington, K.; Matthews, L.; Craig, P.; Simpson, S.; Moore, L. Developing and evaluating complex interventions: Updating Medical Research Council guidance to take account of new methodological and theoretical approaches. *Lancet* **2018**, *392*, S2. [CrossRef]

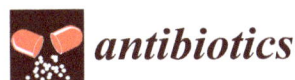

Article

Knowledge, Attitudes and Practices of Veterinarians Towards Antimicrobial Resistance and Stewardship in Nigeria

Usman O. Adekanye [1], Abel B. Ekiri [2,*], Erika Galipó [2], Abubakar Bala Muhammad [3], Ana Mateus [4], Roberto M. La Ragione [2], Aliyu Wakawa [5], Bryony Armson [2], Erik Mijten [6], Ruth Alafiatayo [2], Gabriel Varga [6] and Alasdair J. C. Cook [2]

1. Nigeria Ministry of Defence Health Implementation Programme, 900247 Abuja, Nigeria; adekanyeusmanoladipo@gmail.com
2. School of Veterinary Medicine, University of Surrey, Guildford GU2 7AL, UK; e.galipo@surrey.ac.uk (E.G.); R.Laragione@surrey.ac.uk (R.M.L.R.); b.armson@surrey.ac.uk (B.A.); r.alafiatayo@surrey.ac.uk (R.A.); alasdair.j.cook@surrey.ac.uk (A.J.C.C.)
3. Life Stock Management Services Limited, 900271 Abuja, Nigeria; bala_bubakar2000@yahoo.com
4. Royal Veterinary College, University of London, London AL9 7TA, UK; amateus@rvc.ac.uk
5. Department of Veterinary Surgery and Medicine, Ahmadu Bello University, 810211 Kaduna, Nigeria; asmwakawa@yahoo.com
6. Zoetis-ALPHA Initiative, Zoetis, B-1930 Zaventem, Belgium; erik.mijten@zoetis.com (E.M.); gabriel.varga@zoetis.com (G.V.)
* Correspondence: ab.ekiri@surrey.ac.uk; Tel.: +44-1483-688-779

Received: 7 July 2020; Accepted: 24 July 2020; Published: 28 July 2020

Abstract: Antimicrobial resistance (AMR) is a global health concern and the inappropriate use of antibiotics in animals and humans is considered a contributing factor. A cross-sectional survey to assess the knowledge, attitudes and practices of veterinarians regarding AMR and antimicrobial stewardship was conducted in Nigeria. A total of 241 respondents completed an online survey. Only 21% of respondents correctly defined the term antimicrobial stewardship and 59.8% were unaware of the guidelines provided by the Nigeria AMR National Action Plan. Over half (51%) of the respondents indicated that prophylactic antibiotic use was appropriate when farm biosecurity was poor. Only 20% of the respondents conducted antimicrobial susceptibility testing (AST) frequently, and the unavailability of veterinary laboratory services (82%) and the owner's inability to pay (72%) were reported as key barriers to conducting AST. The study findings suggest strategies focusing on the following areas may be useful in improving appropriate antibiotic use and antimicrobial stewardship among veterinarians in Nigeria: increased awareness of responsible antimicrobial use among practicing and newly graduated veterinarians, increased dissemination of regularly updated antibiotic use guidelines, increased understanding of the role of good biosecurity and vaccination practices in disease prevention, and increased provision of laboratory services and AST at affordable costs.

Keywords: antibiotic; antimicrobial resistance; veterinary; animal health; Africa

1. Introduction

Resistance to antimicrobials is rising worldwide, threatening our ability to treat common infectious diseases of humans and animals [1]. The direct consequences of infection with resistant microorganisms can be severe, including longer and more severe illnesses, increased mortality, prolonged stays in hospital, increased rates of therapeutic failure resulting in loss of protection for patients undergoing operations and other medical procedures, and increased healthcare costs [2]. The overuse and misuse of antibiotics in humans and animals has been linked to the emergence of antimicrobial resistance (AMR) in animals and the environment [1,3–7]. In livestock farming, antibiotics are used for prophylaxis, metaphylaxis (the treatment of a group of animals after the diagnosis of infection and/or clinical disease in part of the group), growth promotion, or are used therapeutically, to maintain health and increase productivity. Interaction between animals, humans and the environment promotes the transfer of resistant genes across different species, making AMR an important One Health challenge emerging on a global scale [3–6,8]. With the dwindling repertoire of antibiotic options available for the control of emerging, life-threatening and multi-drug resistant bacteria, there is a need for proper antibiotic stewardship to preserve the efficacy of existing antibiotics [9].

Antibiotic stewardship programs can play an important role in improving, prescribing and optimizing the use of antibiotics [10–14]. In the human sector, which has made significant strides in this area, antibiotic stewardship programs are defined as hospital-based programs dedicated to improving antibiotic use [15]. These programs increase infection cure rates while reducing treatment failures, adverse effects, hospital costs and lengths of stay, and antibiotic resistance [14,16,17]. Considering the potential benefits of antibiotic stewardship programs, the World Health Organization (WHO) strongly recommends that governments implement them for the containment of AMR [18]. Therefore, it is imperative that governments implement tailored interventions to encourage antimicrobial stewardship among healthcare professionals [19]. Beyond stewardship programs, strategies to tackle other related challenges also need to be considered.

In most sub-Saharan African countries, surveillance programs for antibiotic use and AMR in humans and animals are either lacking or are in their infancy, and the human and animal healthcare sectors at the government or ministry levels tend to work in silos, resulting in a lack of intersectoral collaboration. Furthermore, in Nigeria, the lack of regulation of existing veterinary drug markets and low involvement of pharmacists [20] and veterinarians in the formal drug distribution market [21] may contribute to the issue of substandard drugs in the marketplace. In 2018, the Director General of the Nigeria National Agency for Food and Drug Administration and Control (NAFDAC) held a town hall meeting with all players in the livestock industry, including practicing veterinarians and manufacturers and suppliers of veterinary medicines, and at the meeting announced the ban of use of some antimicrobials and growth promoters in livestock as part of efforts to control AMR and to support the One Health triad [22]. The banned antimicrobials and growth promoters included chloramphenicol, furazolidone, metronidazole, nitrofuran, and carbadox [22]. To address AMR in both humans and animals in sub-Saharan African countries, strong multidisciplinary collaborations are needed; however, these are lacking because of the poor One Health coordination of animal and human national disease surveillance systems [23].

In 2017, the Nigerian Federal Ministry of Agriculture and Rural Development (FMARD), Federal Ministry of Environment and Federal Ministry of Health developed a National Action Plan (NAP) for antimicrobial resistance (the Nigeria Center for Disease Control's five-point action plan) as part of the country's efforts to address the problem of AMR and to promote the responsible use of antimicrobials through a One Health approach [23]. Veterinary surgeons are typically responsible for prescribing and overseeing antimicrobial use in animals. Therefore, the role of the veterinarian in tackling AMR cannot be over-emphasized as they are the custodians of antimicrobials used in animal health [24] and food production. In Nigeria, regulatory authorities like NAFDAC and the Nigeria Centre for Disease Control (NCDC) are involved in creating awareness among veterinarians and veterinary students on the challenge of AMR through campaigns convened by the Veterinary Council of Nigeria (VCN) and the umbrella association for veterinarians in Nigeria, the Nigeria Veterinary Medical Association (NVMA).

Despite the potential negative impact of AMR on animal and public health, there remains a paucity of data concerning the awareness of this problem in sub-Saharan countries [25]. The attitudes of veterinarians towards antibiotic use and determinants influencing prescribing behavior of veterinarians have been investigated elsewhere [26–29]. In Nigeria, a few studies have explored the knowledge, attitude and practices of veterinarians towards antibiotic use, resistance and stewardship. A previous study by Anyanwu and Kolade reported that knowledge about antibiotic stewardship among veterinarians was as low as 21.4% [30]. However, this study was limited to Enugu State and used a non-probability sampling technique, which affected the generalizability of the study findings [30]. A recent study that involved only veterinary students reported that 60% of respondents had unsatisfactory knowledge scores for AMR [31]. To expand on the knowledge base in this area and to inform the development of interventions to promote responsible antibiotic use, a nationwide study of veterinarians in Nigeria was conducted. The objective of this study was to assess the knowledge, attitudes and practices towards AMR and antimicrobial stewardship and to identify factors that influence antibiotic prescription practices of veterinarians in Nigeria.

2. Results

The survey was sent to 5603 participants; there were 488 responses, corresponding to a response rate of 13%. Out of the 488, six did not consent, 59 consented but did not start or attempt the survey, while 128 consented and attempted but did not complete the survey. Thus, 241 respondents consented and completed the survey.

2.1. Demographic Information

Most of the respondents were male (79.7%, 192/241) and almost half were aged 25-34 years (48.1%, 116/241) (Table 1). A majority of respondents reported having a veterinary degree (63.1%, 152/241) as the highest educational qualification. More than a third of respondents had been registered as a veterinarian for 0–5 years (36.1%, 87/241). Mixed practice (defined as any combination of small, large, poultry or other type of practice) was the most frequently reported type of practice (63.5%, 153/241). Five percent of respondents (5.4%, 13/241) did not practice. Most of the respondents were employed in private practice (38.2%, 92/241).

Table 1. Demographics of respondents

Variable	Response	Frequency (n = 241)	Percentage (%)
Gender	Female	49	20.3
	Male	192	79.7
Age group	18–24 years old	1	0.4
	25–34 years old	116	48.1
	35–44 years old	85	35.3
	45–54 years old	27	11.2
	55–64 years old	12	5.0
	65 years and above	0	0
	Prefer not to say	0	0
University of training	Ahmadu Bello University (ABU), Zaria	69	28.6
	University of Maiduguiri	60	24.9
	University of Nigeria Nsukka (UNN)	31	12.9
	Usmanu Danfodiyo University, Sokoto (UDUS)	27	11.2
	University of Ibadan (UI), Ibadan	27	11.2
	Federal University of Agriculture Makurdi (FUAM)	9	3.7
	Federal University of Agriculture, Abeokuta (FUNAAB)	8	3.3
	Other	8	3.3
	University of Abuja	2	0.8
Highest level of education	Veterinary degree (DVM, etc.)	152	63.1
	MSc/MPH	61	25.3
	Fellow, College of Veterinary Surgeon (FCVS)	6	2.5
	PhD	16	6.6
	Other	6	2.5
Type of employment	Private practice	92	38.2
	Government employee	75	31.1
	Teaching	25	10.4
	Non-governmental organization employee	22	9.1
	Research	15	6.2
	Other	12	5.0

Table 1. *Cont.*

Variable	Response	Frequency (n = 241)	Percentage (%)
Years registered as a vet surgeon	0–<5 years	87	36.1
	5–10 years	75	31.1
	10–15 years	30	12.4
	15–20 years	18	7.5
	21 and above	28	11.6
	Prefer not to say	3	1.2
Type of veterinary practice *	Mixed practice (large, small or exotic animals)	97	40.2
	Poultry practice (chicken, turkey)	94	39.0
	Small animal practice (dogs, cats, rabbits)	87	36.1
	Large animal practice (cattle, horse, goat, sheep, pig)	75	31.1
	Fish practice	29	12.0
	Do not practice	15	6.2
	Other practice	11	4.6
	Exotics practice (parrots, tortoise, snakes, etc.)	8	3.3
	Wildlife practice (wild animals)	6	2.5
Location of veterinary practice by geopolitical zone	North Central	69	28.6
	North West	49	20.3
	North East	46	19.1
	South West	39	16.2
	South East	21	8.7
	South South	17	7.1

* The results for this variable are presented as row percentages instead of column percentages, as such the column percentages for this variable do not add up to 100%.

The distribution of respondents based on the location of the vet practice within Nigeria's six geopolitical zones showed that almost half of the respondents were located in the North Central (29%, 69/241) and the North West zones (20%, 49/241) (Table 1). The lowest number of respondents was recorded in the South South zone (7%, 17/241). The distribution of respondents based on the location of the vet practice within Nigeria's 37 states indicated that the Federal Capital Territory, Abuja, had the highest number of respondents (13.7%, 33/241) followed by Kaduna State (10%, 24/241) and Borno State (7.1%, 17/241) (Figure 1). Yobe and Nasarawa States were the only two states without any respondents.

2.2. Knowledge

Eighty-nine (36%) of the 241 respondents had heard of the term antimicrobial stewardship and of these, 69% (61/89) were able to correctly define antimicrobial stewardship (Table S1). Most of the respondents (81.7%, 197/241) were able to differentiate between an antibiotic and an antimicrobial agent. Most of the respondents were aware that antibiotics kill both commensal and pathogenic bacteria (91.3%, 220/241) and 94.6% (228/241) knew that overuse of antibiotics renders them ineffective. Most respondents were aware that antibiotics do not kill viruses (93.4%, 225/241) and all respondents were aware that bacteria can become resistant to antibiotics. Many respondents (93.4%, 225/241) were aware that there was a need to observe withdrawal periods before consuming milk from cows treated with antibiotics, and 97.9% (236/241) were aware that a withdrawal period is necessary before treated poultry can be considered fit for human consumption.

More than half of the respondents (59.8%, 144/241) had not heard of or read the Nigeria Center for Disease Control's five-point action plan for responsible use of antimicrobials. When asked what topics they would like to receive more information on, 75.5% (182/241) of the respondents selected "links between the health of humans, animals and the environment", and 55.6% (134/241) chose "microbial culture and sensitivity testing" (Table S1).

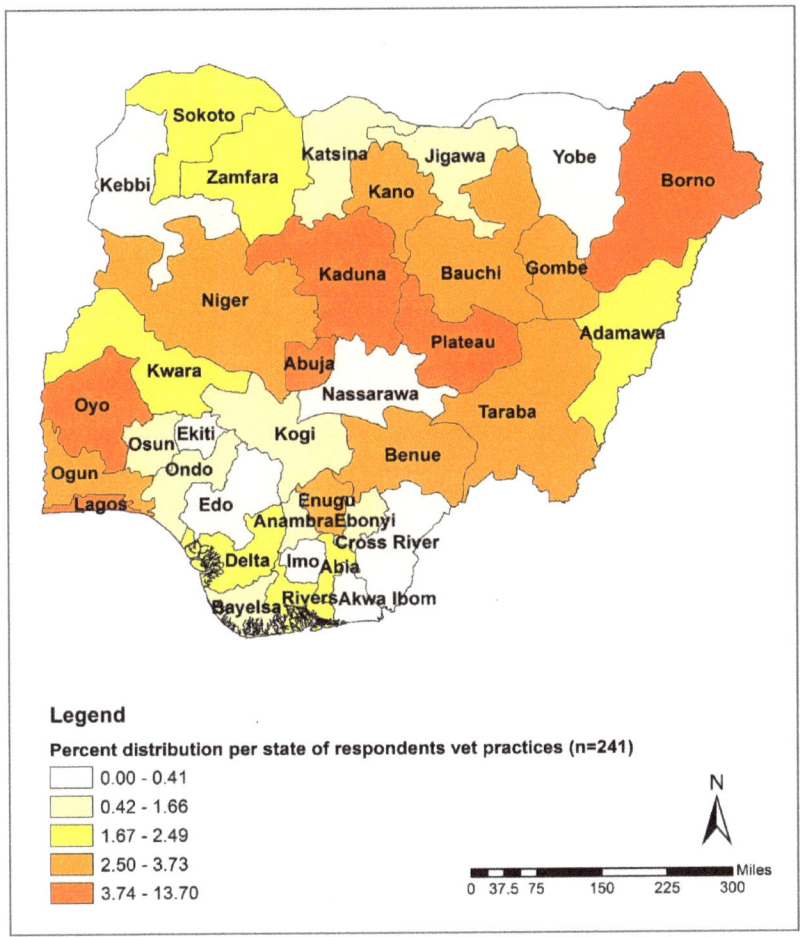

Figure 1. Distribution of survey respondents based on reported location of veterinary practice by state in Nigeria.

2.3. Attitude

All but one (99.6%, 240/241) of the respondents believed that veterinarians have a role to play in preventing public health threats posed by AMR (Table S2). Respondents were asked to indicate if they considered the following as important global challenges and the most frequently reported challenges were: AMR (80.9%, 195/241), food security (74.5%, 180/241) and climate change (60.9%, 146/241). Most respondents (97.9%, 233/238) thought AMR was a national problem in Nigeria, and 96.1% (223/232) of respondents believed AMR will be a greater problem in veterinary practice in the future than it is today. Note the denominators used to calculate the above two percentages, and in the sections below (where relevant), do not add up to 241 because they exclude "unknown" responses (Table S2).

Many of the respondents considered the excessive use of antibiotics in livestock (83.8%, 202/241) and under dosing of antibiotics (78.8%, 185/241) as the most important potential contributors to the development of AMR (Table S3). Most of the respondents agreed that prescribing unnecessary antibiotics was professionally unethical (97.5%, 234/240) and 78.2% (172/220) believed the antibiotics they prescribe may contribute to AMR (Table S2). Most respondents (99.2%, 237/239) agreed with the statement "biosecurity was important in food production" and 28.2% (68/241) considered poor biosecurity practices as a contributor to AMR development. Of concern was that over half of the respondents (56%, 112/200) agreed with the statement "Prophylactic antibiotics are an appropriate alternative to protect animal health when there is poor biosecurity". Almost half of the respondents (42.3%, 102/219) indicated that they lacked enough knowledge on antibiotic use, while 28.9% (59/204) believed there were not enough antibiotics under development to combat the problem of resistance (Table S2).

2.4. Practices Influencing Antibiotic Use

A total of 132/220 (60%) of the respondents reported that they frequently encountered animal owners who had already initiated antibiotic treatment without veterinary supervision (Table S4). Note the denominators used to calculate the percentages for some variables in this section (where relevant) do not add up to 241 because they exclude "don't know" responses (Table S4).

More than half of the respondents (68.4%, 154/225) reported that their practice had a standardized protocol for the treatment of sick animals (Table S4). When asked what guidelines were followed to help select the appropriate antibiotic when a patient was presented for the first time, 53.1% (128/241) of respondents reported using microbiological culture and antimicrobial susceptibility testing (AST) for guidance. More than a half of the respondents (59.8%, 144/241) indicated that they administered empirical treatment while awaiting AST results. A small proportion (14.5%, 35/241) reported selecting antibiotics based on what the client could afford.

With regards to the frequency of AST use before starting antibiotic treatment, 48.7% (112/230) of respondents used AST at a frequency of one to three times in a month while only 21.3% (49/230) used AST more than three times a month. Over a quarter of the respondents (30%, 69/230) never conducted AST (Table S5).

Most respondents (75.5%, 182/241) indicated that poor response to initial antibiotic treatment or treatment failure influenced the veterinarians' decision to request AST. Other reported drivers for AST use included recurrent health conditions (70.5%, 170/241), having no knowledge of the animal or farm's health history (26.6%, 64/241) and owner request (18.3%, 44/241) (Table S5). When asked what were the most important barriers to the use of AST, the majority of respondents selected unavailability of laboratory services (82.2%, 198/241), followed by owners' inability to pay for AST tests (71.8%, 173/241), urgent need for antibiotic therapy (56.8%, 137/241), long waiting time for AST results (35.3%, 85/241) and uncertainty of what to request from the lab to guide antibiotic selection (3.3%, 8/241) (Table S5).

The cost of antibiotics (80.9%, 195/241) and owners' ability to pay (81.3%, 196/241) were reported to influence the respondent's decision when selecting antibiotics. Other cost related influences included: expected profit margin to the veterinarian (27.4%, 66/241), marketing offers (16.6%, 40/241), adverts by pharmaceutical company representatives (12.9%, 31/241) and medicine sellers (8.3%, 20/241) (Table S6).

When asked what antibiotic characteristics had the most influence upon the veterinarian's selection of antibiotics, 85.5% (206/241) of respondents reported the antibiotic's spectrum of activity, 63.1% (152/241) reported AST results, 50.6% (122/241) reported withdrawal period, 44.4% (107/241) reported the ease of administration and 43.2% (104/241) reported the risk of development of AMR (Table S6). Other reported factors that influenced veterinarians' decision to select antibiotics were veterinarians' previous experience (96.3%, 232/241), advice from colleagues (68%, 164/241) and owner preference for a specific antibiotic (9.5%, 23/241) (Table S6).

Finally, when asked what sources of information influenced the veterinarians' decision the most when selecting an antibiotic to use, 79.3% (191/241) of respondents indicated veterinary education and training, followed by prescription guidelines or policies supplied by veterinary hospital or bodies (68.9%, 166/241), product labels or leaflets (64.3%, 155/241), legal restriction of drug to a defined species (38.6%, 93/241) and published scientific literature (35.3%, 85/241) (Table S6).

2.5. Relationship between the Use of AST before Antibiotic Treatment and Select Investigated Parameters

The relationship between the "use of AST before antibiotic treatment" and nine selected variables was assessed (Table S7). The analyses included 230 respondents that responded to the variable "use of AST before antibiotic treatment" and excluded respondents that answered "don't know" (n = 11). The proportion of respondents that reported the "use of AST before antibiotic treatment" was significantly different across the response levels for the following variables: years in practice ($P = 0.049$), knowledge of correct definition of antimicrobial stewardship ($P = 0.032$), knowledge of NCDC five points ($P = 0.003$), agreement with the statement that prophylactic use of antibiotics when farm biosecurity is poor is inappropriate ($P = 0.029$), and having a standard antibiotic treatment protocol in the veterinary practice ($P \leq 0.001$) (Table S7).

2.6. Relationship between Knowledge Level of Appropriate Antibiotic Use and AMR and Select Investigated Parameters

The relationship between "knowledge level on appropriate antibiotic use and AMR" and selected variables was assessed (Table S8). The analyses included 240 respondents that responded to the variable "knowledge level on appropriate antibiotic use and AMR" (assigned to the category "high knowledge" or "low to moderate knowledge") and excluded one respondent that was assigned a knowledge score of zero because they had provided no correct answer. The proportion of respondents with high knowledge was significantly different across the response levels for the following variables: age group ($P = 0.024$), education level ($P = 0.024$), and agreement with the statement that prophylactic use of antibiotics when farm biosecurity is poor is inappropriate ($P = < 0.001$) (Table S8).

3. Discussion

The current study assessed the knowledge, attitudes, and practices towards AMR and antimicrobial stewardship of veterinary professionals in Nigeria. To the best of our knowledge, this is the first nationwide baseline study on the subject. Most of the veterinarians in the current study were between 25 and 44 years old, which probably explains why over 67% of respondents were within 10 years of being registered veterinary surgeons. Most of the respondents were private or government practitioners (69%), followed by teaching (10.4%) and non-governmental organization employees (9.1%); these results likely reflect the distribution of veterinarian employment in Nigeria.

Sixty three percent of the respondents were familiar with the term antimicrobial stewardship, compared to 17% reported in a similar study conducted in Enugu State, Nigeria [30]. The reasons for the observed differences are not clear but the current study can be considered more representative because it targeted participants across the country. However, our study highlights that there is still inadequate awareness of the concept of antimicrobial stewardship among veterinarians. Our study findings also revealed that the proportion of respondents who used AST before antibiotics administration varied among respondents who correctly or incorrectly defined antimicrobial stewardship. This finding suggests that educational strategies aimed at increasing awareness of antimicrobial stewardship among practicing and new veterinarians both at the practice and veterinary school levels may be helpful in promoting the responsible use of antibiotics.

Although most respondents reported that antibiotic resistance occurred in bacteria (98%) and could differentiate between an antibiotic and an antimicrobial (82%), a small percentage of respondents (4%) reported that antibiotics kill viruses, suggesting this proportion of respondents may prescribe antibiotics for viral infections. In comparison, 1% of student healthcare professionals (human and animal health students) surveyed in the United Kingdom thought antibiotics killed viruses [32], suggesting that study population may have been more knowledgeable on this aspect compared to our study population. Additionally, in our study, a small percentage of respondents (6%) reported that a withdrawal period of antibiotics-treated animals is not necessary before milk consumption. Failure to observe appropriate withdrawal periods following antibiotic treatment may result in the introduction of antibiotic residues in animal foods consumed by humans [33,34]. The failure to observe appropriate withdrawal periods has potential human health implications including the development of drug-related allergies and hypersensitivity reactions, especially with beta lactam antibiotics and penicillin [35], and the risk of development of AMR [36,37].

Although most respondents knew that biosecurity is important in food production, this study highlighted a misconception regarding the link between biosecurity and antibiotic use. Over half of the respondents thought that prophylactic antibiotic use was appropriate in situations where biosecurity was poor. The reliance on antibiotics when biosecurity practices are poor has been reported in other studies [38]. Antibiotics can be an integral part of disease preventive methods but should be used only when indicated; they should not be used as the first line of action [39] or as a substitute for poor biosecurity practices [40]. Prophylactic and metaphylactic use of antibiotics administered to animal groups through water and feed may lead to increased environmental concentration of antibiotic residues which can in turn result in exposure of animals and humans alike and elevate the risk of AMR development [41,42]. Based on the current study findings there is a need for an improved understanding among veterinarians of the role of biosecurity practices in preventing and minimizing the risk of infections and reducing the overuse of antibiotics. Biosecurity practices are a key component of animal husbandry and disease prevention measures that can be implemented to improve animal health and welfare, and to reduce the need to use antimicrobials [43].

This study showed that the proportion of respondents with a high knowledge score varied with age group and education level. Although not conclusively established in the current study, this suggests that it is possible that older respondents and those with additional training to a veterinary degree may have a higher knowledge of appropriate antibiotic use and AMR or that the observed differences may be linked to work experiences accrued over time. Further investigation and understanding of the perceptions and barriers to responsible use of antibiotics among this subpopulation would help inform educational efforts.

More than half of the respondents' practices had a standard protocol for the treatment of sick animals to ensure the correct dosages and regimes are administered and to reduce the risk of adverse drug reactions or drug toxicity in the animals. Additionally, the proportion of respondents that reported the use of AST before antibiotic treatment was higher among those with a standard treatment protocol compared to those without. The observed relationship suggests having a standard treatment protocol may contribute to good antimicrobial stewardship. In the human sector, the use of standard treatment guidelines is considered an effective means of improving patient care while enhancing cost savings and changing behavior [44]. The treatment guidelines also reflect data on antimicrobial resistance, recognizing that local patterns of resistance often differ across geographical regions [44]. In the context of the animal health sector in Nigeria, strategies that consider up-to-date antimicrobial stewardship guidelines may be helpful in promoting appropriate antibiotic use among veterinary professionals.

Over half of the respondents (53%) reported conducting microbiological culture and AST before starting treatment, which is higher than the 24% reported in a study conducted in Enugu State, Nigeria [30], and the 38% reported among veterinarians in Europe [45]. The reason for these differences is not clear but may be related to regional differences in the level of awareness of the need to conduct microbiological culture and AST before starting antibiotic treatment or reporting bias which can occur in questionnaire-based studies. However, when asked specifically how often AST was requested before starting antibiotic treatment, only 20% of respondents reported requesting AST frequently (more than three times a month) and a third of the respondents never conducted or requested AST before commencing treatment. The observed drop from 53% to 20% may also be explained by reporting bias. Nevertheless, these findings suggest a considerable number of veterinary professionals do not use AST. There is a need to examine the reasons for the low AST use and identify appropriate interventions.

The respondents in the current study reported that poor response to initial antibiotic treatment (76%) and conditions that recur (71%) were the main factors that influenced their decision to conduct AST, but a lack of information on the animal or farm's health status, and owner requests were also influences, consistent with the findings from a study conducted in Europe [45]. The findings suggest having structured and up-to-date antibiotic use guidelines at the practice level, having access to rapid, cheap diagnostic tools and being able to handle clients' expectations through effective communication, may be helpful in providing guidance to veterinary professionals.

Several barriers to the use of AST were reported in this study. The unavailability of laboratory services and owner's inability to pay were reported as key barriers to the use of AST. The owner's inability to pay is a major concern because it limits the options available for a veterinarian in making decisions that allow for an appropriate diagnosis and treatment and may subsequently negatively influence the veterinarian's decisions and choices regarding antibiotic use. Strategies that explore ways to increase availability of veterinary laboratory services across the country and the provision of AST at affordable costs are necessary. Additionally, respondents reported that there is often an urgent need to administer antibiotics due to the acute onset of severe clinical signs. This is an accepted practice when antibiotics are urgently needed to counteract the disease progression and when delays in administering the therapy can lead to a poor outcome [46]. Nonetheless, veterinarians should take several factors into account to inform their decision on a sound empirical therapy: records from previous AST results in the local area if available, information on local patterns of bacterial resistance if available, previous patient cultural and AST results, the suspected anatomic site affected by infection and etiologic pathogen [47]. The records from previous AST results in the local area and information on local patterns of bacterial resistance were unlikely to be available in the context of Nigeria, emphasizing the need for a national integrated AMR surveillance program, as identified by the Nigeria National Action Plan for Antimicrobial Resistance [23]. The empirical antibiotic treatment should not prevent veterinarians from submitting samples for AST but instead be considered a temporary intervention while waiting for AST results that will inform the final, targeted, antibiotic treatment [46].

Veterinary education or training followed by prescription guidelines and policies were the most frequently selected parameters that influence a veterinarian's decision to select antibiotics. These findings suggest the veterinary curriculum may be a useful means to provide training on appropriate antibiotic use and selection. For example, in the fourth year of study, veterinary students in Nigeria undertake a course in pharmacology and therapeutics, which involves instruction on the types of veterinary pharmacological products and prescription practices. Furthermore, a relationship was observed between having additional education or training on AMR and knowledge of appropriate antibiotic use. Veterinary education or training may present an opportunity to expand and strengthen knowledge on appropriate antibiotic use practices and antimicrobial stewardship, if included in the training curriculum for new animal health professionals. Veterinary education or training also provides an opportunity for practicing veterinarians to update their knowledge, as prescription practices and protocols change over time.

The finding of antibiotic prescription guidelines as one of the most frequently selected parameters that influence a veterinarian's decision to select antibiotics suggests that there is a need for updated and increased dissemination and uptake of antibiotic guidelines. The Nigerian Veterinary formulary [48], provided by the Veterinary Council of Nigeria (VCN) to guide the prescription and administration of veterinary pharmaceuticals in different animal species was produced in 2007 and has not been updated since. In the present study, less than half of the respondents were aware of the Nigeria Center for Disease Control (NCDC) five-point agenda for AMR control, and a relationship was observed between awareness of the NCDC five-point action plan and AST use. These findings suggest regular updating of the VCN guidelines combined with increased awareness of the NCDC five-point action plan may be helpful in promoting antimicrobial stewardship among veterinary professionals.

A concerning, but not surprising, observation was that 86% of respondents reported encountering client-initiated antibiotic therapy without veterinary supervision. Even though the current regulatory policies in Nigeria require that only qualified veterinarians and para-vets can administer medications and treatment, livestock farmers can obtain and administer antibiotics without the requirement of a veterinarian's prescription and this is most likely to occur without regard to antibiotic indication guidelines [49]. This highlights the need for education of not just the veterinary professionals but also the clients, veterinary drug sellers or shop keepers, pharmacies and farmers on appropriate antibiotic use and the risk of antibiotic misuse and AMR. In addition, government interventions such as the formulation and implementation of relevant policies and regulations may also be useful in improving appropriate antibiotic use and stewardship.

In the present study, the proportion of respondents that used AST before antibiotic treatment varied with knowledge of antimicrobial stewardship, knowledge of NCDC's five points, and with agreement with the statement that prophylactic use of antibiotics is inappropriate when biosecurity is poor. These findings suggest that knowledge of antimicrobial stewardship, NCDC's five points and prophylactic use of antibiotics may be related to appropriate antibiotic use. These areas could be targeted when developing strategies to improve antimicrobial stewardship and reduce AMR in veterinary practice in Nigeria.

A few limitations were observed during the conduct of the current study. The response rate of the survey was low, and as such, the study's findings may not be generalizable to the whole of the country. Nevertheless, the gaps identified can still be used to inform discussions by policy makers involved in the development of interventions targeting all veterinarians in Nigeria. The low response rate may have been due to several factors such as unwillingness to participate or lack of internet access in some parts of the country. There may also have been selection bias in the respondent population. For example, it is possible that respondents that completed the survey were more technologically astute or inclined. It could also be that these respondents had a special interest in the subject, hence their participation. Another potential limitation was social desirability bias which might have affected the nature of the responses provided; it is possible that some respondents may have declined to share information they considered inappropriate or erroneous, resulting in an under-reporting of certain aspects on antibiotics and AMR knowledge and practices. Finally, it is important to note that the data analyses performed to assess relationships between selected variables in the current study were exploratory in nature and were not intended to be exhaustive, therefore, no additional inferential analyses such as logistics regression were conducted.

4. Materials and Methods

Ethical review and approval were granted by the Nigeria Ministry of Defense Health Research Ethics Committee, Abuja, via an ethics review application (Ethics approval number: MODHREC/APP/20/12/11/20/1/8/) and by the Research Integrity and Governance Office at the University of Surrey, United Kingdom (Response ID: 353003-352994-41119696).

4.1. Study Area

Nigeria is the most populous nation located in West Africa, with an estimated population of approximately 202 million people [50]. Crude oil, agriculture and solid minerals are the mainstay of the economy. It has 37 states including the Federal Capital Territory, Abuja. There are three major tribes and about 250 ethnic groups. Nigeria has a tropical climate and two distinct weather seasons (rainy and dry seasons). To the north of the country is the Sahel climate, to the west is the tropical savannah while the south and east are characterized by tropical monsoon climates.

4.2. Study Population

There are circa 8000 registered veterinarians in Nigeria involved in livestock/large animal practice, small animal/companion animal practice, poultry practice, public health and academia (personal communication with Interim College secretary, College of Veterinary Surgeons, Nigeria). This study involved veterinarians registered with the Veterinary Council of Nigeria (VCN). For this study, a registered veterinarian was an individual who obtained certification from the VCN as a Doctor of Veterinary Medicine (DVM) upon completion of the six-year university degree program in Nigeria. All registered veterinarians were pooled together irrespective of the type of practice.

4.3. Study Design

This was a cross-sectional study; a questionnaire survey was designed and used to collect data on the knowledge and attitudes towards AMR and antimicrobial stewardship of veterinarians during the period January to February 2019.

4.4. Sample Size

Sample size was estimated as described by Lwanga and Lemeshow (1990) [51] with the prevalence of knowledge of antibiotic resistance set at 50% based on a previous study that investigated the veterinary drugs market in Nigeria [21] and the desired level of precision set at 0.02. The estimated calculated sample size was 2400. A non-response rate of 30% was estimated because studies have shown response rates to web-based surveys are generally low [52] and assumed some respondents would have poor internet access or did not consent. The final estimated minimum sample size considering the non-response rate was 3120 respondents (2400 × 1.3).

4.5. Data Collection

A questionnaire was developed and select questions from previous studies [32,45] were adapted to collect data on demographics, knowledge, attitudes, practices towards antibiotic use and resistance, and awareness of antimicrobial stewardship (Supplementary material S1). The tool was pretested among ten veterinarians in Abuja and thereafter questions were further refined to produce the final survey. The final questionnaire was administered electronically using the Qualtrics® survey platform.

The available list of 5800 registered veterinarians in Nigeria was obtained from the VCN, which was more than the calculated minimum sample size of 3120 respondents. A total of 5603 with phone numbers were randomly selected from this pool of 5800 using a table of random numbers. A link to the survey was sent via a text message to all the 5603 contacts. Of the 5603 contacts, 2662 had email addresses on the VCN register, and the survey link was sent to them via email (in addition to the text message sent to all 5603 contacts). The message inviting contacts to participate in the survey was endorsed by the Nigeria Center for Disease Control (NCDC) and Federal Ministry of Agriculture and Rural Development (FMARD). Further emails and SMS reminders were sent 2, 4 and 6 weeks after the initial message. The survey was made available online for 8 weeks between 2nd January and 28th February 2019.

4.6. Data Analysis

Survey results were downloaded from Qualtrics® to Microsoft Excel. Data collected during the piloting of the survey were excluded from the final analysis. Descriptive statistics were used to summarize the data using R-Studio 1.2.1335.0.

As part of the descriptive analysis, a scoring system was used to assess the knowledge level on antibiotic use and AMR. A set of nine survey questions on knowledge was selected, and for each question, a score of one point was assigned for each correct answer, with a maximum of nine points allowed (Table S9). One respondent that provided no correct answer was assigned a score of zero. Respondents were further regrouped into two categories based on knowledge score; respondents scoring $\geq 7/9$ points were assigned to the category "high knowledge" and those scoring $< 7/9$ points were assigned to the category "low to moderate knowledge".

Following the descriptive analysis, a bivariate analysis was performed using the Chi-square test or Fisher's exact test, as appropriate, to explore the relationship between two selected outcome variables and eleven selected variables. The outcome variables were: "the use of AST before antibiotic treatment" and "knowledge level on appropriate antibiotic use and AMR". The relationships between these two outcome variables and the following 9 variables were assessed: age group of participants, gender, educational level, years in practice, type of practice, practice location, knowledge of the NCDC five-point action plan for correct antibiotic use, prophylactic use of antibiotic when biosecurity is poor, and existing antibiotic treatment protocol in practice. Two further variables, the correct definition of antimicrobial stewardship and owner-initiated treatment, were investigated for the outcome variable "the use of AST before antibiotic treatment". Two additional variables were also investigated for the outcome variable "knowledge level on appropriate antibiotic use and AMR": type of employment and knowledge of antimicrobial stewardship. A two-tailed P-value of ≤0.05 was considered statistically significant. It is important to note that the association analyses were exploratory in nature, used selected variables and were not intended to be exhaustive, therefore, no advanced additional inferential analyses, such as logistics regression, were conducted.

5. Conclusions

Findings from this study provided baseline evidence on the knowledge, attitudes and practices regarding antibiotic use, AMR and antimicrobial stewardship among veterinarians across Nigeria. With respect to knowledge and attitudes on appropriate antibiotic use and AMR, there was little awareness of the concept of antimicrobial stewardship among veterinarians, and the role and use of biosecurity, as well as the prophylactic antibiotic use in the prevention of infection, were not well understood. There is a need for an increased understanding among veterinarians for how the use of biosecurity practices plays a role in the prevention of infection, reducing the burden of disease in animal populations and, therefore, in reducing the need for and use of antibiotics. Education or training strategies aimed at increasing awareness of antimicrobial stewardship among practicing and new veterinarians at the practice and veterinary school levels may be helpful in promoting antimicrobial stewardship.

Regarding practices and factors influencing antibiotic use, the use of AST to inform antibiotic treatment was low, suggesting a need to further examine the reasons for this and identify appropriate interventions. The unavailability of laboratory services and the client's inability to pay were reported as key barriers to AST use. Strategies that explore ways to increase the availability of veterinary laboratory services across the country and the provision of AST at affordable costs are necessary.

Veterinary education or training followed by prescription guidelines and policies were the most frequently selected parameters that influence a veterinarian's decision to select antibiotics. The regular updating of the antibiotic prescription and use guidelines combined with increased awareness and dissemination among veterinarians may be helpful in promoting antimicrobial stewardship. Finally, the reported client-initiated antibiotic therapy was also a concern highlighting the need for education of not just the veterinary professionals, but also their clients and drug shop keepers on appropriate antibiotic use and stewardship.

Supplementary Materials: The following are available online at http://www.mdpi.com/2079-6382/9/8/453/s1, Supplementary material S1: Questionnaire. Table S1. Knowledge of appropriate antibiotics use and AMR among respondents; Table S2. Attitudes of respondents towards antibiotic use and antimicrobial resistance (AMR); Table S3. Contributors to antibiotic resistance, as reported by respondents; Table S4. Factors influencing antibiotic prescription practices and choice; Table S5. Frequency of antimicrobial susceptibility testing (AST) use and barriers to AST use; Table S6. Practices and factors influencing respondents' decisions on selecting antibiotics and antimicrobial susceptibility testing (AST) use; Table S7. Relationship between the use of antimicrobial susceptibility testing (AST) before antibiotic treatment and select investigated variables. Table S8. Relationship between knowledge level on appropriate antibiotic (AB) use and antimicrobial resistance (AMR) and select investigated variables; Table S9. Scoring of knowledge level on appropriate antibiotic (AB) use and antimicrobial resistance (AMR). For each question, a score was assigned based on the response with 0 given for an incorrect response and 1 for a correct response.

Author Contributions: Conceptualization, U.O.A., A.B.M., A.B.E., E.M., G.V.; methodology, U.O.A., E.G., A.B.E., A.M., R.M.L.R.; software, E.G., A.B.E; formal analysis, U.O.A., E.G., A.B.E.; investigation, U.O.A., A.W.; writing—original draft preparation, U.O.A., E.G., A.E.; writing—review and editing, U.O.A., E.G., A.B.E., A.B.M., A.M., R.M.L.R., B.A., A.W., R.A., E.M., G.V., A.J.C.C.; supervision, A.B.E, A.J.C.C.; project administration, U.O.A., A.B.E; funding acquisition, A.J.C.C., G.V. All authors have read and agreed to the published version of the manuscript.

Funding: This research work was delivered by the University of Surrey and funded by Zoetis' Africa Livestock Productivity and Health Advancement (ALPHA) Initiative, co-funded by the Bill and Melinda Gates Foundation (BMGF) and Zoetis. Funding from Zoetis was an unrestricted grant. BMGF Grant number: OPP1165393.

Acknowledgments: The authors would like to express their sincere gratitude to the following people for their support towards this research work. First, thank you to Tetiana Miroshnychenko of Zoetis' ALPHA Initiative Zaventem team and Isaac Odeyemi from Zoetis Outcomes Research team for guidance. We are grateful to the Veterinary Council of Nigeria who assisted with the sharing of the survey and the Nigerian Center for Disease Control for supporting the study. We are also grateful to Adam Trish of the vHive team at the School of Veterinary Medicine, University of Surrey for administrative assistance, and to Ikenna Onoh of the Nigerian Field Epidemiology and Laboratory Training Program and Pharmacist Estelle Mbadiwe of Ducit Blue Solutions for sharing insights on study implementation. Finally, the authors thank the veterinarians who spared their time to complete the questionnaire, without them, this study would not have been possible.

Conflicts of Interest: This study was supported by the Zoetis' Africa Livestock Productivity and Health Advancement (ALPHA) Initiative, co-funded by the Bill and Melinda Gates Foundation and Zoetis. Funding from Zoetis was an unrestricted grant. The Zoetis team (E.M., G.V.) was involved in study conceptualization and the writing of the manuscript. There are no potential areas of bias which may confer any advantage to Zoetis.

References

1. World Health Organization (WHO). Antibiotic Resistance. 2008. Available online: https://www.who.int/news-room/fact-sheets/detail/antibiotic-resistance (accessed on 20 August 2018).
2. World Health Organization (WHO). Global Action Plan on Antimicrobial Resistance. 2015, pp. 8–9. Available online: https://www.who.int/antimicrobial-resistance/publications/global-action-plan/en/ (accessed on 20 September 2018).
3. Fosberg, K.J.; Reyes, A.; Wang, B.; Selleck, E.M.; Sommer, M.O.A.; Danta, G. The shared antibiotic resistome of soil bacteria and human pathogens. *Science* **2012**, *337*, 1107–1111. [CrossRef] [PubMed]
4. Spoor, L.E.; McAdam, P.R.; Weinert, L.A.; Rambaut, A.; Hasman, H.; Aarestrup, F.M.; Kearns, A.M.; Larsen, A.R.; Skov, R.L.; Fitzgerald, J.R. Livestock origin for a human pandemic clone of community associated methicillin-resistant Staphylococcus aureus. *MBio* **2012**, *4*, 1–6. [CrossRef] [PubMed]
5. Ward, M.J.; Gibbons, C.L.; McAdam, P.R.; van Bunnik, B.A.D.; Girvan, E.K.; Edwards, G.F.; Fitzgerald, J.R.; Woolhouse, M.E.J. Time-scaled evolutionary analysis of the transmission and antibiotic resistance dynamics of Staphylococcus aureus CC398. *Appl. Environ. Microbiol.* **2014**, *80*, 7275–7282. [CrossRef]
6. Mather, A.E.; Reid, S.W.J.; Maskell, D.J.; Parkhill, J.; Fookes, M.C.; Harris, S.R.; Brown, D.J.; Coia, J.E.; Mulvey, M.R.; Gilmour, M.W.; et al. Distinguishable epidemics of multidrug-resistant Salmonella Typhimurium DT104 in different hosts. *Science* **2013**, *341*, 1514–1517. [CrossRef]
7. Chantziaras, I.; Boyen, F.; Callens, B.; Dewulf, J. Correlation between veterinary antimicrobial use and antimicrobial resistance in food-producing animals: A report on seven countries. *J. Antimicrob. Chemother.* **2014**, *69*, 827–834. [CrossRef] [PubMed]
8. Van den Bogaard, A.E.; London, N.; Driessen, C.; Stobberingh, E.E. Antibiotic resistance of faecal Escherichia coli in poultry, poultry farmers and poultry slaughterers. *J. Antimicrob. Chemother.* **2001**, *47*, 763–771. [CrossRef] [PubMed]
9. Aslam, B.; Wang, W.; Arshad, M.; Khurshid, M.; Muzammil, S.; Rasool, M.; Nisar, M.A.; Alvi, R.F.; Aslam, M.A.; Qamar, M.U.; et al. Antibiotic resistance: A rundown of a global crisis. *Infect. Drug Resist.* **2018**, *11*, 1645–1658. [CrossRef] [PubMed]
10. Ansari, F.; Gray, K.; Nathwani, D.; Phillips, G.; Ogston, S.; Ramsay, C.; Davey, P. Outcomes of an intervention to improve hospital antibiotic prescribing: Interrupted time series with segmented regression analysis. *J. Antimicrob. Chemother.* **2003**, *52*, 842–848. [CrossRef]
11. Carling, P.; Fung, T.; Killion, A.; Terrin, N.; Barza, M. Favorable impact of a multidisciplinary antibiotic management program conducted during 7 years. *Infect. Control. Hosp. Epidemiol.* **2003**, *24*, 699–706. [CrossRef]
12. Ruttimann, S.; Keck, B.; Hartmeier, C.; Maetzel, A.; Bucher, H.C. Long-term antibiotic cost savings from a comprehensive intervention program in a medical department of a university-affiliated teaching hospital. *Clin. Infect. Dis.* **2004**, *38*, 348–356. [CrossRef]
13. Dellit, T.H.; Owens, R.C.; McGowan, J.E.; Gerding, D.N.; Weinstein, R.A.; Burke, J.P.; Huskins, W.C.; Paterson, D.L.; Fishman, N.O.; Carpenter, C.F.; et al. Infectious Diseases Society of America and the Society for Healthcare Epidemiology of America guidelines for developing an institutional program to enhance antimicrobial stewardship. *Clin. Infect. Dis.* **2007**, *44*, 159–177. [CrossRef]

14. Davey, P.; Brown, E.; Charani, E.; Fenelon, L.; Gould, I.M.; Holmes, A.; Ramsay, C.R.; Wiffen, P.J.; Wilcox, M. Interventions to improve antibiotic prescribing practices for hospital inpatients. *Cochrane Database Syst. Rev.* **2013**, *4*, 2.
15. Centers for Disease Control (CDC). *Core Elements of Hospital Antibiotic Stewardship Programs*; US Department of Health and Human Services, CDC: Atlanta, GA, USA, 2014. Available online: http://www.cdc.gov/getsmart/healthcare/implementation/core-elements.html (accessed on 10 May 2019).
16. Karanika, S.; Paudel, S.; Grigoras, C.; Kalbasi, A.; Mylonakis, E. Systematic Review and Meta-analysis of Clinical and Economic Outcomes from the Implementation of Hospital-Based Antimicrobial Stewardship Programs. *Antimicrob. Agents Chemother.* **2016**, *60*, 4840–4852. [CrossRef]
17. Baur, D.; Gladstone, B.P.; Burkert, F.; Carrara, E.; Foschi, F.; Dobele, S.; Tacconelli, E. Effect of antibiotic stewardship on the incidence of infection and colonisation with antibiotic-resistant bacteria and Clostridium difficile infection: A systematic review and meta-analysis. *Lancet Infect. Dis.* **2017**, *17*, 990–1001. [CrossRef]
18. World Health Organization (WHO). WHO Global Strategy for Containment of Antimicrobial Resistance. Available online: http://www.who.int/csr/resources/publications/drugresist/en/EGlobal_Strat.pdf (accessed on 4 April 2019).
19. Tseng, S.; Lee, C.; Lin, T.; Chang, S. Combating antimicrobial resistance: Antimicrobial stewardship program in Taiwan. *J. Microbiol. Immunol. Infect.* **2012**, *45*, 79–89. [CrossRef]
20. Ogaji, I.; Odumosu, P.; Ngwuluka, C.; Onoja, V. Availability of veterinary pharmaceuticals and the role of pharmacists in health-care delivery services to animal patients in Plateau State. *Niger. J. Pharm. Sci.* **2010**, *9*, 66–72.
21. Kingsley, P. Inscrutable medicines and marginal markets: Tackling substandard veterinary drugs in Nigeria. *Pastor Res. Policy Pract.* **2015**, *5*, 1–13. [CrossRef]
22. National Agency for Food and Drug Administration and Control (NAFDAC). Available online: https://www.nafdac.gov.ng/veterinary-products/ (accessed on 4 July 2020).
23. Federal Ministry of Agriculture and Rural Development, Environment and Health. National Action Plan for Antimicrobial Resistance 2017–2022. 2017; pp. 13–14. Available online: https://ncdc.gov.ng/themes/common/docs/protocols/77_1511368219.pdf (accessed on 4 September 2018).
24. John, F.P. Antimicrobial use in food and companion animals. *Anim. Heal. Res. Rev.* **2008**, *9*, 127–133.
25. Kariuki, S.; Dougan, G. Antibacterial resistance in sub-Saharan Africa: An underestimated emergency. *Ann. N. Y. Acad. Sci.* **2014**, *14*, 1323. [CrossRef]
26. Speksnijder, D.C.; Jaarsma, D.A.C.; Verheij, T.J.M.; Wagenaar, J.A. Attitudes and perceptions of Dutch veterinarians on their role in the reduction of antimicrobial use in farm animals. *Prev. Vet. Med.* **2015**, *121*, 365–373. [CrossRef]
27. Coyne, L.A.; Latham, S.M.; Dawson, S.; Donald, I.J.; Pearson, R.B.; Smith, R.F.; Williams, N.J.; Pinchbeck, G.L. Antimicrobial use practices, attitudes and responsibilities in UK farm animal veterinary surgeons. *Prev. Vet. Med.* **2018**, *161*, 115–126. [CrossRef]
28. Id, J.M.N.; Zhuo, A.; Govendir, M.; Rowbotham, S.J.; Labbate, M.; Degeling, C.; Gilbert, G.L.; Dominey-Howes, D.; Ward, M.P. Factors influencing the behaviour and perceptions of Australian veterinarians towards antibiotic use and antimicrobial resistance. *PLoS ONE* **2019**, *14*, e0223534. [CrossRef]
29. Schneider, S.; Salm, F.; Vincze, S.; Moeser, A.; Petruschke, I.; Schmücker, K.; Ludwig, N.; Hanke, R.; Schröder, C.; Gropmann, A.; et al. Perceptions and attitudes regarding antibiotic resistance in Germany: A cross-sectoral survey amongst physicians, veterinarians, farmers and the general public. *J. Antimicrob. Chemother.* **2018**, *73*, 1984–1988. [CrossRef] [PubMed]
30. Anyanwu, M.U.; Kolade, O.A. Veterinarians' Perception, Knowledge and Practices of Antibiotic Stewardship in Enugu State Southeast, Nigeria. *Notale Sci. Biol.* **2018**, *9*, 321–331. [CrossRef]
31. Odetokun, I.A.; Akpabio, U.; Alhaji, N.B.; Biobaku, K.T.; Oloso, N.O.; Ghali-Mohammed, I.; Biobaku, A.J.; Adetunji, V.O.; Fasina, F.O. Knowledge of Antimicrobial Resistance among Veterinary Students and Their Personal Antibiotic Use Practices: A National Cross-Sectional Survey. *Antibiotics (Basel, Switzerland)* **2019**, *8*, 243. [CrossRef]
32. Dyar, O.J.; Hills, H.; Seitz, L.T.; Perry, A.; Ashiruredope, D. Assessing the Knowledge, Attitudes and Behaviors of Human and Animal Health Students towards Antibiotic Use and Resistance: A Pilot Cross-Sectional Study in the UK. *Antibiotics* **2018**, *7*, 10. [CrossRef]

33. Seymour, E.H.; Jones, G.M.; McGilliard, M.L. Persistence of Residues in Milk Following Antibiotic Treatment of Dairy Cattle. *J. Dairy Sci.* **1988**, *71*, 2292–2296. [CrossRef]
34. Kang'ethe, E.K.; Aboge, G.O.; Arimi, S.M.; Kanja, L.W.; Omore, A.O.; McDermott, J.J. Investigation of the risk of consuming marketed milk with antimicrobial residues in Kenya. *Food Control.* **2005**, *16*, 349–355. [CrossRef]
35. Dewdney, J.M.; Maes, L.; Raynaud, J.P.; Blanc, F.; Scheid, J.P.; Jackson, T.; Lens, S.; Verschueren, C. Risk assessment of antibiotic residues of β-lactams and macrolides in food products with regard to their immuno-allergic potential. *Food Chem. Toxicol.* **1991**, *29*, 477–483. [CrossRef]
36. Vázquez-Moreno, L.; Bermúdez, M.C.; Languré, A.A.; Higuera-Ciapara, I.; Díaz De Aguayo, M.; Flores, E. Antibiotic Residues and Drug Resistant Bacteria in Beef, and Chicken Tissues. *J. Food Sci.* **1990**, *55*, 632–634. [CrossRef]
37. Pena, A.; Serrano, C.; Réu, C.; Baeta, L.; Calderón, V.; Silveira, I.; Sousa, J.C.; Peixe, L. Antibiotic residues in edible tissues and antibiotic resistance of faecal Escherichia coli in pigs from Portugal. *Food Addit. Contam. A* **2007**, *21*, 749–755. [CrossRef]
38. Bokma, J.; Dewulf, J.; Deprez, P.; Pardon, B. Risk factors for antimicrobial use in food-producing animals: Disease prevention and socio-economic factors as the main drivers? *VLAAMS DIERGEN TIJDS* **2018**, *87*, 188–200. [CrossRef]
39. Wierup, M. The control of microbial diseases in animals: Alternatives to the use of antibiotics. *Int. J. Antimicrob. Agents* **2000**, *14*, 315–319. [CrossRef]
40. Robinson, T.P.; Bu, D.P.; Carrique-Mas, J.; Fèvre, E.M. Antibiotic resistance: Mitigation opportunities in livestock sector development. *Camb. Univ. Press* **2017**, *11*, 1–3. [CrossRef] [PubMed]
41. Finley, R.L.; Collignon, P.; Larsson, D.G.J.; McEwen, S.A.; Li, X.; Gaze, W.H.; Reid-Smith, R.; Timinouni, M.; Graham, D.W.; Topp, E. The Scourge of Antibiotic Resistance: The Important Role of the Environment. *Clin. Infect. Dis.* **2013**, *57*, 704–710. [CrossRef] [PubMed]
42. Manyi-Loh, C.; Mamphweli, S.; Meyer, E.; Okoh, A. Antibiotic Use in Agriculture and Its Consequential Resistance in Environmental Sources: Potential Public Health Implications. *Molecules* **2018**, *23*, 795. [CrossRef]
43. European Medicines Agency (EMA) and European Food Safety Authority (EFSA). EMA and EFSA Joint Scientific Opinion on measures to reduce the need to use antimicrobial agents in animal husbandry in the European Union, and the resulting impacts on food safety (RONAFA). [EMA/CVMP/570771/2015]. *EFSA J.* **2017**, *15*, e04666. Available online: https://www.efsa.europa.eu/en/efsajournal/pub/4666 (accessed on 23 March 2020).
44. World Health Organization (WHO), Regional Office for South-East Asia. Step-by-step approach for development and implementation of hospital antibiotic policy and standard treatment guidelines. WHO Regional Office for South-East Asia. 2011, pp. 21–24. Available online: https://apps.who.int/iris/handle/10665/205912 (accessed on 10 January 2020).
45. De Briyne, N.; Atkinson, J.; Pokludová, L.; Borriello, S.P.; Price, S. Factors influencing antibiotic prescribing habits and use of sensitivity testing amongst veterinarians in Europe. *Vet. Rec.* **2013**, *173*, 475. [CrossRef]
46. Leekha, S.; Terrell, C.L.; Edson, R.S. General principles of antimicrobial therapy. *Mayo Clin. Proc.* **2011**, *86*, 156–167. [CrossRef]
47. Beović, B. Emperic Antibiotic Therapy [Internet]. European Society of Clinical Microbiology and Infectious Diseases. 2019. Available online: http://esgap.escmid.org/?page_id=389 (accessed on 7 July 2020).
48. Aliu, Y.O. Nigerian Veterinary formulary. In *Handbook of essential veterinary drugs, biologics, and chemicals*, 1st ed.; Aliu, Y.O., Ed.; Veterinary Council of Nigeria: Abuja, Nigeria, 2007.
49. Luseba, D.; Rwambo, P. Review of the policy, regulatory & administrative framework for delivery of livestock health products and services in West and Central Africa. GALVmed. 2015. Available online: http://www.galvmed.org/wp-content/uploads/2015/09/East-Africa-Review-of-Policy-Regulatory-and-Administrative-Framework-for-Delivery-of-Livestock-Health-Products-and-Services-March-2015.pdf (accessed on 11 November 2019).
50. The World Bank In Nigeria [Internet]. 2019. Available online: https://www.worldbank.org/en/country/nigeria/overview (accessed on 4 July 2019).

51. Lwanga, S.; Lemeshow, S. *Sample Size Determination in Health Studies: A Practical Manual*, 1st ed.; World Health Organization: Geneva, Switzerland, 1991; Available online: https://apps.who.int/iris/bitstream/handle/10665/40062/9241544058_%28p1-p22%29.pdf?sequence=1&isAllowed=y (accessed on 8 December 2018).
52. Pedersen, M.J.; Nielsen, C.V. Improving survey response rates in online panels: Effects of low-cost incentives and cost-free text appeal interventions. *Soc. Sci. Comput. Rev.* **2016**, *34*, 229–243. [CrossRef]

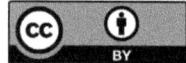

© 2020 by the authors. Licensee MDPI, Basel, Switzerland. This article is an open access article distributed under the terms and conditions of the Creative Commons Attribution (CC BY) license (http://creativecommons.org/licenses/by/4.0/).

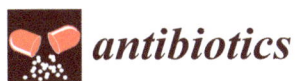

Article

Long-Term Impact of an Educational Antimicrobial Stewardship Program on Management of Patients with Hematological Diseases

Ana Belén Guisado-Gil [1,2], Manuela Aguilar-Guisado [1,*], Germán Peñalva [1], José Antonio Lepe [1], Ildefonso Espigado [3], Eduardo Rodríguez-Arbolí [3], José González-Campos [3], Nancy Rodríguez-Torres [3], María Isabel Montero-Cuadrado [3], José Francisco Falantes-González [3], Juan Luis Reguera-Ortega [3], María Victoria Gil-Navarro [2], José Molina [1], José-Antonio Pérez-Simón [3] and José Miguel Cisneros [1]

[1] Department of Infectious Diseases, Microbiology and Preventive Medicine, Infectious Diseases Research Group, Institute of Biomedicine of Seville (IBiS), University of Seville/CSIC/University Hospital Virgen del Rocio, 41013 Seville, Spain; anaguigil@gmail.com (A.B.G.-G.); german.penalva@gmail.com (G.P.); josea.lepe.sspa@juntadeandalucia.es (J.A.L.); josemolinagb@gmail.com (J.M.); jmcisnerosh@gmail.com (J.M.C.)

[2] Department of Pharmacy, University Hospital Virgen del Rocio, 41013 Seville, Spain; mariav.gil.sspa@juntadeandalucia.es

[3] Department of Hematology, Institute of Biomedicine of Seville (IBiS/CSIC/CIBERONC), University Hospital Virgen del Rocio, University of Seville, 41013 Seville, Spain; ildefonso.espigado.sspa@juntadeandalucia.es (I.E.); edurodarb@gmail.com (E.R.-A.); jose.gonzalez.sspa@juntadeandalucia.es (J.G.-C.); nanarotor@hotmail.com (N.R.-T.); mariai.montero.sspa@juntadeandalucia.es (M.I.M.-C.); josef.falantes.sspa@juntadeandalucia.es (J.F.F.-G.); juanlu_jlr@hotmail.com (J.L.R.-O.); josea.perez.simon.sspa@juntadeandalucia.es (J.-A.P.-S.)

* Correspondence: maguilarguisado@yahoo.es; Tel.: +34-670943816

Abstract: Antimicrobial stewardship programs (ASPs) in hematological patients are especially relevant. However, information about ASPs in this population is scarce. For 11 years, we quarterly assessed antimicrobial consumption and incidence and death rates of multidrug-resistant (MDR) bloodstream infections (BSI) in the hematology Department. Healthcare activity indicators were also monitored yearly. We performed an interrupted time-series analysis. Antimicrobials showed a sustained reduction with a relative effect of −62.3% (95% CI −84.5 to −40.1) nine years after the inception of the ASP, being especially relevant for antifungals (relative effect −80.4%, −90.9 to −69.9), quinolones (relative effect −85.0%, −102.0 to −68.1), and carbapenems (relative effect −68.8%, −126.0 to −10.6). Incidence density of MDR BSI remained low and stable (mean 1.10 vs. 0.82 episodes per 1000 occupied bed days for the pre-intervention and the ASP period, respectively) with a quarterly percentage of change of −0.3% (95% CI −2.0 to 1.4). Early and late mortality of MDR BSI presented a steady trend (quarterly percentage of change −0.7%, 95% CI −1.7 to 0.3 and −0.6%, 95% CI −1.5 to 0.3, respectively). Volume and complexity of healthcare activity increased over the years. The ASP effectively achieved long-term reductions in antimicrobial consumption and improvements in the prescription profile, without increasing the mortality of MDR BSI.

Keywords: antimicrobial stewardship; anti-infective agents; bacteremia; candidemia; hematologic diseases

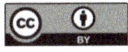

1. Introduction

Antimicrobial stewardship programs (ASPs) have been identified as a valuable tool to optimize the antimicrobial use in healthcare centers, improving patient outcomes and reducing adverse events and the selection pressure related to the use of antimicrobial agents [1].

In hematological patients receiving immunosuppressive therapy, collateral damages of antimicrobial consumption, especially broad-spectrum antibiotic therapy, include the selection of multidrug-resistant (MDR) microorganisms [2], an increased propensity to fungal infections [3], and microbiota dysbiosis [4]. Although, due to these reasons the impact of ASPs in patients with hematological diseases might be especially relevant, information regarding the development of antimicrobial stewardship strategies in these patients is scarce [5–7].

An ASP named Institutional Program for the Optimization of Antimicrobial Treatment (PRIOAM) started in our institution in January 2011. Since then, assessments of antimicrobial use, in-hospital bacterial resistance, and mortality rates associated with nosocomial bloodstream infections (BSI) have decreased significantly [8,9]. This program covers the entire hospital and presents specific interventions focused on hematological patients.

We hypothesized that a comprehensive ASP in hematological patients could also optimize antimicrobial use, reducing the overall consumption and improving the prescription profile without increasing the incidence and mortality rates of BSI produced by MDR microorganisms. Thus, the objective of the present study was to assess the impact of the PRIOAM on antimicrobial consumption and the incidence and death rates caused by MDR BSI in hospitalized adult patients with hematological diseases.

2. Results

Since the inception of the ASP and as part of PRIOAM educative measures (see "Intervention" at the Materials and Methods section), a total number of 218 face-to-face structured educational interviews (EI) were performed (mean 24 ± 19 EI per year). The main reasons for inappropriate antimicrobial therapy were: an incorrect selection of the drug according to the suspected diagnosis (28.4%) or inappropriate duration (28.0%) in the case of empiric treatments, and failing to de-escalate (11.0%) in the case of targeted therapies.

Moreover, 18 clinical sessions (two per year) were performed about practical aspects of common infections in hematological malignancy patients and 45 reports were produced, including one per quarter and an additional annual report to the head of the department, on the level of attainment of pre-agreed objectives.

2.1. Antimicrobial Consumption

The mean consumption of all antimicrobials decreased from 148.2 ± 16.2 defined daily doses (DDD) per 100 occupied bed days (OBD) in the pre-intervention period to 112.0 ± 21.7 DDD per 100 OBD in the ASP period ($p < 0.001$). Detailed data from the pre-post analysis are included in the Supplementary material (Table S1).

The interrupted time-series (ITS) analysis (Table 1, Figures 1–3) showed a sustained reduction in favor of the intervention with a relative effect of −62.3% (95% confidence interval [CI] −84.5 to −40.1) nine years after the inception of the ASP, when compared with the expected antimicrobial consumption based on the pre-intervention trend. As for antibiotics, a prompt change in the level after the inception of the ASP of −17.22 DDD per 100 OBD (95% CI −29.17 to −5.28) was found. Regarding antifungal consumption, a decreasing trend with a change in slope of −3.32 DDD per 100 OBD (95% CI −6.04 to −0.60) and a relative effect −80.4% (95% CI −90.9 to −69.9) was obtained with the intervention. Quinolones were the agents that showed the highest reduction with a change in the level of −18.45 DDD per 100 OBD (95% CI −25.29 to −11.62) after the start of the intervention that led to a relative effect of −85.0% (95% CI −102.0 to −68.1) at the end of the study period. Broad-spectrum antibiotics such as carbapenems and glycopeptides presented significant relative effects of −68.8% (95% CI −126.0 to −10.6) and −70.5% (95% CI −138.9 to −2.1), respectively, compared with the expected consumption based on the pre-intervention trend. The global trend is described in Table S2.

Table 1. Interrupted time-series analysis of changes in trends of antimicrobial consumption.

Outcomes	Pre-Intervention Trend	Change in Level [a]	Change in Trend [b]	Relative Effect [c] %
Total J01+J02	1.83 (−2.14 to 5.80)	−13.98 (−35.65 to 7.69)	−3.52 (−7.57 to 0.52)	−62.3 (−84.5 to −40.1)
Total antibiotics (J01)	−0.65 (−2.84 to 1.54)	−17.22 (−29.17 to −5.28)	−0.27 (−2.49 to 1.95)	−32.4 (−99.2 to 34.5)
Total antifungals (J02)	2.54 (−0.12 to 5.20)	3.31 (−11.12 to 17.74)	−3.32 (−6.04 to −0.60)	−80.4 (−90.9 to −69.9)
Carbapenems	−0.01 (−0.69 to 0.66)	−0.67 (−4.33 to 2.99)	−0.20 (−0.89 to 0.49)	−68.8 (−126.0 to −10.6)
Piperacillin-tazobactam	0.63 (−0.25 to 1.51)	7.78 (3.30 to 12.27)	−0.86 (−1.78 to 0.07)	−67.3 (−96.9 to −38.6)
Antipseudomonal cephalosporins	−0.55 (−1.57 to 0.47)	−10.79 (−16.18 to −5.41)	0.77 (−0.29 to 1.82)	105.1 (−195.6 to 405.8)
Quinolones	0.16 (−1.16 to 1.47)	−18.45 (−25.29 to −11.62)	−0.45 (−1.82 to 0.93)	−85.0 (−102.0 to −68.1)
Amikacin	−0.03 (−0.46 to 0.39)	1.68 (−0.51 to 3.87)	−0.05 (−0.48 to 0.39)	0.1 (−410.8 to 413.6)
Glycopeptides	0.01 (−0.55 to 0.56)	0.68 (−2.27 to 3.62)	−0.17 (−0.74 to 0.40)	−70.5 (−138.9 to −2.1)

Data are presented as quarterly defined daily doses per 100 occupied bed days with a 95% confidence interval, unless otherwise specified. [a] Increase or decrease in the first quarter after the start of the antimicrobial stewardship program (ASP) period with respect to the expected value. [b] Change in slope for the ASP period. [c] Percentage difference between the expected value according to the pre-intervention trend and the trend nine years after the start of the ASP.

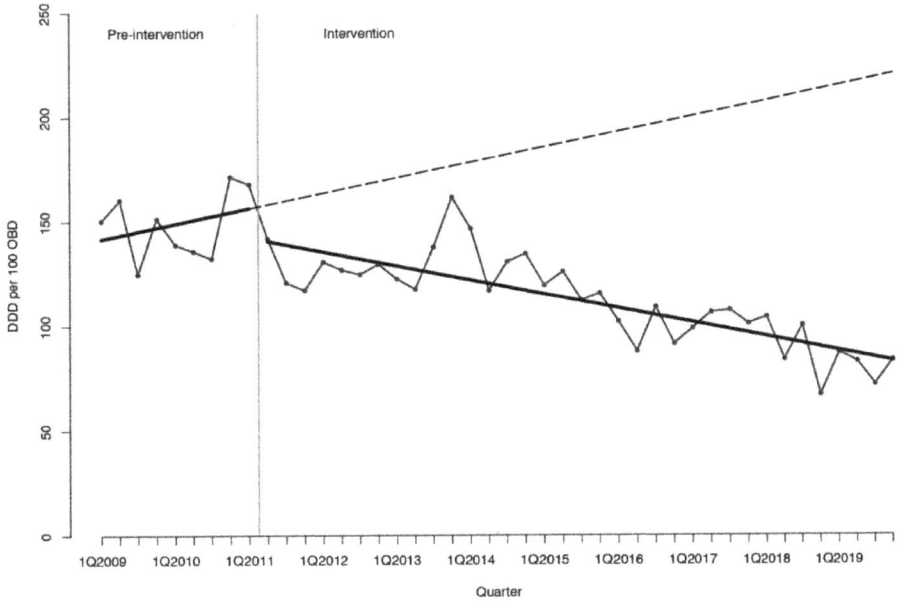

Figure 1. Interrupted time-series analysis of the trends in antimicrobial consumption (antibacterials for systemic use and antifungals) observed before and after the implementation of the antimicrobial stewardship program. Solid lines show the observed trend during the pre-intervention and intervention periods. Dashed lines show the expected trend after the intervention according to the pre-intervention values. DDD, defined daily doses. OBD, occupied bed days. Q, quarter.

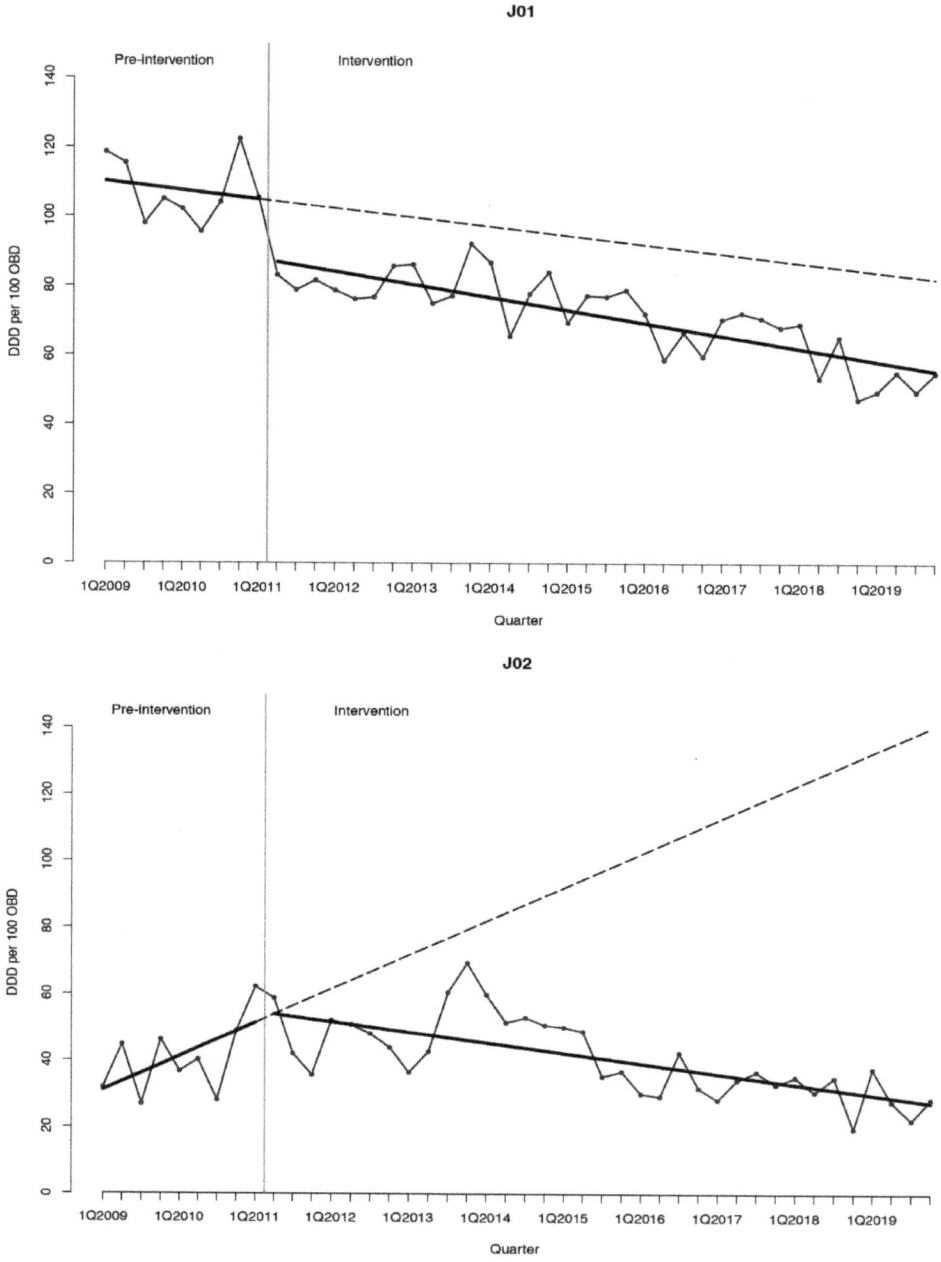

Figure 2. Interrupted time-series analysis of the trends in consumption for antibacterials for systemic use (**J01**) and antifungals (**J02**) observed before and after the implementation of the antimicrobial stewardship program. Solid lines show the observed trend during the pre-intervention and intervention periods. Dashed lines show the expected trend after the intervention according to the pre-intervention values. DDD, defined daily doses. OBD, occupied bed days. Q, quarter.

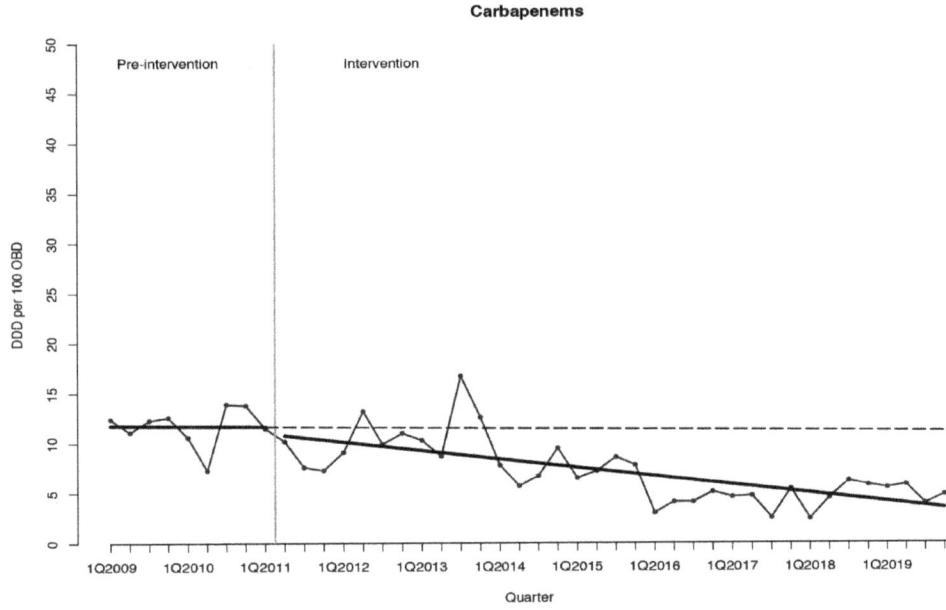

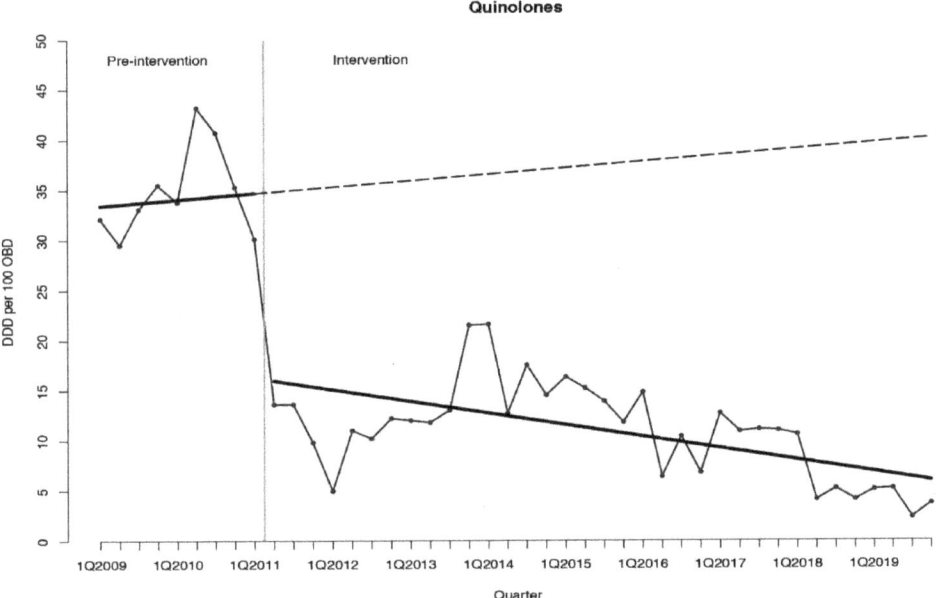

Figure 3. Interrupted time-series analysis of the trends in consumption for carbapenems and quinolones observed before and after the implementation of the antimicrobial stewardship program. Solid lines show the observed trend during the pre-intervention and intervention periods. Dashed lines show the expected trend after the intervention according to the pre-intervention values. DDD, defined daily doses. OBD, occupied bed days. Q, quarter.

2.2. Clinical Outcomes

For the entire study period, the most common gram-negative microorganism causing BSI was non-extended-spectrum beta-lactamase (ESBL) producing *Escherichia coli* (48.1%). MDR gram-negative bacteria and *Candida* spp. caused 14.4% and 5.6% of BSI that were monitored, respectively (Table S3). BSI produced by MDR *Pseudomonas aeruginosa* and *Candida* spp. were responsible for the highest values of early and late mortality rates (Table S4).

For incidence density (ID) and mortality rate, the ITS analysis is shown in Table 2. The pre-post analysis and the trend analysis can be found in Tables S5 and S6, respectively.

Table 2. Interrupted time-series analysis of changes in trends of incidence and mortality rate of multidrug-resistant bloodstream infections.

Outcomes	Pre-Intervention Trend	Change in Level [a]	Change in Trend [b]	Relative Effect [c] %
Incidence density	−0.09 (−0.25 to 0.07)	−0.11 (−1.00 to 0.77)	0.10 (−0.06 to 0.26)	98.9 (−301.4 to 499.2)
Early mortality	0.009 (−0.03 to 0.05)	0.06 (−0.14 to 0.26)	−0.01 (−0.05 to 0.03)	−72.1 (−147.8 to 3.5)
Late mortality	0.01 (−0.06 to 0.08)	−0.03 (−0.42 to 0.36)	−0.005 (−0.08 to 0.07)	−35.55 (−346.9 to 275.8)

Data are presented as quarterly incidence density and all-cause crude death rate per 1000 occupied bed days with a 95% confidence interval, unless otherwise specified. [a] Increase or decrease in the first quarter after the start of the antimicrobial stewardship program (ASP) period with respect to the expected value. [b] Change in slope for the ASP period. [c] Percentage difference between the expected value according to the pre-intervention trend and the trend nine years after the start of the ASP.

The ID of BSI caused by MDR organisms, which kept low during the entire study period, remained stable (mean incidence 1.11 episodes per 1000 OBD for the pre-intervention period and 0.82 episodes per 1000 OBD for the ASP period) with a quarterly percentage change (QPC) of −0.3% (95% CI −2.0 to 1.4, $p = 0.709$). Early and late mortality of MDR BSI presented a steady trend with a QPC of −0.7% (95% CI −1.7 to 0.3, $p = 0.154$) and −0.6% (95% CI −1.5 to 0.3, $p = 0.201$), respectively.

2.3. Changes in Healthcare during the Study Period

Activity indicators related to the volume and complexity of the hematology department such as the number of blood cultures per 1000 OBD, total admissions, OBD, and the number of allogeneic hematopoietic stem-cell transplantation (HSCT) increased during the study period. Other indicators of the department's activity remained stable (Table 3).

Table 3. Indicators related to the volume and complexity of the activity at the hematology department.

Outcomes	2009	2010	2011	2012	2013	2014	2015	2016	2017	2018	2019	APC (95% CI)
Blood cultures per 1000 OBD	72	71	59	71	100	121	92	100	100	133	102	6.014 (2.348 to 9.811)
AML	21	33	35	47	35	37	35	29	43	35	37	4.400 (−6.186 to 16.279)
Admissions	1005	1055	1081	946	1052	1148	1169	1120	1133	1290	1265	2.336 (1.253 to 3.430)
OBD	8966	9128	10,616	10,463	10,343	10,620	10,840	11,135	11,753	11,719	14,463	3.540 (2.358 to 4.735)
Length of stay, mean	16	15	18	17	17	16	16	16	17	14	16	−0.843 (−1.908 to 0.235)
Allogeneic HSCT	19	20	33	40	47	55	56	58	44	43	47	8.609 (4.436 to 12.948)
HSCT−related mortality, %	5.3	5.0	0	0	6.4	1.8	7.1	1.7	0	2.3	2.1	−7.007 (−16.347 to 3.376)

For each year, data are presented as the number of events, unless otherwise specified. In the last column, the annual percentage of change (APC) obtained from joinpoint regression analysis with a 95% confidence interval (CI) is included. OBD, occupied bed days. AML, acute myeloid leukemia. HSCT-related mortality, hematopoietic stem-cell transplantation (HSCT)-related mortality within the first 100 days after allogeneic HSCT from human leukocyte antigen (HLA)-identical siblings.

3. Discussion

The results of our study show that an education-based ASP in the hematology department was able to achieve long-term reductions in overall antimicrobial consumption and improvements in the prescription profile, especially relevant in broad-spectrum antibiotics such as carbapenems, quinolones, and antifungals, without increasing the mortality rates and maintaining a low incidence of MDR BSI. This positive impact was observed in a tertiary care hospital where infectious diseases consultation (IDC) was performed for more than 25 years and up to the PRIOAM implementation. To the best of our knowledge, this is the first study proving nine years' data on the benefits of ASPs in the setting of hematological patients.

Very few previous studies have evaluated the effect of ASPs on antimicrobial consumption in hematological patients with most of them limited by sample size, study period (<2 years before or after intervention), and the absence of data about specific groups of antibiotics. One of the most rigorous is the study performed by So et al. [10] in leukemia units with audit and feedback as the core measures of the ASP. In contrast to our results, the intervention was associated with a significant decrease in antibiotic use (−35.1 DDD per 100 patient-days), but no significant trend in antifungal prescription was observed during a two-year period (−4.0 DDD per 100 patient-days). Two other research works with a one-year evaluation time and including solid and hematological malignancy patients showed favorable results after the beginning of antimicrobial stewardship strategies in terms of global antibiotic consumption [11] and meropenem prescription [7].

The increase of infections caused by MDR bacteria is a major health problem worldwide [12]. This challenge also affects hematological patients [13–15]. However, the percentage of MDR bacteria in our center was lower than previously reported by others [15–18], and notably, remained stable throughout the study period. The low prevalence of ESBL producing *E. coli* and MDR *P. aeruginosa* and, particularly, the absence of carbapenemase-producing *Enterobacteriaceae* was especially important. The sustained reduction of the use of all-class antibiotics associated with the intervention has likely contributed to preventing the generalized increase in MDR infections described in other centers.

In our study, the early and late mortality rates from MDR BSI remained stable during the intervention, showing the absence of deleterious effects for reducing antimicrobial use in these patients. Death rates were higher for BSI caused by MDR organisms as described before [12,18]. Late mortality for ESBL producing *Enterobacteriaceae* was inferior to the 21-day mortality rate reported by Trecarichi et al. [18] for non-susceptible strains (26.2%) and comparable for MDR *P. aeruginosa* (42.4%). Despite the differences in study design, population and antimicrobial utilization due to different local treatment protocols and colonization rates by MDR bacteria, preceding results, similar to ours, illustrated the potential benefits of antimicrobial stewardship approaches. The adherence to ASP recommendation has demonstrated to be an effective and safe strategy with a 64% relative risk reduction in 28-day mortality [19] and a significant decrease in the fatality rate (from 30% to 11%) [5] both in patients with febrile neutropenia and hematological or solid tumors. In patients with hematological diseases and HSCT recipients, stopping antimicrobial therapy early did not significantly increase the incidence of fever relapse and positive blood cultures or the mortality rate, with the advantage of the reduction in the use of antibiotics [20–22].

The results of the current study are even more remarkable if it is taken into consideration that most indicators related to the volume and complexity of the activity at the hematology department increased considerably during the study period. A fact that, in general, is related to a higher frequency of infectious complications and, as a consequence, higher consumption of antibiotics. Only the number of patients diagnosed with acute myeloid leukemia (AML), the length of hospital stay, and the transplant-related mortality within the first 100 days after allogeneic HSCT from human leukocyte antigen (HLA)-identical siblings remained stable. The monitoring of changes in healthcare as an internal control as well as the largest period of study, spanning 11 years in total, are some of the strengths of this work. Additionally, the employment of ITS analyses, the preferential method to assess the impact of health interventions over time [23], and the consistent results throughout the variables evaluated, support a potential causality relation between the ASP implementation and the progressive reduction in the antimicrobial pressure. The stable trend in the mortality by MDR BSI supports the safety of the intervention.

PRIOAM's methods diverge from those ASP performed previously in patients with onco-hematological diseases in which educational initiatives were not incorporated as the core element of the program [11], or they were based on a sole recommendation (de-escalation, discontinuation, antibiotic cycling, etc.) [6,20,21] and/or a specific diagnosis [10], commonly febrile neutropenia [17,19–21]. The educational nature combined with real-time intervention(s) and the inclusion of patients with all types of hematological diseases comprise a differentiating feature of this work.

In patients with hematological diseases, post-chemotherapy febrile neutropenia was one of the most frequent infectious syndromes requiring antimicrobial courses. In this sense, the contribution of the results of the How Long clinical trial [24], led by investigators from our institution, to change the clinical practice and to decrease antibiotic overpressure in hematological patients was considerable. According to the main findings, in high-risk patients with hematological malignancies and febrile neutropenia, empirical antimicrobial therapy can be safely discontinued after 72 h of apyrexia and clinical recovery irrespective of their neutrophil count. It reinforced the previously published recommendation from the 4th European Conference on Infections in Leukaemia (ECIL-4) about empirical treatment of febrile neutropenia [25].

In our center, quinolones were agents commonly selected as an empirical combination therapy in patients with febrile neutropenia, especially in those with a suspected respiratory infection. Quinolones showed the highest reduction after the start of the intervention and the greatest decrease in the relative effect at the end of the study period. It could be explained by the fact that the ASP guidelines highly recommended the withdrawal of combination therapy 48 h after the start if an infection was not confirmed, or if it was presented and narrower spectrum antibiotics could be employed instead of quinolones. The implementation of this recommendation through the ASP has likely contributed to achieving this result.

However, for this study, some limitations should be noted. First, the study design is not exempt from the possibility of ecologic bias, and, consequently, we could not unequivocally associate the results of incidence and mortality of MDR organisms to the ASP implementation. Although the volume and complexity of the activity in the hematology department were monitored, other potential confounding factors such as those related to patients and the center could possibly interfere with the outcomes. In addition, the single-center design limits the external validity of our results and makes it necessary to confirm the reproducibility of the findings in different settings. Second, the close relationship between the IDC in the pre-intervention period and the ASP made it difficult to elucidate the precise weight of each one on the outcomes achieved. Nonetheless, regarding the use of antimicrobials, the stable trends during the pre-intervention period suggest that the implementation of the ASP was necessary to achieve the goals. The sole IDC was insufficient to promote a change in the entire department, as reported in previous studies [26]. Finally, non-MDR BSI, invasive candidiasis (other than candidemia) and aspergillosis have not been examined in this study. The decreasing trend in overall antimicrobial consumption, including voriconazole and liposomal amphotericin B as common treatments for invasive infections caused by molds [27], suggests, at least, a steady frequency of these infections.

4. Materials and Methods

4.1. Study Design and Period

A quasi-experimental before-after study of ITS was performed. The PRIOAM implementation started in January 2011, and, since then, data were prospectively registered for a nine-year period. For the ITS analyses, the study period spanned 44 quarters (11 years) from January 2009 to December 2019.

4.2. Setting

The program was performed at the 39-bed hematology department of the University Hospital Virgen del Rocio (Seville, Spain), which is a teaching hospital providing a tertiary-care service in Southwest Spain. The hospital, with 1177 beds and 72 intensive care unit beds, is a referral-center for solid-organ and HSCT. Adult patients (aged $\geq$ 18 years) receiving treatment for hematological malignancies or undergoing HSCT are treated in this unit. Throughout the last nine years, the hematology department has admitted a mean number of 1134 adult patients per year and has performed a mean of 108 autologous and allogeneic HSCT per year in adults.

4.3. Intervention

The PRIOAM's methods and global outcomes have already been published [8,9]. In brief, it comprises a bundle of educational strategies performed by a multidisciplinary team including infectious diseases physicians, microbiologists, pharmacists, intensive care physicians, pediatricians, and preventivists. The core elements of PRIOAM are summarized in the Supplementary material (Figure S1).

Because most EI were performed when a potentially inappropriate prescription was detected (i.e., use of carbapenems or combination therapy for >48 h, antibiotic duration >7 days or targeted therapies), the main messages tackled in EI were: early identification and management of severe infections, interpretation of microbiologic results, de-escalation and sequential oral treatments whenever possible, diversification of antimicrobial prescriptions, and training in the optimal duration of antimicrobial courses. The form employed for EI is included as Figure S2. No other interventions concerning antimicrobial use (i.e., antimicrobial policies, restrictions, etc.) were performed during the study period. The infection control program in the hematology ward consisted of the isolation in high-efficiency particulate air (HEPA) filters conditioned rooms of neutropenic and HSCT patients, and contact isolation of patients with MDR bacteria or respiratory viruses recovered from clinical samples. Local guidelines for antifungal prophylaxis did not change substantially during the intervention period. No additional measures were implemented regarding infection prevention, and antibiotic prophylaxis was not recommended for hematological patients in our center since 2005.

Before the start of the PRIOAM, a stable IDC program was running at the hematology department, consisting of bedside advice for the management of complex infections, quick report of all BSI, the production and application of local guidelines, updated every two years, for the prevention, diagnosis, and management of infections, and surveillance and analyses of MDR outbreaks. The usual IDC led the implementation of antimicrobial stewardship tasks in the hematology department.

4.4. Study Measures

Antimicrobial use was evaluated through quarterly measures of the antibiotic consumption of the Anatomical Therapeutical Chemical (ATC) group J01 (antibacterials for systemic use) and antifungals ATC group J02. Data about antimicrobial consumption were automatically generated by the electronic prescribing system, which provided information about the units (capsules, injection vials, etc.) used by each department. Consumption was calculated as DDD per 100 OBD, according to the ATC Classification methodology and the 2019 World Health Organization DDD values [28]. Because no DDD was suggested for liposomal amphotericin B, we considered the 210 mg dose as the unit.

For the study period, BSI caused by the most relevant microorganisms in patients with hematological diseases (*E. coli*, *Klebsiella pneumoniae*, *P. aeruginosa*, and *Candida* spp.) were registered. The effect of the intervention on the number of BSI produced by MDR microorganisms (ESBL-producing *Enterobacteriaceae*, MDR *P. aeruginosa*, and *Candida* spp.) was monitored quarterly and presented as ID per 1000 OBD. The German Society for Hygiene and Microbiology criteria [29] was taken into account for MDR categorization. The analysis of antibiotic susceptibility and resistance mechanisms was performed following the European Committee on Antimicrobial Susceptibility Testing (EUCAST) criteria [30,31].

The effect on the mortality rates was assessed as the all-cause crude death rate [9,32] (deaths per 1000 OBD per quarter) on day +7 (early mortality) and +30 (late mortality) after the diagnosis of BSI. Patients dying in less than 24 h after blood sample collection were not considered for the mortality analysis, as previously proposed [26,33,34], for a better selection of patients benefitting from the intervention targeting an optimized use of antimicrobials.

To analyze the effect of changes in the hematology department during the 11-year study period, we monitored yearly indicators related to the volume and complexity of the activity at the department that may influence the antimicrobial use, such as the number of blood cultures per 1000 OBD, new patients diagnosed with AML, admissions, and OBD, as well as the mean length of stay. We also monitored the number of allogeneic HSCT and the transplantation-related mortality within the first 100 days after allogeneic HSCT from HLA-identical siblings.

Because presentation, dissemination, and introduction activities of PRIOAM took place in the different departments of the hospital from January to 31 March 2011, we considered 1 April as the beginning of the intervention period for the analysis.

4.5. Statistical Analysis

For descriptive aims, categorical variables were presented as frequency distribution and percentages, and continuous variables were presented as means $\pm$ standard deviations (SD). The Student's t-test or the Mann-Whitney U test were employed for univariate pre-post analyses, after checking for normality using the Kolmogorov-Smirnov test.

To assess the effect of the ASP, an ITS analysis was performed to estimate changes in the level and trends before and after the inception of the program. We used a generalized least squares regression approach accounting for autocorrelation by autoregressive moving-average (ARMA) models. The final model selection for each variable was based on the Akaike Information Criterion with validation of the autocorrelation structures by likelihood ratio tests [35]. The long-term effect attributable to the ASP for each outcome was estimated by calculating the relative effect, as the percentage difference between the values of the expected pre-intervention trend and the modeled trend at the end of the study. Alternatively, a joinpoint regression analysis was conducted to explore the trends of the time-series [36], calculating the QPC during the 11-year study period by using the Joinpoint software modeling annual percentage change calculation to our log-transformed quarterly data with autocorrelated error models.

Confidence intervals or p-values (p) were included to show statistical significance. Differences were considered statistically significant at $p < 0.05$ (2-tailed tests). Statistical analyses were performed with IBM SPSS Statistics software v. 23.0, R software v. 3.5.2 and Joinpoint Regression Program v. 4.6.0.0.

4.6. Ethics Approval

The study was conducted in accordance with the Declaration of Helsinki, and the protocol was approved by the Ethics Committee of the University Hospital Virgen del Rocio (Project identification code: PI-0361-2010).

5. Conclusions

These results allow us to state that an education-based ASP contributed significantly to the decreasing trend in the use of antimicrobials and, possibly, to maintain the low incidence of MDR BSI despite the increase in the volume and complexity of the activity at the hematology department over the study period. Death rates of BSI caused by MDR organisms were stable, showing that these interventions are safe in this vulnerable population.

Supplementary Materials: The following are available online at https://www.mdpi.com/2079-6382/10/2/136/s1. Table S1: Differences between the pre-intervention period and the antimicrobial stewardship program period regarding pre-post analysis of antimicrobial consumption. Table S2: Trend analysis of antimicrobial consumption (2009–2019). Table S3: Frequency of most relevant gram-negative microorganisms and Candida spp. as causative agents of bloodstream infections (2009–2019). Table S4: Mortality of patients with the most relevant gram-negative microorganisms and Candida spp. causing bloodstream infections (2009–2019). Table S5: Differences between the pre-intervention period and the antimicrobial stewardship program period regarding pre-post analysis of incidence and mortality rate of multidrug-resistant bloodstream infections. Table S6: Trend analysis of the incidence and mortality rate of multidrug-resistant bloodstream infections (2009–2019). Figure S1: Description of the core elements of PRIOAM. Figure S2: Form for PRIOAM educational interviews.

Author Contributions: Conceptualization, M.A.-G. and J.M.C. Methodology, A.B.G.-G. and G.P. Formal analysis, A.B.G.-G. and G.P. Investigation, A.B.G.-G., M.A.-G., G.P., J.A.L., I.E., and M.V.G.-N. Writing—original draft preparation, A.B.G.-G. Writing—review and editing, M.A.-G., G.P., J.A.L., I.E., E.R.-A., J.G.-C., N.R.-T., M.I.M.-C., J.F.F.-G., J.L.R.-O., M.V.G.-N., J.M., J.-A.P.-S., and J.M.C. All authors have read and agreed to the published version of the manuscript.

Funding: This work was supported by public funding from the Regional Health Ministry of Andalucia (grant number PI-0361-2010), which did not participate in the development of the program or the analysis of its results.

Institutional Review Board Statement: The study was conducted according to the guidelines of the Declaration of Helsinki, and approved by the Ethics Committee of the University Hospital Virgen del Rocio (Project identification code: PI-0361-2010).

Informed Consent Statement: Taking into consideration the risks and potential harms involved in the research, the Ethics Committee approved the exemption of informed consent.

Data Availability Statement: The data presented in this study are available on request from the corresponding author.

Acknowledgments: The whole hematology department of the University Hospital Virgen del Rocio, whose close commitment to the program made its results possible. We also acknowledge the invaluable contribution of all the PRIOAM professionals: physicians, clinical microbiologists, pharmacists, nurses, and other members of the hospital. We thank the hospital manager and medical director, and the Andalusian Health Service of the Regional Ministry of Health of Andalucia (Spain) for supporting the ASP.

Conflicts of Interest: J.M.C. has received honoraria as a speaker from Novartis, Astellas Pharma, Pfizer, MSD, Janssen Pharmaceuticals, and AstraZeneca, outside the submitted work. He has also received report grants from Instituto de Salud Carlos III, Spanish Government, co-financed by the European Development Regional Fund "A way to achieve Europe", during the conduct of the study. No potential conflict of interest was reported by all other authors.

References

1. Barlam, T.F.; Cosgrove, S.E.; Abbo, L.M.; MacDougall, C.; Schuetz, A.N.; Septimus, E.J.; Srinivasan, A.; Dellit, T.H.; Falck-Ytter, Y.T.; Fishman, N.O.; et al. Implementing an antibiotic stewardship program: Guidelines by the Infectious Diseases Society of America and the Society for Healthcare Epidemiology of America. *Clin. Infect. Dis.* **2016**, *62*, e51–e77. [CrossRef] [PubMed]
2. Alevizakos, M.; Gaitanidis, A.; Andreatos, N.; Arunachalam, K.; Flokas, M.E.; Mylonakis, E. Bloodstream infections due to extended-spectrum β-lactamase- producing Enterobacteriaceae among patients with malignancy: A systematic review and meta-analysis. *Int. J. Antimicrob. Agents* **2017**, *50*, 657–663. [CrossRef] [PubMed]
3. Das, I.; Nightingale, P.; Patel, M.; Jumaa, P. Epidemiology, clinical characteristics, and outcome of candidemia: Experience in a tertiary referral center in the UK. *Int. J. Infect. Dis.* **2011**, *15*, e759–e763. [CrossRef] [PubMed]
4. Taur, Y.; Jenq, R.R.; Perales, M.A.; Littmann, E.R.; Morjaria, S.; Ling, L.; No, D.; Gobourne, A.; Viale, A.; Dahi, P.B.; et al. The effects of intestinal tract bacterial diversity on mortality following allogeneic hematopoietic stem cell transplantation. *Blood* **2014**, *124*, 1174–1182. [CrossRef] [PubMed]
5. Madran, B.; Keske, Ş.; Tokça, G.; Dönmez, E.; Ferhanoğlu, B.; Çetiner, M.; Mandel, N.M.; Ergönül, Ö. Implementation of an antimicrobial stewardship program for patients with febrile neutropenia. *Am. J. Infect. Control* **2018**, *46*, 420–424. [CrossRef]
6. Webb, B.J.; Majers, J.; Healy, R.; Jones, P.B.; Butler, A.M.; Snow, G.; Forsyth, S.; Lopansri, B.K.; Ford, C.D.; Hoda, D. Antimicrobial Stewardship in a Hematological Malignancy Unit: Carbapenem Reduction and Decreased Vancomycin-Resistant Enterococcus Infection. *Clin. Infect. Dis.* **2020**, *71*, 960–967. [CrossRef]
7. Mardani, M.; Abolghasemi, S.; Shabani, S. Impact of an antimicrobial stewardship program in the antimicrobial-resistant and prevalence of clostridioides difficile infection and amount of antimicrobial consumed in cancer patients. *BMC Res. Notes* **2020**, *13*, 246. [CrossRef]
8. Cisneros, J.M.; Neth, O.; Gil-Navarro, M.V.; Lepe, J.A.; Jiménez-Parrilla, F.; Cordero, E.; Rodríguez-Hernández, M.J.; Amaya-Villar, R.; Cano, J.; Gutiérrez-Pizarraya, A.; et al. Global impact of an educational antimicrobial stewardship program on prescribing practice in a tertiary hospital centre. *Clin. Microbiol. Infect.* **2014**, *20*, 82–88. [CrossRef]
9. Molina, J.; Peñalva, G.; Gil-Navarro, M.V.; Praena, J.; Lepe, J.A.; Pérez-Moreno, M.A.; Ferrándiz, C.; Aldabó, T.; Aguilar, M.; Olbrich, P.; et al. Long-Term Impact of an educational antimicrobial stewardship program on hospital-acquired candidemia and multidrug-resistant bloodstream infections: A quasi-experimental study of interrupted time-series analysis. *Clin. Infect. Dis.* **2017**, *65*, 1992–1999. [CrossRef]
10. So, M.; Mamdani, M.M.; Morris, A.M.; Lau, T.T.Y.; Broady, R.; Deotare, U.; Grant, J.; Kim, D.; Schimmer, A.D.; Schuh, A.C.; et al. Effect of an antimicrobial stewardship programme on antimicrobial utilisation and costs in patients with leukaemia: A retrospective controlled study. *Clin. Microbiol. Infect.* **2018**, *24*, 882–888. [CrossRef]
11. Yeo, C.L.; Chan, D.S.; Earnest, A.; Wu, T.S.; Yeoh, S.F.; Lim, R.; Jureen, R.; Fisher, D.; Hsu, L.Y. Prospective audit and feedback on antibiotic prescription in an adult haematology-oncology unit in Singapore. *Eur. J. Clin. Microbiol. Infect. Dis.* **2012**, *31*, 583–590. [CrossRef] [PubMed]
12. WHO. Antimicrobial Resistance. 2020. Available online: https://www.who.int/news-room/fact-sheets/detail/antimicrobial-resistance (accessed on 12 December 2020).
13. Gudiol, C.; Tubau, F.; Calatayud, L.; Garcia-Vidal, C.; Cisnal, M.; Sánchez-Ortega, I.; Duarte, R.; Calvo, M.; Carratalà, J. Bacteraemia due to multidrug-resistant Gram-negative bacilli in cancer patients: Risk factors, antibiotic therapy and outcomes. *J. Antimicrob. Chemother.* **2011**, *66*, 657–663. [CrossRef] [PubMed]
14. Montassier, E.; Batard, E.; Gastinne, T.; Potel, G.; de La Cochetière, M.F. Recent changes in bacteremia in patients with cancer: A systematic review of epidemiology and antibiotic resistance. *Eur. J. Clin. Microbiol. Infect. Dis.* **2013**, *32*, 841–850. [CrossRef]
15. Garcia-Vidal, C.; Cardozo-Espinola, C.; Puerta-Alcalde, P.; Marco, F.; Tellez, A.; Agüero, D.; Romero-Santana, F.; Díaz-Beyá, M.; Giné, E.; Morata, L.; et al. Risk factors for mortality in patients with acute leukemia and bloodstream infections in the era of multiresistance. *PLoS ONE* **2018**, *13*, e0199531. [CrossRef] [PubMed]

16. Averbuch, D.; Tridello, G.; Hoek, J.; Mikulska, M.; Akan, H.; Yanez San Segundo, L.; Pabst, T.; Özçelik, T.; Klyasova, G.; Donnini, I.; et al. Antimicrobial Resistance in Gram-Negative Rods Causing Bacteremia in Hematopoietic Stem Cell Transplant Recipients: Intercontinental Prospective Study of the Infectious Diseases Working Party of the European Bone Marrow Transplantation Group. *Clin. Infect. Dis.* **2017**, *65*, 1819–1828. [CrossRef] [PubMed]
17. Martinez-Nadal, G.; Puerta-Alcalde, P.; Gudiol, C.; Cardozo, C.; Albasanz-Puig, A.; Marco, F.; Laporte-Amargós, J.; Moreno-García, E.; Domingo-Doménech, E.; Chumbita, M.; et al. Inappropriate Empirical Antibiotic Treatment in High-risk Neutropenic Patients With Bacteremia in the Era of Multidrug Resistance. *Clin. Infect. Dis.* **2020**, *70*, 1068–1074. [CrossRef] [PubMed]
18. Trecarichi, E.M.; Pagano, L.; Candoni, A.; Pastore, D.; Cattaneo, C.; Fanci, R.; Nosari, A.; Caira, M.; Spadea, A.; Busca, A.; et al. Current epidemiology and antimicrobial resistance data for bacterial bloodstream infections in patients with hematologic malignancies: An Italian multicentre prospective survey. *Clin. Microbiol. Infect.* **2015**, *21*, 337–343. [CrossRef] [PubMed]
19. Rosa, R.G.; Goldani, L.Z.; dos Santos, R.P. Association between adherence to an antimicrobial stewardship program and mortality among hospitalised cancer patients with febrile neutropaenia: A prospective cohort study. *BMC Infect. Dis.* **2014**, *14*, 286. [CrossRef]
20. La Martire, G.; Robin, C.; Oubaya, N.; Lepeule, R.; Beckerich, F.; Leclerc, M.; Barhoumi, W.; Toma, A.; Pautas, C.; Maury, S.; et al. De-escalation and discontinuation strategies in high-risk neutropenic patients: An interrupted time series analyses of antimicrobial consumption and impact on outcome. *Eur. J. Clin. Microbiol. Infect. Dis.* **2018**, *37*, 1931–1940. [CrossRef]
21. Petteys, M.M.; Kachur, E.; Pillinger, K.E.; He, J.; Copelan, E.A.; Shahid, Z. Antimicrobial de-escalation in adult haematopoietic cell transplantation recipients with febrile neutropenia of unknown origin. *J. Oncol. Pharm. Pract.* **2020**, *26*, 632–640. [CrossRef]
22. Snyder, M.; Pasikhova, Y.; Baluch, A. Early Antimicrobial De-escalation and Stewardship in Adult Haematopoietic Stem Cell Transplantation Recipients: Retrospective Review. *Open Forum Infect. Dis.* **2017**, *4*, ofx226. [CrossRef] [PubMed]
23. De Kraker, M.E.A.; Abbas, M.; Huttner, B.; Harbarth, S. Good epidemiological practice: A narrative review of appropriate scientific methods to evaluate the impact of antimicrobial stewardship interventions. *Clin. Microbiol. Infect.* **2017**, *23*, 819–825. [CrossRef] [PubMed]
24. Aguilar-Guisado, M.; Espigado, I.; Martín-Peña, A.; Gudiol, C.; Royo-Cebrecos, C.; Falantes, J.; Vázquez-López, L.; Montero, M.I.; Rosso-Fernández, C.; de la Luz Martino, M.; et al. Optimisation of empirical antimicrobial therapy in patients with haematological malignancies and febrile neutropenia (How Long study): An open-label, randomised, controlled phase 4 trial. *Lancet Haematol.* **2017**, *4*, e573–e583. [CrossRef]
25. Averbuch, D.; Orasch, C.; Cordonnier, C.; Livermore, D.M.; Mikulska, M.; Viscoli, C.; Gyssens, I.C.; Kern, W.V.; Klyasova, G.; Marchetti, O.; et al. European guidelines for empirical antibacterial therapy for febrile neutropenic patients in the era of growing resistance: Summary of the 2011 4th European Conference on Infections in Leukemia. *Haematologica* **2013**, *98*, 1826–1835. [CrossRef] [PubMed]
26. Molina, J.; Noguer, M.; Lepe, J.A.; Pérez-Moreno, M.A.; Aguilar-Guisado, M.; de la Vega, R.L.; Peñalva, G.; Crespo-Rivas, J.C.; Gil-Navarro, M.V.; Salvador, J.; et al. Clinical impact of an educational antimicrobial stewardship program associated with infectious diseases consultation targeting patients with cancer: Results of a 9-year quasi-experimental study with an interrupted time-series analysis. *J. Infect.* **2019**, *79*, 206–211. [CrossRef] [PubMed]
27. Tissot, F.; Agrawal, S.; Pagano, L.; Petrikkos, G.; Groll, A.H.; Skiada, A.; Lass-Flörl, C.; Calandra, T.; Viscoli, C.; Herbrecht, R. ECIL-6 guidelines for the treatment of invasive candidiasis, aspergillosis and mucormycosis in leukemia and hematopoietic stem cell transplant patients. *Haematologica* **2017**, *102*, 433–444. [CrossRef]
28. WHO. Collaborating Center for Drug Statistics Methodology. DDD Definition and General Considerations. 2019. Available online: https://www.whocc.no/ddd/ (accessed on 12 December 2020).
29. Mattner, F.; Bange, F.C.; Meyer, E.; Seifert, H.; Wichelhaus, T.A.; Chaberny, I.F. Preventing the spread of multidrug-resistant gram-negative pathogens: Recommendations of an expert panel of the German Society for Hygiene and Microbiology. *Dtsch. Arztebl. Int.* **2012**, *109*, 39–45. [CrossRef]
30. The European Committee on Antimicrobial Susceptibility Testing. EUCAST Guideline for the Detection of Resistance Mechanisms and Specific Resistances of Clinical and/or Epidemiological Importance. Version 2.0. 2017. Available online: https://www.eucast.org/resistance_mechanisms/ (accessed on 12 December 2020).
31. The European Committee on Antimicrobial Susceptibility Testing. Breakpoint Tables for Interpretation of MICs and Zone Diameters. Version 10.0. 2020. Available online: http://www.eucast.org (accessed on 12 December 2020).
32. Porta, M. (Ed.) *A Dictionary of Epidemiology*, 6th ed.; Oxford University Press: New York, NY, USA, 2014.
33. López-Cortés, L.E.; Del Toro, M.D.; Gálvez-Acebal, J.; Bereciartua-Bastarrica, E.; Fariñas, M.C.; Sanz-Franco, M.; Natera, C.; Corzo, J.E.; Lomas, J.M.; Pasquau, J.; et al. Impact of an evidence-based bundle intervention in the quality-of-care management and outcome of Staphylococcus aureus bacteremia. *Clin. Infect. Dis.* **2013**, *57*, 1225–1233. [CrossRef]
34. Lee Rachael, A.; Joanna, Z.; Camins, B.C.; Griffin, R.L.; Martin Rodriguez, J.; McCarty, T.P.; Magadia, J.; Pappas, P.G. Impact of infectious disease consultation on clinical management and mortality in patients with candidemia. *Clin. Infect. Dis.* **2018**, *68*, 1585–1587. [CrossRef]
35. Penfold, R.B.; Zhang, F. Use of interrupted time series analysis in evaluating health care quality improvements. *Acad. Pediatr.* **2013**, *13*, S38–S44. [CrossRef]
36. Kim, H.; Fay, M.P.; Feuer, E.J.; Midthune, D.N. Permutation tests for joinpoint regression with applications to cancer rates. *Stat. Med.* **2000**, *19*, 335–351. [CrossRef]

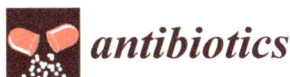

Article

A Qualitative Investigation of the Acceptability and Feasibility of a Urinary Tract Infection Patient Information Leaflet for Older Adults and Their Carers

Leah F. Jones [1], Heidi Williamson [2], Petronella Downing [1], Donna M. Lecky [1], Diana Harcourt [2] and Cliodna McNulty [1,*]

1. Public Health England, Gloucester GL1 1DQ, UK; leah.jones@phe.gov.uk (L.F.J.); pdowning16@gmail.com (P.D.); donna.lecky@phe.gov.uk (D.M.L.)
2. Health and Social Sciences, Frenchay Campus, University of the West of England, Bristol BS16 1QY, UK; Heidi3.williamson@uwe.ac.uk (H.W.); Diana2.Harcourt@uwe.ac.uk (D.H.)
* Correspondence: cliodna.mcnulty@phe.gov.uk

Abstract: Urinary tract infections (UTIs) can be life threatening in older adults. The aim of this study was to primarily understand the acceptability and feasibility of using a UTI leaflet for older adults in care homes and the community. Qualitative interviews and focus groups informed by the Theoretical Domains Framework were conducted in 2019 with 93 participants from two English areas where a UTI leaflet for older adults had been introduced to improve self-care advice. Discussions were conducted with care staff (carers and nurses), older adults, general practice staff (GPs, nurses and health care assistants), and other relevant stakeholders and covered experiences of using the leaflet; its implementation; and barriers and facilitators to use. Participants deemed the leaflet an acceptable tool. Clinicians and care staff believed that having information in writing would reinforce their messages to older adults. Care staff reported that some older adults may find the information overwhelming. Where implemented, care staff used the leaflet as an educational guide. Clinicians requested the leaflet in electronic and paper formats to suit preferences. Implementation barriers included lack of awareness of the leaflet, lack of staffing and resource, and weak working relationships between care homes and general practices. It is recommended that regional strategies must include plans for dissemination to care homes, training, promotion and easy access to the leaflet. Improvements to the leaflet consisted of inclusion of antibiotic course length, D-mannose, atrophic vaginitis and replacement of less alarmist terminology such as 'life threatening'.

Keywords: urinary tract infections (UTI); older adults; qualitative; leaflet; Theoretical Domains Framework; antimicrobial resistance; antibiotics

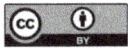

1. Introduction

Urinary tract infections (UTIs) are one of the most common causes of hospitalisation in care home residents, posing a significant threat to life in this age group [1]. Most UTIs are caused by the bacterium *Escherichia coli* (*E. coli*). *E. coli* bloodstream infections (BSIs) rates in the UK have increased by 33.8% since 2012/2013 [2], with the highest rates of *E. coli* bacteraemia observed amongst older adults over the age of 75 [3,4].

The focus of any suspected infection is often difficult to determine in older adults, especially if they have dementia, and therefore clinicians may use point-of-care tests to help determine the focus of infection or use empirical broad-spectrum antibiotics. Despite strong evidence to suggest that antimicrobial therapy to treat asymptomatic bacteriuria (ASB) is unnecessary and potentially harmful [5], urine dipsticks are often used by primary care and care home staff [6]. As a result, a proportion of older adults are misdiagnosed with UTIs rather than ASB and may receive unnecessary antibiotics [7,8].

Combined with improved diagnostic pathways for health care workers, information leaflets can help explain to older adults in the community and in care, clinicians' diagnostic decisions and management plans, providing self-care and prevention advice to patients to improve patients' understanding, and self-care skills. Leaflets can be highly valued by patients and can help reduce unnecessary antibiotic prescribing [9–11]. In 2017, Public Health England (PHE) developed an evidence-based UTI leaflet for older adults and their carers (community and care home carers) to increase patients' and carers' knowledge about ASB, UTIs and antimicrobial resistance (AMR) and increase their skills to recognise, help prevent and self-care for UTIs. The pictorial leaflet can be found in Supplementary Material 1, [12] and provides an anatomical illustration of the urinary system, prevention information, signs and symptoms of UTI, other causes of confusion, self-care advice, what to expect from a clinical consultation, a section on AMR, and safety netting for pyelonephritis and sepsis.

The aim of this study was to:
1. Explore the acceptability and feasibility of using the leaflet.
2. Understand the perceived value of the leaflet.
3. Identify barriers and facilitators to using the leaflet.
4. Understand how the leaflet interacts with UTI diagnostic tools and other resources.
5. Inform further developments to the leaflet.
6. Explore potential indications of behaviour change.

The Theoretical Domains Framework (TDF) [13] is a behavioural model designed to help understand implementation. The TDF was used in the development phase of the leaflet by informing the interview schedules and was used in this study to structure the interview schedules to ensure all behavioural determinants were explored including knowledge, skills, and environmental context.

2. Results

Ninety-three participants took part in either focus groups or interviews from March to September 2019, from a range of urban and rural locations across Gloucestershire and East Kent. For a detailed figure of the recruitment figures and strategy, please see Supplementary Material 2

Of the 93 participants, 53 were carers working in care homes (3 nurses, 2 administrators, and 48 carers), 4 care home residents, 25 general practice staff servicing care homes and the community (13 GPs, 10 nurses and 2 health care assistants), and 8 stakeholders. Stakeholders included representatives from the Royal College of General Practitioners (RCGP; the professional body for general practitioners in the United Kingdom), the National Health Service Improvement (NHSI; responsible for overseeing foundation trusts and NHS trusts, as well as independent providers that provide NHS-funded care), the Care Association Alliance (CAA; a membership association for local Care Associations to exchange best practice), an academic pharmacist, and members of four Clinical Commissioning Groups (CCGs, clinically-led statutory NHS bodies responsible for the planning and commissioning of health care services for their local area), in East Kent (3) and Gloucestershire (1).

2.1. Key Findings

2.1.1. The Acceptability and Feasibility of Leaflet Use in Primary Care and Care Home Settings

All participants reported that the leaflet is a suitable tool for care homes and general practice and that they would like the leaflet to be available in both electronic and hard-copy formats. Suggestions for dissemination included giving the leaflet to residents' families and friends as well as to the residents themselves; displaying the leaflet as a waiting room resource; giving the leaflet to patients during consultations for suspected UTI and providing it at the reception desk or next to urine submission boxes when urine samples are submitted. Most older adults would be happy to receive the leaflet, although some concern was raised by clinicians as to the leaflet's acceptability for older adults who are coping with multiple health issues and who may find the information overwhelming.

2.1.2. Value of the Leaflet

All participants valued the leaflet for various reasons, including

- Written information reinforces their advice to older adults (clinicians and care staff),
- It is an educational guide for care staff (care staff) and friends and family (older adults), and
- It has flexibility for use in other infection prevention and control (IPC) areas (commissioners), with other age groups (clinicians and older adults).

Some participants suggested that the leaflet would be suitable for community pharmacy and out-of-hours (OOH) settings, although one nurse practitioner believed that implementation in OOH settings would be very difficult due to transient staff.

2.1.3. Barriers and Facilitators

Despite reporting local dissemination efforts through the provision of the leaflet, local champions and local hydration campaigns, lack of awareness by GP staff and care staff was the biggest barrier to leaflet use. Although some clinicians believed it was their role to cascade information to care homes, most in this study did not, and therefore weak working relationships between care homes and general practices could contribute to lack of implementation, although this will vary across regions and between facilities. Commissioning teams reported that high turnover of care staff, lack of resources and staffing issues in the CCG meant they are unable to visit every general practice and care home to promote the leaflet and conduct training around UTI diagnosis and management.

In one region, the IPC lead reported utilising 'links practitioners' in every general practice and care facility to promote and disseminate their training and resources, but also believed further work is needed to establish whether this approach is effective, as one link nurse reported attending training but not feeding back about materials.

2.1.4. Comments on the Leaflet

Research findings are represented in Table 1. However, many of the leaflet findings do not directly fit into the TDF domains [14] and are therefore represented below with quotes.

Participants suggested minor improvements to the leaflet content including the use of less alarmist terminology. One participant said *"It might get people panicking about life-threatening ... we currently have two residents with full capacity and the one would be straight on the phone."* Care home staff 3.

Others suggested inclusion of the NICE recommendation of three-day antibiotic courses for proven UTI to address patient expectations for longer antibiotic courses, inclusion of the NICE recommendation of D-mannose (a type of sugar) dietary supplement as a self-care preventative option in recurrent UTI, and mention of atrophic vaginitis as an alternative cause of urinary symptoms in post-menopausal women.

Staff sharing the leaflet liked all sections, reporting that they reinforced the information that they gave to patients. One stated: *"I find them helpful if I'm having a discussion with a patient and they're not really buying into what I'm saying ... it's a little bit of extra evidence that I'm not some weird doctor trying to make up stuff."* General practice staff 3.

A CAA representative recommended increasing leaflet dissemination via the CAA to ensure delivery directly to care homes. The RCGP representative recommended a short RCGP screencast to raise awareness amongst general practitioners (GPs).

Table 1. Key findings and corresponding TDF domains covering use and implementation of the UTI leaflet, UTI diagnosis/identification and UTI management in older adults.

Use and Implementation of the UTI Leaflet	Identifying/Diagnosing a UTI	Managing and/or Treating a UTI
Awareness	**Urine dipsticks**	**Hydration and drinking**
The majority of care staff had not seen the leaflet before. *"I can't even say that I've seen them in the waiting rooms or anything."* Care home staff 1 (**Knowledge**)	A minority of care staff were aware that they should not be using dipsticks. *"I heard that some of them went for the training ... like six months ago, been advised not to follow the urine dip any more."* Care home staff 7 (**Knowledge**)	All older adults knew that hydration could prevent or help manage a UTI. *"I've been drinking water since it's coming out my ears. Yeah, I've been trying to drink as much fluid as I can, so."* Older adult 2 (**Knowledge**)
Leaflet content	One stakeholder reported optimism that their work around UTIs, implementing the leaflet and decreasing dipstick use in their region had reduced the amount of urines being bought in to general practice. *"receptionist love me because I stop that wave of urine that used to come in every morning, and the nurses said it was taking hours of their time."* Stakeholder 8 (**Optimism**)	All care homes actively encouraged residents to keep hydrated. *"I would say actually physically passing the drink to them, so you would encourage them to drink and usually they say, oh you know, I've had a lot today. We say, oh well just a little bit more and try and just sort of encourage them."* Care home staff 3 (**Skills**)
The majority of care staff believed that residents will not understand the content of the leaflet. *"if you want the residents to read, this is too much for them."* Care home staff 7 (**Beliefs about consequences**)	All general practice staff reported that they have had issues with patients bringing in urine samples to reception for dipping. *"lots of patients just dropping in samples that we never knew what they were for or whether to send it off, so we've tightened up on that."* General practice staff 3 (**Social influence**)	All general practice staff encouraged hydration as a preventative and self-care method. *"Hydration is what I focus on."* GP 1 (**Skills**)
Most older adults did not like the title 'older adults' as they do not associate themselves with the label. *"the only thing I didn't like about it was the wording at the top which says it's a leaflet for older adults and carers."* Older adult 2 (**Professional role and identity**)	Care staff decided to use urine dipsticks as a result of noticing other symptoms. *"we usually notice something else which has caused us to do that test anyway ... so we're not just relying on that."* Care home staff 2	Some care homes would decide to encourage drinking before concluding that the resident has a UTI. *"as harsh as it sounds we give them a drink and see if that perks them up and we see how far the confusion goes, we don't automatically think UTI, it could be dehydration."* Care home staff 4 (**Memory, attention and decision processes**)
Stakeholders stated that because the leaflet links with hydration they can link it to many areas of infection prevention such as respiratory infections and AMR. *"I think at a time when people are feeling the pinch, they're very happy for messages that crossed over several goals, really."* Stakeholder 6 (**Reinforcement**)	Care home staff felt pressured by GP staff to use and report dipstick results for suspected UTIs. *"they'll ask if you've done a urine dip, you'll say, yeah, you'll have to tell them what it's showing."* Care home staff 4 (**Social influence**)	One resident described drinking less in order to avoid urinating at night. *"because I keep going at night. Which isn't right . . . I'm not drinking more. I hopefully am drinking less."* Care home resident 2 (**Goals**)
Implementation	Some clinicians feel pressured by care homes to prescribe antibiotics based on a urine dipstick result. *"Sometimes we get a call from the care homes, they dip the urine and if it is positive and then they want antibiotic."* General practice staff 2 (**Social influence**)	Care staff described that residents do not want to drink to avoid visiting the toilet regularly. *"they get worried about drinking too much because they don't want to keep going to the toilet."* Care home staff 7 (**Social influence**)
One OOH practitioner felt that the leaflet would be very difficult to implement in OOH settings. *"so I work in out of hours as well and the, it's not something that I routinely translate across into out of hours ... there are certain things that you have to follow when you do out of hours work."* Nurse practitioner 3 (**Environmental context and resources**)	Some care homes intended to keep using urine dipsticks to identify UTIs. *"Because it's worked for us. It seems to have worked, I think that's the hard thing, because it always has seemed to work that way."* Care home staff 1 (**Intentions**)	**Antibiotics**
CCG stakeholders reported that high turnover of care staff makes implementation difficult. *"It was a two day course and it's like painting the Forth Bridge, due to the turnover. Somebody said to me, what about the rest of (location) and I said, that's a full time job."* Stakeholder 3 (**Environmental context and resources**)		Many general practice staff were prescribing UTI antibiotics over the phone to care home residents. *"in the volume of work it's often, as you quite rightly say it's often over the phone."* GP 1 (**Environmental context and resources**)

Table 1. Cont.

Use and Implementation of the UTI Leaflet	Identifying/Diagnosing a UTI	Managing and/or Treating a UTI
All CCG stakeholders stated that they did not have enough resource to provide education to all care homes and GP practices. "we've got so many care homes I haven't got enough time in the day, as well as 70 odd GP practices." Stakeholder 4 (*Environmental context and resources*) Most general practice staff did not believe it is their role to cascade information to care homes. "if you go to the care homes and you do in care homes one by one it will work very well … Rather than you doing with the GP practice and then you think GP practice will influence the care homes." General practice staff 2 (*Professional role and identity*) One stakeholder suggested that difficulties in implementation in OOH is due to transient staff. "The people who run out of hours say to me, anything that's implemented nationally or best practice, in out of hours is probably 12, 18 months later. Because they work with a bit of a more transient locum population" Stakeholder 3 (*Social influence*) All GP staff expressed the intention to implement or use the leaflet. "I will print it off and I will give, … I definitely will because I do like giving people information … so yeah, that is definitely something I will use." Nurse practitioner 1 (*Intentions*) All CCG stakeholders intended to continue their implementation work of the leaflet and wider complimentary resources. "next year … we're planning to run a day to really train people in how to improve their practice … that's how I really hope to roll it out." Stakeholder 2 (*Intentions*) Commissioner stakeholders stated that they have no way of monitoring leaflet use. "I've got no way of knowing whether they used those leaflets." Stakeholder 3 (*Behavioural regulation*) **Leaflet use** Care staff that had used the leaflet used it as their guide for identifying and managing UTIs. "It's our guide for how we appoint (identify) this UTI." Care home staff 7 (*Environmental context and resources*)	Some care homes intended to stop using urine dipsticks moving forwards. "We feel that if it's not required then it's one less thing that you have to try and get from people." Care home staff 3 (*Intentions*) **Presentation of UTI** Many clinicians expressed that diagnosing UTI in older adults can be very difficult. "often with UTIs, especially in old people … you're not quite sure what's going on … it might be a UTI … they're just given a prescription with no one really finding out what's going on, and it's a nightmare." GP 2 (*Skills*) Some care staff identified that other conditions can present like a UTI. "Some of them will present as if it's a UTI but it's actually constipation." Care home staff 3 (*Knowledge*) Many care home staff expressed that residents will not or are unable to tell them about their symptoms. "A lot of them either don't recognise the symptoms or if you ask them they're going to say yes anyway." Care home staff 7 (*Social influence*) General practice staff stated that care staff sometimes provide vague information. "they say the patient looks a little bit more confused today or a little bit more agitated, it's not unusual, some of the behaviour, but again, that's again vague." General practice staff 2 (*Social influence*) One GP stated that they were mindful that atrophic vaginitis can cause urinary symptoms and present like a UTI. "they've had tummy pain, dysuria, frequency and it's cloudy and they haven't got any itching, then I would treat it as a UTI but … especially in older women, I'm always thinking about have they got atrophic vaginitis, especially if it's a recurrent thing." GP 2 (*Memory, attention and decision processes*)	A few general practice staff reported prescribing antibiotics for UTI as a result of demanding patients. "there is always still that pressure to prescribe. I came here because I've got a urine infection and you are going to prescribe me antibiotics no matter what you think." Nurse practitioner 3 (*Social influence*) Older adults do not mind taking antibiotics as long as it makes them well. "I just want to feel well, and I don't care what I take to feel like me you know." Care home residents 1 (*Goals*) Older adults aware of D-mannose were receptive to trying it as an antibiotic alternative. "I went in and she immediately said I've been looking something up for you and she'd found them, they're expensive but if it's going to work then I'll pay the money." Older adult 3 (*Social influence*) A few general practice staff expressed interest in conducting a UTI antibiotic audit. "Auditing the antibiotic use would be really interesting to do, if we could do that that would be good." General practice staff 1 (*Intentions*) One general practice mentioned auditing their UTI antibiotics. "We've re-audited the antibiotic prescribing … it's kind of improved … my trimethoprim prescribing's halved." General practice staff 3 (*Behavioural regulation*) **Perceived role in UTI management** Care staff and general practice staff were confident in their ability to manage diagnosed UTI. (*Beliefs about capabilities*) All care staff reported changing soiled incontinence pads immediately, even if the resident has a limited pad allowance. "So, the residents are restricted on how many day or night pads that they're assessed or allocated but if we find a resident that is soiled or their pad is wet we automatically change it." Care home staff 5 (*Environmental context and resources*)

Table 1. *Cont.*

Use and Implementation of the UTI Leaflet	Identifying/Diagnosing a UTI	Managing and/or Treating a UTI
The general practice staff using the leaflet tended to also use PHE's national diagnostic and treatment guidelines, or their own adapted version of the guideline as a complementary resource. *"We've all got, the flowcharts we've got them all in colour, they're laminated, they're in all the rooms."* Nurse practitioner 2 (*Environmental context and resources*) One practitioner would not use the leaflet with the over 85s as they feel it could be too much for some. *"it's knowing your patient well enough to think, is this going to add to my consultation or actually are we just better off talking very, very simply and having that as a conversation . . . rather than saying here's some information which backs up what we've talked about. I would spend more time with that older patient so that they feel more comfortable in knowing that information."* Nurse practitioner 3 (*Memory, attention and decision processes*) Two older adults passed the leaflet on to friends and family. *"What I've done is, I've photocopied yours . . . just to give to my daughters because this sort of information is invaluable."* Older adult 1 (*Intentions*) **Accessibility** General practice staff would like the leaflet to be made available electronically and in hard copy to suit their preferences for dissemination, as some prefer texting or emailing leaflets whereas others prefer providing hard copies. *"So, bits of paper get lost in piles but if you've got it electronically, so you can print it off or text it to them, it's easier."* GP 2, telephone interview (*Environmental context and resources*) **Attitudes and intentions** All care staff believed the leaflet will be a useful tool to help staff and relatives identify and manage UTIs. *"I think that might help the relatives understand a little bit more."* Care home staff 3 (*Environmental context and resources*)	**Urine samples for culture** Care staff expressed difficulty in obtaining urine samples, especially if the patient is incontinent or has dementia. *"you try and get a urine sample but that's normally fairly tricky because either they use continence aids . . . Or they'll go to the toilet and then you'll have faeces with the sample."* Care home staff 3 (*Skills*) A few GPs used urine culture results as a diagnostic tool. *"I'm not going to start antibiotics until I have obvious MSU showing there is an infection or not."* General practice staff 2 (*Knowledge*) **Facilitators** Some practices had developed their own diagnostic template to aid UTI diagnosis. *"So we developed this system on protocol which we've not used before, for clinical staff to use like a prompt and help decision making processes."* General practice staff 1 (*Environmental context and resources*) All care staff were confident in their ability to identify early signs of illness. *"We're fairly observant of the symptoms and quite good at noticing changes in people and when they might be unwell."* Care home staff 2 (*Beliefs about capabilities*)	

Table 1. *Cont.*

Use and Implementation of the UTI Leaflet	Identifying/Diagnosing a UTI	Managing and/or Treating a UTI
All older adults believed the leaflet would help with the identification and management of UTIs better. *"I read the leaflet and yes, it's very helpful ... when I looked at the worsening signs of urine infection I've had all those when it's been at its worst and I think people should know what it is and what to expect."* Older adult 3 (**Beliefs about consequences**) Most older adults felt that the leaflet would benefit younger adults too. *"it's not just for older people, is it? I mean it's for, a lot of young people get it as well. So why is it targeted to older people?"* Older adult 2 (**Beliefs about consequences**) One stakeholder believed that the leaflet would reduce the demand for antibiotics. *"one thing that I kept hearing was about GPs feeling pressured by patients for antibiotics. So, what I think .... it will really impact on how health professionals manage and therefore then that will have a knock on."* Stakeholder 1 (**Beliefs about consequences**) Some general practice staff reported that their overall goal was quality improvement. *"the thing is quality improvement ... there's no point in doing stuff if you're not actually making a difference or it's going to be useful to you."* General practice staff 1 (**Goals**) A few general practice staff wanted to use the leaflet to educate those bringing in urine samples to reception. *"to have at reception actually ... for the people that don't get as far as the waiting room and they drop in a sample or want to drop in a sample."* General practice staff 3 (**Intentions**) As detailed in 'beliefs about consequences', all older adults were optimistic that the leaflet could have a positive effect on UTI management, but care staff were pessimistic about the utility of the leaflet with many older adults. (**Optimism**)		

2.1.5. Leaflet Interaction with UTI Diagnostic Tools and Other Resources

GP staff reported that they mostly used the leaflet alongside either PHE or locally developed UTI diagnostic tools as part of quality improvement initiatives within general practice. Some reported that quality improvement was their overall goal.

One stakeholder was optimistic that their work in implementing UTI training, leaflet use and diagnostic guidance had reduced the number of unrequested urines being submitted by patients to several GP practices in their region.

2.1.6. Indications of Behaviour Change Following Use or Implementation of the Leaflet

All commissioners intend to continue their promotion of the leaflet alongside the diagnostic flow charts within their local UTI or infection prevention campaigns.

Care staff are motivated by wanting the best for their residents and improving their wellbeing, and they reported consistent use of genital hygiene and hydration strategies as prevention methods with all residents. Barriers, reported by older adults and care staff, to implementing these prevention strategies for older adults included reluctance to drink in order to avoid regular toilet visits and limited incontinence pad allowance, although care homes also reported buying additional pads to supplement their allocations. One stated: *"because I keep going at night. Which isn't right . . . I'm not drinking more. I hopefully am drinking less."* Care home resident 2

Some care staff intended to cease use of urine dipsticks moving forwards. However, some care staff intended to continue using them and a few GPs were using urine culture to inform diagnostic decision making; dipsticking and culture were perpetuated by unrequested urine samples being dropped off at general practice receptions and perceived pressure from care staff to use urine dipsticks. One stakeholder had reduced unrequested urine submissions in several GP practices in their region through the combined use of training and implementation of the leaflet and diagnostic guidance.

Care staff reported being confident in their ability to identify changes in resident behaviour which indicated illness, but had some difficulty in distinguishing UTIs from other illnesses due to similar presentations. However, despite the leaflet providing signs and symptoms of UTI alongside other causes of confusion, clinicians reported that they had difficulty in diagnosing UTI in patients with dementia. Most clinicians reported that diagnosis of UTI was complicated by atypical presentations, vague symptoms reported by carers, incontinence and other conditions presenting like a UTI. Therefore, clinicians requested further information and resource to support diagnosis in this group.

2.1.7. Key Findings and the Theoretical Domains Framework

To identify important behavioural determinants and using a deductive approach, key themes were placed into the corresponding 14 domains of the TDF listed in Box 1. The first key theme, 'Use and implementation of the UTI leaflet', addresses objectives 1–5 in order to determine the leaflet's acceptability, the feasibility of its use, perceived value, interaction with other resources, barriers to using the leaflet and potential further developments to the leaflet. The second and third key themes(Identifying/diagnosing a UTI' and 'Managing and/or treating a UTI) address objective 6, which explores potential indications of behaviour change by examining current behaviours around UTI diagnosis and management. This process is illustrated in Table 1, with each of the three themes used as column headings.

Box 1. The domains of the Theoretical Domains Framework.

The 14 domains of the Theoretical Domains Framework
1. Knowledge
2. Skills
3. Social/professional role and identity
4. Beliefs about capabilities
5. Optimism
6. Beliefs about Consequences
7. Reinforcement
8. Intentions
9. Goals
10. Memory, attention and decision processes
11. Environmental context and resources
12. Social influences
13. Emotion
14. Behavioural regulation

3. Discussion

3.1. Summary

All participants including care staff, general practice staff, older adults and stakeholders reported that the leaflet is a valuable IPC tool, suitable for care homes and general practice, that can be used alongside diagnostic tools and antibiotic guidance, reinforcing messages to older adults while also providing a useful guide for care staff. Participants believed that younger adults would benefit from the leaflet and it should be provided in other health settings.

Participants provided valuable suggestions for dissemination, such as a provision to families and friends, and placement in clinical waiting rooms, reception areas and next to urine submission boxes.

Lack of awareness of the leaflet was the biggest barrier to its use, and implementation barriers prohibited commissioners from effective dissemination. Suggested changes to the leaflet included use of less alarmist terminology, the inclusion of three-day antibiotic courses, the inclusion of D-mannose, and mention of atrophic vaginitis.

Commissioners reported that they would continue to promote the leaflet locally and some care staff would cease use of urine dipsticks moving forwards. Barriers to preventing UTI which are not easily addressed by the leaflet include difficulties in diagnosing UTI in older adults with dementia, and reluctance by older adults to hydrate sufficiently to help reduce their toilet visits.

3.2. Comparison with Existing Literature

Patient information leaflets on antibiotic prescribing for a variety of conditions have led to reductions in antibiotic use [15,16]. However, process evaluation information, such as the acceptability and feasibility of the patient information leaflets, is rarely reported. In a systematic review of leaflet effectiveness [15], many studies only report clinical outcomes, and are therefore limited by not assessing patient acceptability or feasibility of use in real-world settings outside of controlled trial conditions.

To the best of our knowledge, there have not been any leaflets developed for older adults on the topic of UTI, and therefore drawing comparisons across different leaflets, audiences and conditions was inherently difficult. A qualitative study evaluating an interactive information booklet for parents of young children with respiratory symptoms 'When should I worry?' explored the views and opinions of parents and clinicians as part of a trial measuring the booklet's effectiveness [17]. Francis et al. found that parents and clinicians valued the leaflet and many parents had kept the booklet for future references. They concluded that the role of leaflets and other information resources can help facilitate effective communication, and indeed, the link between effective communication of health information with clinical outcomes is well documented [18]. Despite some similarities to the present study, these findings must be accepted with caution as leaflets can vary in content and quality, and therefore perceived value will vary.

A qualitative study exploring patient views of medication information leaflets found that leaflet font size, paper quality, writing style and size of the paper are important factors for enhancing readability [19]. We addressed these design parameters iteratively during the development of the UTI leaflet, which may explain why there were few criticisms relating to its aesthetics [20].

A similar study by Fleming, et al. [21] explored antibiotic prescribing in long-term care facilities using the TDF and Behaviour Change Wheel (BCW), and recommended the provision of education on the topic of antibiotics, prescribing guidelines and AMR, with the provision of management guidelines and supporting evidence. Even though Fleming et al. [21] explored general antibiotic prescribing across conditions without a UTI focus, a similar recommendation from this study included the provision of education for care homes on UTI diagnosis, management and ASB. The current study further supports the need for additional resources in care homes, specifically around UTI education and the provision of guidance on ASB, diagnosis of UTI and urine dipstick use. Using urine dipsticks to diagnose UTI in older adults is not accurate due to high rates of ASB [22–24]. GP staff reported using the leaflet as part of quality improvement programmes. The leaflet compliments the To Dip or Not To Dip (TDONTD) [8] quality improvement programmes that aim to improve the diagnosis and management of UTI in older patients. Regional evaluations of TDONTD have found significant reductions in UTI antibiotics prescribed in care home residents, unplanned hospital admissions, urosepsis and acute kidney injury [8].

3.3. Strengths and Limitations

This is the first study to explore the acceptability and feasibility of a patient-facing evidence-based UTI leaflet for older adults and their carers in the community, including in care home settings. This study offers valuable insight into implementation and attitudes towards the leaflet as well as current diagnostic and management practices across both settings. To the best of our knowledge, in the UK, there is currently no nationally available patient-facing information leaflets for older adults on the topic of UTI, and there are no evaluation studies assessing acceptability and feasibility, or implementation of patient-facing resources on UTIs for any age group.

The present study included a large number of participants from a range of backgrounds. However, care staff and general practice staff may have had greater interest in UTIs, leading to some selection bias. Selection bias was reduced by inviting care homes and GP practices from two regions, approaching potential participants in random order [25] and by providing an incentive to participate. Our findings indicate a wide variation in management and use of the tools, which indicates that selection bias was minimised. However, many participants had not used or seen the leaflet before and were viewing it for the first time as part of this study. This suggests that either implementation strategies by the CCGs could be improved, or that more time was needed between initial leaflet implementation and participant recruitment [26].

A further sample limitation is that only adults with full capacity were approached to take part, and therefore only older adults who could read and understand the leaflet took part, and no data were captured for those older adults deemed unsuitable to receive the leaflet due to the content being 'overwhelming'. Insights from this group may have proved useful for informing improvements to the leaflet or informing the development of a new leaflet.

Qualitative methodology was employed to gain detailed insight into leaflet use and how it contributes to identifying, managing and preventing UTIs. Using both interviews and focus groups facilitated recruitment as participants could choose the format to suit their preference, and use of both provided breadth of exploration across many individuals, and in-depth exploration with individual experiences and attitudes [27].

3.4. Implications

As the older adult UTI leaflet was reported as "invaluable" by patients and carers, GP staff and CCGs reported that they would continue to implement the leaflet "as a guide for patients and carers to help identify and manage UTIs". We suggest that it should be made available in both electronic and hard-copy formats to suit users' preferences, as part of a quality improvement program to advance the management of UTIs. However, due to reported implementation barriers, commissioners may want to consider electronic dissemination as an inexpensive and potentially easier method of promotion to care homes and general practices. This could include use of QR codes or integration into GP clinical systems for ease of access including use of computer prompts as reminders.

Following minor changes to terminology, and the inclusion of information about a three-day antibiotic course, D-mannose and vaginal atrophy, the leaflet will correspond to the current PHE UTI diagnostic flowcharts and NICE/PHE UTI guidance information [28,29] and should therefore be disseminated in care homes as an educational guide to staff. The leaflets should also be disseminated to older adult care home residents of any age. However, where residents lack capacity or may find the leaflet overwhelming, the leaflet could be given to families and friends of residents to provide education and to reinforce health behaviour messages from staff around hydration, self-care and prevention.

General practices should consider the provision of the leaflet as a waiting room resource or to be given/emailed to patients during or following consultations, or to be given at reception to educate patients bringing in urine samples. Primary care clinicians using the PHE diagnostic flow charts may also want to consider the leaflet as a complementary triaging resource to reinforce and communicate their diagnostic decisions with patients.

As weak working relationships between care homes and general practices could be a contributing factor to lack of implementation, commissioners should consider promoting the leaflet during training sessions for both care homes and general practices as an infection prevention and control resource. Regional strategies must include plans for widespread dissemination to care homes including monitoring of attendees and non-attenders to training sessions, monitoring of leaflet use with TARGET UTI audits. A greater implementation may be needed in OOH and community pharmacy settings.

National promotional strategies through the RCGP and CAA should be considered to ensure national dissemination. Health Education England has a short video explaining the value of the leaflet and diagnostic flowchart [30].

Currently, there is a separate non-pictorial UTI leaflet for younger adults that has been used in GP and pharmacy settings [31]. As participants reported that the information in the older adult leaflet is relevant to people of all ages and some patients did not relate to the label 'older adults', a combined leaflet may be useful. A combined leaflet has been developed, but further work is needed to evaluate this in primary care settings.

4. Materials and Methods

Study design: This is a cross-sectional qualitative study using interviews and focus groups informed by the TDF [13].

Leaflet implementation: To understand implementation and usage in a real-world setting, PHE researchers were not involved in the implementation of the leaflet. As such, those unfamiliar with the leaflet were still eligible to participate to understand their management of UTIs, their reasons for not having seen/used the leaflet, and their assessment of the leaflet's value. All participants were sent the leaflet alongside the study information form to allow reflection prior to the discussions.

Gloucestershire CCGs' plan for implementing the UTI leaflet included posting the leaflet to all general practices; workshops and educational training on the UTI guidance offered to all care homes and GP practices; a hydration campaign in care homes, promoted using merchandise and a touring marketing bus. The East Kent CCG disseminated the leaflet to all practices and care homes electronically or in hard copy depending on preference. Links practitioners were established in every care home and general practice in East

Kent, who were then offered training on the UTI guidance with the view of disseminating it in their respective settings.

Data collection started after the CCGs had implemented the leaflet in each region for a minimum of four months. Each region aimed to saturate their regions with the leaflet but did not monitor uptake to determine whether this had occurred.

4.1. Participant Selection and Eligibility

General practice staff and care staff were invited from two CCG regions in the UK, Gloucestershire CCG and East Kent CCG, which were selected due to their intentions to disseminate the leaflet and willingness to support the study. To avoid recruiting only AMR enthusiasts, regions were selected based on antibiotic prescribing at a primary care level [32], and individual facility prescribing data were not explored. Region size and regional demographic variation were taken into account as these can impact implementation and health literacy [33]. Stratification by rural/urban allowed for a variance in participant demographics.

Lists were formed of all care homes and general practices in each region. All care homes and general practices were contacted with an introductory letter describing the study, and the vast majority of facilities did not respond to the initial letter—only a minority responded expressing an interest. Each list was then randomised using Excel's RAND function, and two weeks following receipt of the letter, care homes and general practices were contacted in random order with a follow-up telephone call.

In accordance with the Enabling Research In Care Homes (ENRICH) guidelines, care homes considered 'inadequate' in the CQC inspection rating were not selected for this study [34]. This only equated to 3 care homes across both regions.

Managers or the point of contact were asked to disseminate the study information to recruit staff and older adults. Managers/contacts were requested to approach older adults with experience of UTI and who were able to provide informed consent.

Stakeholders were identified using known contacts through PHE and previous engagement with professional societies, with the aim to recruit national representatives of primary care clinicians and care staff, as well as commissioners of primary care services to discuss their implementation and regional strategies.

All participants gave written and verbal consent and were offered £20 in vouchers; staff were offered certificates of participation as well as vouchers.

4.2. Data Collection

General practice staff and care staff were offered interviews or focus groups depending on their preference. Focus groups were conducted in a quiet room provided by the facility and were heterogenous i.e., all job roles were permitted to attend. Interviews were either face to face or via telephone, depending on participant preference. Older adults were offered interviews rather than focus groups, as discussing experiences of UTI could be considered personal. However, three older adults from one care home requested a focus group.

Seventeen interviews were conducted and lasted 13–47 min, and 12 focus groups containing between 3 and 10 individuals lasted for 24–57 min. After each, discussion field notes were made of important topics and non-verbal data. All interviews and focus groups were conducted by one researcher (LJ).

4.3. Interview Schedules

Questions were informed by the TDF [13] and the qualitative findings from the needs assessment to develop the leaflet [6].

The schedules were semi-structured and used flexibly (see Supplementary Material 3). Interviews and focus groups with general practice staff and care staff covered their leaflet use, and barriers and facilitators to usage. Discussions with older adults explored their experiences of having UTIs, their attitudes and opinions of receiving the leaflet, its content and its perceived usefulness. Interviews with stakeholders focused on organisational barriers or facilitators to implementation. The interview schedules were piloted with 1–2 people from each group, and pilot data were included in the results as no major amendments were made.

The care home managers viewed the older adult interview schedule in order to ensure they were aware of the questions being asked to their residents and identified older adults with sufficient understanding to participate. However, managers were asked to keep schedules confidential to prevent potential priming.

4.4. Data Analysis

Transcripts were analysed by one researcher (LJ) in Nvivo 11 [35] using Inductive Thematic Analysis (ITA). Following ITA, a deductive approach was adopted by placing key themes into the domains of the TDF to identify important behavioural determinants. A double coder (PD) coded 10% (3) of the transcripts.

4.5. Researcher Context

The primary investigator, LJ, has previous experience of using the TDF, conducting research in this area with care staff, GP staff, and older adults as part of the leaflet development work. Researcher bias in this study has been mitigated by utilising patient input into the interview schedule development, use of a double coder and by presenting the results to both regions and receiving their feedback.

5. Conclusions

This novel study has provided insights into the acceptability and feasibility of using the UTI leaflet for older adults and their carers in general practice and care home settings, including current diagnostic and management practices, variation in implementation, and barriers and facilitators. Consequently, this study highlights the ways in which the leaflet has influenced recognition and treatment behaviours, and also ways to improve the leaflet, implications for successful implementation, and suggestions for ways in which new interventions could overcome the barriers to appropriate UTI diagnosis and management. A combination of new complementary interventions, and improvements to the leaflet and its implementation will be needed in order to further influence behaviour change in this context.

Supplementary Materials: The following are available online at https://www.mdpi.com/2079-6382/10/1/83/s1, Supplementary Material 1: The leaflet 'urinary tract infections; a leaflet for older adults and carers'; Supplementary Material 2: Final recruitment strategy and figures; Supplementary Material 3: Interview schedules

Author Contributions: Conceptualisation, L.F.J. and C.M.; methodology, L.F.J.; formal analysis, L.F.J. and P.D.; investigation, L.F.J.; writing—original draft preparation, L.F.J.; writing—review and editing, H.W., D.H., D.M.L. and C.M.; supervision, H.W., D.H., D.M.L. and C.M.; project administration, L.F.J. All authors have read and agreed to the published version of the manuscript.

Funding: This research received no external funding.

Institutional Review Board Statement: The study was conducted according to the guidelines of the Declaration of Helsinki, and approved by the Ethics Committee of the University of the West of England (UWE REC REF No: HAS.18.10.042 Jones).

Informed Consent Statement: Informed consent was obtained from all subjects involved in the study.

Data Availability Statement: The anonymised data presented in this study are available on request from the corresponding author. The data are not publicly available due to the sensitive nature of the topic.

Acknowledgments: Thank you to Julie Brooke who helped with recruitment and to the local commissioning teams in Gloucestershire and East Kent, especially Leslie MacLeod-Downes and Esther

Taborn who supported this work, and the care staff, general practice staff, older adults and stakeholders who contributed valuable insights.

Conflicts of Interest: L.F.J., P.D., D.M.L. and C.M. work on Public Health England's TARGET Antibiotics programme of work, developing and evaluating antimicrobial stewardship interventions.

References

1. Genao, L.; Buhr, G.T. Urinary tract infections in older adults residing in long-term care facilities. *Ann. Longterm Care* **2012**, *20*, 33–38. [PubMed]
2. Public Health England, Annual Epidemiological Commentary: Gram-Negative, MRSA and MSSA Bacteraemia and C. Difficile Infection Data, Up to and Including Financial Year April 2018 to March 2019. 2019. Available online: https://www.gov.uk/government/statistics/mrsa-mssa-and-e-coli-bacteraemia-and-c-difficile-infection-annual-epidemiological-commentary (accessed on 15 January 2021).
3. Public Health England, Health Protection Report; Infection Report, 17 June 2016. 2016. Available online: https://www.gov.uk/government/publications/health-protection-report-volume-10-2016 (accessed on 15 January 2021).
4. Abernethy, J.; Guy, R.; Sheridan, E.A.; Hopkins, S.; Kiernan, M.; Wilcox, M.H.; Johnson, A.P.; Hope, R. Epidemiology of *Escherichia coli* bacteraemia in England: Results of an enhanced sentinel surveillance programme. *J. Hosp. Infect.* **2017**, *95*, 365–375. [CrossRef] [PubMed]
5. Nicolle, L.E. Asymptomatic bacteriuria in older adults. *Curr. Geriatr. Rep.* **2016**, *5*, 1–8. [CrossRef]
6. Jones, L.F.; Cooper, E.; Joseph, A.; Allison, R.; Gold, N.; Donald, I.; CAM, M. Development of an information leaflet and diagnostic flow chart to improve the management of urinary tract infections in older adults; A qualitative study using the theoretical domains framework. *BJGP Open* **2020**. [CrossRef]
7. Flokas, M.E.; Andreatos, N.; Alevizakos, M.; Kalbasi, A.; Onur, P.; Mylonakis, E. Inappropriate management of asymptomatic patients with positive urine cultures: A systematic review and meta-analysis. *Open Forum Infect. Dis.* **2017**, *4*, 207. [CrossRef]
8. NHS Nottingham. To dip or not to dip—A patient centred approach to improve the management of UTI in the Care Home environment. In Proceedings of the 2017 Federation of Infection Societies Conference, Birmingham, UK, 30 November–2 December 2017.
9. Macfarlane, J.; Holmes, W.; Gard, P.; Thornhill, D.; Macfarlane, R.; Hubbard, R. Reducing antibiotic use for acute bronchitis in primary care: Blinded, randomised controlled trial of patient information leaflet. *Br. Med. J.* **2002**, *324*, 91–94. [CrossRef]
10. Moerenhout, T.; Borgermans, L.; Schol, S.; Vansintejan, J.; Van De Vijver, E.; Devroey, D. Patient health information materials in waiting rooms of family physicians: Do patients care? *Patient Prefer. Adher.* **2013**, *7*, 489–497.
11. Humphris, G.M.; Field, E.A. The immediate effect on knowledge, attitudes and intentions in primary care attenders of a patient information leaflet: A randomized control trial replication and extension. *Br. Dent. J.* **2003**, *194*, 683–688. [CrossRef]
12. Public Health England. UTI Resources Suite. Available online: http://www.rcgp.org.uk/targetantibiotics (accessed on 1 October 2018).
13. Cane, J.; O'Connor, D.; Michie, S. Validation of the theoretical domains framework for use in behaviour change and implementation research. *Implement. Sci.* **2012**, *7*. [CrossRef]
14. Atkins, L.; Francis, J.; Islam, R.; O'Connor, D.; Patey, A.; Ivers, N.; Foy, R.; Duncan, E.M.; Colquhoun, H.; Grimshaw, J.M.; et al. A guide to using the theoretical domains framework of behaviour change to investigate implementation problems. *Implement. Sci.* **2017**, *12*, 77. [CrossRef]
15. De Bont, E.G.; Alink, M.; Falkenberg, F.C.; Dinant, G.J.; Cals, J.W. Patient information leaflets to reduce antibiotic use and reconsultation rates in general practice: A systematic review. *BMJ Open* **2015**, *5*. [CrossRef] [PubMed]
16. Sustersic, M.; Gauchet, A.; Foote, A.; Bosson, J.L. How best to use and evaluate Patient Information Leaflets given during a consultation: A systematic review of literature reviews. *Health Expect.* **2017**, *20*, 531–542. [CrossRef] [PubMed]
17. Francis, N.A.; Phillips, R.; Wood, F.; Hood, K.; Simpson, S.; Butler, C.C. Parents' and clinicians' views of an interactive booklet about respiratory tract infections in children: A qualitative process evaluation of the EQUIP randomised controlled trial. *BMC Fam. Pract.* **2013**, *14*, 1. [CrossRef] [PubMed]
18. Mikesell, L. Medicinal relationships: Caring conversation. *Med. Educ.* **2013**, *47*, 443–452. [CrossRef] [PubMed]
19. Poplas-Susič, T.; Klemenc-Ketis, Z.; Kersnik, J. Usefulness of the patient information leaflet (PIL) and information on medicines from professionals: A patients' view. a qualitative study. *Zdr. Vestn.* **2014**, *83*, 368–375.
20. Jones, L.F.; Cooper, E.; McNulty, C. Urinary tract infections (UTIs); a leaflet for older adults, and carers: The development of a UTI leaflet for older adults and their carers. *Br. J. Gen. Pract.* **2018**, *68*. [CrossRef]
21. Fleming, A.; Bradley, C.; Cullinan, S.; Byrne, S. Antibiotic prescribing in long-term care facilities: A qualitative, multidisciplinary investigation. *BMJ Open* **2014**, *4*, e006442. [CrossRef]
22. Nicolle, L. Symptomatic urinary tract infection or asymptomatic bacteriuria? Improving care for the elderly. *Clin. Microbiol. Infect.* **2019**, *25*, 779–781. [CrossRef]
23. Nicolle, L.E. Asymptomatic bacteriuria in institutionalized elderly people: Evidence and practice. *Can. Med. Assoc. J.* **2000**, *163*, 285.
24. Nicolle, L.E. Asymptomatic bacteriuria. *Curr. Opin. Infect. Dis.* **2014**, *27*, 90–96. [CrossRef]

25. Guest, G.; Namey, E.E.; Mitchell, M.L. Chapter 2: Sampling in qualitative research. In *Collecting Qualitative Data: A Field Manual for Applied Research*; SAGE Publications: New York, NY, USA, 2013.
26. Rogers, E.M. *Diffusion of Innovations*; Simon and Schuster: New York, NY, USA, 2010.
27. Bauer, M.; Gaskell, G. Individual and group interviewing. In *Qualitative Researching with Text, Image and Sound*; Sage Publications: New York, NY, USA, 2000; pp. 39–56.
28. Public Health England. *Diagnosis of Urinary Tract Infections Quick Reference Tool for Primary Care: For Consultation and Local Adaptation*; Public Health England: London, UK, 2018.
29. National Institute for Health and Care Excellence. *Urinary Tract Infection (Lower): Antimicrobial Prescribing*; Public Health England: London, UK, 2018.
30. Health Education England. Antimicrobial Resistance and Infections. Available online: https://www.e-lfh.org.uk/programmes/antimicrobial-resistance-and-infections/ (accessed on 24 November 2020).
31. Lecky, D.M.; Howdle, J.; Butler, C.; McNulty, C.A.M. Women's and general practitionersx experiences and expectations of the consultation for symptoms of uncomplicated urinary tract infection—A qualitative study informing the development of an evidence based, shared decision-making resource. *Br. J. Gen. Pract.* **2020**. [CrossRef]
32. Public Health England. Public Health Profiles. Available online: http://fingertips.phe.org.uk/ (accessed on 24 November 2020).
33. UCL Institute of Health Equity. *Local Action on Health Inequalities; Improving Health Literacy to Reduce Health Inequalities*; Public Health England: London, UK, 2015.
34. ENRICH—Enabling Research in Care Homes Practical Advice. Available online: http://enrich.nihr.ac.uk/page/practical-advice (accessed on 31 May 2017).
35. QSR International Pty Ltd. NVivo Qualitative Data Analysis Software. 2012. Available online: https://www.qsrinternational.com/nvivo-qualitative-data-analysis-software/home (accessed on 24 November 2020).

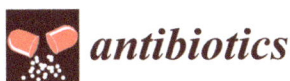

Article

Risk Factors for the Acquisition of *Enterococcus faecium* Infection and Mortality in Patients with Enterococcal Bacteremia: A 5-Year Retrospective Analysis in a Tertiary Care University Hospital

Atsushi Uda [1,2,*], Katsumi Shigemura [1,3,4], Koichi Kitagawa [3,5], Kayo Osawa [6], Kenichiro Onuma [1,7], Yonmin Yan [4], Tatsuya Nishioka [2], Masato Fujisawa [4], Ikuko Yano [2] and Takayuki Miyara [1]

[1] Department of Infection Control and Prevention, Kobe University Hospital, Kobe 650-0017, Japan; katsumi@med.kobe-u.ac.jp (K.S.); onumak@med.kobe-u.ac.jp (K.O.); miyarat@med.kobe-u.ac.jp (T.M.)
[2] Department of Pharmacy, Kobe University Hospital, Kobe 650-0017, Japan; tnishi@med.kobe-u.ac.jp (T.N.); iyano@med.kobe-u.ac.jp (I.Y.)
[3] Division of Infectious Diseases, Department of Public Health, Kobe University Graduate School of Health Sciences, Kobe 654-0142, Japan; ko1.kitgwa@gmail.com
[4] Division of Urology, Kobe University Graduate School of Medicine, Kobe 650-0017, Japan; yym1112@gmail.com (Y.Y.); masato@med.kobe-u.ac.jp (M.F.)
[5] Division of Advanced Medical Science, Kobe University Graduate School of Science, Technology and Innovation, Kobe 657-8501, Japan
[6] Department of Medical Technology, Kobe Tokiwa University, Kobe 653-0838, Japan; osawak@kobe-u.ac.jp
[7] Department of Clinical Laboratory, Kobe University Hospital, Kobe 650-0017, Japan
* Correspondence: a-uda@umin.ac.jp; Tel.: +81-78-382-5111; Fax: +81-78-382-6611

Citation: Uda, A.; Shigemura, K.; Kitagawa, K.; Osawa, K.; Onuma, K.; Yan, Y.; Nishioka, T.; Fujisawa, M.; Yano, I.; Miyara, T. Risk Factors for the Acquisition of *Enterococcus faecium* Infection and Mortality in Patients with Enterococcal Bacteremia: A 5-Year Retrospective Analysis in a Tertiary Care University Hospital. *Antibiotics* **2021**, *10*, 64. https://doi.org/10.3390/antibiotics10010064

Received: 12 December 2020
Accepted: 7 January 2021
Published: 11 January 2021

Publisher's Note: MDPI stays neutral with regard to jurisdictional claims in published maps and institutional affiliations.

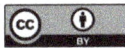

Copyright: © 2021 by the authors. Licensee MDPI, Basel, Switzerland. This article is an open access article distributed under the terms and conditions of the Creative Commons Attribution (CC BY) license (https://creativecommons.org/licenses/by/4.0/).

Abstract: The incidence of bacteremia caused by *Enterococcus faecium*, which is highly resistant to multiple antibiotics, is increasing in Japan. However, risk factors for the acquisition of *E. faecium* infection and mortality due to enterococcal bacteremia are not well known. We compared demographic, microbiological, and clinical characteristics using a Cox regression model and univariate analysis. We performed a multivariate analysis to identify risk factors for patients treated between 2014 and 2018. Among 186 patients with enterococcal bacteremia, two groups included in the Kaplan–Meier analysis (*E. faecalis* (n = 88) and *E. faecium* (n = 94)) showed poor overall survival in the *E. faecium* group (HR: 1.92; 95% confidence interval: 1.01–3.66; $p = 0.048$). The median daily antibiotic cost per patient in the *E. faecium* group was significantly higher than that in the *E. faecalis* group ($23 ($13–$34) vs. $34 ($22–$58), $p < 0.001$). *E. faecium* strains were more frequently identified with previous use of antipseudomonal penicillins (OR = 4.04, $p < 0.001$) and carbapenems (OR = 3.33, $p = 0.003$). Bacteremia from an unknown source (OR = 2.79, $p = 0.025$) and acute kidney injury (OR = 4.51, $p = 0.004$) were associated with higher risks of 30-day mortality in patients with enterococcal bacteremia. Therefore, clinicians should provide improved medical management, with support from specialized teams such as those assisting antimicrobial stewardship programs.

Keywords: enterococcal; bacteremia; epidemiology; risk factors; mortality; antimicrobial stewardship

1. Introduction

Enterococcus species are Gram-positive, facultative anaerobic cocci that constitute the normal bacterial flora in human and animal intestines. Enterococcal bacteremia is associated with a high mortality rate and prolonged hospitalization [1–3]. *Enterococcus faecalis*, followed by *E. faecium* are the most frequent *Enterococcal* species that cause bacteremia [4]. *Enterococcus* species are intrinsically cephalosporins-resistant, which inhibit bacterial cell wall synthesis. Primarily, infections caused by vancomycin-resistant enterococci are associated with higher mortality and are a major problem in the United States and Western countries [3,5,6]. However, the prevalence of vancomycin-resistant *Enterococcus* infections in Japan is markedly lower than that in other countries [4,7,8]. In contrast, most *E. faecalis* are susceptible to penicillins, although *E. faecium* tends to have resistance to some antimicrobial agents, including penicillins, aminoglycosides, and carbapenems [4]. The hospital cost and mortality for patients with multidrug-resistant pathogens were higher than those with antimicrobial-susceptible pathogens [9–11]. Many studies have reported that previous use of broad-spectrum antibiotics is a risk factor for acquiring the multidrug-resistant pathogens [12–14]; however, few studies have been done to identify the correlation between the previous antibiotic exposure and the acquisition of *E. faecium* strains [15]. In the United States and Western countries, the enterococcal isolates of *E. faecalis* (80–90%) and *E. faecium* (5–20%) [8,16] are considerably different than those in Japan (*E. faecium* strains account for 40%) [4]. Although there are many studies on enterococcal bacteremia, the clinical outcomes, epidemiological features, and risk factors for nosocomial infection produced different results depending on the country, hospitalization ward, or patient characteristics. Only few studies have described the situation in Japan [17,18], and the conclusions are inconsistent. Therefore, we aimed to investigate the clinico-epidemiological features and risk factors predisposing to the acquisition of *E. faecium* strains and mortality due to nosocomial enterococcal bacteremia.

2. Results

2.1. Patient Data

During the 5-year study period (2014–2018), 186 patients had bacteremia caused by *Enterococcus* species. The most common *Enterococcus* species were *E. faecium* (n = 94, 51%), followed by *E. faecalis* (n = 88, 47%), *E. avium* (n = 1, 0.5%), *E. casseliflavus* (n = 1, 0.5%), *E. raffinosus* (n = 1, 0.5%), and *E. gallinarum* (n = 1, 0.5%). As few patients had bacteremia caused by *E. avium*, *E. casseliflavus*, *E. raffinosus*, and *E. gallinarum*, only the clinical characteristics of bacteremia with *E. faecalis* and *E. faecium* were further investigated among two subgroups. After excluding four cases of bacteremia caused by strains other than *E. faecalis* or *E. faecium*, 182 patients were eligible for inclusion in this study. The survival rates for both study groups are shown in the Kaplan–Meier curves in Figure 1, showing a significant decrease in overall survival rates among the patients with *E. faecium* bacteremia (hazard ratio (HR): 1.92; 95% confidence interval (CI): 1.01–3.66; p = 0.048).

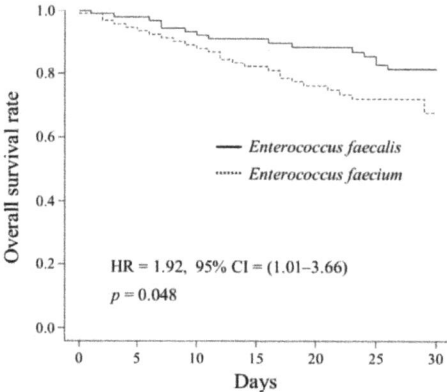

Figure 1. Kaplan–Meier survival curves of patients with *E. faecalis* and *E. faecium* bacteremia.

2.2. Demographic and Clinical Characteristics

The demographic and clinical characteristics of the study participants are shown in Table 1. There was no significant difference between groups regarding sex, age, hospitalization ward, length of hospitalization before the onset of bacteremia, quick Sequential Organ Failure Assessment (qSOFA) score $\geq$ 2, use of invasive devices, or surgical history. The coexistence of hepatobiliary (p = 0.005) and hematologic (p = 0.027) tumors were more frequently observed in patients with *E. faecium* bacteremia. The most common primary source of infection arose from an insertion of a central venous catheter (n = 41, 23%), followed by cholecystocholangitis (n = 38, 21%), urinary tract infection (n = 18, 9.9%), and intra-abdominal infection (n = 12, 6.6%). *E. faecium* bacteremia originated more frequently from cholecystocholangitis ($p < 0.001$) and febrile neutropenia ($p = 0.015$) than in the *E. faecalis* group. However, the *E. faecalis* group had an unknown source of infection more frequently ($p = 0.041$). The incidence of urinary tract infections was lower in the *E. faecium* group than in the *E. faecalis* group ($p = 0.017$). A history of antibiotic therapy with antipseudomonal penicillins ($p < 0.001$) and carbapenems ($p < 0.001$) was more frequently observed in the *E. faecium* group. Based on the analysis by a logistic regression model, preexisting hematologic tumors (adjusted OR = 7.85, $p = 0.004$), cholecystocholangitis (adjusted OR = 5.21, $p = 0.001$), and previous use of both antipseudomonal penicillins (adjusted OR = 4.04, $p < 0.001$) and carbapenems (adjusted OR = 3.33, $p = 0.003$) were independent risk factors for the acquisition of an *E. faecium* infection.

Table 1. Intergroup comparison of demographic and clinical characteristics of patients with enterococcal bacteremia and risk factors for the acquisition of *E. faecalis* and *E. faecium*.

	E. faecalis (n = 88)	*E. faecium* (n = 94)	p	Adjusted OR (95% CI)	p
Age (years), median (IQR)	73.5 (66–80)	72 (65–75)	0.073		
Male sex, n (%)	53 (60)	54 (58)	0.82		
Hospitalization ward, n (%)					
Medical ward	24 (27)	30 (32)	0.60		
Surgical ward	41 (47)	33 (35)	0.15		
Intensive Care Unit	23 (26)	31 (33)	0.40		
Comorbidities, n (%)					
Chronic renal failure	35 (40)	32 (34)	0.52		
Dialysis	8 (9.1)	10 (11)	0.9		
Diabetes mellitus	21 (24)	18 (19)	0.55		
Cardiovascular disease	23 (26)	12 (13)	0.058		
Previous cardiac valve replacement	11 (13)	9 (9.6)	0.69		
Coronary artery bypass grafting	3 (3.4)	3 (3.2)	0.9		
Hepatobiliary tumor	5 (5.7)	20 (21)	0.005	3.01 (0.87–10.5)	0.083
Other solid tumors	15 (17)	13 (14)	0.69		
Hematologic tumor	3 (3.4)	13 (14)	0.027	7.85 (1.96–31.4)	0.004
Solid organ transplant recipient	1 (1.1)	1 (1.1)	1		
Bone marrow transplant recipient	1 (1.1)	2 (2.1)	1		
Neutropenia	0 (0.0)	9 (9.6)	0.008		
Hepatobiliary disease	6 (6.8)	3 (3.2)	0.43		
Collagen disease	1 (1.1)	10 (11)	0.018	8.41 (0.91–77.7)	0.061
Source of infections, n (%)					
Central venous catheter	18 (21)	23 (25)	0.64		
Cholecystocholangitis	8 (9.1)	30 (32)	<0.001	5.21 (1.89–14.3)	0.001
Urinary tract infection	14 (16)	4 (4.3)	0.017		
Intra-abdominal infection	3 (3.4)	9 (9.6)	0.17		
Febrile neutropenia	0 (0.0)	8 (8.5)	0.015		
Infectious endocarditis	4 (4.6)	0 (0.0)	0.11		
Wound infection	2 (2.3)	1 (1.1)	0.95		
Unknown	24 (27)	14 (15)	0.041		
Others	6 (6.8)	2 (2.1)	0.24		
Hospital stay before the onset of bacteremia (days), median (IQR)	23.5 (8–56.5)	31 (13.3–75.8)	0.13		
qSOFA score $\geq$ 2, n (%)	27 (31)	29 (31)	1		
Recent surgery, n (%)	32 (36)	31 (33)	0.75		
Invasive devices, n (%)					

Table 1. Cont.

	E. faecalis (n = 88)	E. faecium (n = 94)	p	Adjusted OR (95% CI)	p
Central intravenous catheter	39 (44)	50 (53)	0.29		
Urinary catheter	43 (49)	39 (42)	0.40		
Immunosuppression (within 30 days), n (%)					
Immunosuppressive treatment	2 (2.3)	9 (9.6)	0.079		
Corticosteroid treatment	13 (15)	26 (28)	0.053		
Chemotherapy	5 (5.7)	13 (14)	0.11		
Previous antibiotic therapy (within 30 days)					
Non-antipseudomonal penicillins					
Number of patients (%)	16 (18)	27 (29)	0.13		
Duration of use, median (IQR)	6 (3–9)	5 (2.5–8.5)	0.68		
Antipseudomonal penicillins					
Number of patients (%)	14 (16)	42 (45)	<0.001	4.04 (1.81–9.0)	<0.001
Duration of use, median (IQR)	7 (4.3–9.5)	6 (4–8)	0.89		
Cephalosporins					
Number of patients (%)	51 (58)	53 (56)	0.95		
Duration of use, median (IQR)	5 (3–7)	5 (2–10)	1		
Carbapenems					
Number of patients (%)	16 (18)	42 (45)	<0.001	3.33 (1.51–7.36)	0.003
Duration of use, median (IQR)	7 (3.8–9)	6.5 (4.3–10.8)	0.24		
Quinolones					
Number of patients (%)	9 (10)	19 (20)	0.097		
Duration of use, median (IQR)	4 (4–6)	7 (4–9)	0.69		
Aminoglycosides					
Number of patients (%)	0 (0.0)	3 (3.2)	0.27		
Duration of use, median (IQR)	0 (0–0)	3 (2.5–3.5)	<0.001		
Anti-MRSA agents (VCM)					
Number of patients (%)	15 (17)	28 (30)	0.065		
Duration of use, median (IQR)	5 (2.5–9.5)	4 (2–5.3)	0.26		
Anti-MRSA agents (DAP, LZD)					
Number of patients (%)	6 (6.8)	10 (11)	0.52		
Duration of use, median (IQR)	3.5 (2.3–7)	2.5 (1.3–6)	0.51		

IQR: interquartile range, qSOFA: quick Sequential Organ Failure Assessment, MRSA: methicillin-resistant *Staphylococcus aureus*, VCM: vancomycin, DAP: daptomycin, LZD: linezolid.

2.3. Microbiological Data

Table 2 shows the microbiological characteristics of patients with enterococcal bacteremia. There was no significant intergroup difference in polymicrobial cultures; all isolates of *E. faecalis* and 15% (14/94) strains of *E. faecium* were susceptible to ampicillin. We found no vancomycin-resistant isolates among the enterococci. No imipenem-resistant *E. faecalis* strain was isolated; however, all *E. faecium* isolates were imipenem-resistant. Susceptibility to levofloxacin was detected in 91% (80/88) and 12% (11/94) of *E. faecalis* and *E. faecium* isolates, respectively.

2.4. Clinical Management and Outcomes

Table 3 shows the clinical management and outcomes of patients with bacteremia caused by *E. faecalis* and *E. faecium* infections. The rate of source control with drainage in the *E. faecium* group was ~1.7 times higher than that in the *E. faecalis* group, although the difference was not significant ($p = 0.15$). Non-antipseudomonal penicillins (n = 55, 63%) was the most common antibiotic used for *E. faecalis* bacteremia, whereas vancomycin (n = 74, 79%) was most frequently prescribed in *E. faecium* bacteremia. Compared with the *E. faecium* group, the *E. faecalis* group more frequently received penicillins ($p < 0.001$) and aminoglycosides ($p = 0.031$). Vancomycin ($p < 0.001$) and other anti-methicillin-resistant *Staphylococcus aureus* (MRSA) agents ($p = 0.028$) were more frequently administered in the *E. faecium* group. Non-antipseudomonal penicillins ($p = 0.022$) and quinolones ($p = 0.022$)

were prescribed for longer durations in the E. faecalis group, whereas the median duration of vancomycin use was longer in the E. faecium group ($p < 0.001$). When vancomycin treatment took more than three days, all patients underwent therapeutic drug monitoring. The E. faecalis group showed a shorter median duration to the commencement of initial antibiotic therapy against enterococci ($p = 0.049$), although there was no significant intergroup difference in the total duration of antibiotic treatment ($p = 0.99$). The median daily antibiotic cost per patient in the E. faecium group was significantly higher than that in the E. faecalis group (\$23 [\$13–\$34] vs. \$34 [\$22–\$58], $p < 0.001$). Patients in the E. faecium group more frequently attained a vancomycin median serum trough concentration ≥ 20 mg/L ($p = 0.007$) than in the E. faecalis group. Acute kidney injury (AKI) was observed in both groups but was more frequent in the E. faecium group ($p = 0.02$). The clinical outcome for patients with enterococcal bacteremia was analyzed based on the length of hospitalization; however, no significant between-group difference ($p = 0.34$) was observed.

Table 2. Microbiological characteristics of enterococcal bacteremia.

	E. faecalis (n = 88)	E. faecium (n = 94)	p
Polymicrobial culture, n (%)	22 (25)	29 (31)	0.48
Antibiotic susceptibility, n (%)			
Ampicillin	88 (100)	14 (15)	<0.001
Vancomycin	88 (100)	94 (100)	0.66
Imipenem	88 (100)	0 (0.0)	<0.001
Levofloxacin	80 (91)	11 (12)	<0.001

Table 3. Clinical treatments and outcomes of patients with enterococcal bacteremia.

	E. faecalis (n = 88)	E. faecium (n = 94)	p
Source control with drainage, n (%)	13 (15)	23 (25)	0.15
Antibiotic therapy against enterococci			
Non–antipseudomonal penicillins			
Number of patients (%)	55 (63)	4 (4.3)	<0.001
Duration of use, median (IQR)	10 (6–14)	5 (3–8)	0.022
Antipseudomonal penicillins			
Number of patients (%)	25 (28)	1 (1.1)	<0.001
Duration of use, median (IQR)	7 (3–10)	5 (5–5)	0.74
Cephalosporins			
Number of patients (%)	2 (2.3)	2 (2.1)	1
Duration of use, median (IQR)	14 (12–15)	11 (10–12)	0.41
Carbapenems			
Number of patients (%)	2 (2.3)	0 (0.0)	0.16
Duration of use, median (IQR)	11 (9–13)	0 (0–0)	0.74
Quinolones			
Number of patients (%)	4 (4.6)	0 (0.0)	0.046
Duration of use, median (IQR)	9 (7–11)	0 (0–0)	0.022
Aminoglycosides			
Number of patients (%)	6 (6.8)	0 (0.0)	0.031
Duration of use, median (IQR)	14 (11–35)	0 (0–0)	1
Anti–MRSA agent (VCM)			
Number of patients (%)	33 (38)	74 (79)	<0.001
Duration of use, median (IQR)	4 (2–11)	12 (7–16)	<0.001
Anti–MRSA agents (DAP, LZD)			
Number of patients (%)	13 (15)	28 (30)	0.028
Duration of use, median (IQR)	5 (4–15)	4 (3–8)	0.12
Time to antibiotic therapy against enterococci (days), median (IQR)	0 (0–1)	1 (0–1)	0.049
Total duration of antibiotic therapy (days), median (IQR)	14 (8–19.3)	13 (8–17)	0.99
Daily antimicrobial cost ($), median (IQR)	23 (13–34)	34 (22–58)	<0.001
Vancomycin median serum trough concentrations (≥ 20 mg/L), n (%)	5 (5.7)	19 (20)	0.007
AKI after the onset of bacteremia, n (%)	7 (8.0)	20 (21)	0.02
Hospital length after the onset of bacteremia until discharge (days), median (IQR)	33 (14.8–69.5)	29 (15.3–58.5)	0.34

IQR: interquartile range, MRSA: methicillin-resistant *Staphylococcus aureus*, VCM: vancomycin, DAP: daptomycin, LZD: linezolid, AKI: acute kidney injury.

In this study cohort, the overall 30-day mortality rate was 23% (41/182). Table 4 shows the risk factors associated with the overall 30-day mortality in patients with enterococcal bacteremia. Patient groups with variables such as admission to an intensive care unit, an unknown source of infection, qSOFA score ≥ 2, previous immunosuppressive and corticosteroid treatment, or encountered AKI were associated more frequently with 30-day death. These variables were included in the multivariate logistic regression analysis revealing the following independent risk factors for mortality: unknown source of infection (OR = 2.79, p = 0.025), qSOFA score ≥ 2 (OR = 2.96, p = 0.024), previous corticosteroid treatment (OR = 2.84, p = 0.034), and AKI (OR = 4.51, p = 0.004).

Table 4. Risk factors that were associated with 30-day mortality due to enterococcal bacteremia.

	Survived (n = 141)	Died (n = 41)	p	Adjusted OR (95% CI)	p
Admission to intensive care unit, n (%)	32 (23)	22 (54)	<0.001	1.65 (0.61–4.47)	0.33
Comorbidities at bacteremia, n (%)					
Chronic renal failure	52 (37)	18 (44)	0.38		
Dialysis	16 (11)	3 (7.3)	0.74		
Diabetes mellitus	27 (19)	9 (22)	0.46		
Cardiovascular disease	19 (14)	6 (15)	0.54		
Cardiac valve replacement	11 (7.8)	8 (20)	0.089		
Source of infections, n (%)					
Central venous catheter	34 (25)	7 (17)	0.003		
Cholecystocholangitis	29 (21)	9 (22)	1		
Unknown	24 (17)	16 (39)	0.014	2.79 (1.14–6.85)	0.025
Hospital stay before the onset of bacteremia (days), median (IQR)	25 (10–55)	39 (14–80)	0.16		
qSOFA score ≥ 2 at bacteremia, n (%)	33 (23)	23 (56)	<0.001	2.96 (1.15–7.62)	0.024
Previous immunosuppression (within 30 days), n (%)					
Immunosuppressive treatment	5 (3.6)	6 (15)	0.024	2.31 (0.46–11.5)	0.31
Corticosteroid treatment	24 (17)	15 (37)	0.014	2.84 (1.08–7.46)	0.034
Chemotherapy	16 (11)	2 (4.9)	0.36		
Acute kidney injury after the onset of bacteremia, n (%)	15 (11)	12 (29)	<0.001	4.51 (1.61–12.7)	0.004
E. faecium bacteremia, n (%)	67 (48)	27 (66)	0.059		
Antibiotic susceptibility, n (%)					
Ampicillin	57 (40)	24 (59)	0.11		
Imipenem	67 (48)	27 (66)	0.059		
Levofloxacin	65 (46)	26 (63)	0.076		

IQR: interquartile range, qSOFA: quick Sequential Organ Failure Assessment.

3. Discussion

This observational retrospective study analyzed the epidemiological and clinical outcomes of enterococcal bacteremia and evaluated the risk factors for the acquisition of *E. faecium* and *E. faecalis* infection and mortality in enterococcal bacteremia. We found a significant increase in *E. faecium* bacteremia among patients with enterococcal bacteremia, especially those who were previously treated with antipseudomonal penicillins and carbapenems. We also found that severely ill patients, those with an unknown source of infection, and AKI during treatment conferred higher risks of mortality in enterococcal bacteremia. The results of our analyses suggest the need for greater efforts to provide accurate medical treatment, including appropriate antimicrobial use in patients with enterococcal bacteremia.

As a leading cause of nosocomial bacteremia, enterococci have become more prevalent worldwide. In particular, the spread of vancomycin-resistant *Enterococcus* has become a major public health problem in the United States and in Western Europe [3,5,6]. However, we found no vancomycin-resistant strains of enterococci in our hospital during the 5-year study period. *E. faecalis* and *E. faecium* are two major *Enterococcus* species that can cause various complicated infectious diseases [3,4,16] and were the most common strains in our cohort. In agreement with the results of an earlier study [19], we observed significantly lower survival rates with *E. faecium* than with *E. faecalis*, as determined using the Kaplan–Meier survival curves. Furthermore, the *E. faecium* group showed a higher daily antibiotic cost than the *E. faecalis* group. Infections with drug-resistant pathogens are typically associated with increased hospitalization costs [9]. De-escalation therapy to narrower spectrum antibiotics is a cost-saving strategy [20,21]. After bacterial identification, antibiotics should be changed, if needed, to administer appropriate targeted antibiotic therapy in accordance with bacterial culture and susceptibility data. In general, patients infected with enterococcal bacteremia are older and more likely to develop renal failure; thus, less toxic regimens such as penicillins may be preferred. In this study, because all the *E. faecalis* remained susceptible to penicillins, the *E. faecalis* group received narrower spectrum antibiotics, such as non-antipseudomonal penicillins. Whereas the *E. faecium* group, which had a higher resistance to penicillins, was most frequently prescribed vancomycin. Non-antipseudomonal penicillins, which constitute the most prescribed antibiotics in the *E. faecalis* group, were of a lower price in Japan than anti-MRSA agents [22], which resulted in a lower median daily antibiotic cost in the *E. faecalis* group. We demonstrated that *E. faecium* bacteremia caused more serious problems regarding therapeutic outcomes.

Previous studies have focused on risk factors for the acquisition of *E. faecium* infections among various ethnic groups [15,23], but little is known about the risk factors in Japan [17]. In this study, multivariate analysis revealed that the risk factors for bacteremia due to *E. faecium* included preexisting illness (hematologic tumor), source of infection (cholecystocholangitis), and previous use of broad-spectrum antibiotics (antipseudomonal penicillins and carbapenems). For patients with nosocomial or intra-abdominal infections, broad-spectrum antibiotics were often prescribed to treat anaerobic bacteria and Gram-negative bacteria such as *Pseudomonas aeruginosa*. In a previous report, carbapenems were reported as the only independent risk factor associated with *E. faecium* bloodstream infections [15]. However, this study is the first to characterize antipseudomonal penicillins as a predictive risk factor for the acquisition of *E. faecium*. In Japanese national and public university hospitals, the consumption of antipseudomonal penicillins increased five times from 2008 to 2015 [24], and the rates of *E. faecium* among enterococcal bacteremia patients increased from 36% to 43% in the same period [4]. The higher rates of *E. faecium* isolation might correlate with the increased use of antipseudomonal penicillins in Japan. Broad-spectrum antibiotics might destroy the normal anaerobic flora of the gastrointestinal tract by selective elimination of enterococci due to the bactericidal activity against these organisms, which might subsequently induce infectious diseases. A case-control study revealed that broad-spectrum antibiotic therapy, including antipseudomonal penicillins, was a risk factor for *P. aeruginosa* resistance among hospitalized patients [25]. The Infectious Diseases Society of America guidelines recommend the implementation of antibiotic stewardship programs to restrict the prevalence of antimicrobial-resistant pathogens [26]. Overuse of broad-spectrum antibiotics leads to the selective growth of resistant bacteria; thus, one of the aims of antimicrobial stewardship is to promote appropriate antibiotic use. Our hospital has practiced antimicrobial stewardship since 2010 to optimize antibiotic usage [27–29]; however, the consumption of antipseudomonal penicillins significantly increased between 2009 and 2016 [27]. Thus, narrower spectrum antibiotics should be prescribed to avoid the development and prevalence of bacterial resistance as much as possible with consideration to preexisting infectious diseases and patient conditions even before the onset of bacteremia.

Empirical antibiotic therapy is often commenced before pathogen identification and without susceptibility data. *E. faecium* is typically resistant to penicillins [4]; thus, when enterococcal infection is suspected, initial empiric therapy often requires the prescription of anti-MRSA agents, especially vancomycin. We found that the *E. faecium* group showed a longer duration of vancomycin use, higher vancomycin trough levels, and higher rates of AKI. Higher vancomycin trough levels have been previously identified as a risk factor for nephrotoxicity [30], and thus, the longer duration of vancomycin use in the *E. faecium* group might have elevated the vancomycin trough levels leading to renal injury. Furthermore, glycopeptide use is associated with higher mortality in patients with *E. faecalis* bacteremia [31]. These findings suggest that vancomycin doses need to be considered carefully for patients with enterococcal bacteremia to prevent AKI.

Risk factors for mortality due to enterococcal bloodstream infections may include malignancy, admission to the intensive care unit, severity of illness, and high-level resistance to ampicillin and ciprofloxacin [1,15,18,32,33]. In this study, we identified AKI, unknown source of infection, previous corticosteroid treatment, and qSOFA score ≥ 2 as independent risk factors associated with mortality due to enterococcal bacteremia. These findings may be clinically plausible because impairment of kidney function and consequent multiorgan dysfunction syndrome, which likely leads to mortality, occurs in critically ill patients [34,35]. Moreover, severely ill patients, such as those with collagenase disease, nephrotic syndrome, and advanced cancer, receive corticosteroid therapy. However, corticosteroids not only decrease inflammation but also have side effects, including a reduction in the activity of the immune system, as well as hyperglycemia. A previous study reported that an unknown focus of bacteremia was associated with inappropriate antibiotic therapy and poor clinical outcome [36]. These findings suggest that the risk factors associated with mortality provide useful information for clinicians to avoid treatment failure, thereby enabling appropriate medical therapy after the onset of bacteremia. Specialized personnel, such as antimicrobial stewardship teams, can support clinical management through appropriate antibiotic use and early diagnosis.

This study has some limitations. First, we conducted a retrospective study in a single university hospital, and the data were gathered by reviewing electronic medical records, relying on other investigators for data collection; hence, a measurement bias could not be ignored. Second, this study investigated only *E. faecalis* and *E. faecium* bacteremia. To evaluate the characteristics of enterococci, we must assess the clinical outcomes of patients with bacteremia caused by *Enterococcus* species, including *E. avium*, *E. casseliflavus*, and *E. raffinosus*, other than *E. faecalis* and *E. faecium*.

4. Materials and Methods

4.1. Setting and Patients

We conducted an observational retrospective study between 1 January 2014, and 31 December 2018, at Kobe University Hospital. We defined nosocomial enterococcal bacteremia as positive blood cultures obtained after 48 h of hospitalization. We investigated all adult patients (age > 18 years) with only the first episode of at least one positive blood culture for *Enterococcus* species. In patients with two or more blood cultures for the same organism, only one was included in the analysis. Patient data were obtained from electronic medical records.

4.2. Definitions

The demographic information included age and sex. The clinical and microbiological data for each case were carefully reviewed. The hospitalization ward, comorbidities, the source of infection, qSOFA score, and use of invasive devices were evaluated on the day of bacteremia onset. Data pertaining to recent surgery, immunosuppressive treatment, and previous antibiotic therapy within 30 days prior to the first positive blood culture were collected. The polymicrobial culture was defined as the isolation of more than one organism, excluding contaminated pathogens, which were defined if the following pathogens (coagulase-negative staphylococci, *Bacillus* species, *Corynebacterium* species, *Propionibacterium* species, Viridans-group *streptococci*, and *Micrococcus* species) were detected in one of two or more blood culture sets on the same day. Antibiotic therapy against enterococci was defined as the prescription of antibiotics to which the isolated enterococci were susceptible to bacteremia. Source control with surgical drainage, time to the initiation of antibiotic therapy against enterococci, and total duration of antibiotic treatment was reviewed from the onset of bacteremia. Daily antimicrobial cost during antibiotic therapy for enterococcal bacteremia was calculated by multiplying the drug prices per dose by the total number of given doses and dividing the product by the total number of days of antibiotic therapy. All costs are shown in US dollars ($; exchange rate, 1 $ = 104.30 yen in 1 December 2020). We counted the number of patients whose vancomycin median serum trough concentration was ≥20 mg/L. AKI was defined as an absolute increase in the serum creatinine level to >0.3 mg/dL or a >1.5-fold increase from the baseline value within 7 days. We defined the 30-day mortality as death due to any cause within 30 days after the onset of bacteremia.

4.3. Identification and Antibiotic Susceptibility Testing

The BACTEC FX system (Becton and Dickinson, Tokyo, Japan) was used to process the blood cultures. Enterococci were isolated according to standard microbiological procedures. The isolates were identified using matrix-assisted laser desorption/ionization time-of-flight mass spectrometry (MALDI-TOF MS; Bruker, Tokyo, Japan). The minimum inhibitory concentrations of ampicillin, vancomycin, imipenem, and levofloxacin were determined by a broth microdilution method using Microscan Walk Away 96plus (Beckman Coulter, Tokyo, Japan) and interpreted according to the breakpoints proposed by the Clinical and Laboratory Standards Institute guidelines. *Staphylococcus aureus* (ATCC 29213, VA, USA) was used as the quality control strain.

4.4. Statistical Analysis

Continuous variables are expressed as medians with interquartile ranges (IQRs) and categorical variables as frequency counts with percentages. Continuous variables were compared using the Mann–Whitney U test. Categorical variables were compared using the Chi-square test. Multivariate conditional logistic regression analysis of factors that were potentially associated with *E. faecium* acquisition and mortality included clinically important variables of the statistically significant variables in the univariate analysis. We assessed the in-hospital mortality by using Kaplan–Meier analysis and estimated HR and 95% CI using multivariate Cox proportional hazard regression models. All statistical analyses were performed using the statistical software EZR (Saitama Medical Center, Jichi Medical University, Saitama, Japan).

4.5. Ethics Approval

This study was approved by the Kobe University Graduate School of Health Sciences Institutional Review Board (approval no. 472-6) and was performed in accordance with the ethical standards of the Institutional Research Committee and the tenets of the Declaration of Helsinki (1964).

5. Conclusions

In summary, we conducted an observational retrospective study to compare the clinical features and outcomes of bacteremia caused by *E. faecalis* and *E. faecium*. Multivariate analysis was used to identify the risk factors for the acquisition of *E. faecium* bacteremia and mortality due to enterococcal bacteremia. This study demonstrated that the *E. faecium* group had a shorter survival period and higher antimicrobial cost than the *E. faecalis* group. *E. faecium* bacteremia occurred more frequently among patients treated with broad-spectrum antibiotics, especially patients with hematologic tumors and cholecystocholangitis. Furthermore, we identified that severe illness, which tends to be associated with a worse renal function without an infectious focus, was an independent risk factor for mortality due to enterococcal bacteremia. These findings suggest that clinicians should provide a rational treatment strategy supported by specialized teams, such as those assisting antimicrobial stewardship programs, even before the onset of bacteremia in hospitalized patients.

Author Contributions: Conceptualization, A.U.; methodology, A.U., K.O. (Kayo Osawa) and K.O. (Kenichiro Onuma); software, A.U.; validation, A.U.; formal analysis, A.U. and K.O. (Kayo Osawa); investigation, A.U.; resources, A.U. and K.O. (Kenichiro Onuma); data curation, A.U. and K.O. (Kayo Osawa); writing—original draft preparation, A.U. and K.S.; writing—review and editing, A.U., K.S., and I.Y.; visualization, A.U.; supervision, K.K., Y.Y., T.N., M.F., and I.Y.; project administration, T.M.; funding acquisition, T.M. All authors have read and agreed to the published version of the manuscript.

Funding: This research received no external funding.

Informed Consent Statement: The requirement of patient consent was waived owing to the retrospective nature of the study.

Data Availability Statement: Data sharing is not applicable to this article.

Conflicts of Interest: The authors declare no conflict of interest.

References

1. Caballero-Granado, F.J.; Becerril, B.; Cuberos, L.; Bernabeu, M.; Cisneros, J.M.; Pachón, J. Attributable mortality rate and duration of hospital stay associated with enterococcal bacteremia. *Clin. Infect. Dis.* **2001**, *32*, 587–594. [CrossRef] [PubMed]
2. Moses, V.; Jerobin, J.; Nair, A.; Sathyendara, S.; Balaji, V.; George, I.A.; Peter, J.V. Enterococcal bacteremia is associated with prolonged stay in the medical intensive care unit. *J. Glob. Infect. Dis.* **2012**, *4*, 26–30. [CrossRef] [PubMed]
3. Chiang, H.-Y.; Perencevich, E.N.; Nair, R.; Nelson, R.E.; Samore, M.; Khader, K.; Chorazy, M.L.; Herwaldt, L.A.; Blevins, A.; Ward, M.A.; et al. Incidence and Outcomes Associated with Infections Caused by Vancomycin-Resistant Enterococci in the United States: Systematic Literature Review and Meta-Analysis. *Infect. Control Hosp. Epidemiol.* **2017**, *38*, 203–215. [CrossRef] [PubMed]
4. Ministry of Health, Labour and Welfare. Japan Nosocomial Infections Surveillance. Available online: https://janis.mhlw.go.jp/english/index.asp (accessed on 1 December 2020).
5. Weber, S.; Hogardt, M.; Reinheimer, C.; Wichelhaus, T.A.; Kempf, V.A.J.; Kessel, J.; Wolf, S.; Serve, H.; Steffen, B.; Scheich, S. Bloodstream Infections with Vancomycin-Resistant Enterococci Are Associated with a Decreased Survival in Patients with Hematological Diseases. *Ann. Hematol.* **2019**, *98*, 763–773. [CrossRef] [PubMed]
6. Vincent, J.-L.; Sakr, Y.; Singer, M.; Martin-Loeches, I.; Machado, F.R.; Marshall, J.C.; Finfer, S.; Pelosi, P.; Brazzi, L.; Aditianingsih, D.; et al. Prevalence and Outcomes of Infection among Patients in Intensive Care Units in 2017. *JAMA* **2020**, *323*, 1478. [CrossRef]
7. Harbarth, S.; Cosgrove, S.; Carmeli, Y. Effects of Antibiotics on Nosocomial Epidemiology of Vancomycin-Resistant Enterococci. *Antimicrob. Agents Chemother.* **2002**, *46*, 1619–1628. [CrossRef]
8. Data from the ECDC Surveillance Atlas—Antimicrobial Resistance. Available online: https://www.ecdc.europa.eu/en/antimicrobial-resistance/surveillance-and-disease-data/data-ecdc (accessed on 1 January 2021).
9. Webb, M.; Riley, L.; Roberts, R.B. Cost of Hospitalization for and Risk Factors Associated with Vancomycin-Resistant Enterococcus Faecium Infection and Colonization. *Clin. Infect. Dis. Off. Publ. Infect. Dis. Soc. Am.* **2001**, *33*, 445–452. [CrossRef]
10. Morales, E.; Cots, F.; Sala, M.; Comas, M.; Belvis, F.; Riu, M.; Salvadó, M.; Grau, S.; Horcajada, J.P.; Montero, M.M.; et al. Hospital Costs of Nosocomial Multi-Drug Resistant Pseudomonas Aeruginosa Acquisition. *BMC Health Serv. Res.* **2012**, *12*, 122. [CrossRef]
11. Mauldin, P.D.; Salgado, C.D.; Hansen, I.S.; Durup, D.T.; Bosso, J.A. Attributable Hospital Cost and Length of Stay Associated with Health Care-Associated Infections Caused by Antibiotic-Resistant Gram-Negative Bacteria. *Antimicrob. Agents Chemother.* **2010**, *54*, 109–115. [CrossRef]
12. Tenney, J.; Hudson, N.; Alnifaidy, H.; Li, J.T.C.; Fung, K.H. Risk Factors for Aquiring Multidrug-Resistant Organisms in Urinary Tract Infections: A Systematic Literature Review. *Saudi Pharm. J.* **2018**, *26*, 678–684. [CrossRef]
13. Kaye, K.S.; Cosgrove, S.; Harris, A.; Eliopoulos, G.M.; Carmeli, Y. Risk Factors for Emergence of Resistance to Broad-Spectrum Cephalosporins among *Enterobacter* Spp. *Antimicrob. Agents Chemother.* **2001**, *45*, 2628–2630. [CrossRef] [PubMed]
14. Falagas, M.E.; Kopterides, P. Risk Factors for the Isolation of Multi-Drug-Resistant *Acinetobacter baumannii* and *Pseudomonas aeruginosa*: A Systematic Review of the Literature. *J. Hosp. Infect.* **2006**, *64*, 7–15. [CrossRef] [PubMed]
15. Gudiol, C.; Ayats, J.; Camoez, M.; Domínguez, M.Á.; García-Vidal, C.; Bodro, M.; Ardanuy, C.; Obed, M.; Arnan, M.; Antonio, M.; et al. Increase in bloodstream infection due to vancomycin-susceptible *Enterococcus faecium* in cancer patients: Risk factors, molecular epidemiology and outcomes. *PLoS ONE* **2013**, *8*, e74734. [CrossRef] [PubMed]
16. Treitman, A.N.; Yarnold, P.R.; Warren, J.; Noskin, G.A. Emerging Incidence of *Enterococcus faecium* among hospital isolates (1993 to 2002). *J. Clin. Microbiol.* **2005**, *43*, 462–463. [CrossRef] [PubMed]
17. Kajihara, T.; Nakamura, S.; Iwanaga, N.; Oshima, K.; Takazono, T.; Miyazaki, T.; Izumikawa, K.; Yanagihara, K.; Kohno, N.; Kohno, S. Clinical Characteristics and Risk Factors of Enterococcal Infections in Nagasaki, Japan: A Retrospective Study. *BMC Infect. Dis.* **2015**, *15*, 426. [CrossRef] [PubMed]
18. Suzuki, H.; Hase, R.; Otsuka, Y.; Hosokawa, N. A 10-Year Profile of Enterococcal Bloodstream Infections at a Tertiary-Care Hospital in Japan. *J. Infect. Chemother.* **2017**, *23*, 390–393. [CrossRef]
19. Morvan, A.C.; Hengy, B.; Garrouste-Orgeas, M.; Ruckly, S.; Forel, J.M.; Argaud, L.; Rimmelé, T.; Bedos, J.P.; Azoulay, E.; Dupuis, C.; et al. Impact of species and antibiotic therapy of enterococcal peritonitis on 30-day mortality in critical care—An analysis of the OUTCOMEREA database. *Crit. Care* **2019**, *23*, 307. [CrossRef]
20. Garnacho-Montero, J.; Gutiérrez-Pizarraya, A.; Escoresca-Ortega, A.; Corcia-Palomo, Y.; Fernández-Delgado, E.; Herrera-Melero, I.; Ortiz-Leyba, C.; Márquez-Vácaro, J.A. De-escalation of empirical therapy is associated with lower mortality in patients with severe sepsis and septic shock. *Intensive Care Med.* **2014**, *40*, 32–40. [CrossRef]
21. Uda, A.; Tokimatsu, I.; Koike, C.; Osawa, K.; Shigemura, K.; Kimura, T.; Miyara, T.; Yano, I. Antibiotic de-escalation therapy in patients with community-acquired nonbacteremic pneumococcal pneumonia. *Int. J. Clin. Pharm.* **2019**, *41*, 1611–1617. [CrossRef]

22. Ministry of Health, Labour and Welfare. Available online: https://www.mhlw.go.jp/topics/2020/04/tp20200401-01.html (accessed on 1 December 2020).
23. Noskin, G.A.; Peterson, L.R.; Warren, J.R. *Enterococcus faecium* and *Enterococcus faecalis* bacteremia: Acquisition and outcome. *Clin. Infect. Dis.* **1995**, *20*, 296–301. [CrossRef]
24. Izumikawa, K.; Tomita, T.; Nishimura, N.; Niwa, T.; Takayama, K.; Ohana, N.; Kusama, F.; Hida, Y.; Negayama, K.; Matsuda, J.; et al. The current status and issue of usage of intravenous antimicrobial agents in national and public university hospitals in Japan. *Jpn. J. Chemother.* **2018**, *66*, 738–748. (In Japanese)
25. Harris, A.D.; Perencevich, E.; Roghmann, M.-C.; Morris, G.; Kaye, K.S.; Johnson, J.A. Risk factors for piperacillin-tazobactam-resistant *Pseudomonas aeruginosa* among hospitalized patients. *Antimicrob. Agents Chemother.* **2002**, *46*, 854–858. [CrossRef]
26. Barlam, T.F.; Cosgrove, S.E.; Abbo, L.M.; MacDougall, C.; Schuetz, A.N.; Septimus, E.J.; Srinivasan, A.; Dellit, T.H.; Falck-Ytter, Y.T.; Fishman, N.O.; et al. Implementing an antibiotic stewardship program: Guidelines by the Infectious Diseases Society of America and the Society for Healthcare Epidemiology of America. *Clin. Infect. Dis.* **2016**, *62*, e51–e77. [CrossRef] [PubMed]
27. Kimura, T.; Uda, A.; Sakaue, T.; Yamashita, K.; Nishioka, T.; Nishimura, S.; Ebisawa, K.; Nagata, M.; Ohji, G.; Nakamura, T.; et al. Long-term efficacy of comprehensive multidisciplinary antibiotic stewardship programs centered on weekly prospective audit and feedback. *Infection* **2018**, *46*, 215–224. [CrossRef] [PubMed]
28. Uda, A.; Shigemura, K.; Kitagawa, K.; Osawa, K.; Onuma, K.; Inoue, S.; Kotani, J.; Yan, Y.; Nakano, Y.; Nishioka, T.; et al. How does antimicrobial stewardship affect inappropriate antibiotic therapy in urological patients? *Antibiotics* **2020**, *9*, 63. [CrossRef] [PubMed]
29. Uda, A.; Kimura, T.; Nishimura, S.; Ebisawa, K.; Ohji, G.; Kusuki, M.; Yahata, M.; Izuta, R.; Sakaue, T.; Nakamura, T.; et al. Efficacy of educational intervention on reducing the inappropriate use of oral third-generation cephalosporins. *Infection* **2019**, *47*, 1037–1045. [CrossRef]
30. Kullar, R.; Davis, S.L.; Levine, D.P.; Rybak, M.J. Impact of vancomycin exposure on outcomes in patients with methicillin-resistant *Staphylococcus aureus* bacteremia: Support for consensus guidelines suggested targets. *Clin. Infect. Dis.* **2011**, *52*, 975–981. [CrossRef]
31. Foo, H.; Chater, M.; Maley, M.; van Hal, S.J. Glycopeptide use is associated with increased mortality in *Enterococcus faecalis* bacteraemia. *J. Antimicrob. Chemother.* **2014**, *69*, 2252–2257. [CrossRef]
32. Zheng, J.; Li, H.; Pu, Z.; Wang, H.; Deng, X.; Liu, X.; Deng, Q.; Yu, Z. Bloodstream infections caused by *Enterococcus* spp: A 10-year retrospective analysis at a tertiary hospital in China. *J. Huazhong Univ. Sci. Technolog. Med. Sci.* **2017**, *37*, 257–263. [CrossRef]
33. McBride, S.J.; Upton, A.; Roberts, S.A. Clinical characteristics and outcomes of patients with vancomycin-susceptible *Enterococcus faecalis* and *Enterococcus faecium* bacteraemia—A five-year retrospective review. *Eur. J. Clin. Microbiol. Infect. Dis.* **2010**, *29*, 107–114. [CrossRef]
34. Uchino, S.; Kellum, J.A.; Bellomo, R.; Doig, G.S.; Morimatsu, H.; Morgera, S.; Schetz, M.; Tan, I.; Bouman, C.; Macedo, E.; et al. Acute renal failure in critically ill patients: A multinational, multicenter study. *JAMA* **2005**, *29*, 813–818. [CrossRef] [PubMed]
35. Zhang, Y.; Du, M.; Chang, Y.; Chen, L.; Zhang, Q. Incidence, clinical characteristics, and outcomes of nosocomial *Enterococcus* spp. bloodstream infections in a tertiary-care hospital in Beijing, China: A four-year retrospective study. *Antimicrob. Resist. Infect. Control* **2017**, *6*, 73. [CrossRef] [PubMed]
36. Courjon, J.; Demonchy, E.; Degand, N.; Risso, K.; Ruimy, R.; Roger, P.-M. Patients with community-acquired bacteremia of unknown origin: Clinical characteristics and usefulness of microbiological results for therapeutic issues: A single-center cohort study. *Ann. Clin. Microbiol. Antimicrob.* **2017**, *16*, 40. [CrossRef] [PubMed]

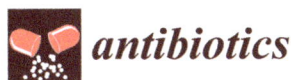

Article

Antimicrobial Stewardship: Development and Pilot of an Organisational Peer-to-Peer Review Tool to Improve Service Provision in Line with National Guidance

Olaolu Oloyede [1], Emma Cramp [2] and Diane Ashiru-Oredope [1,*]

1 Public Health England, London SE1 8UG, UK; Olaolu.oloyede@phe.gov.uk
2 Patient Safety, NHS Improvement, London SE1 6LH, UK; emma.cramp@nhs.net
* Correspondence: diane.ashiru-oredope@phe.gov.uk

Abstract: Antimicrobial resistance continues to be a considerable threat to global public health due to the persistent inappropriate use of antibiotics. Antimicrobial stewardship (AMS) programs are essential in reducing the growth and spread of antibiotic resistance, in an environment which lacks incentives for the development of new antibiotics. Over the years, a variety of resources have been developed to strengthen antimicrobial stewardship. However, the differences in resources available present a challenge for organisations/teams to establish the best resources to utilise for service provision. A peer review tool was formulated using four national documents on AMS and tested through three phases with feedback. A survey method was used to collect feedback on the validity, feasibility, and impact of the AMS peer review tool. Feedback received was positive from the earlier pilots. The tool was found to be useful at identifying areas of good practice and gaps in antimicrobial stewardship across various pilot sites. Feedback suggests the tool is useful for promoting improvements to AMS programs and highlights that the content and features of the tool are appropriate for evaluating stewardship.

Keywords: AMS; antimicrobial resistance; antimicrobial stewardship intervention; PDSA cycle

1. Introduction

Antimicrobial stewardship (AMS) is an organisational or healthcare system-wide approach to improving and optimising antimicrobial therapy through the promotion and monitoring of the appropriate use of antimicrobials to prevent the development of resistance. Evidence suggests that a coordinated and comprehensive AMS programme is vital in tackling the emergence of antimicrobial resistance [1].

Several national AMS guidance and toolkits have been developed to support and encourage best practice in acute National Health Service (NHS) hospitals in England, as well as the goals outlined in the UK 5-year National Action Plan 2019–2024. These collections of resources, produced by different expert groups and at different time points, present a challenge for organisations/teams to establish the best resources to improve service provision. In response to this, the consolidation of recommendations from these national resources into one complete AMS tool can provide clarity to enable adherence to national guidance, thus consistent and better stewardship. The Health Foundation defines peer review as the professional assessment against standards of the organisation on healthcare processes and quality of work, to foster improvement [2]. The peer review tool developed aims to support hospitals to systematically review their processes for appropriate antimicrobial prescribing, stewardship and improving patient outcomes. The tool is intended for use at the host site with an external peer reviewer, to allow for an impartial assessment of AMS practices and development of an improvement plan [3].

Organisational peer-to-peer reviews offer an objective assessment to drive internal improvement through the evaluation of a provider by another organisation without the

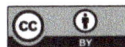

need for formal regulatory authority involvement. Cases of organisational peer-to-peer review are rare in healthcare; an example of this approach includes the UK National Chronic Obstructive Pulmonary Disease (COPD) Resources and Outcomes Project and the regional intervention to improve the hospital mortality associated with coronary artery bypass graft surgery (The Northern New England Cardiovascular Disease Study Group) [4].

To prevent the growing issue of antimicrobial resistance (AMR), NHS England (now NHS England & Improvement) launched the world's largest healthcare incentive scheme for hospitals and other health service providers. The programmed offered NHS Trusts incentive funding valued up to £150 million to support expert clinicians and pharmacist's assessment and reduction of inappropriate antimicrobial prescription [5]. The development of the AMS peer review tool with a plan-do-study-act (PDSA) cycle approach aims to support national investment in tackling AMR issues through organisational peer-to-peer reviews.

2. Results

PDSA Cycle 1:

In 2016, positive feedback was received from all participants from the East of England pilot using the first version of the tool [6]. The tool was found to be beneficial at identifying areas of good practice and gaps in antimicrobial stewardship at each pilot site, as well as presenting opportunities to learn from peers. The participants found that the tool was relatively easy to use and indicated peer review visits annually would be adequate.

The average length of time to undertake the peer review was five hours in total. These five hours where made up of approximately 2 h for reviewing necessary documents prior to visiting the host organisation and 3 h to conduct the site visit which included attendance at the AMS committee meeting and visiting a ward area to interview healthcare workers.

PDSA Cycle 2:

In 2018, following the presentation of the peer review tool to the national multi-disciplinary group on antimicrobial resistance and utilisation, the English surveillance programme for antimicrobial utilisation and resistance (ESPAUR) group; the number of indicators in the tool was reduced from 101 to 37 following a two stage process and updated to include indicators from the current antimicrobial stewardship guidance and toolkits. Similar indicators were merged so that repetition was minimised, and themes were grouped together. Table 1 summarises the number of indicators from each stage of the toolkit development during cycle 2.

PDSA Cycle 3:

In 2019, feedback on the revised shortened tool from another pilot of five participating acute hospitals (three teaching and two non-teaching trusts) in two regions of England suggested a two-week lead time for submission of the hospitals' documented evidence of the AMS programme was appropriate and the documents shared were found to be "mostly relevant". It was also viewed that the tool could be beneficial in "promoting shared learning across the hospital stewardship programmes" and the peer review should be repeated every three years. One of the challenges highlighted was arranging a suitable date for the peer review on-site visit for both parties.

Despite the revision of the tool and reduction in the number of questions, the time taken to complete the peer review did not decrease from the initial pilot, with an average of 5 h (1.6 h to review the document before the site visit and 3.4 h for the on-site visit). The reason for this was because although the indicators were merged to form fewer questions for the reviewer, the themes required an in-depth review which did not change the overall amount of time needed for the review. In circumstances where the NHS Trust's AMS programme is satisfactory, the tool was considered time-consuming, but the outcome of the visit provided assurance for the AMS team. All participants agreed that the benefit from the tool included its application to reinforce good practice and benchmarking against peers.

The majority of respondents highlighted that all domains assessing the NHS Trust's antimicrobial stewardship programme were either "very relevant" or "relevant" with the exception of the "Patient and Carers" domain in which some responded "neutral". The consensus was that the tool would be best used by healthcare professionals with an infection specialist background, as well as an excellent resource to promote shared learning across the hospital stewardship programme. Some of the planned actions by the host organisations following the peer review were:

- Review of the antimicrobial team at a future ASC meeting,
- Analysis of detailed data at consultant and ward level data,
- To re-visit the area highlighted that require strengthening,
- Develop an education plan, and
- Develop audit and feedback plan.

Table 1. Number of indicators at each stage of the toolkit development.

Section	Area	Original Tool	Stage 1	Stage 2
1	AMS management team/antimicrobial stewardship committee (ASC)	15	10	6
2	AM Prescribing management	48	20	18
3	Surveillance, resistance, and standards	12	7	1
4	Risk assessment for antimicrobials	7	7	5
5	Patients and carers	5	5	4
6	Education and training on the use of antimicrobials	6	4	3
-	Antimicrobial pharmacist	8	6	Moved *
	Total number of indicators	101	59	37

* Moved to the AMS management team/ASC.

3. Discussion

The development of the AMS peer review tool focussed on establishing a resource that amalgamates the variety of national guidance and tools on good antimicrobial stewardship into a single resource. Thus, providing a comprehensive and structured instrument to strengthen an NHS Trust antimicrobial stewardship programme. However, selecting a sample of acute NHS Trusts conveniently located within the same geography to pilot the tool at various stages of development proved to be quite challenging. With the variation across NHS Trusts with different processes, cultures, capacity, and attitudes on tackling antimicrobial resistance, there is a need to broaden the geographical spread sample that will provide a more detailed insight to the feasibility of the tool. Thus, it was intended that the tool would be piloted across at least two hospital trusts in all the NHS regions to have a representative sample in the development of the tool. However, having a broad and large sample of secondary care institutions (National Health Service Trusts) willing to participate in the pilot proved to be a significant challenge as coordinating the on-site visit between both organisations was dependent on the dates the antimicrobial stewardship committee meetings were due to take place, as well as the pharmacist's clinical commitments, and annual leave. During the pilot, it was highlighted that having a central team to coordinate organisation of on-site visit across the hospitals is important and beneficial; however, this strategy will require additional resources within each regional health system. To support widespread uptake of such measuring instruments and opportunity for regional or national perspective on the variation of stewardship programmes, implementation of future organisational peer-to-peer review tools could benefit from a central resource to coordinate dates and visits to reduce burden on individual teams.

The feedback from the pilot showed that participants found the tool to be a useful resource that encourages shared learning between peers and identifying gaps within their antimicrobial stewardship programme. However, the results of the pilots may be biased towards individuals with a keen specialist interest in improvement measuresand actively involved in promoting and implementing good stewardship practices across the hospital. Furthermore, there is the potential for selection bias from the pilots, as there was an overrepresentation of pharmacists conducting the peer review (all reviews completed by pharmacists). Although it is hoped that through the feedback from the ESPAUR oversight group (which includes members from a wide range of backgrounds such as microbiology consultants, members of the dental profession, and nurses) who provided critical review of the tool, some of the selection bias may have been addressed. The use of the tool is not intended to be exclusive to a specific profession, but rather to be used by any healthcare professional with an antimicrobial stewardship/infection management background.

In addition, the evidence across various medical areas suggests that following a peer review, improvements to services can sometimes occur slowly with inconsistent outcomes. It has been suggested, to achieve better results that will deliver change and improved services, that a multidisciplinary peer review visit may be a more attractive mechanism as a collective and agreed strategy to implement the recommendations is likely to breed success [7]. Organisation-wide support on antimicrobial stewardship is considered crucial to addressing AMR, thus without this, minimal impact may be expected following visits.

The iterations of developing the tool demonstrated that the content and elements of the assessment tool are suitable for evaluating stewardship, thus providing a robust and systematic approach. The challenge from the outset was coordinating a system-wide simultaneous uptake within regions of the AMS peer review tool, with a proposed annual visit to reassess and support consistent improvement in stewardship programmes.

4. Materials and Methods

The AMS peer review tool was originally developed and piloted by East of England Antimicrobial Pharmacists Network in 2016 across eight NHS acute Trusts. The tool includes consolidated recommendations from a number of national AMS guidance and toolkits [8–11] into one easy-to-use document, assessing an organisation's stewardship programme on the following domains:

- AMS leadership and management,
- Antimicrobial prescribing management,
- Surveillance, resistance and standards,
- Risk assessments for antimicrobials,
- Patient and carers, and
- Education and training on the use of antimicrobials

The intention was to develop a voluntary tool (available to download as a Supplementary Material) to strengthen antimicrobial stewardship in acute hospitals through the facilitation of organisational peer reviews within the regional health systems in England. The tool was tested through three phases with the feedback and outcome shared with the English surveillance programme for antimicrobial utilisation and resistance (ESPAUR) group, consisting of experts from various backgrounds (microbiologist, paediatricians, infection disease specialist, and pharmacists). Through the phases of developing the AMS peer review tool, a survey method was used to collect feedback on the validity, feasibility, and impact.

The findings of the pilot were first presented to ESPAUR oversight group in January 2017. The average length of time to perform a peer review was five hours (two hours to review key documents before the site visit and three hours to carry out the site visit which included attending an AMS committee meeting). Feedback from the ESPAUR members was to simplify the tool by reducing the number of indicators before the next piloting stage. The tool was further updated in January 2019 and validated using the checklist outlined by Pulcini et al. [12] in their publication on developing a global checklist for hospital AMS programmes. The updated version of the tool was shared via the AMR network leads with antimicrobial pharmacists across some acute hospitals in England to request their participation to pilot. Incorporated into the updated peer-review process was a pre-visit stage, to encourage more focussed and productive on-site visits. Volunteering hospitals were paired within their region to avoid long-distance travel to conduct the peer-review.

The three iterations of testing and evaluating feedback were used to validate and refine the tool, with time to completion measured, and participants' experience of utilising the tool collected (Table 2).

Table 2. Summary of the plan-do-study-act (PDSA) cycles.

Cycle	Completed by:	Intervention
1	January 2016	Pilot of original tool and feedback by eight organisations within one region of England through the East of England Antimicrobial Pharmacists Network.
	January 2017	Results of pilot presented to the English surveillance programme for antimicrobial utilisation and resistance (ESPAUR).
2	March 2018	Tool updated in line with latest national guidance and toolkits.
	July 2018	Updated tool including indicators from national guidance and toolkits presented to EPSAUR.
	December 2018	Two stages of review and feedback to reduce number of indicators assessed through the tool.
	January 2019	Shortened version presented to ESPAUR group.
3	April/May 2019	Pilot of updated peer review tool with five NHS Trusts across 2 regions.
	July 2019	Pilot output presented to ESPAUR and final tool endorsed with recommendations methods for cascade.

Using the AMS Peer Review Tool

It was recommended that those wishing to pilot the tool (available as supplementary material) consider choosing peer hospitals based on geographical location to minimise the amount of travel time, and that the whole review process may take one full working day to complete and that peer review process can be considered every two to three years (as this allows enough time to lapse to accrue the benefits of the peer review and appropriate time for reassessment), or more frequently if an improvement plan is implemented. The peer review may be carried out by an individual or team from an external organisation, which is not limited to the list below, and may include one or more of the following:

- Antimicrobial pharmacist
- Infection prevention control/AMS Nurse
- Director (lead) of infection prevention and control (DIPC)
- Commissioner
- Clinical microbiologist or ID physician
- Other member of AMS committee
- National or regional antimicrobial stewardship leads/committee members

The AMS peer review tool outlines key aspects across the six AMS domains mentioned earlier to be critically reviewed and assessed by the host organisation and peer reviewer. The recommended process for conducting the peer review is outlined below:

Step 1

Plan and schedule the onsite visit to occur ideally on the day the Antimicrobial Stewardship Committee (ASC) is held. This would allow the reviewer to witness first-hand the attendance, management, and leadership at the meetings. The host organisation should schedule an opportunity for the peer review team to meet with senior clinicians and managers. The date and time of visit should be scheduled during less busy periods and where possible consider staff availability due to annual leave.

Step 2

Host organisation to prepare documents listed in the tool for submission to peer reviewer two weeks ahead of scheduled visit and self-assess AMS prior to peer reviewer visit.

Peer reviewer to review documents submitted by host organisation and prepare approach prior to visit.

Step 3

During the onsite visit, the reviewers should speak with clinical staff on the ward. In addition, where it is considered necessary or additional benefit for the review process, reviewers may also consider having discussions with senior clinicians, and managers including the medical director, lead for infection prevention and control (e.g., the director for IPC in the UK (DIPC)), director of nursing, microbiologist lead for AMS and chief pharmacist within the NHS Trust, the director of nursing and quality, AMR/AMS lead pharmacist and chief pharmacist within the CCG, and the system AMR lead.

Step 4

Peer review report to be submitted within the agreed time frame at the onsite visit. The report should outline the areas of success and opportunities for improvement.

5. Conclusions

The pilots were important in assessing the feasibility of the tool and outlining the barriers for use. The feedback from participants and expert group suggest that the tool is best used where a gap or issue has been identified within a hospital stewardship programme, with the tool providing a comprehensive review to help develop strategies for improvements. The tool also presents an opportunity for regional antimicrobial groups to voluntarily lead on coordinating the visits to share best practices amongst hospital within the region. Overall, this quality improvement project showed there was a need for tools that support organisational peer-to-peer review. However, future work on developing such a quality improvement model need to build in considerations that will reduce the time burden and pressure for the reviewers.

Supplementary Materials: The following are available online at https://www.mdpi.com/2079-6382/10/1/44/s1, Antimicrobial Stewardship (AMS) Peer Review Tool as PDF and editable excel document.

Author Contributions: Conceptualization, E.C. and, D.A.-O.; data curation, O.O.; formal analysis, O.O.; methodology, O.O., E.C., and, D.A.-O.; project administration, O.O.; resources, D.A.-O.; supervision, D.A.-O.; writing—original draft, O.O.; writing—review and editing, E.C. and, D.A.-O. All authors have read and agreed to the published version of the manuscript.

Funding: This project received no external funding.

Institutional Review Board Statement: Not applicable.

Informed Consent Statement: Not applicable.

Data Availability Statement: Data is contained within the article or supplementary material.

Acknowledgments: All participating hospitals and infection leads are acknowledged for their support in piloting the tool. In particular, the authors would like to acknowledge the East of England Antimicrobial Pharmacy Network for their initial support with shaping the original version of the peer review tool and piloting it across the region.

Conflicts of Interest: The authors declare no conflict of interest.

References

1. Akpan, M.R.; Ahmad, R.; Shebl, N.A.; Ashiru-Oredope, D. A Review of Quality Measures for Assessing the Impact of Antimicrobial Stewardship Programs in Hospitals. *Antibiotics* **2016**, *5*, 5. [CrossRef]
2. McCormick, B. *Pathway Peer Review to Improve Quality: Health Foundation*; Health Foundation: London, UK, 2012.
3. Public Health England. *English Surveillance Programme for Antimicrobial Utilisation and Resistance (ESPAUR) Report 2018–2019*; Public Health England: London, UK, 2019.
4. Pronovost, P.J.; Hudson, D.W. Improving healthcare quality through organisational peer-to-peer assessment: Lessons from the nuclear power industry. *BMJ Qual. Saf.* **2012**, *21*, 872. [CrossRef] [PubMed]

5. NHS England. NHS England Launches National Programme to Combat Antibiotic Overusage. 2016. Available online: https://www.england.nhs.uk/2016/03/antibiotic-overusage/ (accessed on 20 October 2020).
6. East of England Pharmacy Infection Network. Antimicrobial Stewardship (AMS) Peer Review Inspection Tool. 2016. Available online: https://www.networks.nhs.uk/nhs-networks/thames-valley-wessex-regional-antimicrobial/documents/e-of-england-ams-pharmacy-peer-review-tool (accessed on 20 October 2020).
7. Roberts, C.M.; Buckingham, R.J.; Stone, R.A.; Lowe, D.; Pearson, M.G. The UK National Chronic Obstructive Pulmonary Disease Resources and Outcomes Project—A feasibility study of large-scale clinical service peer review. *J. Eval. Clin. Pract.* **2010**, *16*, 927–932. [CrossRef]
8. Public Health England. *Start Smart—Then Focus: Antimicrobial Stewardship Toolkit for English Hospitals*; Public Health England: London, UK, 2015.
9. Excellence NIfHaC NICE. *Guidance Antimicrobial Stewardship: Systems and Processes for Effective Antimicrobial Medicine Use*; NICE: London, UK, 2015.
10. Antimicrobial Resistance and Healthcare Associated Infections (ARHAI) icwtDoHD. *Antimicrobial Self-Assessment Toolkit (ASAT) for Acute Hospitals*; ARHAI: London, UK, 2012.
11. Department of Health. *Health and Social Care Act 2008: Code of Practice on the Prevention and Control of Infections*; Department of Health: Hong Kong, China, 2015.
12. Pulcini, C.; Binda, F.; Lamkang, A.S.; Trett, A.; Charani, E.; Goff, D.A. Developing core elements and checklist items for global hospital antimicrobial stewardship programmes: A consensus approach. *Clin. Microbiol. Infect.* **2019**, *25*, 20–25. [CrossRef] [PubMed]

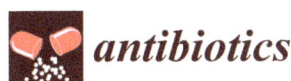
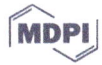

Article

Evaluation of an Antimicrobial Stewardship Program for Wound and Burn Care in Three Hospitals in Nepal

Varidhi Nauriyal [1,*], Shankar Man Rai [2], Rajesh Dhoj Joshi [3], Buddhi Bahadur Thapa [4], Linda Kaljee [5,*], Tyler Prentiss [5], Gina Maki [1], Basudha Shrestha [3], Deepak C. Bajracharya [6], Kshitij Karki [6], Nilesh Joshi [6], Arjun Acharya [4], Laxman Banstola [4], Suresh Raj Poudel [4], Anip Joshi [4], Abhinav Dahal [3], Niranjan Palikhe [3], Sachin Khadka [3], Piyush Giri [2], Apar Lamichhane [2] and Marcus Zervos [1]

[1] Division of Infectious Disease, Henry Ford Health System, Detroit, MI 48202, USA; gmaki1@hfhs.org (G.M.); mzervos1@hfhs.org (M.Z.)
[2] Kirtipur Hospital, Kathmandu 44600, Nepal; shankarrai1956@gmail.com (S.M.R.); dr.piyushgiri@gmail.com (P.G.); aparlamichhane@gmail.com (A.L.)
[3] Kathmandu Model Hospital, Kathmandu 44600, Nepal; rdhojrajesh@gmail.com (R.D.J.); basudha111@gmail.com (B.S.); dahal.abhinav@hotmail.com (A.D.); niranjanpalikhe@gmail.com (N.P.); sachin_khadka18@hotmail.com (S.K.)
[4] Pokhara Academy of Health Science, Pokhara 33700, Nepal; pahspokhara@gmail.com (B.B.T.); drarjunacharya@gmail.com (A.A.); lbanstola@hotmail.com (L.B.); poudelsuresh6@gmail.com (S.R.P.); anipjoshi@yahoo.com (A.J.)
[5] Global Health Initiative, Henry Ford Health System, Detroit, MI 48202, USA; tprenti1@hfhs.org
[6] Group for Technical Assistance, Kathmandu 44600, Nepal; bajra.deepak@gmail.com (D.C.B.); k49karki@gmail.com (K.K.); jos_nil@live.com (N.J.)
* Correspondence: vnauriy1@hfhs.org (V.N.); lkaljee1@hfhs.org (L.K.); Tel.: +1-203-909-4111 (V.N.); +1-301-873-1203 (L.K.)

Received: 9 November 2020; Accepted: 12 December 2020; Published: 16 December 2020

Abstract: Antimicrobial stewardship (AMS) programs can decrease non-optimal use of antibiotics in hospital settings. There are limited data on AMS programs in burn and chronic wound centers in low- and middle-income countries (LMIC). A post-prescription review and feedback (PPRF) program was implemented in three hospitals in Nepal with a focus on wound and burn care. A total of 241 baseline and 236 post-intervention patient chart data were collected from three hospitals. There was a significant decrease in utilizing days of therapy per 1000 patient days (DOT/1000 PD) of penicillin ($p = 0.02$), aminoglycoside ($p < 0.001$), and cephalosporin ($p = 0.04$). Increases in DOT/1000 PD at post-intervention were significant for metronidazole ($p < 0.001$), quinolone ($p = 0.01$), and other antibiotics ($p < 0.001$). Changes in use of antibiotics varied across hospitals, e.g., cephalosporin use decreased significantly at Kirtipur Hospital ($p < 0.001$) and Pokhara Academy of Health Sciences ($p = 0.02$), but not at Kathmandu Model Hospital ($p = 0.59$). An independent review conducted by infectious disease specialists at the Henry Ford Health System revealed significant changes in antibiotic prescribing practices both overall and by hospital. There was a decrease in mean number of intravenous antibiotic days between baseline (10.1 (SD 8.8)) and post-intervention (8.8 (SD 6.5)) ($t = 3.56$; $p < 0.001$), but no difference for oral antibiotics. Compared to baseline, over the 6-month post-intervention period, we found an increase in justified use of antibiotics ($p < 0.001$), de-escalation ($p < 0.001$), accurate documentation ($p < 0.001$), and adherence to the study antibiotic prescribing guidelines at 72 h ($p < 0.001$) and after diagnoses ($p < 0.001$). The evaluation data presented provide evidence that PPRF training and program implementation can contribute to hospital-based antibiotic stewardship for wound and burn care in Nepal.

Keywords: antibiotic resistance; stewardship; wound care; burn care; Nepal

1. Introduction

Antimicrobial resistance (AMR) has been recognized as a complex global health challenge lacking a universal solution. In 2015, the World Health Organization (WHO) released a global action plan (GAP) on AMR which provides a framework for developing national action plans on a country-by-country basis. The burden of health care associated infection is higher in low- and middle-income countries (LMIC) compared to higher income countries [1]. Inappropriate antimicrobial prescribing practices, lack of adequate antibiotic tracking systems, and limited healthcare funding to facilitate surveillance and laboratory infrastructure are some of the factors that have contributed to rising antimicrobial resistance in LMIC. There is evidence that antimicrobial stewardship (AMS) interventions are effective in increasing compliance with antibiotic policy, reducing duration of antibiotic treatment and potentially reducing hospital length of stay [2].

Post-prescription review and feedback (PPRF) programs include expert review of antibiotic prescribing decisions and feedback to the attending physician [3]. PPRF programs have been shown to be effective in U.S. hospitals, and on the basis of four studies reviewed by Dijck et al., there was a decrease in antibiotic days noted with audit and feedback in LMIC [4]. In addition, comparison of baseline and post-intervention data of a PPRF program in medical, obstetrics and gynecology, and general surgery wards at Kathmandu Model Hospital indicated decreased days of therapy per 1000 patient-days for courses of aminoglycoside and cephalosporin, increased justified use of antibiotics, de-escalation, and rational use of antibiotics [5].

To date, there are very limited data on the potential impact of AMS programs on antibiotic prescribing practices in burn and wound care centers in LMIC. Annually, an estimated 5 million deaths occur in LMIC due to injuries, with 10 to 50 times more individuals living with associated permanent disabilities [6]. Fire-related burns alone account for about 300,000 deaths annually, 95% percent of those occurring in LMIC. The highest rates of burns occur in Asia. In rural Nepal, burns are the second most common injury, accounting for 5% of disabilities. Overall, burns are the third most common injury after fall and road traffic accidents in the country [7]. Lack of a national burn registry makes estimating burden of disease difficult, however, a recent systematic review suggested the average hospital stay among burn victims ranged from 13 to 60 days in Nepal, with mortality estimates of 4.5 to 23.5% [8].

Studies have estimated infection-related mortality in burn victims to range from 40 to 60% [9–11]. Within LMIC, chronic wounds are commonly colonized and infected with antibiotic-resistant bacteria both during hospitalization and after discharge [12,13]. Inadequate hospital and clinic infection control protocols, delay in treatment, and use of self-treatment are some of the factors contributing to prevalence of infection in this population [14,15]. A primary concern is the increasing prevalence of antibiotic resistance in LMIC [16–18].

High morbidity and mortality associated with wounds and burns in Nepal and other LMIC has incentivized an urgent need to develop infection prevention practices and improve treatment. The aim of this study was to implement and evaluate the role of a hospital-based AMS program to support optimal antibiotic use for wounds and burns and in the longer-term decrease risks of infection from resistant pathogens.

2. Results

2.1. Patient Chart Data: Demographics

A total of 241 baseline and 236 post-intervention patient chart data were collected from the three study hospitals. At both baseline and post-intervention, a majority of patients were male and the mean age was less than 40 years. Number of study patients were evenly distributed across the three hospitals at both baseline and post-intervention. At post-intervention, there were more patient charts from the burn and less from the plastic and reconstructive surgery wards compared to baseline ($p < 0.001$). Length of stay decreased significantly within the burn unit ($p < 0.001$), as well as overall ($p = 0.006$) (see Table 1). There were no reported deaths among study patients.

Table 1. Baseline and post-intervention patient characteristics, length of hospital stay, and distribution across hospital sites and wards.

Demographic Characteristics		Baseline	Post-Intervention	p-Value
Gender	Female	38.6% (93)	38.6% (91)	0.995
Mean age (SD)		39.2 (17.6) Range: 16–83	37.4 (17.4) Range: 15–88	0.252
Hospital	Kathmandu Model	33.2% (80)	31.5% (74)	0.837
	Kirtipur	32.4% (78)	34.9% (82)	
	Pokhara	34.4% (83)	33.6% (79)	
Ward	Surgery	67.4% (161)	65.5% (154)	<0.001
	Plastic and reconstructive surgery	22.6% (54)	8.9% (21)	
	Burn unit	10.0% (24)	25.5% (60)	
Mean length of hospital stay (days) (SD) by ward	Total	8.0 (5.9) Range: 3–48	6.4 (6.2) Range: 3–70	0.006
	Surgery	6.7 (3.7) Range: 3–27	6.6 (7.0) Range: 3–70	0.788
	Plastic and reconstructive surgery	8.3 (5.4) Range: 3–24	6.3 (6.0) Range: 3–27	0.181
	Burn unit	15.2 (11.2) Range: 3–48	6.1 (4.1) Range: 3–16	<0.001

2.2. Patient Chart Data: Antibiotic Use at Baseline and Post-Intervention

Overall, there was a decrease in mean number of intravenous (IV) antibiotic days between baseline (10.1 (SD 8.8)) and post-intervention (8.8 (SD 6.5)) ($t = 3.56$; $p < 0.001$). There was no significant change for mean number of oral (PO) antibiotic days between baseline (4.2 (SD 3.3)) and post-intervention (3.7 (SD 3.5)) ($t = 0.66$; $p = 0.510$).

Across the three sites, there was a significant decrease in mean days of therapy between baseline and post-intervention for both aminoglycoside (6.1 (SD 4.3) vs 4.6 (SD 2.1)) ($t = 2.08$, $p = 0.04$) and cephalosporin (6.0 (SD 6.1) vs. 4.1 (SD 3.4)) ($t = 3.54$, $p < 0.001$). There were no significant changes in mean days of therapy for quinolines, penicillin, metronidazole, and other prescribed antibiotics.

Utilizing days of therapy per 1000 patient days (DOT/1000 patient-days (PD)) for data across the three study sites, we found no change in administering antibiotics either IV ($p = 0.67$) or PO ($p = 0.09$). There was a significant decrease in use of penicillin ($p = 0.02$), aminoglycoside ($p < 0.001$), and cephalosporin ($p = 0.04$). Increases in DOT/1000 PD at post-intervention were significant for metronidazole ($p < 0.001$), quinolone ($p = 0.01$), and other antibiotics ($p < 0.001$) (Figure 1 and Table 2).

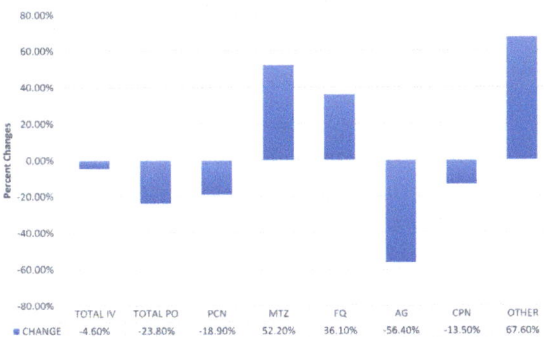

Figure 1. Changes in days of therapy (DOT) per 1000 patient-days (PD) between baseline and post-intervention in three hospitals in Nepal (Kirtipur, Kathmandu Model, and Pokhara hospitals). PCN = penicillin; MTZ = metronidazole; FQ: fluoroquinolone; AG: aminoglycosides; CPN: cephalosporin.

Table 2. Days of therapy (DOT) per 1000 patient-days (PD) of prescribed antibiotics at baseline and post-intervention periods total and by study sites (Kirtipur, Kathmandu Model, and Pokhara hospitals).

Site	Antibiotic Delivery & Class	Baseline DOT/1000 PD (N)	Post-Intervention DOT/1000 PD (N)	p-Value
TOTAL SITES	Intravenous antibiotics	1165 (222)	1114 (227)	0.67
	Oral antibiotics	101 (46)	75 (31)	0.09
	Penicillin	301 (91)	241 (70)	0.02
	Cephalosporin	525 (167)	454 (167)	0.04
	Metronidazole	75 (30)	160 (56)	<0.001
	Quinolone	46 (17)	72 (24)	0.01
	Aminoglycoside	266 (84)	117 (39)	<0.001
	Other course	57 (16)	177 (53)	<0.001
KIRTIPUR	Intravenous antibiotics	292 (70)	304 (77)	0.56
	Oral antibiotics	64 (27)	37 (10)	0.004
	Penicillin	49 (15)	61 (19)	0.30
	Cephalosporin	264 (71)	228 (71)	<0.001
	Metronidazole	10 (4)	30 (10)	0.002
	Quinolone	9 (30)	14 (5)	0.40
	Aminoglycoside	8 (40	16 (4)	0.15
	Other course	18 (5)	16 (4)	0.73
KATHMANDU MODEL	Intravenous antibiotics	289 (70)	354 (72)	0.80
	Oral antibiotics	29 (17)	32 (18)	0.80
	Penicillin	63 (18)	54 (17)	0.04
	Cephalosporin	125 (63)	144 (61)	0.59
	Metronidazole	42 (18)	112 (42)	<0.001
	Quinolone	37 (14)	24 (9)	0.02
	Aminoglycoside	34 (21)	40 (16)	0.90
	Other course	20 (6)	16 (9)	0.23
POKHARA	Intravenous antibiotics	584 (82)	436 (77)	0.12
	Oral antibiotics	8 (2)	5 (3)	0.37
	Penicillin	189 (58)	127 (34)	0.22
	Cephalosporin	136 (33)	76 (35)	0.02
	Metronidazole	24 (8)	15 (4)	0.62
	Quinolone	0	33 (9)	<0.001
	Aminoglycoside	224 (59)	56 (18)	<0.001
	Other course	19 (5)	142 (41)	<0.001

Looking at these data by site, we found no change in IV administration of antibiotics, but there was a decrease in administering PO antibiotics at Kirtipur Hospital ($p = 0.004$). Moreover, at Kirtipur Hospital, there was a significant decrease in use of cephalosporin ($p < 0.001$) but an increase in use of metronidazole ($p = 0.002$). At Kathmandu Model Hospital, there were significant decreases in use of penicillin ($p = 0.04$) and quinolones ($p = 0.02$), but a significant increase in use of metronidazole ($p < 0.001$). At Pokhara Academy of Health Science, there was a decrease in both cephalosporin ($p = 0.02$) and aminoglycoside ($p < 0.001$), but increases in quinolones ($p < 0.001$) and other antibiotics ($p < 0.001$). (Table 2).

An independent review conducted by infectious disease specialists at the Henry Ford Health System revealed significant changes in antibiotic prescribing practices both overall and by hospital. Over the 6-month post-intervention period, there was a noted increase in justified use of antibiotics, de-escalation, accurate documentation, and adherence to the study antibiotic prescribing guidelines at 72 h and after diagnoses (definitive) (Table 3).

Table 3. Justification, de-escalation, treatment rationale, and fidelity to guidelines at baseline and post-intervention by total sites and individual hospitals (Kirtipur, Kathmandu Model, and Pokhara).

Site	Review Criteria	Baseline	Post-Intervention	p-Value
TOTAL SITES	Was the antibiotics course justified? (Yes)	34.9% (84)	78.0% (184)	<0.001
	Were antibiotics de-escalated? (Yes)	28.0% (51)	85.9% (167)	<0.001
	Was the treatment rationale documented correctly? (Yes)	33.3% (62)	77.7% (146)	<0.001
	Were guidelines followed within the first 72 h of therapy? (Yes)	37.9% (67)	82.2% (143)	<0.001
	Were recommendations followed for definitive therapy? (Yes)	29.4% (50)	82.8% (154)	<0.001
KIRTIPUR	Was the antibiotics course justified? (Yes)	33.3% (26)	70.7% (58)	<0.001
	Were antibiotics de-escalated? (Yes)	41.8% (28)	87.5% (56)	<0.001
	Was the treatment rationale documented correctly? (Yes)	27.4% (20)	68.6% (48)	<0.001
	Were guidelines followed within the first 72 h of therapy? (Yes)	30.8% (20)	78.6% (44)	<0.001
	Were recommendations followed for definitive therapy? (Yes)	27.8% (20)	77.2% (44)	<0.001
KATHMANDU MODEL	Was the antibiotics course justified? (Yes)	46.3% (37)	77.0% (57)	<0.001
	Were antibiotics de-escalated? (Yes)	30.4% (21)	78.6% (55)	<0.001
	Was the treatment rationale documented correctly? (Yes)	53.5% (38)	81.4% (57)	<0.001
	Were guidelines followed within the first 72 h of therapy? (Yes)	63.0% (46)	80.6% (54)	0.016
	Were recommendations followed for definitive therapy? (Yes)	46.2% (30)	79.4% (54)	<0.001
POKHARA	Was the antibiotics course justified? (Yes)	25.3% (21)	86.1% (68)	<0.001
	Were antibiotics de-escalated? (Yes)	4.3% (2)	91.7% (55)	<0.001
	Was the treatment rationale documented correctly? (Yes)	9.5% (4)	85.4% (41)	<0.001
	Were guidelines followed within the first 72 h of therapy? (Yes)	2.6% (1)	88.2% (45)	<0.001
	Were recommendations followed for definitive therapy? (Yes)	0	91.7% (55)	<0.001

Physician champions recorded information on recommendations made during the post-intervention period. Across the three study sites, there were a total of 249 logbook entries with 71 recommendations (28.5%). Among the recommendations, there were 53 cases (74.6%) in which the physician champion recommended a change in the antibiotic and 18 cases (25.4%) in which the recommendation was to stop antibiotics. Overall, 41/71 (57.7%) recommendations were followed by the prescribing physician. Among 47 entries with the reason listed for the recommendation, 25 cases (53.2%) were related to obtaining data on resistance/sensitivity patterns, 6 cases (12.8%) due to no definitive evidence of infection, and 5 cases (10.6%) were related to extended duration of antibiotic use. Other reasons included use of multiple antibiotics, IV to oral conversion, patient symptoms, and change from a broader to a narrower spectrum antibiotic.

3. Discussion

The World Health Organization Global Action Plan (GAP) for AMR includes five strategic objectives that must be addressed to decrease pathogen resistance to available pharmaceutical therapeutics. These objectives include to (1) increase awareness and understanding of AMR, (2) strengthen knowledge through surveillance and research, (3) reduce the incidence of infection, (4) optimize the use of antimicrobial medicines, and (5) ensure sustainable investment in countering antimicrobial resistance [18]. Over the past 5 years, the partnership between the Henry Ford Health System, Nepali private, public, and non-profit hospital systems, and the Group for Technical Assistance in Kathmandu has supported AMR stewardship education and programs. The data presented in this paper represent an important step for implementation of hospital-based stewardship programs with an emphasis on the urgent need in LMIC to reduce risks of infection in wound and burn care. The hospitals selected included the non-profit and government health sectors. Both Kathmandu Model and Kirtipur hospitals were part of a previous post-prescription review and feedback (PPRF) project, and all three hospitals remain connected to ongoing education and training through a new web-based program Global Learning in Antimicrobial Resistance (GLAMR).

The data presented provide evidence that PPRF training and program implementation can contribute to hospital-based stewardship in Nepal. Across all three hospitals, there is a clear indication that prescribing practices at post-intervention were more likely justified and followed antibiotic prescribing guidelines. Utilizing DOT/1000 PD analytics, we found that across the three hospitals there were significant decreases in the use of penicillin, cephalosporins, and aminoglycosides. Within each individual hospital, there was some variation in prescribing practices, however, there was evidence of decreased use of penicillin, aminoglycosides, quinolones, and cephalosporins. Variations may be attributable to differences in prescribing practices at baseline within the various study wards. A recent study published on bacteriological profile of burn wound infections in Nepal suggested predominance of resistant Gram-negative organisms such as *Acinetobacter* spp., *Pseudomonas* spp., and *Enterobacter* spp. [19]. The decrease in use of penicillin, cephalosporins, and quinolones is hence an encouraging signal towards recognition of bacterial epidemiology and appropriate use of antimicrobials. While there was an increase in metronidazole use at post-intervention, the overall increase in "justified use" of antibiotics in our post-intervention group indicates an overall improvement in prescribing practices. The use of metronidazole with another agent would have been deemed "unjustified".

The changes across three hospitals within two separate locations in Nepal (Kathmandu and Pokhara) indicate that PPRF programs can be successfully implemented under different hospital administration and supports further dissemination as a part of hospital-based stewardship elsewhere in Nepal. Our evaluation of the previous implementation of the PPRF program at Kathmandu Model Hospital indicated decreases in use of cephalosporins and aminoglycosides. While there was no further decrease in these two antibiotics in the current study at Kathmandu Model Hospital, this may have been due to less use of these antibiotics at baseline.

The review of the prescribing practices shows significant improvements across all three study sites in terms of justified use, following guidelines, and documentation. Therefore, even as use of some antibiotics increased, these data suggest that prescribing practices at post-intervention were more likely appropriate to the diagnosis in terms of type and duration. Furthermore, the logbook data indicate that physician champions were actively reviewing patient charts within their wards and making recommendations. More than half of those recommendations were followed by the prescribing physician, with a majority of those recommendations due to information on pathogen resistance/sensitivity, lack of evidence of infection, and long duration of use of a single antibiotic.

The study strengths include the potential for introducing antimicrobial stewardship programs in low-resource hospital settings with comprehensive training and locally salient antibiotic prescribing guidelines. In addition, non-infectious disease physicians were successfully trained as physician champions and supported prescribing changes within their wards. Utilizing the existing training materials and guidelines reflective of potential regional differences in resistance and availability of antibiotics, the program can be duplicated elsewhere in Nepal. There are some limitations to the study. Data collection was dependent on manual review of handwritten notes given the lack of electronic medical record in Nepal. "Other courses" is an un-identified pool of antibiotics since the focus was on obtaining usage data on the most commonly prescribed antibiotics. Physician champions had to manually fill out log-books, which added to their workload, and hence not all data points were consistently entered. Out of a total of 249 log-book entries, only 47 outlined rationale for recommendations. The study length did not provide time to determine if there were any changes in resistance levels among pathogens.

4. Materials and Methods

The study was part of a larger AMR and AMS collaboration between the Henry Ford Health System Division of Infectious Diseases and Global Health Initiative (Detroit, MI, USA); the Group for Technical Assistance (Kathmandu, Nepal); and various non-profit, public, and private hospitals in Nepal. PPRF programs include expert review of antibiotic prescribing decisions and feedback to the prescribing physician. One strength of the current study is the focus of the PPRF program on wound and burn care. In many LMIC, there are inadequate numbers of infectious disease specialists, and therefore a key element of the adapted PPRF program in Nepal includes training "physician champions" in AMR and AMS. More details about the adaptation of the PPRF intervention for use in Nepal is described in detail elsewhere [5]. Variations for the current study included revisions to the antibiotic prescribing guidebook to include information on wound and burn care and a training-of-trainers approach, whereby the AMR "physician champions" were both trained in the PPRF program and provided with information and tools to train other healthcare providers within their wards. The antibiotic prescribing guidebook included 5 sections: (1) empiric guidelines, (2) suggested definitive guidelines with options depending on susceptabilities, (3) suggested duration of antibiotic therapy based on indications, (4) intravenous to oral conversions, and (5) renal dosing (Table 4). A total of 52 healthcare providers and hospital administrators including 6 physician champions from 3 study sites (Kathmandu Model, Kirtipur, and Pokhara hospitals) were trained over 2 days (11–12 July 2018).

Table 4. Examples of empiric, definitive, and duration antibiotic prescribing guidelines.

Empiric Guidelines			
Diagnosis	Suspected Pathogen	Empiric Therapy	Duration of Therapy
Abdominal infection, community-acquired (e.g., cholecystitis, cholangitis, diverticulitis, abscess); NOTE: add gentamicin if MDRO suspected or identified	Enterobacteriaceae *Bacteroides* sp. Enterococci Streptococci	Preferred: • Ceftriaxone IV 1 g q24h + metronidazole IV or PO 500 mg q8h • +/− gentamicin IV 5 mg/kg q24h Alternative: • piperacillin/tazobactam IV 4.5 g q6h • cefepime IV 2 g q12h + metronidazole IV or PO 500 mg q8h + IV 5mg/kg q24hr • imipenem IV 1g q8h Oral options for outpatient therapy: • ofloxacin PO 400 mg q12h + metronidazole PO 500 mg q12h • moxifloxacin PO 400 mg q24h	4 days with adequate source control
Suggested Definitive Guidelines			
Organism	Preferred Therapy	Alternative Therapy (Depending on Allergies and Susceptibilities)	
Enterobacter spp. (AmpC-producing organism)	Cefepime	Meropenem, colistin, tigecycline, trimethoprim/sulfamethoxazole, gentamicin, amikacin Consider combination therapy for extensively drug-resistant *Acinetobacter*	
Suggested Duration of Antimicrobial Therapy Based on Indication			
Diagnosis	Duration of Therapy	Key References	
Complicated intra-abdominal infection, community-acquired (appendicitis, cholecystitis, diverticulitis)	4 to 7 days after adequate source control	Infectious Diseases Society of America Guidelines: http://www.idsociety.org/uploadedFiles/ IDSA/GuidelinesPatient_Care/PDF_ Library/Intraabdominal%20Infectin.pdf Other resources: http://www.nejm.org/doi/ pdf/10.1056/NEJMoa1411162	

4.1. Study Sites

The research took place in 2 hospitals in Kathmandu (Kathmandu Model Hospital and Kirtipur Hospital) and 1 hospital in Pokhara (Pokhara Academy of Health Science). Kathmandu is located in central Nepal and Pokhara is further toward the western region (Figure 2).

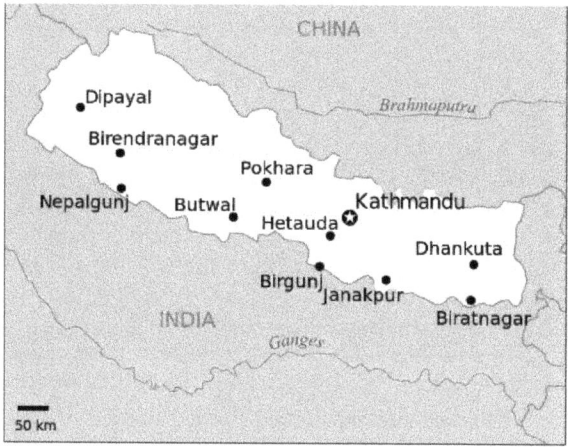

Figure 2. Map of major cities in Nepal.

Both Kathmandu Model and Kirtipur hospitals are a part of a larger non-profit health organization, the Public Health Concern Trust (Phect, Nepal). Kathmandu Model is a 125-bed hospital that opened in 1993. Kathmandu Model Hospital provides a range of in-patient and out-patient services. The current study was focused in the general and specialized surgical wards. Kirtipur Hospital is a 100-bed hospital with additional specialized services including a 24 h emergency department. Kirtipur Hospital has a reconstructive surgery ward and the only burn intensive care unit in Nepal, which were the study sites for the current project. Kirtipur Hospital receives burn patients from throughout the country, and is part of the Resurge International Surgical Outreach Program that provides training and support to local hospitals and surgeons engaged in reconstructive and burn-related surgeries. Pokhara Academy of Health Science is a government facility and the second largest hospital in Nepal. The 500-bed hospital offers a broad range of services including a trauma center, burn unit, and surgical ward. These 3 wards were the study sites for the current project.

4.2. Study Population

The 3 study hospitals provide services to a range of socio-economic groups from both urban and rural areas in Nepal. Eligibility criteria for the patient chart review evaluation data included (1) inpatient within the study wards, (2) aged 15 + years, and (3) prescribed antibiotics for at least 72 h within the hospital.

4.3. Data Collection

4.3.1. Patient Chart Data

Eligible patient chart data were collected for 6 months baseline (pre-PPRF training) from January 2018 to June 2018 and 6 months post-intervention between August 2018 and January 2019. The gap month (July 2018) was the implementation of the intervention. Data collection was coordinated and conducted by trained staff at a local nongovernmental agency (Group for Technical Assistance) located in Kathmandu.

Sample size was based on published data on duration of injectable drug use from Nepali hospitals [20]. Using a two-sided comparison of a continuous variable (days of therapy per 1000 study patient days, DOT/1000PD), we calculated that a sample size of 211 patients per group (baseline and post-intervention) was necessary to detect a difference of 20% between time periods (90% CI, $\alpha = 05$).

Patient chart data included: (1) demographics (gender and age), (2) hospital/ward, (3) length of stay, (4) source of infection, (5) patient height/weight, (6) conditions present at study enrollment, (7) systemic antibiotic use during prior 72 h, (8) origin of onset of infection, (9) working and final diagnosis, (10) systemic antibiotic use throughout the hospital stay period, (11) therapy prescribed at discharge, (12) infection-related complications, (13) factors associated with persistent infection, and (14) disposition at end of hospital stay (if deceased, date and cause).

After data collection, patient chart data were reviewed by infectious disease specialists at the Henry Ford Health System to determine whether prescribed antibiotics were justified. Justification was determined by diagnosis, pathogen (when available), duration, and route (IV or PO) as described within the antibiotic prescribing guidelines (Table 4). Reviews included both initial therapy and therapy changes after recommendations by the physician champions.

4.3.2. Physician Logbook Data

Physician champions were provided with antibiotic prescribing guidelines, which included a logbook. Through the logbooks, physicians documented chart reviews, recommendations made, and acceptance of recommendations by the prescribing physician. Recommendations were made verbally to the prescribing physician and/or as written notes. Logbooks were collected on a monthly basis to ensure that they were completed as required by the evaluation protocol.

4.4. Data Management and Analysis

Patient chart data were entered into REDCap (Research Electronic Data Capture) [21] by trained staff at the Group for Technical Assistance in Nepal. REDCap is a secure web application for building and managing online databases. REDCap allowed immediate access to the data both at the Henry Ford Health System and the project data team in Nepal. Data were reviewed and cleaned, which included deleting 2 cases that were under 15 years and 4 cases that were collected after the end of the 6-month post-intervention period. Continuous data were described using means and standard deviations, and univariate two group comparisons used independent two-group t-tests to assess significance. Categorical data were described using counts and percentages, and chi-squared tests were used to assess significance. Days of therapy DOT/1000 PD was calculated at baseline and intervention periods for IV and PO delivery and specific antibiotics. Days of therapy was calculated as 1921 at baseline ($N = 241$) and 1520 ($N = 236$) at post-intervention across the 3 sites. Days of therapy at baseline and post-intervention were calculated by site at 321 and 390 (Kathmandu Model), 358 and 365 (Kirtipur), and 592 and 449 (Pokhara), respectively. The proportion of DOT/1000 PD was compared between baseline and intervention time points using tests of proportion and Fisher's exact test to determine significance. Statistical significance was set at $p < 0.05$.

Logbooks were collected by the project data team on a monthly basis and scanned. Scanned logbook data were sent to the evaluation team at the Henry Ford Health System for review. Scanned data were entered into Excel and analyzed using descriptive statistics. All statistical analysis was performed using SPSS 25.0 (Version 25.0. Armonk, NY, USA).

4.5. Ethical Review

The study was approved by the Institutional Review Board at the Henry Ford Health System, Detroit, MI (#11732), and the Nepal Health Research Council, Kathmandu, Nepal (#1523).

5. Conclusions

This study demonstrates successful implementation of PPRF as an antimicrobial stewardship tool at burn and wound in-patient centers in Nepal. There is an encouraging trend towards change in antimicrobial prescribing practice with more thoughtful and justified use.

Author Contributions: Conceptualization, S.M.R., L.K., and M.Z.; data curation, V.N., T.P., and B.S.; formal analysis, V.N. and L.K.; funding acquisition, L.K. and T.P.; investigation, T.P., G.M., D.C.B., K.K., L.B., S.R.P., A.J., A.D., N.P., S.K., P.G., and A.L.; methodology, L.K.; project administration, V.N., S.M.R., R.D.J., T.P., D.C.B., K.K., N.J., and A.A.; supervision, S.M.R., R.D.J., B.B.T., G.M., A.A., and M.Z.; writing—original draft, V.N. and L.K.; writing—review and editing, G.M. All authors have read and agreed to the published version of the manuscript.

Funding: This research was funded by the MERCK INVESTIGATOR STUDIES PROGRAM (MISP), grant number 57055.

Acknowledgments: We would like to thank the physician champions from Kathmandu Model and Kirtipur hospitals and the Pokhara Academy of Health Science for their commitment to the intervention and the research. We would also like to thank the support staff at the Group for Technical Assistance (Kathmandu) who contributed significantly to the organization of the physician training program logistics and day-to-day tasks associated with the program.

Conflicts of Interest: The authors declare no conflict of interest. The funders had no role in the design of the study; in the collection, analyses, or interpretation of data; in the writing of the manuscript; or in the decision to publish the results.

References

1. Allegranzi, B.; Nejad, S.B.; Combescure, C.; Graafmans, W.; Attar, H.; Donaldson, L.; Pittet, D. Burden of endemic health-care-associated infection in developing countries: Systematic review and meta-analysis. *Lancet* **2011**, *377*, 228–241. [CrossRef]
2. Davey, P.; Brown, E.; Fenelon, L.; Finch, R.; Gould, I.; Hartman, G.; Holmes, A.; Ramsay, C.; Taylor, E.; Wilcox, M.; et al. Interventions to improve antibiotic prescribing practices for hospital inpatients. *Cochrane Database Syst. Rev.* **2005**, *4*, CD003543. [CrossRef]
3. Arnold, F.W.; McDonald, L.C.; Smith, R.S.; Newman, D.; Ramirez, J.A. Improving Antimicrobial Use in the Hospital Setting by Providing Usage Feedback to Prescribing Physicians. *Infect. Control. Hosp. Epidemiol.* **2006**, *27*, 378–382. [CrossRef] [PubMed]
4. Van Dijck, C.; Vlieghe, E.; Cox, J.A. Antibiotic stewardship interventions in hospitals in low-and middle-income countries: A systematic review. *Bull. World Health Organ.* **2018**, *96*, 266–280. [CrossRef] [PubMed]
5. Joshi, R.D.; Zervos, M.; Kaljee, L.; Shrestha, B.; Maki, G.; Prentiss, T.; Bajracharya, D.C.; Karki, K.; Joshi, N.; Rai, S.M. Evaluation of a Hospital-Based Post-Prescription Review and Feedback Pilot in Kathmandu, Nepal. *Am. J. Trop. Med. Hyg.* **2019**, *101*, 923–928. [CrossRef] [PubMed]
6. Gosselin, R.A. Injuries: The neglected burden in developing countries. *Bull. World Health Organ.* **2009**, *87*, 246. [CrossRef] [PubMed]
7. Gupta, S.; Wong, E.G.; Nepal, S.; Shrestha, S.; Kushner, A.L.; Nwomeh, B.C.; Wren, S.M. Injury prevalence and causality in developing nations: Results from a countrywide population-based survey in Nepal. *Surgery* **2015**, *157*, 843–849. [CrossRef] [PubMed]
8. Tripathee, S.; Basnet, S.J. Epidemiology of burn injuries in Nepal: A systemic review. *Burn. Trauma* **2017**, *5*, 10. [CrossRef]
9. Krishnan, P.L.; Frew, Q.; Green, A.; Martin, R.; Dziewulski, P. Cause of death and correlation with autopsy findings in burns patients. *Burns* **2013**, *39*, 583–588. [CrossRef] [PubMed]
10. Bloemsma, G.; Dokter, J.; Boxma, H.; Oen, I. Mortality and causes of death in a burn centre. *Burns* **2008**, *34*, 1103–1107. [CrossRef] [PubMed]
11. Lachiewicz, A.M.; Hauck, C.G.; Weber, D.J.; Cairns, B.A.; Van Duin, D. Bacterial Infections After Burn Injuries: Impact of Multidrug Resistance. *Clin. Infect. Dis.* **2017**, *65*, 2130–2136. [CrossRef] [PubMed]
12. Sharma, K.; Thanbuana, B.T.; Gupta, A.K.; Rajkumari, N.; Mathur, P.; Gunjiyal, J.; Misra, M.C. A prospective study of wound infection among post-discharge patients at a level 1 trauma centre of India. *Indian J. Med. Microbiol.* **2016**, *34*, 198–201. [CrossRef] [PubMed]

13. Bhangu, A.; Ademuyiwa, A.O.; Aguilera, M.L.; Alexander, P.; Al-Saqqa, S.W.; Borda-Luque, G.; Costas-Chavarri, A.; Drake, T.M.; Ntirenganya, F.; Fitzgerald, J.E.; et al. Surgical site infection after gastrointestinal surgery in high-income, middle-income, and low-income countries: A prospective, international, multicentre cohort study. *Lancet Infect. Dis.* **2018**, *18*, 516–525. [CrossRef]
14. Phuyal, K.; Ogada, E.A.; Bendell, R.; Price, P.E.; Potokar, T. Burns in Nepal: A participatory, community survey of burn cases and knowledge, attitudes and practices to burn care and prevention in three rural municipalities. *BMJ Open* **2020**, *10*, e033071. [CrossRef] [PubMed]
15. Karki, B.; Rai, S.M.; Nakarmi, K.K.; Basnet, S.J.; Magar, M.G.; Nagarkoti, K.K.; Thapa, S. Clinical Epidemiology of Acute Burn Injuries at Nepal Cleft and Burn Centre, Kathmandu, Nepal. *Ann. Plast. Surg.* **2018**, *80*, S95–S97. [CrossRef] [PubMed]
16. Viswanathan, V.; Pendsey, S.; Radhakrishnan, C.; Rege, T.D.; Ahdal, J.; Jain, R. Methicillin-Resistant Staphylococcus aureus in Diabetic Foot Infection in India: A Growing Menace. *Int. J. Low. Extrem. Wounds* **2019**, *18*, 236–246. [CrossRef] [PubMed]
17. Bahemia, I.; Muganza, A.; Moore, R.E.; Sahid, F.; Menezes, C. Microbiology and antibiotic resistance in severe burns patients: A 5 year review in an adult burns unit. *Burns* **2015**, *41*, 1536–1542. [CrossRef] [PubMed]
18. WHO. Global Action Plan on Antimicrobial Resistance. Available online: https://www.who.int/antimicrobial-resistance/global-action-plan/en/ (accessed on 6 October 2020).
19. Pujji, O.J.S.; Nakarmi, K.K.; Shrestha, B.; Rai, S.M.; Jeffery, S.L.A. The Bacteriological Profile of Burn Wound Infections at a Tertiary Burns Center in Nepal. *J. Burn. Care Res.* **2019**, *40*, 838–845. [CrossRef] [PubMed]
20. Gyawali, S.; Shandar Ravi, P.; Saha, A.; Mohan, L. Study of prescription injectable drugs and intravenous fluids to inpatients in a teaching hospital in Nepal. *McGill J. Med.* **2009**, *12*, 13–20. [PubMed]
21. Harris, P.A.; Taylor, R.; Minor, B.L.; Elliott, V.; Fernandez, M.; O'Neal, L.; McLeod, L.; Delacqua, G.; Delacqua, F.; Kirby, J.; et al. The REDCap consortium: Building an international community of software platform partners. *J. Biomed. Inform.* **2019**, *95*, 103208. [CrossRef] [PubMed]

Publisher's Note: MDPI stays neutral with regard to jurisdictional claims in published maps and institutional affiliations.

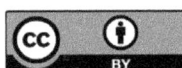

© 2020 by the authors. Licensee MDPI, Basel, Switzerland. This article is an open access article distributed under the terms and conditions of the Creative Commons Attribution (CC BY) license (http://creativecommons.org/licenses/by/4.0/).

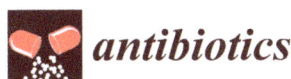

Article

Feasibility and Validity of a Framework for Antimicrobial Stewardship in General Practice: Key Stakeholder Interviews

Lesley A. Hawes [1,2,*], **Jaclyn Bishop** [2,3,4], **Kirsty Buising** [2,5,6] **and Danielle Mazza** [1,2]

1. Department of General Practice, School of Primary and Allied Health Care, Monash University, Level 1, 270 Ferntree Gully Road, Notting Hill, Victoria 3168, Australia; Danielle.Mazza@monash.edu
2. National Centre for Antimicrobial Stewardship, The Peter Doherty Institute for Infection and Immunity, University of Melbourne, Level 5, 792 Elizabeth Street, Melbourne, Victoria 3000, Australia; jaclynb@student.unimelb.edu.au (J.B.); Kirsty.Buising@mh.org.au (K.B.)
3. Department of Medicine—Royal Melbourne Hospital, Faculty of Medicine, Dentistry and Health Sciences, The University of Melbourne, Royal Parade, Melbourne, Victoria 3050, Australia
4. Pharmacy Department, Ballarat Health Services, Drummond Street, Ballarat, Victoria 3350, Australia
5. Victorian Infectious Diseases Service, Royal Melbourne Hospital, 300 Grattan St, Parkville, Victoria 3050, Australia
6. Department of Infectious Diseases, Peter Doherty Institute for Infection and Immunity, University of Melbourne, Melbourne, Victoria 3010, Australia
* Correspondence: Lesley.Hawes@monash.edu

Received: 26 October 2020; Accepted: 10 December 2020; Published: 13 December 2020

Abstract: There is little guidance about developing systems for antimicrobial stewardship (AMS) for general practice. A literature review identified six key components: governance, monitoring of antibiotic prescribing and resistance with feedback to prescribers, consultation support, education of the public and general practitioners, pharmacist and nurse involvement, and research, which were incorporated into a potential framework for the general practice context. Objectives: to determine the feasibility and validity of the proposed AMS framework. A secondary objective was to identify likely bodies responsible for implementation in Australia. We undertook interviews with 12 key stakeholders from government, research, and professional groups. Data were analysed with a thematic approach. The framework was considered valid and feasible. No clear organisation was identified to lead AMS implementation in general practice. The current volume-based antibiotic prescription monitoring system was considered insufficient. AMS education for the public, further development of GP education, and improved consultation support were strongly recommended. The role of community-based pharmacists and nurses is largely unexplored, but their involvement was recommended. A clear leader to drive AMS in general practice is essential for an action framework to gain traction. Monitoring and feedback of antibiotic prescribing require urgent development to include monitoring of prescribing appropriateness and patient outcomes.

Keywords: antimicrobial stewardship; general practice; family practice; antibiotic; health policy; quality of health care; antibiotics; public health; pharmacist; nurse

1. Introduction

Antimicrobial resistance is a global problem with a major impact on health care and associated costs [1]. Exposure of microbes to antimicrobials contributes to the problem [2,3]; unnecessary use of antimicrobials must be minimised. The consumption of antibiotics in the Australian community is high in comparison with similar countries [4], with most antibiotics prescribed by general practitioners [4].

There is a high rate of prescribing of moderate- (66% of use) and broad-spectrum antibiotics (25%) [5], and inappropriate use is still common for conditions such as upper respiratory tract infections [4]. For these conditions, antibiotics are prescribed at rates 4–9 times that recommended by the Australian national antibiotic prescribing guidelines Therapeutic Guidelines—Antibiotic [6]. Australia's National Antimicrobial Resistance Strategy calls for the introduction of antimicrobial stewardship (AMS) to address inappropriate antibiotic prescribing [7]. However, there is little guidance for how to implement AMS across Australian general practice.

Through a review of international health system approaches to AMS in general practice [8–23], a potential framework to guide AMS in general practice was formulated. This framework contains six key components: governance, monitoring of antimicrobial resistance and prescribing with feedback to GPs, education for general practitioners (GPs) and the public, consultation support, the involvement of community-based pharmacists and nurses, and research [24]. Details of the framework are provided in Appendix A.

The aim of this study was to interview key stakeholders to determine the likely feasibility and validity of the proposed AMS framework and a secondary aim was to identify any existing organisations who may take on responsibility for implementation in Australia.

2. Results

Of the 24 invited stakeholders, 13 accepted. Two declined, another was on extended leave, and eight did not respond to two emails. One of those who declined—despite being invited to participate as an expert, not as a representative—replied, "[name of organisation] is not in the best place to help with your query regarding AMS in general practice and we recommend you contact [another named organisation]." We already had stakeholders from the organisation recommended. One respondent accepted but could not be interviewed in the timeframe. The 12 interviewed stakeholders' background, relevant expertise, and location are outlined in Table 1. The COREQ checklist is available in Supplementary Table S1.

Table 1. The professional background, antimicrobial stewardship (AMS) involvement, and location of the 12 interviewed stakeholders.

Professional Background (Not Necessarily Current Employment)	Number
General practitioner	6
Pharmacist	5
Medical Microbiologist	1
TOTAL	12
AMS Involvement (Stakeholders may have multiple roles)	
Clinical Quality Improvement/AMS committee/professional organisation representative	9
Researcher in general practice AMS	4
Health Department (including Public Health)	2
Primary Health Network	2
Microbiology Laboratory	1
Location	
New South Wales and/or Australian Capital Territory	4
Victoria	4
Queensland	3
Tasmania	1
TOTAL	12

Overall, stakeholders reported that the proposed AMS framework for general practice and its components were feasible and valid; and that it provided a link between the objectives of Australia's National AMR Strategy and action. However, most stakeholders highlighted that it would require leadership and prioritisation for implementation to have the desired impact. Importantly, the stakeholders had difficulty nominating the best organisation to oversee this implementation. (Representative quotes are supplied; additional quotes are available in Supplementary Table S2).

It seems very comprehensive to me ... able to be implemented ... I think we need to have an agreed upon governance structure and agreed upon priorities ... I don't think there is one clear person or group who is responsible for the whole caboodle of this. (Participant (P) 6)

Asked how they would define success, stakeholders nominated short- and long-term goals. Short-term goals were increased adherence to prescribing guidelines and improved patient outcomes with no increase in harm. Stakeholders also commented that increased professional support provided by such a framework may lead to improved professional satisfaction for GPs. The long-term goals that they stated were a decrease, or at least, no increase in antimicrobial resistance (AMR).

Governance was reported by the stakeholders to be important to set strategic priorities and harmonize approaches. The importance of aligning work in primary care with work in other sectors was highlighted. A national action plan for AMS in general practice was regarded as a Commonwealth responsibility, with the Office of Health Protection (within the Department of Health) suggested to lead stakeholder engagement.

I think within the implementation plan the Office of Health Protection has an important role ... I mean they have the remit of the strategy. In terms of the organisations that will have a responsibility some of them are probably clear, and some of them just need coordination. The important part of that is to work in a collaborative way, coordinated way ... We shouldn't be ... isolating sectors such as hospital, aged care ... primary care. (P5)

There were calls to make practice accreditation mandatory and to include AMS activities such as antibiotic monitoring or education in this. Suggestions were made for financial incentives to encourage AMS activity in general practice.

Stakeholders also generally supported greater regulatory controls on prescriptions, the removal of automatic repeats, and promotion of unit dispensing (dispensed quantities match antibiotic guideline recommendations, not pack sizes).

People you can educate as much as you like, but until you actually restrict the antibiotics people aren't going to stop using them ... (P6)

Monitoring and feedback on antibiotic prescribing was perceived as effective for changing behaviour, but the current process was viewed as problematic. Unresolved practical considerations included that complete datasets are not available, the possible defensiveness of GPs about their data being reviewed, questions about who would analyse and provide feedback to GPs, and whether collection should be mandatory or incentivised. The government was regarded as responsible for obtaining complete datasets. Stakeholders saw potential for the Practice Incentives Program—Quality Improvement Incentive [25] (GP data collected by the Primary Health Networks (PHNs) for process measures) to include antibiotic monitoring. Stakeholders said that feedback should include peer comparisons, and ideally link in with education and consultation support. The potential use of positive variance was described, that is, investigating the strategies used by those who prescribe fewer antibiotics than their peers.

Government needs to incentivize, to capture [antibiotic prescribing] information. You know organisations like the PHNs are really well suited to that. (P11)

In terms of investigating what works, one thing that we do poorly is to look for positive variance. (P7)

Community education in the form of ongoing tailored public health campaigns was considered important and viewed as a government responsibility. There were suggestions that health literacy education for antibiotic awareness should start at school.

We do need the consumer to come on board to ... not have that expectation [for antibiotics], which then does make the consultation very difficult. (P8)

GP education endorsed by the Royal Australian College of General Practitioners (RACGP) or supplied by PHNs or medical specialists was well regarded and trusted. NPS MedicineWise (an independent organisation supporting quality use of medicines) was acknowledged as an existing channel for GP education, but it was questioned as to whether what was currently provided was at the depth necessary to have the largest impact. There were concerns that pharmaceutical marketing may undermine AMS messages.

What type of education do GPs trust? And often that'll be one that comes from kind of RACGP-branded things, or PHNs, and sometimes specialist. (P4)

Stakeholders wanted improved clinical software that integrated prescribing guidelines, patient information resources, and alerts. There was a suggestion that some GPs are using product information rather than guidelines to inform decision making because unlike guidelines, product information is integrated into the clinical software. Government-funded health services (e.g., NPS MedicineWise, PHNs) were suggested as potential developers of patient information resources with PHN Health Pathways as another potential host to make the resources widely available. Keeping the resources current was identified as a challenge.

I think electronic decision support can work well if it's in real time .... the first line choices of antibiotics are ... if you couple that with patient information that will be ... made available to the patient, that's helpful. (P7)

Rapid and point-of-care tests elicited mixed comments. Some thought these could be useful if subsidised. Others thought they should only be available if it would change the decision to prescribe an antibiotic. Selective reporting of antibiotic susceptibilities was suggested as a priority along with standardised information for GPs about the use of microbiology testing, particularly around specimen collection and interpretation of results. It was suggested that the Royal College of Pathologists of Australasia (RCPA) should oversee this.

Not all labs do selective reporting of antibiotics; it should be implemented ... we need one official form rather than lots of different ones—they are not as strong as one consistent message. (P12)

Expert advice sought from hospital specialists (including infectious diseases consultants) was often based on relationships developed during training. There were calls for a central advice line, or lines of communication to enable consistent messages or access to the local hospital specialist's guidance.

Expert advice for me is very dependent on relationships that I built when I was in the hospital system. So if you've got a good network of experts you can call on but you know from an infection perspective it's ... reliant on the goodness of ... them giving you their time ... (P6)

... whether or not the government would be interested in having access lines for antibiotic resistance ... if someone could ring them up ... and get advice, probably wouldn't be a bad thing. (P8)

Respondents suggested that adding the reason-for-prescription (subject to privacy requirements) and providing an exact duration of antibiotic therapy to the prescription would help community pharmacists be more engaged in AMS. It was perceived that to successfully implement delayed prescriptions (where the patient is told when and under what conditions antibiotics should be dispensed), better communication between GPs and community pharmacists is needed. Pharmacists employed by the general practice were identified as an opportunity for practice-level AMS support.

[pharmacists] *put a sticker on the box of antibiotics that says finish the course ... we should change the stickers to 'take as long as prescribed' ...* (P8)

Allergy testing was regarded as beneficial for individual patients but not a system issue. Handover of antimicrobial prescribing on patient transfer was considered part of the larger issue of handover of all information.

Stakeholders thought that nurses may have a role in AMS, e.g., patient triage and education in the community and in the practice, but there was a perceived lack of funding.

I think [nurse triage is] fantastic in an ideal world, but we don't have the funding. (P8)

Stakeholders agreed that research into general practice AMS with translation of the evidence into practice was required. Research areas suggested included understanding the potentially negative effects of antibiotics on the gut microbiome, and better understanding of the use of delayed antibiotic prescription *"whether an illness that's been present for more days is more likely to respond to antibiotics"* (P7). Stakeholders also suggested more research to understand low prescribing GPs:

Those who seem to manage to preserve this resource [antibiotics] really well and apparently not with any problems in terms of the health of their patients. Yeah. How does it work for them? What helps them, what supports them? What can we put in place to enable others to not prescribe? (P9)

3. Discussion

Stakeholders agreed that the proposed framework was valid and feasible, and provided a suitable action framework for the introduction of AMS into Australian general practice. Central coordination was identified as a priority, but the lack of clarity around who would provide this leadership was surprising, particularly given the seniority of the participating stakeholders. The Office of Health Protection (OHP) was suggested to lead and coordinate the introduction of AMS into Australian general practice. Whether the OHP has the capacity for this was not investigated. Sweden's Strama program offers an example of leadership at county and national levels [17,18,26].

Monitoring of and feedback on antibiotic prescribing will enable targeting and evaluation of AMS interventions. Several issues were highlighted including GP trust in a transparent external audit process [27] and a need to obtain complete datasets (including the reason-for-prescription in a standardised format). Inclusion of information on any adverse patient outcomes, e.g., hospitalisations, would require linkage of datasets [27]. There was a view that monitoring and feedback needs urgent development beyond the current volume-based feedback so that it better meets clinical need. No current monitoring system was identified that could provide the information required. An example of monitoring and reporting are the annual reports published by the English Surveillance Programme for Antimicrobial Utilisation and Resistance (ESPAUR) [28].

Regulatory changes were supported. Manufacturer's pack sizes rarely match the recommended duration for common conditions [29], and when antibiotics were supplied by the pack, patients were thought to be likely to save leftovers for future use [30]. Restrictions on repeat prescriptions for five of the most commonly prescribed antibiotics in Australia were introduced on 1 April 2020 [31], illustrating that regulatory changes are achievable.

Electronic decision support was strongly supported and should be further examined in Australia. It has been used to guide prescribing in hospitals, and has been effective at reducing antibiotic prescribing when combined with other AMS interventions [32]. Work is required to develop and pilot suitable electronic decision support to ensure that the tools meet prescriber needs in Australian primary care, are usable, fit in with workflow [33], and have the desired impact.

Stakeholders were unanimous that community education is required to support general practice AMS. Evidence suggests that campaigns may work best when developed in partnership with consumer organisations, are coordinated with health professionals, and promoted at local and national levels [34]. Community awareness of a common colds campaign reflected changes in the frequency of the campaign [35], suggesting that community education should be ongoing. School-based programs, such as Europe's eBug [36] and Canada's Do Bugs need Drugs? [37], have introduced AMS to children. Alongside community education, the provision of written patient information was widely supported by stakeholders and has been associated with reduced antibiotic prescribing in common infections [38]. However, the issues of updating the information, which languages and cultural information are required, and the most appropriate place to host these have not yet been well addressed in the literature.

Ongoing work on selective reporting of antibiotic susceptibilities by microbiology services, which has been shown to be effective in influencing prescribing behaviour [39], should be pursued as a priority in Australia [40].

Increased access to expert advice has been utilized internationally as a method to influence antibiotic prescribing choices. Telephone advice has been provided to GPs in France for patient management [22] and in Sweden, experts provide advice on interpretation of audit results [18]. While stakeholders supported the provision of centralised expert advice, there was no clarity on who should provide it beyond the suggestion that local hospital specialists might participate.

Internationally, pharmacists have participated effectively in activities to help reduce antibiotic prescribing and increase prescribing guideline concordance [41], but Australian community pharmacists may require additional support for this expanded role [42]. Non-dispensing pharmacists in general practice may be suitable for an AMS role. Research to explore the role of pharmacists in general practice AMS is recommended. The role in AMS of practice nurses and that of nurses in the community (e.g., phone triage lines) and their need for formal AMS education remains largely unexplored.

Allergy testing and handover of antimicrobial prescribing on patient transfer will be removed from the framework as the former is an individual issue and the latter part a broader issue. No other changes were recommended.

There are limitations to this research: the recruited practice nurse stakeholder was unavailable for interview in the timeframe, so there may be additional insights to be gained regarding the involvement of practice-based nurses. There were only 12 interviews conducted and stakeholder identification was partly reliant on the authors' networks. Areas covered in less detail were the roles for specific organisations in implementation. The RCPA and the Office of Health Protection were specifically named by one stakeholder for each. However, other stakeholders referred more generally to the "professional colleges" and "Department of Health", respectively. Components in which only three stakeholders commented were: planning for new antibiotics, the role of allergy testing, handover of patient information, unit prescribing, and knowledge about other AMS models. Components discussed by four stakeholders included: pharmaceutical company marketing, nurse involvement, monitoring of AMR. All other components were discussed with at least five stakeholders.

The views of the expert stakeholders may not reflect those of the wider GP community. Experts are likely to be early adopters or innovators in a field [43], whereas the wider community will include those who fear the consequences of not having antibiotics and those who may not perceive that AMR affects them. The stakeholders were speaking as experts, not as representatives of their organisations, thus it is unknown if the organisations have the current capacity to implement the framework.

I should just say ... I'm not doing this from [a named organisation] policy view. (P3)

This is a health system-wide framework developed from a review of the international literature [24] which identified components that may play an interdependent role affecting GP antimicrobial prescribing. A systematic review of interventions found that "No single intervention can be recommended for all behaviours in any setting" and that "local barriers should be removed before implementation" [44]. Examination of these components may help to explain why an intervention may be successful in one setting but fail in another [44,45]. This research highlights that AMS in general practice needs a health system leader, the involvement of health departments, especially One Health AMS committees, with input from professional colleges and health professional representatives.

Implementation science and behaviour change principles [46–48] with GP and relevant professional input are recommended to pilot, implement, and evaluate changes.

4. Materials and Methods

4.1. Study Design and Participants

A qualitative approach was used. Australian-based senior expert stakeholders in AMS in general practice were identified through the authors' AMS networks (8), relevant organisations' websites (3), and via contact with government and professional organisations (2). Stakeholders were provided with a study information sheet and purposively invited to participate in a telephone interview. Gift cards to the value of AUD 150 were offered as compensation for their time.

4.2. Data Collection and Qualitative Analysis

Consented participants received an outline of the proposed AMS framework prior to the interview (Appendix A).

In-depth telephone interviews using a semi-structured interview guide (Appendix B) were conducted and recorded between September and December 2019. Stakeholders were purposively invited until key components had been discussed with at least one stakeholder. Feasibility and validity were assessed by asking participants the extent to which components and subcomponents were being done or if plausible, what needed to be done to make them implementable; their priorities; and if they could identify any gaps. Data collection was completed before analysis commenced. Interview recordings were transcribed and returned to stakeholders with a 10–14-day window for amendments. Transcripts underwent thematic analysis using deductive coding targeting comments about the proposed framework and its components, and by open coding for other comments [49]. Two transcripts were independently coded by two authors and an agreed coding framework was developed. Three more interviews were dual coded using the agreed framework and adjustments made. Seven transcripts were coded by one author. NVivo 12 qualitative data analysis software (QSR International Pty Ltd. Chadstone, Australia) was used to manage the transcripts and coding.

Ethics approval was granted by the Monash University Human Research Ethics Committee, number 20721.

5. Conclusions

The stakeholders regarded this AMS framework as feasible and valid for Australian general practice. The individual subcomponents were viewed as providing a link between the objectives of Australia's National AMR Strategy and action. However, stakeholders considered that the framework required an implementation process with priorities and an integrated approach. The identification of a clear leader to drive AMS in general practice is essential for AMS to gain traction. Monitoring and feedback of antibiotic prescribing require urgent development beyond the current volume-based system and should include monitoring of appropriateness of the prescriptions and patient outcomes. AMS education for the public, further development of GP education, and improved consultation support were strongly recommended. The role of community-based pharmacists and nurses is largely unexplored but their involvement, particularly for patient education, was recommended. Several areas for research were suggested.

Supplementary Materials: The following are available online at http://www.mdpi.com/2079-6382/9/12/900/s1, Table S1: The COREQ checklist, Table S2 Representative quotes for AMS components.

Author Contributions: Conceptualization, L.A.H.; methodology, L.A.H.; formal analysis, L.A.H., J.B., K.B., D.M.; resources, D.M.; data curation, L.A.H.; writing—original draft preparation, L.A.H.; writing—review and editing, L.A.H., J.B., K.B., D.M.; supervision, K.B., D.M.; project administration, L.A.H.; funding acquisition, K.B., D.M. All authors have read and agreed to the published version of the manuscript.

Funding: This work was supported by a National Health and Medical Research Council Centre for Research Excellence Grant for the National Centre for Antimicrobial Stewardship (APP1079625), and a PhD stipend from the National Centre for Antimicrobial Stewardship for L.A.H. and J.B.

Conflicts of Interest: The authors declare no conflict of interest. The funders had no role in the design of the study; in the collection, analyses, or interpretation of data; in the writing of the manuscript, or in the decision to publish the results.

Appendix A. Component List Used during the Interviews

The detailed list of the subcomponents for antimicrobial stewardship in general practice. This list was sent to each Stakeholder before interview and referred to during the interview.

1. Governance

    a. National action plan;
    b. Antimicrobial resistance included on national risk register;
    c. Multi-level and/or multi-disciplinary response;
    d. Regulations around antimicrobial stewardship and antibiotic prescribing;
    e. Accreditation of prescribers;
    f. Funding for antimicrobial resistance and stewardship activities;
    g. Planning for release of new antibiotics;
    h. Practice level antimicrobial stewardship policy/program/activities;
    i. Handover of antibiotic information.

2. Education

    a. Community and patient education;
    b. GP continuing education in antimicrobial stewardship;
    c. GP education on communication skills, patient-centred approaches and shared decision making;
    d. GP education on non-antibiotic management of self-limiting infection;
    e. GP education on delayed prescribing;
    f. General practice team member education;
    g. Independent education (restrict pharma marketing).

3. Consultation support

    a. Prescribing guidelines;
    b. Point of care tests;
    c. Microbiology testing and reporting;
    d. Allergy testing;
    e. Electronic decision support for prescribers;
    f. Expert advice;
    g. Decision support for use with patients.

4. Allied health support for antimicrobial stewardship

    a. Unit dispensing;
    b. Supply and timely access to antibiotics;
    c. Pharmacy review and advice;
    d. Appropriate disposal of leftover antibiotics;
    e. Nurse triage, patient assessment and education.

5. Data monitoring

   a. Monitoring of antibiotic prescriptions;
   b. Monitoring of antimicrobial resistance;
   c. Feedback to prescribers and reporting.

6. Research

   a. Research into AMR/AMS gaps, translation into practice.

Appendix B. The Semi-Structured Interview Guide

1. What can you tell me about your interest or experience in antimicrobial stewardship?
2. What do you think is required to improve antibiotic prescribing in general practice?

Now I will take 2–3 min to explain the model framework and then I will ask you for your comments on it.

3. What is your overall impression of this framework?
4. How well does each component reflect what you understand about AMS?
5. Is it plausible?
6. Does anything not ring true?
7. Do you know of any other models?

   a. How do they differ from this model?

8. To what extent are each of these components currently being done?
9. To what extent do you think the other components are implementable?

   a. What needs to be done to make it happen?

10. Who is, or should be, responsible for each of these components?
11. What do you think may happen if all this came to be?
12. Are there any gaps in this framework?
13. What would you prioritise?
14. How do we measure success? (Interviews 6–12 only)
15. Is there anything missing that we haven't discussed?

References

1. O'Neill, J. *Antimicrobial Resistance: Tackling a Crisis for the Health and Wealth of Nations*; HM Government and Wellcome Trust London: London, UK, 2014; pp. 1–20.
2. Bell, B.G.; Schellevis, F.; Stobberingh, E.; Goossens, H.; Pringle, M. A systematic review and meta-analysis of the effects of antibiotic consumption on antibiotic resistance. *BMC Infect. Dis.* **2014**, *14*, 13. [CrossRef] [PubMed]
3. Holmes, A.H.; Moore, L.S.; Sundsfjord, A.; Steinbakk, M.; Regmi, S.; Karkey, A.; Guerin, P.J.; Piddock, L.J. Understanding the mechanisms and drivers of antimicrobial resistance. *Lancet* **2016**, *387*, 176–187. [CrossRef]
4. Australian Commission on Safety and Quality in Health Care. *AURA 2019: Third Australian Report on Antimicrobial Use and Resistance in Human Health*; ACSQHC: Sydney, Australia, 2019.
5. Pharmaceutical Benefits Advisory Committee, Drug Utilisation Sub-Committee. *Antibiotics: PBS/RPBS Utilisation, October 2014 and February 2015*; Department of Health: Canberra, Australia, 2015.
6. McCullough, A.R.; Pollack, A.J.; Plejdrup Hansen, M.; Glasziou, P.P.; Looke, D.F.; Britt, H.C.; Del Mar, C.B. Antibiotics for acute respiratory infections in general practice: Comparison of prescribing rates with guideline recommendations. *Med. J. Aust.* **2017**, *207*, 65–69. [CrossRef] [PubMed]
7. Australian Department of Health; Australian Department of Agriculture, Water and the Environment. *Australia's National Antimicrobial Resistance Strategy 2020 and beyond*; DH: Canberra, Australia, 2020.

8. Ashiru-Oredope, D.; Sharland, M.; Charani, E.; McNulty, C.; Cooke, J.; ARHAI Antimicrobial Stewardship Group. Improving the quality of antibiotic prescribing in the NHS by developing a new Antimicrobial Stewardship Programme: Start Smart—Then Focus. *J. Antimicrob. Chemother.* **2012**, *67* (Suppl. 1), i51–i63. [CrossRef]
9. Ashiru-Oredope, D.; Hopkins, S.; English Surveillance Programme for Antimicrobial Utilization Resistance Oversight Group. Antimicrobial stewardship: English Surveillance Programme for Antimicrobial Utilization and Resistance (ESPAUR). *J. Antimicrob. Chemother.* **2013**, *68*, 2421–2423. [CrossRef]
10. Australian Commission on Safety and Quality in Health Care. *Antimicrobial Stewardship in Australian Health Care*; ACSQHC: Sydney, Australia, 2018.
11. British Society for Antimicrobial Chemotherapy; ESCMID Study Group for Antimicrobial Stewardship; European Society of Clinical Microbiology and Infectious Diseases. *Antimicrobial Stewardship: From Principles to Practice*; BSAC: Birmingham, Alabama, 2018.
12. Del Mar, C.B.; Scott, A.M.; Gla sziou, P.P.; Hoffmann, T.; van Driel, M.L.; Beller, E.; Phillips, S.M.; Dartnell, J. Reducing antibiotic prescribing in Australian general practice: Time for a national strategy. *Med. J. Aust.* **2017**, *207*, 401–406. [CrossRef]
13. Essack, S.; Pignatari, A.C. A framework for the non-antibiotic management of upper respiratory tract infections: Towards a global change in antibiotic resistance. *Int. J. Clin. Pract. Suppl.* **2013**, *67*, 4–9. [CrossRef]
14. European Commission. *EU Guidelines for the Prudent Use of Antimicrobials in Human Health*; ECDC: Solna, Sweden, 2017.
15. Keller, S.C.; Tamma, P.D.; Cosgrove, S.E.; Miller, M.A.; Sateia, H.; Szymczak, J.; Gurses, A.P.; Linder, J.A. Ambulatory antibiotic stewardship through a human factors engineering approach: A systematic review. *J. Am. Board Fam. Med.* **2018**, *31*, 417–430. [CrossRef]
16. McNulty, C.A. Optimising antibiotic prescribing in primary care. *Int. J. Antimicrob. Agents* **2001**, *18*, 329–333. [CrossRef]
17. Molstad, S.; Erntell, M.; Hanberger, H.; Melander, E.; Norman, C.; Skoog, G.; Lundborg, C.S.; Söderström, A.; Torell, E.; Cars, O. Sustained reduction of antibiotic use and low bacterial resistance: 10-year follow-up of the Swedish Strama programme. *Lancet Infect. Dis.* **2008**, *8*, 125–132. [CrossRef]
18. Molstad, S.; Lofmark, S.; Carlin, K.; Erntell, M.; Aspevall, O.; Blad, L.; Hanberger, H.; Hedin, K.; Hellman, J.; Norman, C.; et al. Lessons learnt during 20 years of the Swedish strategic programme against antibiotic resistance. *Bull. World Health Organ.* **2017**, *95*, 764–773. [CrossRef] [PubMed]
19. National Institute for Health and Care Excellence. Antimicrobial stewardship: Systems and processes for effective antimicrobial medicine use. Full guideline: Methods, evidence and recommendations. In *NICE Guideline*; NICE: London, UK, 2015.
20. Sanchez, G.V.; Fleming-Dutra, K.E.; Roberts, R.M.; Hicks, L.A. Core elements of outpatient antibiotic stewardship. *MMWR Recomm. Rep.* **2016**, *65*, 1–12. [CrossRef] [PubMed]
21. The UK Faculty of Public Health; The Royal College of Physicians; The Royal Pharmaceutical Society; The Royal College of Nursing; The Royal College of General Practitioners. *Joint Statement on Antimicrobial Resistance*; FPH, RCP, RPS, RCN, RCGP: London, UK, 2014.
22. Wang, S.; Pulcini, C.; Rabaud, C.; Boivin, J.M.; Birge, J. Inventory of antibiotic stewardship programs in general practice in France and abroad. *Med. Mal. Infect.* **2015**, *45*, 111–123. [CrossRef] [PubMed]
23. World Health Organization. *Global Action Plan on Antimicrobial Resistance*; WHO: Geneva, Switzerland, 2015.
24. Hawes, L.; Buising, K.; Mazza, D. Antimicrobial stewardship in general practice: A scoping review of the component parts. *Antibiotics* **2020**, *9*, 498. [CrossRef] [PubMed]
25. Australian Department of Health. Practice Incentives Program Quality Improvement Incentive Guidelines. Available online: https://www1.health.gov.au/internet/main/publishing.nsf/Content/PIP-QI_Incentive_guidance (accessed on 26 October 2020).
26. Mölstad, S.; Cars, O.; Struwe, J. Strama—A Swedish working model for containment of antibiotic resistance. *Eurosurveillance* **2008**, *13*, 19041. [PubMed]
27. Canaway, R.; Boyle, D.I.; Manski-Nankervis, J.E.; Bell, J.; Hocking, J.S.; Clarke, K.; Clark, M.; Gunn, J.M.; Emery, J.D. Gathering data for decisions: Best practice use of primary care electronic records for research. *Med. J. Aust.* **2019**, *210* (Suppl. 6), S12–S16. [CrossRef]
28. Public Health England. *English Surveillance Programme for Antimicrobial Utilisation and Resistance (ESPAUR): Report 2019 to 2020*; PHE: London, UK, 2020.

29. McGuire, T.M.; Smith, J.; Del Mar, C. The match between common antibiotics packaging and guidelines for their use in Australia. *Aust. N. Z. J. Public Health* **2015**, *39*, 569–572. [CrossRef]
30. Kardas, P.; Pechere, J.C.; Hughes, D.A.; Cornaglia, G. A global survey of antibiotic leftovers in the outpatient setting. *Int. J. Antimicrob. Agents* **2007**, *30*, 530–536. [CrossRef]
31. Pharmaceutical Benefits Scheme. Revised PBS Listings for Antibiotic Use from 1 April 2020. Available online: http://www.pbs.gov.au/info/news/2020/03/revised_pbs_listings_for_antibiotic_use_from_1_april_2020 (accessed on 1 June 2020).
32. Rawson, T.M.; Moore, L.S.P.; Hernandez, B.; Charani, E.; Castro-Sanchez, E.; Herrero, P.; Hayhoe, B.; Hope, W.; Georgiou, P.; Holmes, A.H. A systematic review of clinical decision support systems for antimicrobial management: Are we failing to investigate these interventions appropriately? *Clin. Microbiol. Infect.* **2017**, *23*, 524–532. [CrossRef]
33. Ahearn, M.D.; Kerr, S.J. General practitioners' perceptions of the pharmaceutical decision-support tools in their prescribing software. *Med. J. Aust.* **2003**, *179*, 34–37. [CrossRef]
34. Donovan, J.; Australian Pharmaceutical Advisory Council. Consumer activities on antimicrobial resistance in Australia. *Commun. Dis. Intell. Q. Rep.* **2003**, *27*, S42–S46. [PubMed]
35. Wutzke, S.E.; Artist, M.A.; Kehoe, L.A.; Fletcher, M.; Mackson, J.M.; Weekes, L.M. Evaluation of a national programme to reduce inappropriate use of antibiotics for upper respiratory tract infections: Effects on consumer awareness, beliefs, attitudes and behaviour in Australia. *Health Promot. Int.* **2007**, *22*, 53–64. [CrossRef] [PubMed]
36. Lecky, D.M.; McNulty, C.A.; Touboul, P.; Herotova, T.K.; Beneš, J.; Dellamonica, P.; Verlander, N.Q.; Kostkova, P.; Weinberg, J.; Goossens, H.; et al. Evaluation of e-Bug, an educational pack, teaching about prudent antibiotic use and hygiene, in the Czech Republic, France and England. *J. Antimicrob. Chemother.* **2010**, *65*, 2674–2684. [CrossRef] [PubMed]
37. Carson, M.; Patrick, D.M. "Do Bugs Need Drugs?" A community education program for the wise use of antibiotics. *Can. Commun. Dis. Rep.* **2015**, *41*, 5–8. [CrossRef] [PubMed]
38. de Bont, E.G.; Alink, M.; Falkenberg, F.C.; Dinant, G.J.; Cals, J.W. Patient information leaflets to reduce antibiotic use and reconsultation rates in general practice: A systematic review. *BMJ Open* **2015**, *5*, e007612. [CrossRef] [PubMed]
39. McNulty, C.A.; Lasseter, G.M.; Charlett, A.; Lovering, A.; Howell-Jones, R.; Macgowan, A.; Thomas, M. Does laboratory antibiotic susceptibility reporting influence primary care prescribing in urinary tract infection and other infections? *J. Antimicrob. Chemother.* **2011**, *66*, 1396–1404. [CrossRef]
40. Graham, M.; Walker, D.A.; Haremza, E.; Morris, A.J. RCPAQAP audit of antimicrobial reporting in Australian and New Zealand laboratories: Opportunities for laboratory contribution to antimicrobial stewardship. *J. Antimicrob. Chemother.* **2019**, *74*, 251–255. [CrossRef]
41. Saha, S.K.; Hawes, L.; Mazza, D. Effectiveness of interventions involving pharmacists on antibiotic prescribing by general practitioners: A systematic review and meta-analysis. *J. Antimicrob. Chemother.* **2019**, *74*, 1173–1181. [CrossRef]
42. Rizvi, T.; Thompson, A.; Williams, M.; Zaidi, S.T.R. Perceptions and current practices of community pharmacists regarding antimicrobial stewardship in Tasmania. *Int. J. Clin. Pharm.* **2018**, *40*, 1380–1387. [CrossRef]
43. Rogers, E.M. *Diffusion of Innovations*, 5th ed.; Free Press: New York, NY, USA, 2003.
44. Arnold, S.R.; Straus, S.E. Interventions to improve antibiotic prescribing practices in ambulatory care. *Cochrane Database Syst. Rev.* **2005**, CD003539. [CrossRef]
45. Ranji, S.R.; Steinman, M.A.; Shojania, K.G.; Gonzales, R. Interventions to reduce unnecessary antibiotic prescribing: A systematic review and quantitative analysis. *Med. Care* **2008**, *46*, 847–862. [CrossRef] [PubMed]
46. Grimshaw, J.M.; Eccles, M.P.; Lavis, J.N.; Hill, S.J.; Squires, J.E. Knowledge translation of research findings. *Implement. Sci.* **2012**, *7*, 50. [CrossRef] [PubMed]
47. Michie, S.; Atkins, L.; West, R. *The Behaviour Change Wheel: A Guide to Designing Interventions*; Silverback Publishing: London, UK, 2014.

48. Craig, P.; Dieppe, P.; Macintyre, S.; Michie, S.; Nazzareth, I.; Pettigrew, M. *Developing and Evaluating Complex Interventions*; Medical Research Council: London, UK, 2019.
49. Ryan, G.W.; Bernard, H.R. Techniques to identify themes. *Field Methods* **2003**, *15*, 85–109. [CrossRef]

Publisher's Note: MDPI stays neutral with regard to jurisdictional claims in published maps and institutional affiliations.

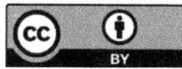
© 2020 by the authors. Licensee MDPI, Basel, Switzerland. This article is an open access article distributed under the terms and conditions of the Creative Commons Attribution (CC BY) license (http://creativecommons.org/licenses/by/4.0/).

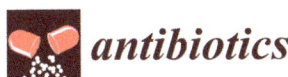

Review

Are Follow-Up Blood Cultures Useful in the Antimicrobial Management of Gram Negative Bacteremia? A Reappraisal of Their Role Based on Current Knowledge

Francesco Cogliati Dezza [†], Ambrogio Curtolo [†], Lorenzo Volpicelli [†], Giancarlo Ceccarelli, Alessandra Oliva and Mario Venditti *

Department of Public Health and Infectious Diseases, University "Sapienza" of Rome, 00185 Rome, Italy; francesco.cogliatidezza@uniroma1.it (F.C.D.); ambrogio.curt@uniroma1.it (A.C.); lorenzo.volpicelli@uniroma1.it (L.V.); giancarlo.ceccarelli@uniroma1.it (G.C.); alessandra.oliva@uniroma1.it (A.O.)
* Correspondence: mario.venditti@uniroma1.it
† These authors contributed equally to the paper.

Received: 6 November 2020; Accepted: 9 December 2020; Published: 11 December 2020

Abstract: Bloodstream infections still constitute an outstanding cause of in-hospital morbidity and mortality, especially among critically ill patients. Follow up blood cultures (FUBCs) are widely recommended for proper management of *Staphylococcus aureus* and *Candida* spp. infections. On the other hand, their role is still a matter of controversy as far as Gram negative bacteremias are concerned. We revised, analyzed, and commented on the literature addressing this issue, to define the clinical settings in which the application of FUBCs could better reveal its value. The results of this review show that critically ill patients, endovascular and/or non-eradicable source of infection, isolation of a multi-drug resistant pathogen, end-stage renal disease, and immunodeficiencies are some factors that may predispose patients to persistent Gram negative bacteremia. An analysis of the different burdens that each of these factors have in this clinical setting allowed us to suggest which patients' FUBCs have the potential to modify treatment choices, prompt an early source control, and finally, improve clinical outcome.

Keywords: follow-up blood cultures; Gram negative bacteremia; critically ill patients; antibiotic therapy

1. Introduction

Bloodstream infections (BSIs) represent a leading cause of death in industrialized countries, with an estimate of two million episodes and 250,000 deaths annually in North America and Europe, despite the availability of new potent antimicrobial therapies and advances in supportive care. In particular, hospital-acquired BSIs are a major cause of morbidity and mortality in intensive care units (ICU), and septic shock still represents the first cause of ICU total mortality [1]. This burden is likely to grow over the next few decades due to the increase in life-expectancy and in median number of patient comorbidity [2]. Unlike Gram positive (GP) BSIs, whose incidence rate has declined over the last few decades, Gram negative (GN) BSIs have markedly increased overtime and nowadays account for up to half of BSIs, with a mortality rate of 20–40% [3–5].

When considering GP-BSIs, international guidelines and consolidated evidence-based procedure bundles are available for the management of the leading pathogen species, *Staphylococcus aureus*. In this setting, follow-up blood cultures (FUBCs) are regarded as essential to document clearance of bacteremia after treatment initiation and exclude seeding [6–8]. On the other hand, FUBCs are mandatory in the case of *Candida* spp. BSIs in order to determine the end of candidemia and optimize treatment duration [9].

As for GN-BSIs, relevant advances in management strategies have been made in the last few years, such as the non-inferiority demonstration of 7 vs 14 day antibiotic courses [10] and of oral step-down vs continued parental therapy [11] in uncomplicated GN-BSIs. Recently, a combined approach of rapid diagnostic testing with a bundle of antimicrobial stewardship found a decrease in readmission rate and in cost per case [12]. Anyway, the management of GN-BSIs remains poorly codified and thus prone to personal clinician judgement, as compared to Gram positive settings. In a recently published scoping review, Fabre et al. proposed an algorithm for bacterial blood culture (BC) recommendations. They found that in bacteremias due to *Enterobacterales*, FUBCs are unlikely to grow unless the source of infection is endovascular or there is inadequate source control. Although with small numbers, similar results were found in *Pseudomonas* infections. The authors suggest clinical judgment to evaluate the need of FUBCs for GN. Of note, this review considered studies published from 1 January 2004 to 1 June 2019 [13], but the majority of studies addressing the topic of FUBCs in GN infections are actually subsequent to this time frame. At the time of writing, the role of FUBCs in Gram negative bacteremia (GNB) still represents an important matter of debate, with controversial results [14].

The early studies conducted have focused on the disadvantages of FUBCs, mainly represented by the risk of false positive results, prolonged hospitalization, inappropriate antibiotic use and increased cost [15,16]. Recently, the issue of FUBCs came out on top through the availability of new evidence that may have tipped the balance in favor. In this review, we aimed to examine and summarize the current knowledge on the usefulness of FUBCs in GNB, especially in the light of the reassessment of this management tool by recent studies. Moreover, we propose two guidance tools (clinical and microbiological) that summarize and graduate the recommendations for FUBCs.

2. Results: Review of the Literature

In 2004, Tabriz et al. published the first study where FUBCs in GNB were suggested. The authors conducted a retrospective single center study of 96 patients with at least one FUBC over 1 month (199 BC episodes without differences between GP and GN). Most FUBCs were performed within 4 days from first positive blood culture (FPBC) and during antimicrobial therapy (AT) (both 158, 79.4%). The common reasons to repeat BCs were fever, follow-up of positive BCs, and persistent leukocytosis. Positive FUBCs after FPBC were 21 (25.9%) and after a negative BC were 1.7% of cases. The conclusions were that persistent leukocytosis and fever are poor predictors of bacteremia. Then, the authors gave some general indications about when to perform FUBCs correctly, even if no definition of FUBCs was provided. They suggested FUBCs in these circumstances: 1. new septic episode, 2. suspected endocarditis, 3. follow-up of a positive BC in certain conditions that may have diagnostic and therapeutic implications, such as *S. aureus*, GNB and candidemia, 4. confirmation of response to therapy for endocarditis or other endovascular infections caused by *S. aureus*, *Enterococcus* spp., GN or other difficult-to-treat organisms because the only use of clinical data may not be reliable, 5. confirmation of diagnosis of intravascular catheter-associated bacteremia. Even if the data presented do not seem to support the above cited conclusions, this was the first time that the question of FUBCs in GNB was dealt with [17].

A summary of the main subsequent studies on the role of FUBCs in the management of GNB is reported in Table 1.

Table 1. Summary of the main studies on follow up blood cultures (FUBCs) in Gram negative bacteremia.

Study: First Author, Year Design	Inclusion Criteria ✓ Exclusion Criteria ✗	FUBC Definition N of FUBCs/N of Patients (%)	Positive FUBC/N of FUBCs (%)	Positive ICU FUBCs/ICU Patients (%)	Results and Conclusions	Limitations
Kang, 2013 retrospective case-control [18]	✓ Age ≥ 18 ✓ First episode of KpB ✗ Polymicrobial ✗ Recurrent KpB	BC drawn after more than 2 days from the index BC 862/1068 (81)	62/862 (7.2)	NA	Risk factors for persistent KpB included in a clinical score: unfavorable treatment response - intra-abdominal infection - high CCI - SOT Routine FUBCs not justified.	• Retrospective • Only one pathogen considered • No ICU data • No multivariate for mortality risk factors
Wiggers, 2016 retrospective cohort [19]	✓ Age ≥ 18 ✓ First episode of GNB ✗ Recurrent GNB	BC drawn 2–7 days from the index BC 247/901 (27.4) [GN only considered]	27/247 (10.9) [GNB only considered]	NA	Increased 30 days mortality in patients undergoing FUBCs, regardless of the result Repeated BC in GN bacteremia offer low yield	• Retrospective • Mixed population of GP and GN • No ICU data • Small sample with PB (defined as positive BC 2–7 days after the index BC
Canzoneri, 2017 retrospective case-control [15]	✓ Age ≥ 18 ✓ One positive BC ✗ Fungemia ✗ Potential contaminants	BC drawn after at least 24 h from the index BC 383/500 (77) [GP + GN considered]	8/140 (6) [GNB only considered]	18/165 (10.9) [GP + GN considered]	PB more common for GPs (21%), than polymicrobial (10%), than GNs (6%) FUBCs have little utility in patients with GNB	• Retrospective • Mixed population of GP and GN • Polymicrobial infections included • Small number of patients with PB
Shi, 2019 retrospective case-control [20]	✓ Age ≥ 18 ✓ Bacteremic UTI ✓ At least one FUBC ✗ Non-urinary source of bacteremia	More than one separate BC taken more than 24 h after the index BC 306/333 (92) [GP + GN considered]	39/264 (14.8) [GN only considered]	20/55 (36.4)	Not recommended routine FUBC Predictors for positive FUBC in bacteremic UTI: malignancy, initial ICU admission, high CRP level and longer time to defervescence	• Retrospective • Mixed population with GP and GN • Only UTIs considered
Uehara, 2019 retrospective observational [21]	✓ Age ≤ 18 ✓ GN B ✗ Polymicrobial ✗ FUBCs ≤ 24 h from the index BC ✗ AT started ≥ 48 h from the index BC	BCs taken over 24 h from the index BC 99/137 (72.3)	21/99 (21.2)	NA	FUBC may still be useful in the management of GNB in children Presence of a CVC and resistance to empirical antibiotics were risks for positive FUBCs	• Retrospective • Small sample • Possible selection bias

Table 1. *Cont.*

Study: First Author, Year Design	Inclusion Criteria Exclusion Criteria	FUBC Definition N of FUBCs/N of Patients (%)	Positive FUBC/N of FUBCs (%)	Positive ICU FUBCs/ICU Patients (%)	Results and Conclusions	Limitations
Giannella, 2020 retrospective cohort [22]	✓ Age ≥ 18 ✓ GNB × Polymicrobial × Potential contaminants × Death ≤ 72 h after index BC × Unavailable clinical data	• BCs drawn between 24 h and 7 days after the index BC • 278/1576 (17.6)	• 107/278 (38.5)	• 21/126 (16.6)	• FUBCs drawn in more severe, high risk, antibiotic resistant and initially inappropriately treated patients • In this context, FUBCs execution associated to higher rate of source control, ID consultation and lower 30-day mortality	• Retrospective • Single center
Maskarinec, 2020 prospectively enrolled cohort [23]	✓ Age ≥ 18 ✓ GNB × Polymicrobial × Death ≤ 24 h after index BC	• BCs drawn from 24 h to 7 days from index BC • 1164/1702 (68.4)	• 228/1164 (19.6)	• 4/41 (9.8)	• FUBCs drawn in high risk patients • Obtaining FUBCs associated with decreased all-cause and attributable mortality • Positive FUBCs associated with increased all-cause and attributable mortality	• Poor data on patients' clinical status at FUBCs collection • No data on management changes based on FUBC results
Jung, 2020 retrospective observational cohort [24]	24GNB × Age < 18 × Death ≤ 48 h after index BC × Polymicrobial × Different species from the index BC identified by FUBC	• BCs drawn 2–7 days from index BC • 1276/1481 (86.2)	• 122/1276 (9.6)	NA	• FUBCs can be avoided in most uncomplicated cases of GNB and could be considered selectively in high risk patients • Two clinical scores for patients with eradicable and non-eradicable source of infection	• Retrospective • Not evaluated the impact of FUBCs on patient outcome
Mitaka, 2020 retrospective multicenter observational [25]	✓ Age ≥ 18 ✓ GNB × Potential contaminants	• BC draws after at least 24h of AT • 306/463 (66.1)	• 28/306 (9.2)	• 18/130 (13.9)	• RF for positive FUBCs: ESRD on hemodialysis, intravascular device, ESBL or carbapenemase-producing organism • Higher yield of positive FUBCs in patients with ≥ 1 RF • Routine FUBCs are not necessary	• Retrospective • Only the first FUBC analyzed • 26% FUBCs not performed without standardizing the decision

Table 1. Cont.

Study: First Author, Year Design	Inclusion Criteria Exclusion Criteria	FUBC Definition N of FUBCs/N of Patients (%)	Positive FUBC/N of FUBCs (%)	Positive ICU FUBCs/ICU Patients (%)	Results and Conclusions	Limitations
Spaziante, 2020 retrospective observational study [26]	✓ Inclusion: • Age ≥ 18 • GNB • FUBC ≤ 24–72 h from the FUBC or ≤ 48 h from the beginning of AAT ✗ Exclusion: • Polymicrobial	• BCs done within 48 h from the beginning of AT and then every 24–72 h after FUBCs • 78/107 (73) [GNB episodes from 69 patients]	• 28/78 (35.9) [patients]	• [All patients were in ICU]	• Septic thrombus infection was the source in 14 (50%) cases of GNB-PB. • A MDR isolate was in 60 BCs (76.9%) • FUBCs represent a useful tool in the management of GN-PB, especially if caused by STI	• Retrospective • Only ICU patients from polytrauma ICU • Small sample

Abbreviations: AT, antimicrobial therapy; BC, blood culture; BSI, blood stream infection; CCI, Charlson comorbidity index; CRP, C-reactive protein; CVC, central venous catheter; ESBL, extended spectrum β-lactamase; ESRD, end stage renal disease; FUBC, follow-up blood cultures; GN, Gram negative; GNB, Gram negative bacteremia; GP, Gram positive; ICU, intensive care unit; KpB, *Klebsiella pneumoniae* bacteremia; MDR, multidrug resistant; NA, not available/not applicable; PB, persistent bacteremia; RF, risk factor; SOT, solid organ transplant; UTI, urinary tract infection.

In a retrospective multicenter case-control study of 2013 [18], the authors analyzed 1068 individuals with *Klebsiella pneumoniae* bacteremia (KpB) and showed a wide prescription of FUBCs as these were performed in 80.7% of cases, while only 7.2% were found to be positive. Moreover, 53.2% of patients with non-persistent KpB underwent more than two consecutive BCs. The routine use of FUBCs was considered not justified because of the low incidence of persistent bacteremia (PB) detected. Unfavorable treatment response on the second day after the initial BCs, intra-abdominal infection, high weighted Charlson comorbidity index, and prior solid organ transplantation (SOT) were recognized as independent risk factors for persistent KpB. The authors stated that the retrospective analysis, the small sample size, and the lack of a multivariable analysis of mortality-related factors represented possible limitations of their study. Furthermore, they focused only on a specific pathogen (*K. pneumoniae*) and, although transfer to ICU was considered as an outcome, no data were available concerning the original patient allocation (ICU vs non-ICU ward) [18].

In 2016, Wiggers et al. conducted a retrospective monocentric cohort SCRIBE study on a mixed population of 1801 patients with a first episode of bacteremia caused by GP, GN or anaerobic bacteria. FUBCs were executed in 701 patients (38.9%) and PB was demonstrated in only 118 (6.6%) of the whole population. As expected, an endovascular source of infection, *S. aureus* and the inability to achieve source control in 48 h were associated with higher risk of PB. Analyzing the data provided, there were 901 GNBs (50% of the whole cohort) and 247 of them had FUBCs taken (27.4%), of which 27 (10.9%) tested positive, compared to GP bacteremias (GPBs) where BCs were repeated in 457 out of 882 patients (51.8%), with a positive yield in 90 (19.7%). Male sex, admission to a medical service, *S. aureus* bacteremia and endovascular or epidural focus were identified as risk factors for PB, but unfortunately this multivariate analysis was conducted on the whole population, rather than only on patients with GNB. Authors concluded that bacteremias caused by GNs, viridans group or beta-hemolytic streptococci are common situations in which repeat BCs offer low yield, with the related inappropriate expense. When possible, a revision of the charts regarding physician's impression on clinical status was made and authors inferred that only 30.3% of FUBCs were drawn because of patients' instability, a situation in which FUBCs could be suitable. Regardless of the result, 30 day mortality was significantly higher (27%) among patients undergoing repeated BCs [19].

Until 2020, the most relevant and influential article addressing the topic of FUBCs in GNBs was that conducted by Canzoneri et al. in 2017. They retrospectively analyzed 500 episodes of bacteremia, of which 383 (77%) had at least one FUBC taken. Among these 383, 206 (54%) had initial bacteremia caused by a GP organism and 140 (37%) by a GN, with an average of 2.37 FUBCs per patient. The FUBCs yielded positive in 55 (14%) of the overall population, 43 (78%) of those with GP cocci and eight (15%) with GN bacilli. The incidence of PB, defined as positive FUBC for the same original organism, was 21% in GPBs, 10% in polymicrobial bacteremias and 6% only in GNBs. Fever on the day of FUBC sampling, presence of an intravenous (IV) central catheter and end-stage renal disease (ESRD) were associated with a higher probability of PB in the whole cohort. Subgroup analysis confirmed these factors, with the adjunct of diabetes mellitus, as predictors of positive FUBC, only among subjects with GPB, while fever was the only factor associated with PB in GNB. No impact of positive FUBC on ICU admission or mortality was detectable. No clue concerning the clinical reasons for drawing FUBCs was available. The authors concluded that FUBCs may have little utility in patients with GNB, as compared to the serious negative implications of unrestrained use, represented by false positive results, longer hospital stays and increased healthcare costs [15].

In 2019, Shi et al. reported the results of a monocentric case-control study in 333 patients with bacteremic urinary tract infection (UTI): 306 (91.9%) of them had FUBCs drawn, of which 55 (18%) tested positive. Among all those that underwent FUBCs, 264 (86.3%) had a GN-related UTI with positivity in 39 (14.8%), compared to 14 (4.6%) with a GP UTI that yielded positive FUBCs in six (42.9%). Of note, four out of six of this latter group were caused by *S. aureus*. PB, defined as more than seven days of positive BCs, occurred in only six (3.3%) out of 306 patients. Several clinical and biochemical factors were associated with higher probability of PB. Eventually, four factors were selected and confirmed through multivariate analysis as independent predictors: malignancy, initial ICU admission, high c-reactive protein (CRP) level and longer time to defervescence. Among the subgroup of patients without any of these risk factors, no one had a positive FUBC. The authors concluded that, due to the low positivity rate, liberally prescribed FUBCs have little utility in the management of bacteremic UTI [20]. However, the results of this study might be limited by the design focused on only one clinical syndrome (UTI), the mixed causative agents considered (including a not negligible proportion of *S. aureus*) and the lack of data regarding the effect of pathogen antibiotic susceptibilities on FUBC results, clinical reasons for drawing FUBCs and original admission service of the patients.

In the same year, a study conducted in a pediatric hospital of Tokyo firstly questioned the conception of the usefulness of FUBC in the setting of GNB. Uehara et al. enrolled 99 children with GNB, with a median age of two years. The most frequent underlying diseases were SOT (21.2%), malignant neoplasm (17.2%) and kidney/urinary tract malformation (15.2%); a central venous catheter (CVC) was in place in 57% of patients. Twenty-one patients (21.2%) had positive FUBCs, with *Klebsiella* spp. and *Escherichia coli* being the most represented pathogens. Interestingly, no cases of positive FUBCs emerged among patients with UTI. Multivariate analysis revealed the presence of CVC and resistance to empirical therapy as significantly associated with PB. More importantly, the authors reviewed clinical charts and reported that the positive yield of FUBCs promoted a treatment modification in 57% of patients, which included optimization of antibiotic therapy and/or removal of medical devices [21].

In 2020, the prior view of FUBCs as a tool of little utility in patients with GNB, counterpoised to many clinical and economical drawbacks, underwent a systematic reassessment. Completely different results from those obtained by Canzoneri et al. [15] were in fact reported by Giannella et al. in a single center, retrospective cohort analysis of 1576 patients with GNB [22]. As in previous studies, FUBCs were prescribed based on personal clinical judgement rather than systematically. Nevertheless, FUBCs were performed in only 278 (17.6%) patients but demonstrated a high rate of PB: 107 (38.5%). Patients that underwent FUBCs were younger, with a lower Charlson comorbidity index, but more frequently immunocompromised, admitted to ICU, with a hospital-acquired GNB, and with a non-urinary source of infection, compared to those without FUBCs performed. Furthermore, patients with FUBC taken had higher initial severity of GNB clinical pictures according to SOFA (Sequential Organ Failure Assessment) score and septic shock criteria, higher frequency of carbapenem-resistant enterobacteriaceae (CRE) isolation and of inappropriate empirical therapy. Thus, as a matter of fact, the patient complexity seemed to progressively rise from those without FUBCs drawn, those with FUBCs, to those with positive FUBCs. That is to say that, for the first time since the topic of FUBCs in the setting of GNB has been debated, the authors provided elements to interpret the mechanism by which physicians currently use FUBCs. Interestingly, taking into account the higher complexity of patients that underwent FUBCs, the execution of FUBCs was followed by increased rate of source control, infectious disease consultation and longer treatment duration. Thus, performance of FUBCs appeared to act for physicians as an incitement to more careful management. At the same time, Giannella et al. demonstrated that FUBCs had a favorable impact on patient outcome, an effect probably linked to prompt source control. In fact, through multivariate analysis, FUBCs, along with UTI origin of BSI, source control and active empiric therapy, resulted as independent factors protective from all-cause 30 day mortality. The authors concluded that future prospective studies with a systematic use of FUBCs in GNB are necessary in order to better identify the settings where FUBCs could be cost-effective [22].

Similar favorable results of FUBC use were obtained by Maskarinec et al. in an observational study of 1702 prospectively enrolled inpatients with monomicrobial GNB [23]. FUBCs were drawn in 1164 patients (68%) and more commonly in patients with *Pseudomonas aeruginosa* and *Serratia* spp. (80%). PB was detected in 228 (20%). Patients with PB had a lower probability of having under effective antibiotic treatment (with higher rates of fluoroquinolone and/or carbapenem-resistant isolates in FUBCs) and higher probability of being a transplant recipient, hemodialysis dependent, having a cardiac device, recent corticosteroid use, a malignancy, or an endovascular source of infection. Bacteremias caused by *Serratia* (32%, 95% CI 24–44%) and *Stenotrophomonas maltophilia* (52%, 95% CI

32–72%) had the higher rate of persistence. Patients' clinical outcomes were also evaluated. Relevantly, the regression model showed that obtaining FUBCs was associated with decreased rates of both all-cause and attributable mortality. This result was also confirmed in a species-specific analysis performed for *E. coli* and *K. pneumoniae* and in a sensitivity analysis that excluded all deaths occurring in the first 48 h. On the contrary, PB implied a nearly double all-cause and attributable mortality relative to those with negative FUBCs, and similar to those without FUBCs drawn. The probability of PB was estimated through a risk scoring system and finally, an endovascular source of infection was identified as the only breakpoint separating high and low rates of FUBC positivity. The authors concluded that FUBCs have clinical utility in detecting patients with increased risk of poor outcome, and that could benefit from additional diagnostic and therapeutic interventions. Considering the low rate (2%) of false positivity FUBCs and the little difference in duration of antibiotic treatment (2 days), this study also scaled back the traditional concerns of increased healthcare costs and antimicrobial prescription usually attributed to FUBCs [23].

On the other hand, Jung et al. from South Korea recently presented a retrospective observational cohort study conducted on 1481 cases of GNB. FUBCs were widely performed (86.2%), while positivity resulted in 122 (9.6%) [24]. Comparing the clinical characteristics of those that underwent FUBCs and those that did not, female gender, neutropenia, hematologic malignancy, presence of an intravascular device and of an extended spectrum β-lactamase (ESBL)-producing organism were more represented in the first group, while a biliary source was more common in the latter. No difference was detected in terms of incident mortality between FUBCs drawn and not. The comparison between patients with positive and negative FUBC yield was made by sub-stratification according to eradicable and non-eradicable source of infection. Several factors were identified and included in a predictive scoring model if independently associated with FUBC positivity through a multivariate logistic regression. Results indicated that, in the case of a removable source of infection, if there is appropriate management (early source control and appropriate therapy) followed by a favorable clinical response (quick SOFA score <2), performing FUBCs adds little value. Furthermore, even in a non-eradicable setting, the administration of effective treatment corresponded to 95% probability of negative conversion, regardless of the underlying disease, offending pathogen, or treatment response. Author conclusions were that FUBCs can be avoided in most uncomplicated cases of GNB and could be considered selectively in high-risk patients. In addition to the retrospective nature of the study, it should be underlined that neither the patients' outcome nor the relative impact of FUBCs' execution/results were evaluated. In addition, mortality was not taken into consideration in the comparison between positive and negative results of FUBCs and no data concerning ICU vs non-ICU ward allocation were provided [24].

Mitaka et al. conducted a retrospective multicenter observational study in all adults with at least one BC positive for GNs admitted between January 2017 and December 2018 [25]. A total of 463 patients were included; of these, 306 (66%) had FUBCs performed at least once. The results showed positive FUBCs in only 10% of patients. The authors found a correlation between positive FUBCs and the following risk factors: ESRD, presence of intravascular devices, and bacteremia due to ESBL-producing organism or CRE. The yield of positive FUBCs in patients without the risk factors was 1.6%, compared to 14.8% in the presence of ≥1 risk factor. The authors concluded that FUBCs may not be necessary for all GNBs, but only in the presence of risk factors [25]. In addition to the retrospective design and the lack of standardization of decision making regarding FUBCs, other limitations of the study included that authors only analyzed the positivity or negativity of the first FUBC without checking the possibility of intermittent bacteremia and no information about clinical outcomes and therapeutic change based on the results of FUBCs was provided.

In 2020, Spaziante et al. conducted a retrospective single center observational study on 307 patients admitted to a multidisciplinary ICU in 2017 [26]. Sixty-nine patients (22.4%) presenting with at least one GNB episode for a total of 107 episodes were included in the study. Exclusion criteria were the occurrence of fungemia, GP or mixed GP/GN bacteremic episodes. FUBCs were defined as BC performed within 48 h from the beginning of antimicrobial therapy (AT) and then every 24–72 h after FPBCs. PB was defined as repeatedly positive BCs for GNs after ≥96 h of appropriate AT and ≥48 h after removal of all potentially infected endovascular indwelling devices. Twenty-nine GNB episodes (27.1%) were excluded from the study because no FUBCs were performed. Eventually, 28 (35.9%) out of 78 GNB episodes were diagnosed as PB. Under these circumstances, septic thrombosis (ST) was the hematogenous source of infection in approximately half of the cases, resulting in a significant association with positive FUBCs ($p < 0.001$). On the other hand, negative FUBCs were associated with primary bacteremia ($p < 0.001$). As part of the retrospective design, this is the only paper entirely focused on critically ill patients. In particular, the study was conducted in an ICU that is a reference center for polytrauma and, based on the aforementioned results, the authors hypothesized that frequent deep venous thrombosis occurring near to bone fractures may provide a suitable medium for microbial seeding for GNB originating from other body sites [26].

3. Discussion

GNB still represents an extremely relevant cause of morbidity and mortality in hospitalized patients, especially in ICU settings. Therefore, it is crucial to achieve an optimization of patient care, which, at the same time, could reduce mortality rates and meet the growing demands of antimicrobial stewardship and cost control. In this regard, the use of FUBCs in patients with GNB has represented a contentious topic in the past few years and especially in the very last period.

Indeed, unnecessary FUBCs may cause patient discomfort and carry the risk of false positive results. According to previous reports, as many as 90% of all BCs grow no organisms and of the approximate 10% that do grow organisms, almost half are considered contaminants (false positives) [27]. Thus, given a constant rate of contamination, performing more FUBCs may result in a higher chance of encountering contaminant organisms, and consequently, in increased costs and patients discomfort, longer hospital stays, unnecessary consultations, and inappropriate antimicrobial therapy [15,16]. Of note, this reasoning includes an inherent fallacy. Although theoretically acceptable in cases of GP yield, the growth of GN bacteria in BCs should always be regarded as relevant and never, or just anecdotally, be considered as a contamination [28].

On the other side, performing FUBCs may have a relevant impact on patient management and outcome, reducing mortality rates. When FUBCs are performed in more severe patients with comorbidities and without adequate infection source control, in cases of bacteremia due to multidrug resistant (MDR) GNs and without an appropriate empiric therapy, the positive or negative results may guide the clinician to the correct decision about type and duration of antibiotic therapy [22,23].

Not surprisingly, the evidence concerning the usefulness of FUBCs underwent a progressive shift in the last few years, going from a restrictive to a selective approach. Taking a look at Table 1, it appears that papers with a higher rate of FUBCs performed, more frequently found no evidence of benefit in contrast to those that applied FUBCs more selectively. In fact, Kang et al. [18] and Jung et al. [24] performed FUBCs in GNB in 81% and 86% of the cases, respectively, as compared to Maskarinec and Giannella that used this tool only in 68% and 17% of cases, respectively. Likely, Spaziante et al. [26] found a high rate of PB by only performing FUBCs in high-risk ICU patients with GNB. Furthermore, the inclusion in the analysis of a mixed GP and GN population was also associated with pessimistic results. Therefore, it seems that the more refined the selection of patients in which to draw FUBCs, the more evident the benefits they bring. Indeed, the results of our literature review show that, while in some subgroups of patients the use of FUBCs may not translate into a clear benefit, it is possible to identify several situations where the application of this tool may steer the clinical decision making in the correct way. Thus, selection is a sticking point in this topic.

For the purposes of performing rational FUBCs, physicians well trained in infectious diseases should be available in all settings where risk factors for positive FUBCs are present. For this reason, ICU patients might be evaluated from dedicated infectious disease consultants in order to avoid unnecessary BCs [22,26]. The study written by Ceccarelli et al. shows an example of this management [29]. In fact, they reported some cases of GN-related septic thrombosis (ST) with indolent clinical course and long-term positive BCs despite adequate antibiotic treatment as one possible exception to the restricted use of FUBCs. In these cases, FUBCs allowed the determination of the correct treatment duration, representing a tool of critical importance for patient management [29]. The same group of authors further stressed this concept in a case series of 13 critical care patients with ST caused by GN bacilli (Figure 1): this disease was characterized by PB despite prompt source control and appropriate antibiotic treatment, an indolent clinical course and, even more important, a rapid defervescence with normalization of procalcitonin (PCT) values preceding bacteremia clearance. This phenomenon was interpreted as a mechanism of immune tolerance [30].

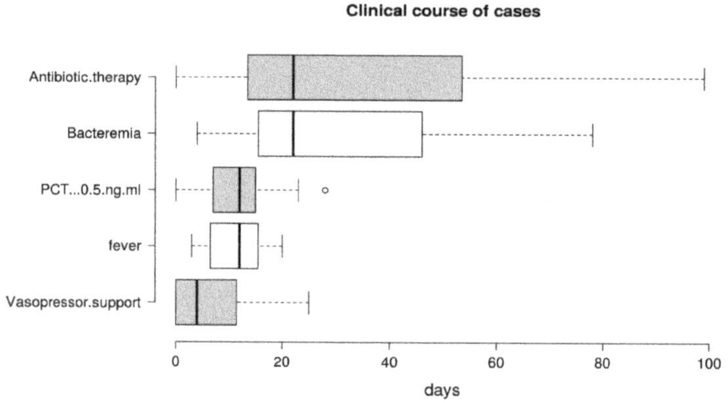

Figure 1. Duration of bacteremia and clinical course features of Gram negative septic thrombosis in critically ill patients, modified from Spaziante et al. [30]. This figure shows that bacteremia may persist despite clinical improvement (fever disappearance, negative procalcitonin (PCT) values and no vasopressor support); under these circumstances, FUBCs may remain the only driver of antibiotic therapy.

Based on the fascinating hypothesis that FUBCs in BSIs due to GNs could be part of clinical practice, we tried to investigate which conditions make FUBCs either necessary or unfounded. Figures 2 and 3 show clinical and microbiological risk factors for PB, respectively. Rows and columns of each figure intersect in a colored square and every color means a risk threshold of PB, from green (FUBCs highly recommended), light green (moderate recommendation), yellow (weak recommendation) to red (avoid FUBCs), of various combinations of all risk factors recognized in this review.

In order to point out the right setting where FUBCs should be prescribed (otherwise when they are not warranted), we created Figures 2 and 3 analyzing the risk factors for persistent bacteremia found in the revised articles. On the other hand, we identified settings where FUBCs are moderate or even weakly recommended based on risk factors cited by less authors/articles and our judgment. For these reasons, a clinical decision on a case-by-case basis is needed to judge when to perform FUBCs.

In general, FUBCs should be always considered in critically ill patients because they frequently present multiple risk factors that may account for resistant or persistent GNB: intravascular catheter, antibiotic resistant pathogen or an occult source of infection that requires control. As an example, FUBCs are warranted in patients with an endovascular source of GNB that represents the single most important indication to this procedure, even in some instances where a biomarker of active infection, such as PCT, is decreased to negative values. In fact, Spaziante et al. stressed this point by analyzing Gram negative ST where positive FUBCs played a crucial role in patient outcomes (Figure 1). Along the same line, the presence of a non-eradicable infection source appears to be a condition in which FUBCs should be performed, especially in patients that require ICU, with persistent fever or as a moderate recommendation (light green) in individuals afflicted with ESRD on hemodialysis [23–25]. FUBCs might also be indicated in persistently febrile patients with primary bacteremia, long term intravascular catheter or urinary tract infection, to a lower degree of evidence. Additionally, we suggest that even in some instances of a lower positivity rate of FUBCs, a clinical decision might be reached in cases of light green and yellow squares both in Figures 2 and 3. For this reason, in the case of patients without a clear clinical indication to perform FUBCs as shown in Figure 2, they should be checked for microbiological risk factors, as shown in Figure 3. To this end, in our opinion, FUBCs might be performed even in instances of microbiological risk factors alone. In fact, taking clinically stable patients with UTI as an example (yellow to red squares in Figure 2), instances where the column of MDR microorganisms' etiology and the row of ineffective therapy intersect in a green square might represent a recommendation to perform FUBCs [20,21,24,25].

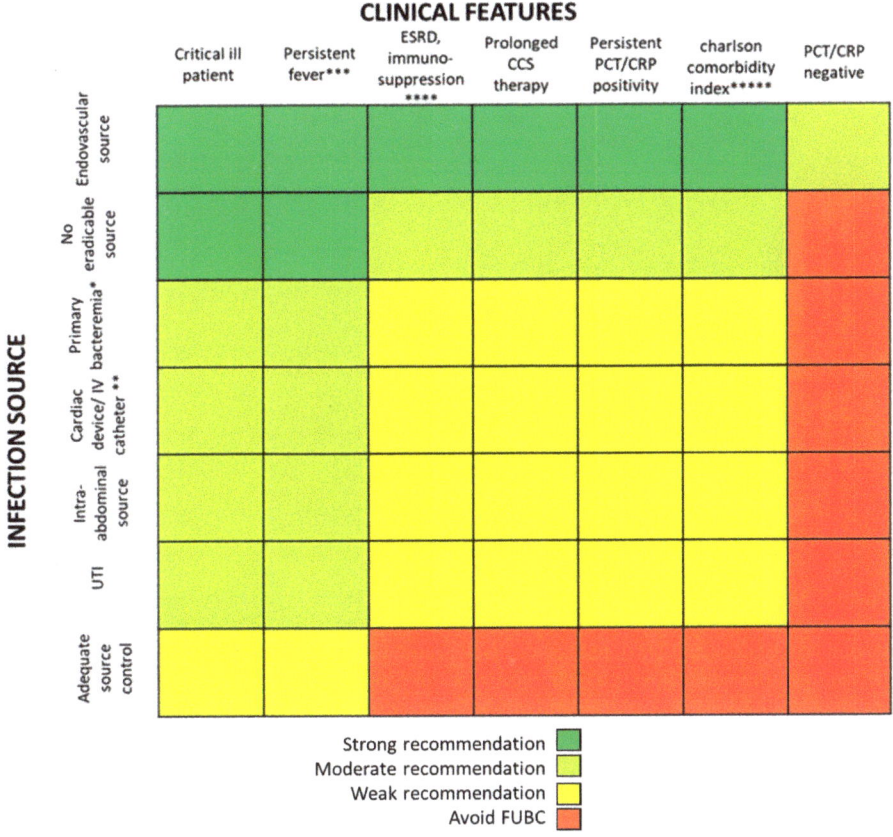

Figure 2. Analysis of recommendations for FUBC sampling in the setting of Gram negative bacteremia on the basis of clinical features and source of infection. **Note:** infection source: * when apparently there is not an infection source; ** if another infection source is presented; *** fever for more than 72–96 h; **** malignancy, solid organ transplantation; ***** Charlson comorbidity index ≥ 6. References: critical ill patient [20,22,23,25,26]; persistent fever [15,20,26]; ESRD, immuno-suppression [15,18,20,23–25]; prolonged corticosteroid (CCS) therapy [23]; persistent PCT/C-reactive protein (CRP) positivity [20]; Charlson comorbidity index [18]; PCT/CRP negative [20]; endovascular source [19,23,24,26]; no eradicable source [22,24,25]; primary bacteremia [26]; cardiac device/intravenous (IV) catheter [15,21, 23–25]; intra-abdominal source [18]; UTI [20,23,25]; adequate source control [24]. **Abbreviations:** UTI, urinary tract infections; ICU, intensive care unit; ESRD, end stage renal disease; CCS, corticosteroids; PCT, procalcitonin; CRP, C-reactive protein.

Getting to the point, if Figure 2 recommends FUBCs, it deals with a "green light" and they should be performed in any case. Additionally, when FUBCs are not indicated by clinical risk factors, clinicians should check the presence of microbiological risk factors, as shown in Figure 3. In the case of neither clinical nor microbiological risk factors, we are in front of a "red light" and FUBCs are not warranted.

A possible limitation of Figures 2 and 3 is that the definitions of risk factors are often different between studies or even not provided at all. For instance, the dosage and duration of corticosteroid treatment with a significant immunosuppressive effect are not clearly defined in the literature as they are considered to depend on the characteristics of the patient and underlying disease [31].

Finally, progressive acquisition of resistance during antimicrobial therapy through the selection of a hidden resistant subpopulation (named hetero-resistance) is a growing concern in the case of persistent bacteremia [32]. Future studies should elucidate the possible role of FUBCs in early detection and management of this increasingly appreciated mechanism of resistance.

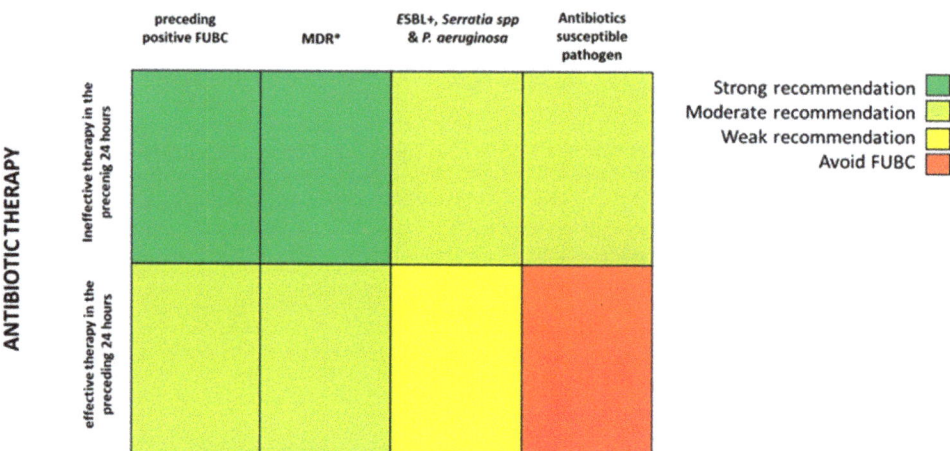

Figure 3. Analysis of recommendations for FUBC sampling in the setting of Gram negative bacteremia on the basis of microbiological factors and efficacy of antibiotic therapy. **Note:** * MDR definition by Magiorakos AP et al., 2012 [33]; ESBL, extended-spectrum beta-lactamases. References: ineffective therapy in the preceding 24 h [18,21–23]; effective therapy in the preceding 24 h [18,21–24]; preceding positive FUBC [26]; MDR [22,23,25,26]; ESBL+, Serratia spp. and P. aeruginosa [23–25]; antibiotic susceptible pathogen [22,23,25,26].

4. Materials and Methods

We searched in the Pubmed database for articles addressing the use of FUBCs in patients with GNB. The following search strategy was adopted: "((FUBCs) or (Follow-up blood cultures) or (follow-up blood culture) or (repeat blood cultures)) and ((gram-negative) or (gram negative rod)) and ((bacteremia) or (BSI) or (bloodstream infection))". The research yielded 102 results. Two reviewers independently assessed the titles and abstracts to identify papers that fulfilled the inclusion criteria: (1) clinical studies; (2) studies that included human subjects; and (3) studies that evaluated the utility of FUBCs in patients with GNB. Full texts of studies assessed as relevant or unclear were evaluated. Studies that only discussed either GNB or FUBCs were excluded. We also examined the bibliographic references of articles to identify any relevant studies that were not identified in the initial literature search. Eleven articles were selected, compared, and critically evaluated (Figure 4).

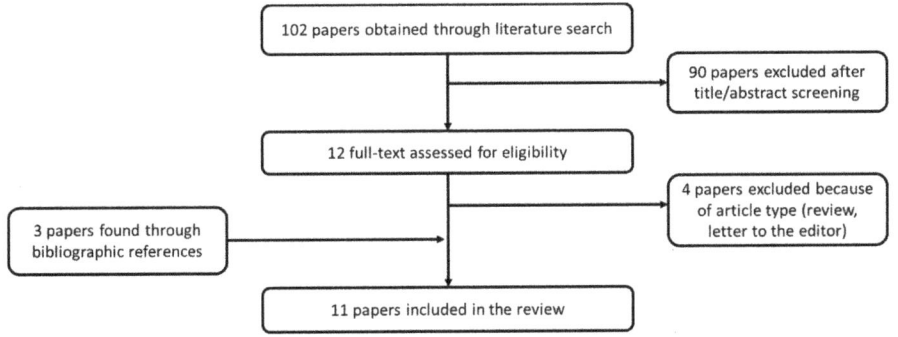

Figure 4. Flow chart of article selection process. References of eleven selected articles: [15,17–26].

5. Conclusions

The usefulness and the drawbacks of FUBCs in GNBs have been largely investigated in the last few years. Of course, some clinical and microbiological factors define the settings where FUBCs exert their maximum capacity to detect PB. Expert clinicians and a correct selection of high-risk patients could make the difference in terms of the efficiency of this diagnostic tool. Furthermore, a targeted and optimized selection of the occasions where to draw FUBCs may also provide a positive impact on patients' management and outcomes. Of note, valuable insights about outcomes of patients where FUBCs were performed remain poor and should be further investigated.

Author Contributions: Conceptualization, M.V.; methodology, M.V., F.C.D., A.C., L.V.; formal analysis, F.C.D., A.C., L.V., A.O.; investigation, F.C.D., A.C., L.V.; writing—original draft preparation, F.C.D., A.C, L.V.; writing—review and editing, G.C., A.O., M.V.; supervision, A.O., M.V. All authors have read and agreed to the published version of the manuscript.

Funding: This research received no external funding.

Conflicts of Interest: The authors declare no conflict of interest.

References

1. Siddiqui, S. Mortality profile across our Intensive Care Units: A 5-year database report from a Singapore restructured hospital. *Indian J. Crit. Care Med.* **2015**, *19*, 726–727. [CrossRef]
2. Goto, M.; Al-Hasan, M.N. Overall burden of bloodstream infection and nosocomial bloodstream infection in North America and Europe. *Clin. Microbiol. Infect.* **2013**, *19*, 501–509. [CrossRef]
3. Kang, C.-I.; Song, J.-H.; Chung, D.R.; Peck, K.R.; Yeom, J.-S.; Ki, H.K.; Son, J.S.; Lee, S.S.; Kim, Y.-S. Risk factors and pathogenic significance of severe sepsis and septic shock in 2286 patients with gram-negative bacteremia. *J. Infect.* **2011**, *62*, 26–33. [CrossRef]
4. Sligl, W.I.; Dragan, T.; Smith, S.W. Nosocomial Gram-negative bacteremia in intensive care: Epidemiology, antimicrobial susceptibilities, and outcomes. *Int. J. Infect. Dis.* **2015**, *37*, 129–134. [CrossRef]
5. Islas-Muñoz, B.; Volkow, P.; Ibanes-Gutiérrez, C.; Villamar-Ramírez, A.; Vilar-Compte, D.; Cornejo-Juárez, P. Bloodstream infections in cancer patients. Risk factors associated with mortality. *Int. J. Infect. Dis.* **2018**, *71*, 59–64. [CrossRef]
6. Liu, C.; Bayer, A.; Cosgrove, S.E.; Daum, R.S.; Fridkin, S.K.; Gorwitz, R.J.; Kaplan, S.L.; Karchmer, A.W.; Levine, D.P.; Murray, B.E.; et al. Clinical Practice Guidelines by the Infectious Diseases Society of America for the Treatment of Methicillin-Resistant *Staphylococcus aureus* Infections in Adults and Children. *Clin. Infect. Dis.* **2011**, *52*, e18–e55. [CrossRef]
7. López-Cortés, L.E.; Del Toro, M.D.; Gálvez-Acebal, J.; Bereciartua-Bastarrica, E.; Fariñas, M.C.; Sanz-Franco, M.; Natera, C.; Corzo, J.E.; Lomas, J.M.; Pasquau, J.; et al. Impact of an Evidence-Based Bundle Intervention in the Quality-of-Care Management and Outcome of *Staphylococcus aureus* Bacteremia. *Clin. Infect. Dis.* **2013**, *57*, 1225–1233. [CrossRef]

8. Holland, T.L.; Arnold, C.J.; Fowler, V.G. Clinical Management of *Staphylococcus aureus* Bacteremia. *JAMA* **2014**, *312*, 1330–1341. [CrossRef]
9. Cornely, O.A.; Bassetti, M.; Calandra, T.; Garbino, J.; Kullberg, B.; Lortholary, O.; Meersseman, W.; Akova, M.; Arendrup, M.; Arikan-Akdagli, S.; et al. ESCMID** This guideline was presented in part at ECCMID 2011. European Society for Clinical Microbiology and Infectious Diseases. Guideline for the diagnosis and management of Candida diseases 2012: Non-neutropenic adult patients. *Clin. Microbiol. Infect.* **2012**, *18*, 19–37. [CrossRef]
10. Yahav, D.; Franceschini, E.; Koppel, F.; Turjeman, A.; Babich, T.; Bitterman, R.; Neuberger, A.; Ghanem-Zoubi, N.; Santoro, A.; Eliakim-Raz, N.; et al. Seven Versus 14 Days of Antibiotic Therapy for Uncomplicated Gram-negative Bacteremia: A Noninferiority Randomized Controlled Trial. *Clin. Infect. Dis.* **2019**, *69*, 1091–1098. [CrossRef]
11. Tamma, P.D.; Conley, A.T.; Cosgrove, S.E.; Harris, A.D.; Lautenbach, E.; Amoah, J.; Avdic, E.; Tolomeo, P.; Wise, J.; Subudhi, S.; et al. Association of 30-Day Mortality With Oral Step-Down vs Continued Intravenous Therapy in Patients Hospitalized With Enterobacteriaceae Bacteremia. *JAMA Intern. Med.* **2019**, *179*, 316–323. [CrossRef]
12. Erickson, R.M.; Tritle, B.J.; Spivak, E.S.; Timbrook, T.T. Impact of an antimicrobial stewardship bundle for uncomplicated gram-negative bacteremia. *Open Forum Infect. Dis.* **2019**, *6*, ofz490. [CrossRef]
13. Fabre, V.; Sharara, S.L.; Salinas, A.B.; Carroll, K.C.; Desai, S.; E Cosgrove, S. Does This Patient Need Blood Cultures? A Scoping Review of Indications for Blood Cultures in Adult Nonneutropenic Inpatients. *Clin. Infect. Dis.* **2020**, *71*, 1339–1347. [CrossRef]
14. Chan, J.D.; Bryson-Cahn, C.; Kassamali-Escobar, Z.; Lynch, J.B.; Schleyer, A.M. The Changing Landscape of Uncomplicated Gram-Negative Bacteremia: A Narrative Review to Guide Inpatient Management. *J. Hosp. Med.* **2020**, *15*, 746–753. [CrossRef]
15. Canzoneri, C.N.; Akhavan, B.J.; Tosur, Z.; Andrade, P.E.A.; Aisenberg, G.M. Follow-up Blood Cultures in Gram-Negative Bacteremia: Are They Needed? *Clin. Infect. Dis.* **2017**, *65*, 1776–1779. [CrossRef]
16. Dempsey, C.; Skoglund, E.; Muldrew, K.L.; Garey, K.W. Economic health care costs of blood culture contamination: A systematic review. *Am. J. Infect. Control.* **2019**, *47*, 963–967. [CrossRef]
17. Tabriz, M.; Riederer, K.; Jr, J.B.; Khatib, R. Repeating blood cultures during hospital stay: Practice pattern at a teaching hospital and a proposal for guidelines. *Clin. Microbiol. Infect.* **2004**, *10*, 624–627. [CrossRef]
18. Kang, C.K.; Kim, E.S.; Song, K.-H.; Kim, W.; Kim, T.S.; Kim, N.-H.; Kim, C.-J.; Choe, P.G.; Bang, J.H.; Park, W.B.; et al. Can a routine follow-up blood culture be justified in Klebsiella pneumoniaebacteremia? A retrospective case–control study. *BMC Infect. Dis.* **2013**, *13*, 365. [CrossRef]
19. Wiggers, J.B.; Xiong, W.; Daneman, N. Sending repeat cultures: Is there a role in the management of bacteremic episodes? (SCRIBE study). *BMC Infect. Dis.* **2016**, *16*, 286. [CrossRef]
20. Shi, H.; Kang, C.-I.; Cho, S.Y.; Huh, K.; Chung, D.R.; Peck, K.R. Follow-up blood cultures add little value in the management of bacteremic urinary tract infections. *Eur. J. Clin. Microbiol. Infect. Dis.* **2019**, *38*, 695–702. [CrossRef]
21. Uehara, E.; Shoji, K.; Mikami, M.; Ishiguro, A.; Miyairi, I. Utility of follow-up blood cultures for Gram-negative rod bacteremia in children. *J. Infect. Chemother.* **2019**, *25*, 738–741. [CrossRef]
22. Giannella, M.; Pascale, R.; Pancaldi, L.; Monari, C.; Ianniruberto, S.; Malosso, P.; Bussini, L.; Bartoletti, M.; Tedeschi, S.; Ambretti, S.; et al. Follow-up blood cultures are associated with improved outcome of patients with gram-negative bloodstream infections: Retrospective observational cohort study. *Clin. Microbiol. Infect.* **2020**, *26*, 897–903. [CrossRef]
23. Maskarinec, S.; Park, L.; Ruffin, F.; Turner, N.; Patel, N.; Eichenberger, E.; Van Duin, D.; Lodise, T.; Fowler, V.G.; Thaden, J. Positive follow-up blood cultures identify high mortality risk among patients with Gram-negative bacteraemia. *Clin. Microbiol. Infect.* **2020**, *26*, 904–910. [CrossRef]
24. Jung, J.; Song, K.-H.; Jun, K.I.; Kang, C.K.; Kim, N.-H.; Choe, P.G.; Park, W.B.; Bang, J.H.; Kim, E.S.; Park, S.-W.; et al. Predictive scoring models for persistent gram-negative bacteremia that reduce the need for follow-up blood cultures: A retrospective observational cohort study. *BMC Infect. Dis.* **2020**, *20*, 1–10. [CrossRef]
25. Mitaka, H.; Gomez, T.; Lee, Y.I.; Perlman, D.C. Risk Factors for Positive Follow-up Blood Cultures in Gram-Negative Bacilli Bacteremia: Implications for Selecting Who Needs Follow-up Blood Cultures. *Open Forum Infect. Dis.* **2020**, *7*. [CrossRef]

26. Spaziante, M.; Oliva, A.; Ceccarelli, G.; Alessandri, F.; Pugliese, F.; Venditti, M. Follow up blood cultures in Gram-negative bacilli bacteremia: Are they needed for critically ill patients? *Minerva Anestesiol.* **2020**, *86*, 498–506. [CrossRef]
27. Weinstein, M.P.; Towns, M.L.; Quartey, S.M.; Mirrett, S.; Reimer, L.G.; Parmigiani, G.; Reller, L.B. The Clinical Significance of Positive Blood Cultures in the 1990s: A Prospective Comprehensive Evaluation of the Microbiology, Epidemiology, and Outcome of Bacteremia and Fungemia in Adults. *Clin. Infect. Dis.* **1997**, *24*, 584–602. [CrossRef]
28. Dargère, S.; Cormier, H.; Verdon, R. Contaminants in blood cultures: Importance, implications, interpretation and prevention. *Clin. Microbiol. Infect.* **2018**, *24*, 964–969. [CrossRef]
29. Ceccarelli, G.; Giuliano, S.; Falcone, M.; Venditti, M. Follow-up Blood Cultures: A 2.0 Diagnostic Tool in Patients with Gram-Negative Bacteremia and Septic Thrombophlebitis. *Clin. Infect. Dis.* **2017**, *66*, 1154–1155. [CrossRef]
30. Spaziante, M.; Giuliano, S.; Ceccarelli, G.; Alessandri, F.; Borrazzo, C.; Russo, A.; Venditti, M. Gram-negative septic thrombosis in critically ill patients: A retrospective case–control study. *Int. J. Infect. Dis.* **2020**, *94*, 110–115. [CrossRef]
31. Youssef, J.; Novosad, S.A.; Winthrop, K.L. Infection Risk and Safety of Corticosteroid Use. *Rheum. Dis. Clin. N. Am.* **2016**, *42*, 157–176. [CrossRef]
32. Brukner, I.; Oughton, M.T. A Fundamental Change in Antibiotic Susceptibility Testing Would Better Prevent Therapeutic Failure: From Individual to Population-Based Analysis. *Front. Microbiol.* **2020**, *11*. [CrossRef]
33. Magiorakos, A.-P.; Srinivasan, A.; Carey, R.; Carmeli, Y.; Falagas, M.; Giske, C.; Harbarth, S.; Hindler, J.; Kahlmeter, G.; Olsson-Liljequist, B.; et al. Multidrug-resistant, extensively drug-resistant and pandrug-resistant bacteria: An international expert proposal for interim standard definitions for acquired resistance. *Clin. Microbiol. Infect.* **2012**, *18*, 268–281. [CrossRef]

Publisher's Note: MDPI stays neutral with regard to jurisdictional claims in published maps and institutional affiliations.

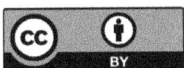

© 2020 by the authors. Licensee MDPI, Basel, Switzerland. This article is an open access article distributed under the terms and conditions of the Creative Commons Attribution (CC BY) license (http://creativecommons.org/licenses/by/4.0/).

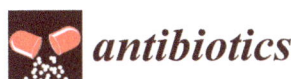 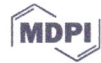

Article

Impact and Sustainability of Antibiotic Stewardship in Pediatric Emergency Departments: Why Persistence Is the Key to Success

Elisa Barbieri [1],*, Maia De Luca [2], Marta Minute [3], Carmen D'Amore [4], Marta Luisa Ciofi Degli Atti [4], Stefano Martelossi [3], Carlo Giaquinto [1], Liviana Da Dalt [5], Theoklis Zaoutis [6] and Daniele Dona [1]

[1] Division of Pediatric Infectious Diseases, Department of Women's and Children's Health, University of Padova, 35131 Padova, Italy; carlo.giaquinto@unipd.it (C.G.); daniele.dona@unipd.it (D.D.)
[2] Unit of Immune and Infectious Diseases, Academic Department of Pediatrics, Bambino Gesù Children's Hospital, IRCCS, 00165 Rome, Italy; maia.deluca@opbg.net
[3] Pediatric Unit, Ca' Foncello's Hospital, 31100 Treviso, Italy; marta.minute@aulss2.veneto.it (M.M.); stefano.martelossi@aulss2.veneto.it (S.M.)
[4] Unit of Clinical Epidemiology, Bambino Gesù Children's Hospital, IRCCS, 00165 Rome, Italy; carmen.damore@opbg.net (C.D.); marta.ciofidegliatti@opbg.net (M.L.C.D.A.)
[5] Pediatric Emergency Department, Department of Women's and Children's Health, University Hospital of Padua, 2-35128 Padova, Italy; liviana.dadalt@unipd.it
[6] Division of Infectious Diseases and the Center for Pediatric Clinical Effectiveness, Children's Hospital of Philadelphia, Philadelphia, PA 19104, USA; zaoutis@email.chop.edu
* Correspondence: elisa.barbieri.5@phd.unipd.it

Received: 15 October 2020; Accepted: 30 November 2020; Published: 4 December 2020

Abstract: Antibiotic stewardship programs proved to be effective in improving prescribing appropriateness. This multicenter quasi-experimental study, aimed to assesses the stewardship impact on antibiotics prescribing in different semesters from 2014 to 2019 in three pediatric emergency departments (Center A, B, and C) in Italy. All consecutive patients diagnosed with acute otitis media or pharyngitis were evaluated for inclusion. Two different stewardship were adopted: for Center A and B, clinical pathways were implemented and disseminated, and yearly lectures were held, for Center C, only pathways were implemented. Broad-spectrum prescription rates decreased significantly by 80% for pharyngitis and 29.5 to 55.2% for otitis after the implementation. In Center C, rates gradually increased from the year after the implementation. Amoxicillin dosage adjusted to pharyngitis recommendations in Center C (53.7 vs. 51.6 mg/kg/die; $p = 0.011$) and otitis recommendations in Center A increasing from 50.0 to 75.0 mg/kg/die ($p < 0.001$). Days of therapy in children < 24 months with otitis increased from 8.0 to 10.0 in Center A, while in older children decreased in Center A (8.0 vs. 7.0; $p < 0.001$) and Center B (10.0 vs. 8.0; $p < 0.001$). Clinical pathways combined with educational lectures is a feasible and sustainable program in reducing broad-spectrum antibiotic prescribing with stable rates over time.

Keywords: antibiotic stewardship; pharyngitis; acute otitis media; clinical pathways; children; emergency departments; antibiotic use; prescribing appropriateness

1. Introduction

Antibiotics remain the most commonly prescribed drugs in the pediatric population [1], with pharyngitis and acute otitis media (AOM) accounting for more than half of the prescriptions in the emergency departments and primary care practices [2,3], with an overprescribing of broad-spectrum antibiotics.

Both conditions have a viral and a bacterial etiology: AOM is mostly caused by Streptococcus pneumoniae, non-typeable *Haemophilus influenzae*, and *Moraxella catarrhalis* [4], while around 20% of pharyngitis are caused by Group A β-hemolytic streptococcus [5].

Although most of the pathogens remain sensible to first line amoxicillin, co-amoxiclav and III-gen cephalosporins are, respectively, prescribed in around 30% and 15% of AOM primary care cases, and in more than 24% and 15% of Group A streptococcus pharyngitis cases [3].

To decrease or reverse this trend, various antibiotic stewardship programs (ASPs) have been implemented worldwide, focusing on different approaches [6].

Clinical pathways have proven to be a feasible and efficient first step in improving prescribing appropriateness, especially in settings where funding is limited [7–10]. A clinical pathway is a task-oriented plan designed to support the implementation of clinical guidelines and protocols in primary care and inpatient settings.

In October 2015, an ASP based on clinical pathways was implemented in the pediatric emergency department of Padova University Hospital. Preliminary results reported an increase in "wait-and-see" approach rate for AOM (21.7% vs. 33.1%) and an increase in narrow-spectrum antibiotics treatments for both AOM (32.0% vs. 51.6%) and pharyngitis (53.6% vs. 93.4%), with no variation in treatment failures [10].

While there is not yet a consensus on the most effective ASP—especially in terms of settings and costs—we aimed to evaluate the efficacy and sustainability over time of ASPs based on clinical pathways with and without yearly educational lectures in three pediatric emergency departments.

2. Results

2.1. Pharyngitis

During the study, 4534 pharyngitis episodes were evaluated, accounting for around 3% of total pediatric emergency department visits. In total, 3249 episodes were included; the demographic characteristics of children included were similar with respect to sex, with a higher prevalence among older children in both Center B and C (Supplementary Materials, Table S2).

In Center A and B amoxicillin prescriptions rate increased (Center A: from 53.6% to 98.5%; $p < 0.001$, Center B: from 69.7% to 96.0%, $p < 0.001$) with a consequent decrease in broad-spectrum-antibiotic prescription rates (broad-spectrum antibiotic prescriptions) (Table 1).

The interrupted time series model strongly suggest a broad-spectrum antibiotic prescriptions reduction following the introduction of the clinical pathways by 81.6% (relative risk (RR) 0.184 (95% CI: 0.072–0.471); $p = 0.002$) for Center A and by 88.6% (RR 0.114 (95% CI: 0.016–0.816); $p = 0.0471$) for Center B, as illustrated in Figure 1.

The interrupted time series model shows a 77% reduction (RR 0.230 (95% CI: 0.167–0.316); $p < 0.001$) in broad-spectrum antibiotic prescriptions rates after the intervention with rates increasing monthly by 3.5% (RR 1.035 (95% CI: 1.025–1.045); $p < 0.001$) in the post periods in Center C.

Amoxicillin dosage adjusted from 53.7 (IQR:7.0) to 51.6 mg/kg/die (IQR:3.8) in Center B (Table 1 and pair-wise comparison in Supplementary Materials, Figure S1) and the median days of therapy (DOT) met the recommended 10 days (8.0 vs. 10.0; $p < 0.001$) after clinical pathways implementation in Center A (Table 1 and pair-wise comparison in Supplementary Materials, Figure S2).

Table 1. Treatment option for pharyngitis in the different periods in the three Centers.

Period	Center A					Center B				Center C				
	Pre	Post 1	Post 2	Post 3	p-Value	Pre	Post 1	Post 2	p-Value	Pre	Post 1	Post 2	Post 3	p-Value
	298	364	326	264		290	241	251		363	217	316	319	
No antibiotic, N (%)	147 (49.3)	198 (54.4)	120 (36.8)	129 (48.9)	<0.001	135 (46.6)	140 (58.1)	122 (48.6)	0.021	23 (6.3)	15 (6.9)	44 (13.9)	23 (7.2)	0.002
Antibiotic therapy, N (%)	151 (50.7)	166 (45.6)	206 (63.2)	135 (51.1)		155 (53.4)	101 (41.9)	129 (51.4)		340 (93.7)	202 (93.1)	272 (86.1)	296 (92.8)	
Amoxicillin, N (%)	81 (53.6)	155 (93.4)	192 (93.2)	133 (98.5)	<0.001	108 (69.7)	97 (96.0)	114 (88.4)	<0.001	42 (12.4)	144 (71.3)	133 (48.9)	84 (28.4)	<0.001
Broad spectrum, N (%)	70 (46.4)	11 (6.6)	14 (6.8)	2 (1.5)	<0.001	47 (30.3)	4 (4.0)	15 (11.6)	<0.001	298 (87.6)	58 (28.7)	139 (51.1)	212 (71.6)	<0.001
Co-amoxiclav, N (%)	60 (39.7)	5 (3.0)	9 (4.4)	1 (0.7)	<0.001	28 (18.1)	1 (1.0)	5 (3.9)	<0.001	249 (73.2)	45 (22.3)	102 (37.5)	170 (57.4)	<0.001
Cephalosporins, N (%)	10 (6.6)	6 (3.6)	4 (1.9)	1 (0.7)	0.029	14 (9.0)	3 (3.0)	7 (5.4)	0.131	17 (5.0)	4 (2.0)	25 (9.2)	33 (11.1)	<0.001
Macrolides, N (%)	0 (0.0)	0 (0.0)	1 (0.5)	0 (0.0)		5 (3.2)	0 (0.0)	3 (2.3)	0.203	32 (9.4)	9 (4.5)	12 (4.4)	9 (3.0)	0.004
Amoxicillin dosage, Median [IQR], mg/kg/die	50.0 [0.0]	50.0 [0.0]	50.0 [1.0]	50.0 [0.0]	0.288	53.7 [7.0]	50.6 [3.5]	51.6 [3.8]	<0.001	/	/	/	/	/
Days of therapy, Median [IQR]	8.0 [3.0]	10.0 [0.0]	10.0 [0.0]	10.0 [0.0]	<0.001	10.0 [1.0]	10.0 [0.0]	10.0 [0.0]	0.622	7.0 [0.0]	7.0 [3.0]	8.00 [1.0]	7.0 [1.0]	<0.001

IQR = Interquartile range.

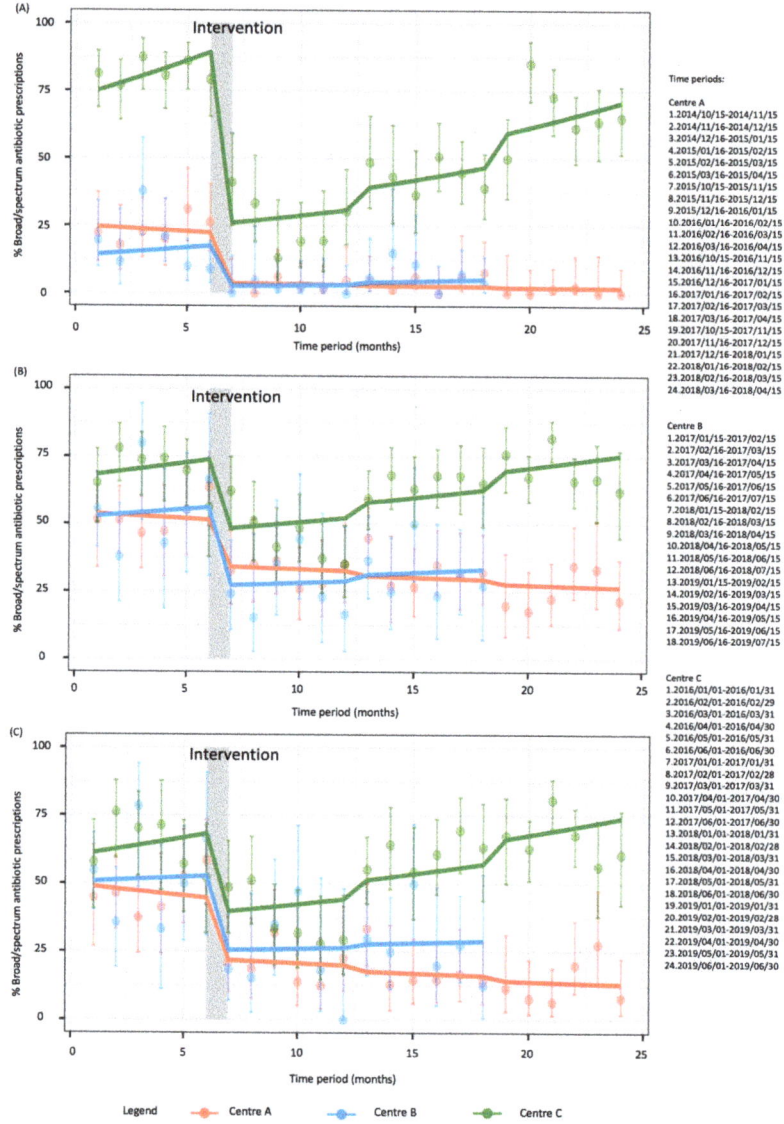

Figure 1. Interrupted time series of monthly broad-spectrum antibiotics prescriptions (dots) expressed as percentages with 95% confidence intervals (bars) for (**A**) pharyngitis, (**B**) acute otitis media, and (**C**) non-complicated acute otitis media in the three centers. The lines represent the broad-spectrum prescriptions trend in the different centers.

2.2. Acute Otitis Media—Total

Overall, 3980 AOM visits were assessed, and 3039 met the inclusion criteria. In Center A and C, a significant difference was reported in age class in the various periods (Supplementary Materials, Table S2).

After ASP implementation, "wait-and-see" approach rates were higher in Center A (from 21.6% to 34.1%; $p = 0.006$) and amoxicillin prescriptions rates increased in Center A and B, with a concomitant decrease in broad-spectrum antibiotic prescriptions rates (Center A: from 67.3% to 38.1%; $p < 0.001$, Center B: from 56.6% to 33.6%; $p < 0.001$), especially cephalosporins prescriptions (Table 2).

In Center C, the highest "wait-and-see" approach rate (32.7%) and the lowest broad-spectrum antibiotic prescriptions rate (68.3%) were reported in the semester following the ASP. Initially, the intervention doubled the "wait-and-see" approach rates (RR 2.510 (95% CI: 1.832–3.349); $p < 0.001$), even if rates did not remain stable, but decreased by 3.6% monthly (RR 0.036 (95% CI: 0.964–0.955); $p < 0.001$).

The broad-spectrum antibiotic prescriptions rates decreased by 29.5% (RR 0.705 (95% CI: 0.538–0.923); $p = 0.011$) in Center A and by 55.2% (RR 0.448 (95% CI: 0.235–0.856); $p = 0.015$) in Center B after the clinical pathways implementation. In Center C, the intervention reduced broad-spectrum antibiotic prescriptions by 41.1% (RR 0.589 (95% CI: 0.470–0.737); $p < 0.001$), but in the following semesters, the broad-spectrum antibiotic prescriptions rates increased by 1.5% monthly (RR 1.015 (95% CI 1.009–1.022); $p < 0.001$). The interrupted time series are shown in Figure 1.

Amoxicillin dosage increased from 50.0 (IQR:0.0) to 75.0 (IQR:5.0) mg/kg/die in Center A ($p < 0.001$), similarly to Center B (from 56.7 (IQR:14.3) to 75.0 (IQR:7.1) mg/kg/die). Co-amoxiclav dosage increase was also significant for both centers (Supplementary Materials, Figure S3).

DOT in children <24 months varied significantly from 8.0 (IQR:2.0) to 10.0 (IQR:0.0) just in Center A (Figure 2).

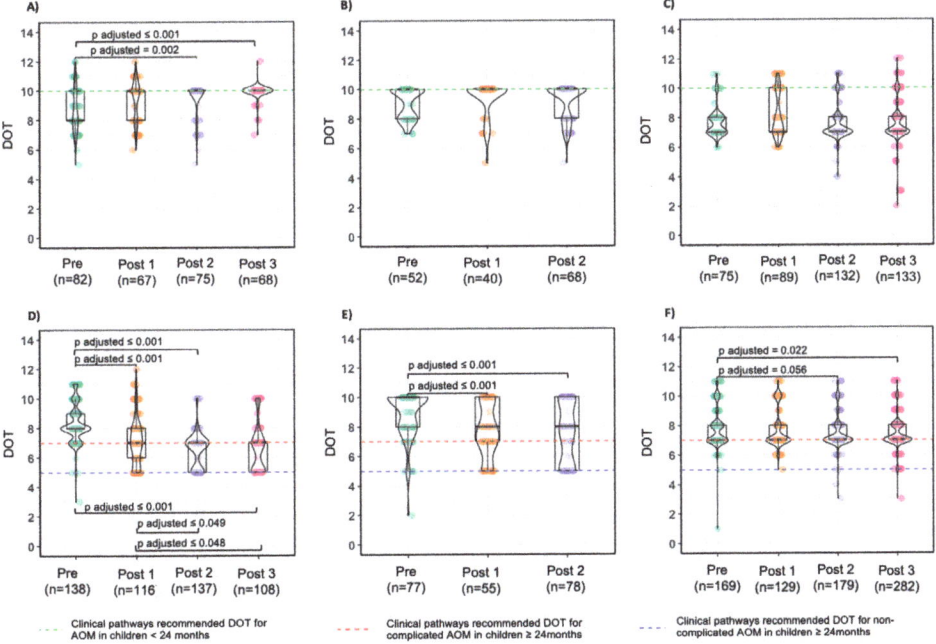

Figure 2. Distribution of days of therapy for non-complicated acute otitis media in the different periods in Center A (**A,D**), Center B (**B,E**), and Center C (**C,F**) stratified by age class (<24 months: **A–C**; ≥24 months: **D–F**) with pair-wise comparison. The dots represent the granular data, horizontal lines are median and IQR; whiskers extend to the minimum and maximum within 1.5 times the IQR. Violin plots present quantifications. The dotted green line represents the DOT recommended in the clinical pathways for acute otitis media in children <24 months, while the dotted blue line represents clinical pathways recommended DOT for non-complicated AOM in children ≥24 months and the dotted red line represents clinical pathways recommended DOT for complicated AOM in children ≥24 months.

Table 2. Treatment option for acute otitis media in the different periods in the three centers.

Period	Center A					Center B					Center C				
	Pre	Post 1	Post 2	Post 3	p-Value	Pre	Post 1	Post 2	p-Value		Pre	Post 1	Post 2	Post 3	p-Value
	281	273	299	267		139	105	151			302	324	387	481	
Wait and see, N (%)	61 (21.7)	90 (33.0)	87 (29.1)	91 (34.1)	0.006	10 (7.2)	10 (9.5)	5 (3.3)	0.116		58 (19.2)	106 (32.7)	76 (19.6)	66 (13.7)	<0.001
Antibiotic treatment, N (%)	220 (78.3)	183 (67.0)	212 (70.9)	176 (65.9)		129 (92.8)	95 (90.5)	146 (96.7)			244 (80.8)	218 (67.3)	311 (80.4)	415 (86.3)	
Amoxicillin, N (%)	72 (32.7)	95 (51.9)	113 (53.3)	109 (61.9)	<0.001	56 (43.4)	66 (69.5)	97 (66.4)	<0.001		30 (12.3)	69 (31.7)	59 (19.0)	73 (17.6)	<0.001
Broad spectrum, N (%)	148 (67.3)	88 (48.1)	99 (46.7)	67 (38.1)	<0.001	73 (56.6)	29 (30.5)	49 (33.6)	<0.001		214 (87.7)	149 (68.3)	252 (81.0)	342 (82.4)	<0.001
Co-amoxiclav, N (%)	100 (45.5)	68 (37.2)	83 (39.2)	62 (35.2)	0.169	44 (34.1)	22 (23.2)	34 (23.3)	0.081		165 (67.6)	121 (55.5)	184 (59.2)	293 (70.6)	<0.001
Cephalosporins, N (%)	44 (20.0)	16 (8.7)	14 (6.6)	5 (2.8)	<0.001	28 (21.7)	5 (5.3)	15 (10.3)	<0.001		43 (17.6)	26 (11.9)	62 (19.9)	45 (10.8)	0.002
Macrolides, N (%)	4 (1.8)	4 (2.2)	1 (0.5)	0 (0.0)	0.119	1 (0.8)	2 (2.1)	0 (0.0)	0.187		6 (2.5)	2 (0.9)	6 (1.9)	4 (1.0)	0.364
Fluoroquinolones, N (%)	0 (0.0)	0 (0.0)	1 (0.5)	0 (0.0)		0 (0.0)	0 (0.0)	0 (0.0)			0 (0.0)	0 (0.0)	0 (0.0)	0 (0.0)	
Amoxicillin dosage, Median [IQR], mg/kg/die	50.0 [0.0]	75.0 [25.0]	75.0 [14.0]	75.0 [0.0]	<0.001	57.6 [14.3]	73.0 [8.6]	75.0 [7.1]	<0.001		/	/	/	/	
Co-amoxiclav dosage, Median [IQR], mg/kg/die	50.0 [10.0]	75.0 [25.0]	73.0 [15.2]	75.0 [5.0]	<0.001	56.7 [7.9]	63.1 [23.9]	68.6 [15.2]	<0.001		/	/	/	/	
Days of therapy, Median [IQR], 2–23 months	8.0 [2.0]	10.0 [2.0]	10.0 [0.0]	10.0 [0.0]	<0.001	10.0 [2.0]	10.0 [0.0]	10.0 [2.0]	0.170		7.0 [1.0]	7.0 [3.0]	7.0 [1.0]	7.0 [1.0]	0.024
Days of therapy, Median [IQR], ≥24 months	8.0 [1.0]	7.0 [2.0]	7.0 [2.0]	7.0 [2.0]	<0.001	10.0 [2.0]	8.0 [3.0]	8.0 [5.0]	<0.001		7.0 [1.0]	7.0 [1.0]	7.0 [1.0]	7.0 [1.0]	<0.001

IQR = Interquartile range.

In older children, a variation was noted in Center A (from 8.0 (IQR:1.0) to 7.0 (IQR:2.0) DOT; $p < 0.001$) and in Center B (from 10.0 (IQR:2.0) to 8.0 (IQR:5.0) DOT; $p < 0.001$), while in Center C the median DOT remained 7.0 for the all periods in both age class.

2.3. Acute Otitis Media—Sensitivity Analysis

In 58.0% (2310/3980) of the AOM diagnoses, there was no sign of otorrhea reported.

In Center A and Center B, co-amoxiclav prescriptions decreased after clinical pathway introduction (Center A: from 43.6% to18.6%; $p < 0.001$, Center B: from 33.3% to 19.7%; $p = 0.035$), whereas a pattern similar to total AOM prescription was noted for Center C (Supplementary Materials, Table S3).

The "wait-and-see" approach rates increased by 68.8% after the intervention and stabilized in Center A (RR 1.688 (95% CI: 1.116–2.552); $p = 0.013$), while in Center C, the intervention was significant in increasing the "wait-and-see" approach rates immediately after the intervention (RR: 2.363 (95% CI: 1.774–3.148); $p < 0.001$); then, rates decreased monthly by 3.3% (RR: 0.967 (95% CI: 0.959–0.976); $p < 0.001$)).

The interrupted time series analysis (Figure 1) confirmed previous findings for Center A and Center C on broad-spectrum antibiotic prescriptions rates, but the reduction by 54.1% (RR 0.459 (95% CI: 0.198–1.060)) in Center B was non-significant ($p = 0.068$).

Amoxicillin and co-amoxiclav dosages did not differ from total AOM findings (Supplementary Materials, Figure S4), whereas median DOT for older children decreased significantly from 8.0 (IQR:2.5) to 5.0 (IQR:2.0) DOT (Supplementary Materials Figure S5) in Center A.

3. Discussion

In this multicentric study, clinical pathways combined with educational lectures proved to be a feasible ASP in decreasing and maintaining broad-spectrum antibiotic prescriptions rates over time for both AOM and pharyngitis (Center A and B). On the other hand, clinical pathways alone failed to maintain the low broad-spectrum prescription rates achieved after the intervention (Center C).

The ASPs reduced co-amoxiclav and cephalosporins prescription rates for pharyngitis by around 80% in all centers. In Center C, the reduction was not maintained after the first semester, possibly due to prescribers' fear of coinfection in Group A Streptococcus carriers [11]. DOT changes reflected prescriptions variation in Center A and Center C, reaching the 10 DOT suggested for amoxicillin in order to decolonize the oropharynx in the Center A. It is unlikely that the recommended duration of amoxicillin is less than the clinical pathway indications, even if penicillin V administered four times daily for five days could represent an alternative regimen in older children with Group A Streptococcus pharyngitis, where commercially available [12,13].

"Wait-and-see" approach rates increased significantly in non-complicated AOM with stable rates after the ASPs implementation. The "wait-and-see" approach was introduced in the early 2000s and was included in most guidelines for the treatment of AOM [14,15] with variation in its applicability. The clinical pathways suggested a "wait-and-see" approach in children with non-severe AOM: if aged 6–24 months just with the unilateral form. In all cases, parents' compliance and the possibility of a follow-up 48–72 h after was needed. The lack of rate variation in Center B could imply that emergency physicians did not feel that it was an appropriate strategy for their setting [16]. Similar to pharyngitis, ASPs were effective in broad-spectrum antibiotic prescriptions rate reduction for AOM. Nonetheless, in Center C, broad-spectrum antibiotic prescriptions rates for non-complicated AOM raised in the last semesters, increasing the possibility to cause more adverse events (i.e., vomiting, diarrhea, rash), in a country where only fixed 7:1 ratio packages are marketed, and the risk of selection of resistant bacteria in the community [17–19]. The same might be the reason why in Center B a more cautious behavior was noted for administering co-amoxiclav, especially at high dosage. Literature findings suggest that a higher co-amoxiclav ratio seems to be associated with fewer side effects without reducing clinical efficacy, but clinical pathways are based on the available medicine formulary to be easily adaptable.

In non-complicated AOM, five median DOT for older children was achieved in Center A's final semester, reflecting prescribers' initial discomfort with short-course treatment. Overall median DOT might not be the most suitable indicator in assessing ASP efficacy on treatment duration when higher rates of second-line therapy (i.e., cephalosporins) are observed, such as in Center C. A possible solution is calculating the median DOT stratified by different drugs.

Our study has several caveats: first, its retrospective nature and difficulties in assessing the reasons why broad-spectrum antibiotics were prescribed. However, the same study nature allowed us to exclude the Hawthorne effect that sometimes could be argued to play a major role in the ASP success. Second, no control groups were selected; hence, we cannot conclude with a high degree of certainty that the variation in broad-spectrum antibiotic prescriptions rates is caused by the ASP implementation without considering other possible explanations. On the other hand, no policy restricting antibiotic prescriptions was implemented in the different centers during the study period, nor were there any shortages in Group A Streptococcus-rapid tests. Third, patient follow-up was beyond the aim of the study and was, therefore, not performed. Although it is possible that patients receiving broad-spectrum antibiotic prescriptions had better clinical outcomes, preliminary results reported that there was no difference in treatment failure rate nor in adverse event rate in the first and second semesters [10]. Fourth, even if the first part of clinical pathways was focused on diagnosis, with a particular emphasis on signs to be considered, clinicians were not tested on the use of pneumatic otoscope nor Group A Streptococcus -rapid tests. Finally, it can be argued that differences in prescriptions may reflect variations in local bacteria resistance, but clinical pathways were developed with microbiologists from different centers, and clinicians were able to adapt them according to local microbiological data.

Despite clinical pathways proving to be a feasible ASP tool with rapid implementation and reduced applicability cost, this study revealed that without combining it with continuous education, it might have no lasting effect. In fact, the Infectious Disease Society of America recommends two core strategies to be implemented together, even if most pediatric ASPs consist of just one intervention. According to a recent systematic review, most of the studies do not report a long follow up, and few report negative results, though publication bias might contribute to this [6].

A study trial where an ASP based on continuous clinician-specific education combined with audit and feedback was implemented in the USA outpatients setting found that following the removal of the audit and feedback, the initial reduction in broad-spectrum antibiotic prescriptions to children with acute respiratory tract infection was lost [20]. The authors believed that audit and feedback was a vital element of the ASP and continuous, active efforts are required to sustain initial improvements in prescribing attitude. Moreover, another trial in a similar setting, comparing different ASPs, found out that only the peer-comparison approach maintained prescription rates lower than the control group after stopping the interventions [21].

Clinicians and researchers interested in implementing an ASP should carefully consider their options in order to avoid inefficiency. A possible improvement in the ASPs proposed lay on the analysis timing. Data were manually collected in condition-specific data collection forms, requiring ad hoc specialists to perform data entry. One solution could be conducting random day-point prevalence surveys every couple of weeks or months in setting with rapid patients turn-over, thus limiting the time dedicated to the collection and providing more rapid estimates on prescribing behaviors [22–24]. Secondly, having IT support to aid in developing real-time indicators will allow for rapid intervention and identification of root causes in cases of prescriber non-adherence to the ASPs [25]. Lastly, in our study, we assessed ASPs' impact and sustainability for conditions with a higher incidence in the cold season, and for this reason, lectures were specifically held in the first months of the season; in the case of developing an ASP for a condition with no such seasonal variation (i.e., sepsis), the ASP team could opt for lectures closer together in time.

4. Materials and Methods

4.1. Study Design

This multicenter quasi-experimental study assesses the ASPs impact on antibiotics prescribing in the pediatric emergency department of three different hospitals: two tertiary-level university hospitals (Azienda Ospedale-Università, Padova and Ospedale Pediatrico Bambino Gesù, Rome, having around 24,000 and 56,000 yearly emergency room visits, respectively) and one secondary-level hospital (Ospedale Ca' Foncello, Treviso, having around 14,000 yearly emergency room visits). Each institution was randomly named with a capital letter (Center A, B, C) to keep them intentionally anonymous.

The different periods considered were: one semester before and three semesters after implementation for Center A and C (Center A: 15 October 2014–15 April 2015; 15 October 2015–15 April 2016; 15 October 2016–15 April 2017; 15 October 2017–15 April 2018; Center C: 1 January 2016–30 June 2016; 1 January 2017–30 June 2017; 1 January 2018–30 June 2018; 1 January 2019–30 June 2019) and one semester before and two semesters after implementation for Center B (1 January 2017–30 June 2017; 1 January 2018–30 June 2018; 1 January 2019–30 June 2019). The study flowchart is shown in Figure 3.

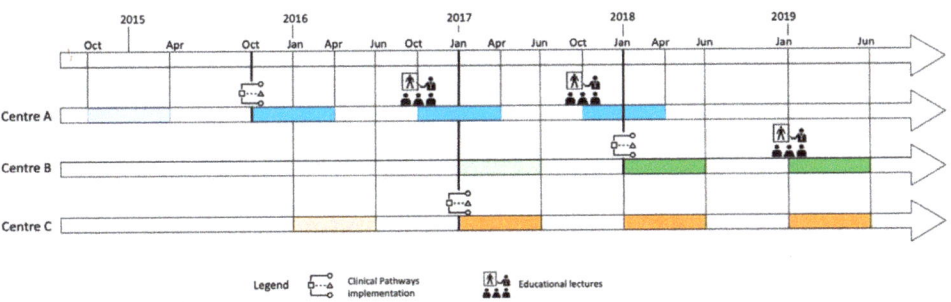

Figure 3. Study flow chart of the ASPs' implementation in the three centers.

During the study period, in the pediatric emergency departments of the three hospitals, there were physicians that worked on a daily basis, specialist consultants that worked depending on the requests and residents that worked on a daily basis but changed every couple of months.

4.2. Intervention

Two different ASPs were adopted: for Center A and B, the intervention consisted of clinical pathway implementation and dissemination as laminated pocket-cards with yearly educational lectures for residents and pediatricians, and for Center C, the intervention consisted only of the implementation of clinical pathways with the possibility of consulting in the hospital intranet.

A multidisciplinary group of experts from each center, in collaboration with the Division of Pediatric Infectious Diseases of the Children's Hospital of Philadelphia, developed the clinical pathways for pharyngitis and AOM that were adapted to the centers' standard of care with no changes in the algorithm (Appendix A Figure A1 and Appendix B Figure A2).

The educational lectures addressed to residents, structured physicians and specialists and held by the center ASP team, consisted of two hours of training on the diagnosis and treatments of AOM and pharyngitis with a focus on the rational for antibiotic prescribing.

4.3. Population and Case Definition

All consecutive patients aged two months to 14 years with an International Classification of Diseases, 9th Revision, Clinical Modification code, or descriptive diagnosis of AOM or pharyngitis admitted to the pediatric emergency department in one of the three centers were included.

General exclusion criteria were immunodeficiency or immunosuppressive therapy, concomitant bacterial infections or systemic bacterial infection, craniofacial abnormalities, chronic diseases (i.e., diabetes, cystic fibrosis), and ongoing antibiotic therapy at admission. Pharyngitis exclusion criteria were previous tonsillectomy, periodic fever, aphthous stomatitis, pharyngitis and adenitis syndrome, and admission to the pediatric emergency department for feeding difficulties. AOM exclusion criteria were tympanostomy tubes at the time of diagnosis, chronic otitis media, and AOM complicated by mastoiditis.

Pediatric emergency department visits occurring for the same patient greater than 30 days apart were analyzed as separate events.

All AOM episodes with otorrhea were considered as complicated AOM; the remaining episodes were considered as non-complicated.

Broad-spectrum antibiotics were defined as β-lactam and β-lactamase inhibitor combinations, second- and third-generation cephalosporins, fluoroquinolones, and macrolides. Topic antibiotics (i.e., ciprofloxacin ear drops) were not considered.

4.4. Outcomes

The following aspects of antibiotic prescriptions for pharyngitis and AOM were assessed:

1. "Wait-and-see" approach rates (AOM only);
2. Broad-spectrum antibiotic prescriptions rates;
3. Rates by active agent;
4. Amoxicillin and co-amoxiclav dosage, expressed in mg/kg/day (Center A and Center B only);
5. Duration of therapy expressed in DOT.

The "wait-and-see" approach was defined as AOM episodes with no antibiotic prescription.

4.5. Data Collection and Sample Size Calculation

All clinical, demographic, diagnostic, and prescription data were manually collected from electronic medical records, using a password protected REDCap 10.0.1-© 2020 (Vanderbilt University) data collection form and stored on a secured server at the University of Padova. Privacy was guaranteed by assigning each patient a unique study-specific number and not collecting personally identifying data.

Assuming that before ASP implementation, (i) in 10% of AOM episodes a "wait-and-see" approach would be chosen and in 45% of pharyngitis episodes no antibiotic would be prescribed, (ii) the broad-spectrum antibiotic prescriptions rates would be 50%, (iii) broad-spectrum antibiotic prescriptions would decrease by 25%, (iv) 15% of the episodes did not fulfill the inclusion criteria, (v) a two-tailed Type I error of 0.05 is used, and (vi) the study is required to have at least a power of 70%, we estimated a minimum sample size of 330 pharyngitis and 260 AOM episodes per period per center to detect a significant decrease in broad-spectrum antibiotic prescriptions. The power for estimating the difference between independent proportions was calculated using G Power 3.1.9.4-© 1992–2019 (Universitat Kiel, Germany) [26].

The investigations were carried out following the rules of the Declaration of Helsinki of 1975 (https://www.wma.net/what-we-do/medical-ethics/declaration-of-helsinki/), revised in 2013. This study was approved by the Ethical Committees of all Centers (3737/AO/16). Due to the nature of the study (observational retrospective), no informed consent was required from the patients.

4.6. Data Analysis

Single center results in the different periods were summarized as numbers and percentages (categorical variables) and as median and interquartile range (continuous variables). Categorical variables were compared with χ^2 or Fisher's 2-tailed exact test in a contingency table $r \times c$; a Fisher test was used when the value in any of the cells of the contingency table was below five. Continuous variables were compared with a non-parametric Kruskal-Wallis rank sum test; for pair-wise comparisons, we used

Dwass-Steele-Critchlow-Fligner all-pairs test adjusted with Holm method. Since different DOT are recommended depending on child age, DOT analysis was stratified according to age class (2–23 months of age vs. 2–14 years of age).

An interrupted time series analysis supposing an abrupt step change in monthly significative outcomes (1 and 2) using quasi-Poisson regression models was used to determine the effect of the intervention. [27]"Wait-and-see" approach, log-transformed total AOM episodes, a variable representing the frequency in months in which observations were taken, and a dummy variable indicating the pre- and post-intervention periods were considered. For outcome (2), broad-spectrum antibiotic prescriptions and log-transformed total antibiotic prescriptions were considered together with a frequency variable and a dummy variable previously specified. A seasonal adjustment was not necessary since the same calendar months were considered to control for effects. Autocorrelation was assessed, examining the plot for residuals and the partial autocorrelation function. The corresponding relative risk and 95% confidence interval (95% CI) according to normal approximation were calculated.

Outcome data were sometimes missing (0–20%, Supplementary Materials, Table S1). If variable data were missing completely at random [28] and restricting the analysis would not have resulted in a significant loss of information or biased estimation, listwise deletion was performed (i.e., dosage); in the opposite case (i.e., DOT), group-wise predictive mean matching within the fully conditional specification algorithm was used to fit the missing data [29].

A sensitivity analysis was conducted for non-complicated AOM episodes. Data were analyzed using R statistical software (version 3.6.3, Vienna, Austria) for Windows [30]. The multiple imputation was performed with the "mice" and "miceadds" packages [31]. Figures were created with the packages "ggplot2" [32] and "ggstatsplot" [33]. For brevity, statistical parameters were included in figures displaying pair-wise comparisons. Statistical significance was set at the 0.05 level and p values were two-sided.

5. Conclusions

To the best of our knowledge, this is the first attempt to study the efficacy and sustainability of ASPs over time based on clinical pathways in pediatric emergency departments. Our findings suggest that clinical pathways paired with continuous education can be effective in reducing broad-spectrum antibiotic prescription and in reaching target treatment duration. Researchers should push for efficient assessment and publication of intervention sustainability in order to help other clinicians in choosing the most suitable ASP for their setting.

Supplementary Materials: The following are available online at http://www.mdpi.com/2079-6382/9/12/867/s1, Table S1. Missing data in the different periods in the three centers (A, B, C); Table S2. Demographic characteristics of the included and excluded patients with pharyngitis and AOM in the different periods in the three centers (A, B, C); Table S3. Treatment option for non-complicated AOM in the different periods in the three centers (A, B, C); Figure S1. Distribution of amoxicillin dosage for pharyngitis among different periods in Center A and B with pairwise comparison; Figure S2. Distribution of days of therapy for pharyngitis among different periods in the three centers (A, B, C) with pairwise comparison; Figure S3. Distribution of co-amoxiclav (A, B) and amoxicillin (C, D) dosage for acute otitis media among different periods in Center A (A, C) and Center B (B, D) with pairwise comparison; Figure S4. Distribution of co-amoxiclav (A, B) and amoxicillin (C, D) dosage for non-complicated acute otitis media among different periods in Center A (A, C) and Center B (B, D) with pairwise comparison; Figure S5. Distribution of days of therapy (DOT) for acute otitis media in the different periods in Centre A (A, D), Centre B (B, E) and Centre C (C, F) stratified by age class (<24 months: A, B, C; ≥24 months: D, E, F) with pair wise comparison.

Author Contributions: Conceptualization, D.D., T.Z., L.D.D., and C.G.; methodology, D.D., T.Z., L.D.D., and C.G.; software, E.B.; validation, E.B., M.D.L., and M.M.; formal analysis, E.B.; investigation, D.D., M.D.L., and M.M.; resources, C.G., L.D.D., C.D., M.L.C.D.A., and S.M.; data curation, E.B., M.D.L., and M.M.; writing—original draft preparation, E.B.; writing—review and editing, D.D., T.Z., M.D.L., and M.M.; visualization, E.B. and D.D.; supervision, T.Z., L.D.D., C.D., M.L.C.D.A., S.M., and C.G. All authors have read and agreed to the published version of the manuscript.

Funding: This research received no external funding.

Acknowledgments: The authors would like to thank Giulia Brigadoi, Giulia Cesca, Sofia Mezzalira, Antonino Reale, Livia Gargiullo, Lorenza Romani, Simona Pipino, Nicole Colantoni, and Anna Maselli for collecting the data, and Lindsey Hunter for helping to edit the manuscript.

Conflicts of Interest: The authors declare no conflict of interest.

Appendix A

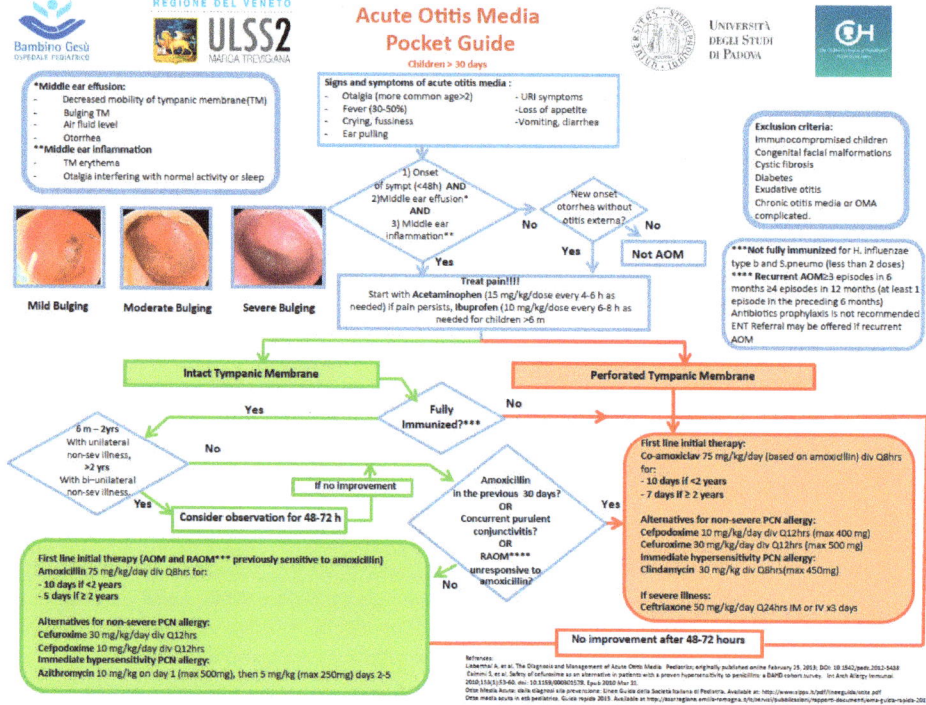

Figure A1. Clinical pathway for acute otitis media for children older than 30 days of age.

Appendix B

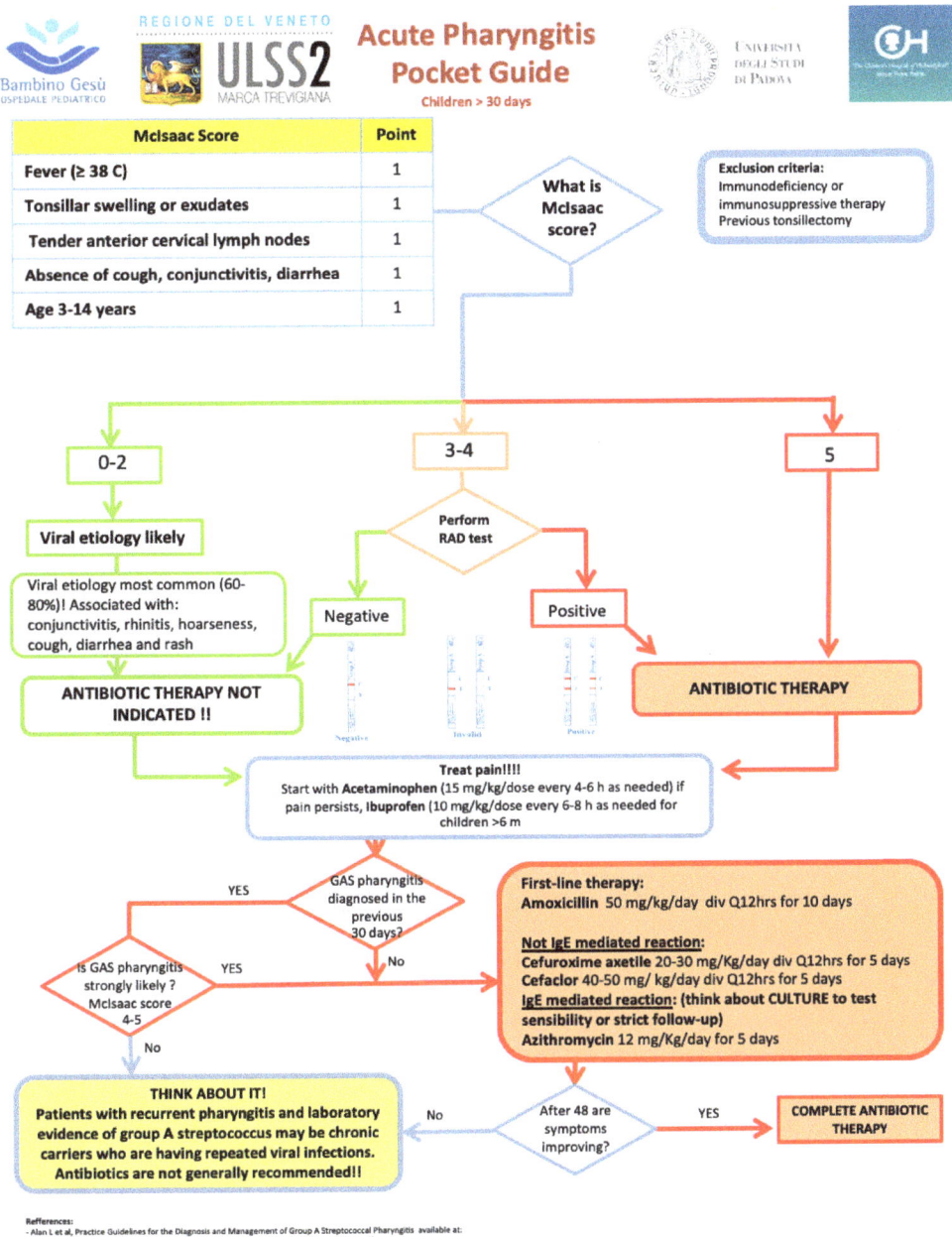

Figure A2. Clinical pathway for acute acute pharyngitis for children older than 30 days of age.

References

1. Sturkenboom, M.C.J.M.; Verhamme, K.M.C.; Nicolosi, A.; Murray, M.L.; Neubert, A.; Caudri, D.; Picelli, G.; Sen, E.F.; Giaquinto, C.; Cantarutti, L.; et al. Drug use in children: Cohort study in three European countries. *BMJ* **2008**, *337*, 2245. [CrossRef] [PubMed]
2. Messina, F.; Clavenna, A.; Cartabia, M.; Piovani, D.; Bortolotti, A.; Fortino, I.; Merlino, L.; Bonati, M. Antibiotic prescription in the outpatient paediatric population attending emergency departments in Lombardy, Italy: A retrospective database review. *BMJ Paediatr. Open* **2019**, *3*, e000546. [CrossRef] [PubMed]
3. Barbieri, E.; Donà, D.; Cantarutti, A.; Lundin, R.; Scamarcia, A.; Corrao, G.; Giaquinto, C. Antibiotic prescriptions in acute otitis media and pharyngitis in Italian pediatric outpatients. *Italy J. Pediatr.* **2019**, *45*, 103. [CrossRef] [PubMed]
4. Marchisio, P.; Esposito, S.; Picca, M.; Baggi, E.; Terranova, L.; Orenti, A.; Biganzoli, E.; Principi, N.; Gallia, P.; Mazzucchi, E.; et al. Prospective evaluation of the aetiology of acute otitis media with spontaneous tympanic membrane perforation. *Clin. Microbiol. Infect.* **2017**, *23*, 486.e1–486.e6. [CrossRef]
5. Kronman, M.P.; Zhou, C.; Mangione-Smith, R. Bacterial prevalence and antimicrobial prescribing trends for acute respiratory tract infections. *Pediatrics* **2014**, *134*, e956–e965. [CrossRef]
6. Donà, D.; Barbieri, E.; Daverio, M.; Lundin, R.; Giaquinto, C.; Zaoutis, T.; Sharland, M. Implementation and impact of pediatric antimicrobial stewardship programs: A systematic scoping review. *Antimicrob Resist. Infect Control* **2020**, *9*, 3. [CrossRef]
7. Samore, M.H.; Bateman, K.; Alder, S.C.; Hannah, E.; Donnelly, S.; Stoddard, G.J.; Haddadin, B.; Rubin, M.A.; Williamson, J.; Stults, B.; et al. Clinical decision support and appropriateness of antimicrobial prescribing: A randomized trial. *JAMA* **2005**, *294*, 2305–2314. [CrossRef]
8. Donà, D.; Zingarella, S.; Gastaldi, A.; Lundin, R.; Perilongo, G.; Frigo, A.C.; Hamdy, R.F.; Zaoutis, T.; Da Dalt, L.; Giaquinto, C. Effects of clinical pathway implementation on antibiotic prescriptions for pediatric community-acquired pneumonia. *PLoS ONE* **2018**, *13*, e0193581. [CrossRef]
9. Donà, D.; Luise, D.; Barbieri, E.; Masiero, N.; Maita, S.; Antoniello, L.; Zaoutis, T.; Giaquinto, C.; Gamba, P. Effectiveness and Sustainability of an Antimicrobial Stewardship Program for Perioperative Prophylaxis in Pediatric Surgery. *Pathogens* **2020**, *9*, 490. [CrossRef]
10. Dona, D.; Baraldi, M.; Brigadoi, G.; Lundin, R.; Perilongo, G.; Hamdy, R.F.; Zaoutis, T.; Da Dalt, L.; Giaquinto, C. The Impact of Clinical Pathways on Antibiotic Prescribing for Acute Otitis Media and Pharyngitis in the Emergency Department. *Pediatr. Infect Dis. J.* **2018**, *37*, 901–907. [CrossRef]
11. Spuesens, E.B.M.; Fraaij, P.L.A.; Visser, E.G.; Hoogenboezem, T.; Hop, W.C.J.; Van Adrichem, L.N.A.; Weber, F.; Moll, H.A.; Broekman, B.; Berger, M.Y.; et al. Carriage of Mycoplasma pneumoniae in the upper respiratory tract of symptomatic and asymptomatic children: An observational study. *PLoS Med.* **2013**, *10*, e1001444. [CrossRef] [PubMed]
12. Ståhlgren, G.S.; Tyrstrup, M.; Edlund, C.; Giske, C.G.; Mölstad, S.; Norman, C.; Rystedt, K.; Sundvall, P.-D.; Hedin, K. Penicillin V four times daily for five days versus three times daily for 10 days in patients with pharyngotonsillitis caused by group A streptococci: Randomised controlled, open label, non-inferiority study. *BMJ* **2019**, *367*, l5337. [CrossRef] [PubMed]
13. Pichichero, M.E. Treatment and prevention of streptococcal pharyngitis. In *Up to Date*; Post, T.W., Ed.; UpToDate: Waltham, MA, USA, 2015.
14. Lieberthal, A.S.; Carroll, A.E.; Chonmaitree, T.; Ganiats, T.G.; Hoberman, A.; Jackson, M.A.; Joffe, M.D.; Miller, D.T.; Rosenfeld, R.M.; Sevilla, X.D.; et al. The diagnosis and management of acute otitis media. *Pediatrics* **2013**, *131*, e964–e999. [CrossRef]
15. SIP Guidelines. Available online: https://sip.it/2019/06/17/gestione-otite-media-acuta-linee-guida/ (accessed on 1 December 2020). (In Italian).
16. Fischer, T.; Singer, A.J.; Lee, C.; Thode, H.C., Jr. National trends in emergency department antibiotic prescribing for children with acute otitis media, 1996–2005. *Acad. Emerg. Med.* **2007**, *14*, 1172–1175. [CrossRef]
17. Arguedas, A.; Dagan, R.; Leibovitz, E.; Hoberman, A.; Pichichero, M.; Paris, M. A multicenter, open label, double tympanocentesis study of high dose cefdinir in children with acute otitis media at high risk of persistent or recurrent infection. *Pediatr. Infect Dis. J.* **2006**, *25*, 211–218. [CrossRef]

18. Agenzia Italiana del Farmaco—Italian Medicine Agency. Available online: https://farmaci.agenziafarmaco.gov.it/bancadatifarmaci/cerca-per-principioattivo?princ_att=Amoxicillina%20e%20inibitori%20enzimatici (accessed on 31 July 2020).
19. Hoberman, A.; Paradise, J.L.; Rockette, H.E.; Jeong, J.-H.; Kearney, D.H.; Bhatnagar, S.; Shope, T.R.; Muñiz, G.; Martin, J.M.; Kurs-Lasky, M.; et al. Reduced-Concentration Clavulanate for Young Children with Acute Otitis Media. *Antimicrob. Agents Chemother.* **2017**, *61*, e00238-17. [CrossRef]
20. Gerber, J.S.; Prasad, P.A.; Fiks, A.G.; Localio, A.R.; Bell, L.M.; Keren, R.; Zaoutis, T.E. Durability of benefits of an outpatient antimicrobial stewardship intervention after discontinuation of audit and feedback. *JAMA* **2014**, *312*, 2569–2570. [CrossRef] [PubMed]
21. Linder, J.A.; Meeker, D.; Fox, C.R.; Friedberg, M.W.; Persell, S.D.; Goldstein, N.J.; Doctor, J.N. Effects of Behavioral Interventions on Inappropriate Antibiotic Prescribing in Primary Care 12 Months After Stopping Interventions. *JAMA* **2017**, *318*, 1391–1392. [CrossRef] [PubMed]
22. Velasco-Arnaiz, E.; Simó-Nebot, S.; Ríos-Barnés, M.; Ramos, M.G.L.; Monsonís, M.; Urrea-Ayala, M.; Jordan, I.; Mas-Comas, A.; Casadevall-Llandrich, R.; Ormazábal-Kirchner, D.; et al. Benefits of a Pediatric Antimicrobial Stewardship Program in Antimicrobial Use and Quality of Prescriptions in a Referral Children's Hospital. *J. Pediatr.* **2020**, *225*, 222–230.e1. [CrossRef] [PubMed]
23. De Luca, M.; Donà, D.; Montagnani, C.; Vecchio, A.L.; Romanengo, M.; Tagliabue, C.; Centenari, C.; D'Argenio, P.; Lundin, R.; Giaquinto, C.; et al. Antibiotic Prescriptions and Prophylaxis in Italian Children. Is It Time to Change? Data from the ARPEC Project. *PLoS ONE* **2016**, *11*, e0154662. [CrossRef] [PubMed]
24. Hsia, Y.; Lee, B.R.; Versporten, A.; Yang, Y.; Bielicki, J.; Jackson, C.; Newland, J.; Goossens, H.; Magrini, N.; Sharland, M. Use of the WHO Access, Watch, and Reserve classification to define patterns of hospital antibiotic use (AWaRe): An analysis of paediatric survey data from 56 countries. *Lancet Glob. Health* **2019**, *7*, e861–e871. [CrossRef]
25. Bremmer, D.N.; Trienski, T.L.; Walsh, T.L.; Moffa, M.A. Role of Technology in Antimicrobial Stewardship. *Med. Clin. N. Am.* **2018**, *102*, 955–963. [CrossRef] [PubMed]
26. Faul, F.; Erdfelder, E.; Buchner, A.; Lang, A.-G. Statistical power analyses using G*Power 3.1: Tests for correlation and regression analyses. *Behav. Res. Methods* **2009**, *41*, 1149–1160. [CrossRef] [PubMed]
27. Bernal, J.L.; Cummins, S.; Gasparrini, A. Interrupted time series regression for the evaluation of public health interventions: A tutorial. *Int. J. Epidemiol.* **2017**, *46*, 348–355. [CrossRef]
28. Kang, H. The prevention and handling of the missing data. *Korean J. Anesthesiol.* **2013**, *64*, 402–406. [CrossRef]
29. Kleinke, K. Multiple imputation by predictive mean matching when sample size is small. *Methodol. Eur. J. Res. Methods Behav. Soc. Sci.* **2018**, *14*, 3–15. [CrossRef]
30. R Core Team. *R: A Language and Environment for Statistical Computing*; R Foundation for Statistical Computing: Vienna, Austria, 2019; Available online: https://www.R-project.org/ (accessed on 1 December 2020).
31. Van Buuren, S.; Groothuis-Oudshoorn, K. Mice: Multivariate Imputation by Chained Equations in R. *J. Stat. Softw.* **2011**, *45*. [CrossRef]
32. Wickham, H. *Ggplot2: Elegant Graphics for Data Analysis*; Springer: New York, NY, USA, 2016; Available online: https://ggplot2-book.org/ (accessed on 1 December 2020).
33. Patil, I. Ggstatsplot: "ggplot2" Based Plots with Statistical Details. *CRAN* **2018**. [CrossRef]

Publisher's Note: MDPI stays neutral with regard to jurisdictional claims in published maps and institutional affiliations.

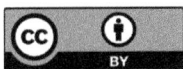

© 2020 by the authors. Licensee MDPI, Basel, Switzerland. This article is an open access article distributed under the terms and conditions of the Creative Commons Attribution (CC BY) license (http://creativecommons.org/licenses/by/4.0/).

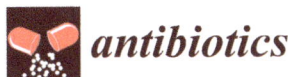

Article

Effectiveness and Acceptance of Multimodal Antibiotic Stewardship Program: Considering Progressive Implementation and Complementary Strategies

Flavien Bouchet [1,2,*], Vincent Le Moing [1], Delphine Dirand [2], François Cros [3], Alexi Lienard [4], Jacques Reynes [1], Laurent Giraudon [2] and David Morquin [1]

1. Service de Maladies Infectieuses et Tropicales, Centre Hospitalier Universitaire de Montpellier, Université de Montpellier, 34000 Montpellier, France; v-le_moing@chu-montpellier.fr (V.L.M.); j-reynes@chu-montpellier.fr (J.R.); d-morquin@chu-montpellier.fr (D.M.)
2. Pôle Appui aux Fonctions Cliniques, Département de la Pharmacie, Hôpitaux du Bassin de Thau, 34200 Sète, France; ddirand@ch-bassindethau.fr (D.D.); lgiraudon@ch-bassindethau.fr (L.G.)
3. Département Informatique, Hôpitaux du Bassin de Thau, 34200 Sète, France; fcros@ch-bassindethau.fr
4. Département de Biologie Médicale, Hôpitaux du Bassin de Thau, 34200 Sète, France; alienard@ch-bassindethau.fr
* Correspondence: fbouchet@ch-bassindethau.fr

Received: 31 October 2020; Accepted: 25 November 2020; Published: 27 November 2020

Abstract: Multiple modes of interventions are available when implementing an antibiotic stewardship program (ASP), however, their complementarity has not yet been assessed. In a 938-bed hospital, we sequentially implemented four combined modes of interventions over one year, centralized by one infectious diseases specialist (IDS): (1) on-request infectious diseases specialist consulting service (IDSCS), (2) participation in intensive care unit meetings, (3) IDS intervention triggered by microbiological laboratory meetings, and (4) IDS intervention triggered by pharmacist alert. We assessed the complementarity of the different cumulative actions through quantitative and qualitative analysis of all interventions traced in the electronic medical record. We observed a quantitative and qualitative complementarity between interventions directly correlating to a decrease in antibiotic use. Quantitatively, the number of interventions has doubled after implementation of IDS intervention triggered by pharmacist alert. Qualitatively, these kinds of interventions led mainly to de-escalation or stopping of antibiotic therapy (63%) as opposed to on-request IDSCS (32%). An overall decrease of 14.6% in antibiotic use was observed ($p = 0.03$). Progressive implementation of the different interventions showed a concrete complementarity of these actions. Combined actions in ASPs could lead to a significant decrease in antibiotic use, especially regarding critical antibiotic prescriptions, while being well accepted by prescribers.

Keywords: antibiotic stewardship program; complementarity; prospective audit and feedback

1. Introduction

In 2015 in Europe, 671,689 cases of infections with antibiotic-resistant bacteria features occurred, leading to 33,110 deaths, corresponding to 6.44 deaths per 100,000 population and 874,541 disability adjusted life-years (DALYs) [1]. Without any practical measures, the current state could worsen exponentially with 390,000 deaths every year expected in Europe by 2050. Moreover, this concerning healthcare issue also represents a dramatic economic burden; that is, if the antibiotic-resistant bacteria infection rate remains at the same level as today, this could lead to a loss of 100 trillion of USD worldwide [2,3]. Implementing antibiotic stewardship programs (ASPs) in hospitals is a major way to improve this issue [4–7]. Many studies have shown the positive impact of antibiotic stewardship programs (ASPs) on antibiotic use and antibiotic resistance, improvement of morbidity and mortality, reduction of *Clostridium difficile* infections incidence, and health costs savings [7–13]. One of the key points of ASP success is to gather a multidisciplinary team including pharmacists, microbiologists, and infectious diseases physicians with a specific time dedicated to this task [5,14,15].

Nowadays, cross-disciplinary medical project funding is limited by the current economic healthcare situation. Despite many warnings from French and European infectious diseases societies about the crucial need for ASPs, raising funds and dedicating time to implement these strategies are still difficult, especially when the short-term economic benefit is not obvious [16–18].

In France, ASPs are not fully implemented and the current system relies on supporting prescribers mainly through training and on-request infectious diseases specialist consulting [19]. Training may be a key point to improve antibiotics prescription, yet a recent multicenter web-based survey brings to light that most final-year European medical students feel they still need more education on antibiotic use for their future practice as junior doctors [20]. In this context, the association of the improvement of medical student training and a more interventionist strategy including microbiological laboratory alerts and prospective audit and feedback (PAF) interventions, such as prescription review with assistance by pharmacists, could be useful [6,21,22]. Indeed, PAF allows clinicians to prescribe any empiric antibiotic regimen, then the ASP can advise the clinician on discontinuing or adjusting therapy after prescription analysis. Although feedback further increased the intervention effect, it is used in only a minority of enabling interventions, as shown in a Cochrane meta-analysis [23]. This study raises the need for new studies to assess different stewardship interventions and to explore the facilitators to implementation.

Indeed, the practical way to link together these interventions is not clear and neither the complementarity of these actions nor the acceptance of physicians towards unsolicited advice have yet been evaluated. Based on recent publications [24–27], we progressively implemented an innovative multimodal ASP in 2018 in a secondary care hospital. The aim of this study was to evaluate the complementarity of different interventions in an ASP and the impact on antibiotic use. We also analyzed the impact on mean of length of stay (LOS), 30-day readmission rate (30-DRR), and mortality. Prescribers' acceptance was also assessed in the perspective of long-term system development.

2. Results

2.1. Interventions Complementarity

Over the entire analysis period, 7508 stays involved the administration of antibiotic therapy, of which 1316 received an intervention. At least one intervention was carried out for 1430 stays, corresponding to 2046 interventions noted in the electronic medical records (EMRs) (Figure 1).

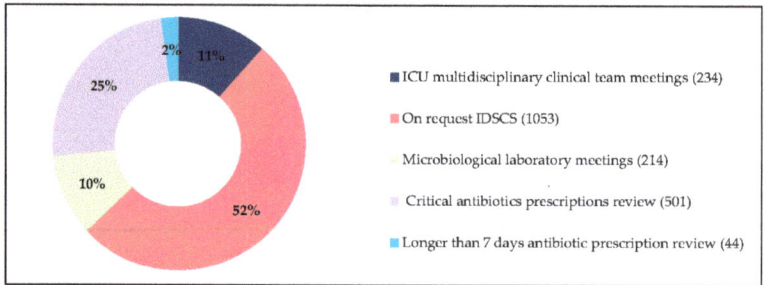

Figure 1. Interventions' distribution. Distribution of the 2046 interventions noted in the electronic patient record related to 1430 hospital stays and 1243 patients. Abbreviations: ICU, intensive care unit; IDSCS, infectious diseases specialist consulting service.

The overall acceptance rate for the proposals was 88%, with a variation according to intervention types ranging from 68 to 92% (Figure 2). The distribution analysis of intervention-types normalized to working days on site highlights a true complementarity between interventions (Figure 3). In summary, the implementation of PAF interventions in a second phase widens the ASP field of action without impacting other types of intervention.

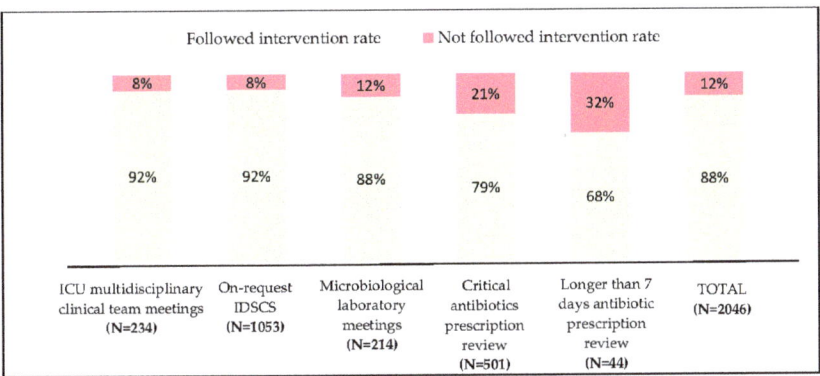

Figure 2. Compliance depending on intervention type. Compliance rate of the 2046 interventions noted in electronic patient record. Abbreviations: ICU, intensive care unit; IDSCS, infectious diseases specialist consulting service; N = number of interventions.

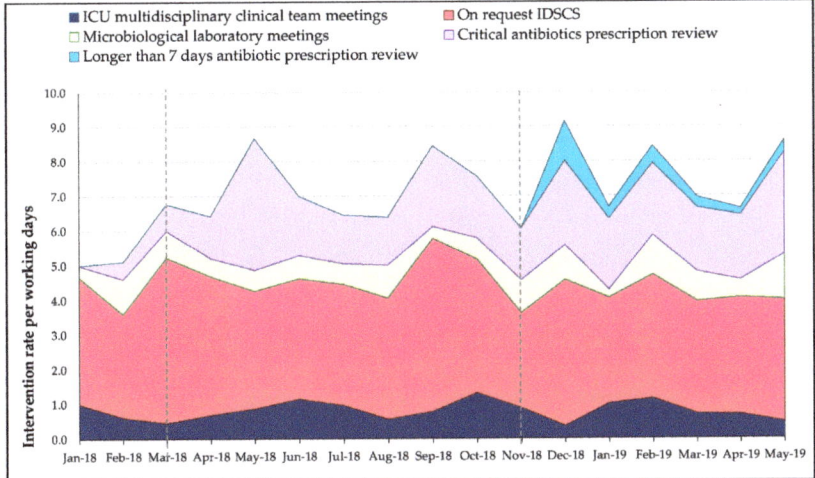

Figure 3. Interventions' distribution per working days. Dotted lines represent initiation of prospective audit and feedback interventions in association with pharmacy unit members (critical antibiotics prescription review and longer than 7 days antibiotic prescription review, respectively). Abbreviations: ICU, intensive care unit; IDSCS, infectious diseases specialist consulting service.

This complementarity is also illustrated when comparing advice type according to different kinds of interventions. Regarding IDSCS interventions, 341 of 1053 interventions (32%) were either a lack of antibiotic initiation, a therapeutic de-escalation, a cessation of all antibiotics, or a reduction in treatment duration with a 92% acceptance rate. On the other hand, 535 proposals (51%) were either a therapeutic escalation or an extension of antibiotic therapy with a 92% acceptance rate.

Of the 501 proposals made during PHARM-cATB interventions, 316 (63%) were either a therapeutic de-escalation, a cessation of all antibiotics, or a reduction in the duration of treatment with a 76% acceptance rate. Only 69 proposals (14%) consisted of a therapeutic escalation or an extension of antibiotic therapy with an 84% acceptance rate (Figure 4).

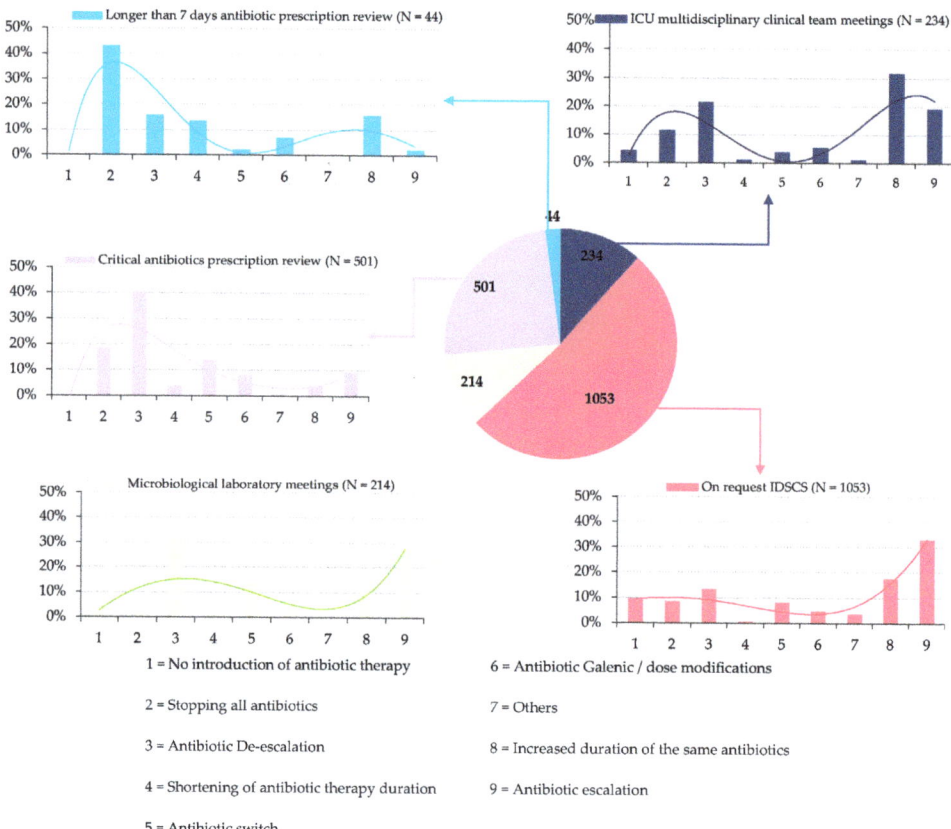

1 = No introduction of antibiotic therapy
2 = Stopping all antibiotics
3 = Antibiotic De-escalation
4 = Shortening of antibiotic therapy duration
5 = Antibiotic switch
6 = Antibiotic Galenic / dose modifications
7 = Others
8 = Increased duration of the same antibiotics
9 = Antibiotic escalation

Figure 4. Advice type according to different kind of interventions. Distribution of the 2046 interventions noted in the electronic patient record related to 1430 hospital stays and rate of propositions according to different kind of interventions. N = number of interventions. IDSCS = infectious diseases specialist consulting service.

2.2. Impact on Mortality, 30-Day Readmission Rate, and Mean Length of Stay

There were 3561 inpatients with deep infections hospitalized in the eight wards who benefited from the whole ASP from January 2016 to May 2017 versus 3839 from January 2018 to May 2019. The clinical and demographic characteristics of these patients are summarized in Table 1. There was a downward trend in the mean LOS in patients with deep infections, from an LOS of 11.03 days before the implementation of the system to a LOS of 10.44 days after implementation, but this difference was not statistically significant ($p = 0.096$). Nor was there any significant difference regarding in-hospital mortality in patients with deep infections (267 (7.31%) versus 266 (6.9%); $p = 0.37$) or 30-DRR (8.2% (293) versus 7.7% (296) in 2019, $p = 0.44$).

Table 1. Demographic characteristics and pre-existing medical conditions of patients with a diagnosis of deep infection before and after implementation of the antibiotic stewardship program in the eight wards that benefited from all types of interventions.

	Before Implementation	After Implementation	p-Value
	1/1/2016 to 31/5/2017	1/1/2018 to 31/5/2019	
Number of stays	3561	3839	
Gender			
Female	1646 (46%)	1848 (48%)	
Male	1915 (54%)	1991 (52%)	
Age (years)			
Mean (Min–Max)	73.13 (17–108)	73.30 (17–103)	
ICU stays	600 (17%)	567 (15%)	0.015
Pre-existing medical conditions			
Solid organ transplant	7 (0.2%)	14 (0.4%)	0.25
Immunomodulatory therapy	1 (0.03%)	9 (0.2%)	0.036
End stages renal disease (IV–V)	30 (0.8%)	72 (1.9%)	0.0002
Chronic liver disease	47 (1.3%)	39 (1%)	0.27
Chronic respiratory failure	187 (5.3%)	250 (6.5%)	0.025
Agranulocytosis	10 (0.3%)	15 (0.4%)	0.54
Chemotherapy during the stay	2 (0.06%)	9 (0.2%)	0.09
Diabetes	724 (20%)	874 (23%)	0.01
HIV	33 (0.9%)	24 (0.6%)	0.18
Infection types			
Pyelonephritis	1124	1013	
Intra-abdominal infections	651	673	
Cellulitis and skin abscess	233	253	
Meningitis	5	7	
Endocarditis	9	10	
Pulmonary infection	1834	1809	
Osteomyelitis and prosthetic joint infection	62	70	

Results are presented as No (and rate %). All patients with a diagnosis of deep infection regarding the International Classification of Diseases were included. Abbreviation: HIV, human immunodeficiency virus; ICU, intensive care unit.

2.3. Impact on Antibiotic Consumption

Overall, antibiotic use was significantly decreased by 14.6% in the whole hospital after ASP implementation (336 daily dose of antibiotics per 1000 patient-days (DDD_{1000PD}) in 2017 versus 287 DDD_{1000PD} in 2019; $p = 0.03$). Carbapenems use was moderate and stable over time (from 5 DDD_{1000PD} in 2017 to 4 DDD_{1000PD} in 2019; $p = 0.82$). A slight increase in injectable third-generation cephalosporins use was observed (from 53 DDD_{1000PD} in 2017 to 60 DDD_{1000PD} in 2019; $p = 0.12$). There was a significant decrease of fluoroquinolones use of 63% (51 DDD_{1000PD} in 2017 versus 19 DDD_{1000PD} in 2019; $p = 0.03$) (Figure 5). We also observed a significant decrease in overall antibiotic use for the eight departments included in PAF interventions from 543 DDD_{1000PD} in 2017 versus 474 DDD_{1000PD} in 2019 ($p = 0.016$). Moreover, the reduction in fluoroquinolones use was more noticeable between April and December 2018 (60 DDD_{1000PD} versus 34 DDD_{1000PD}, respectively). This decrease continued until the end of the analysis. An effect on carbapenems use took longer to appear, but a clear decrease was observed from January to June 2019 (13 DDD_{1000PD} versus 7 DDD_{1000PD}, respectively) (Figure 6).

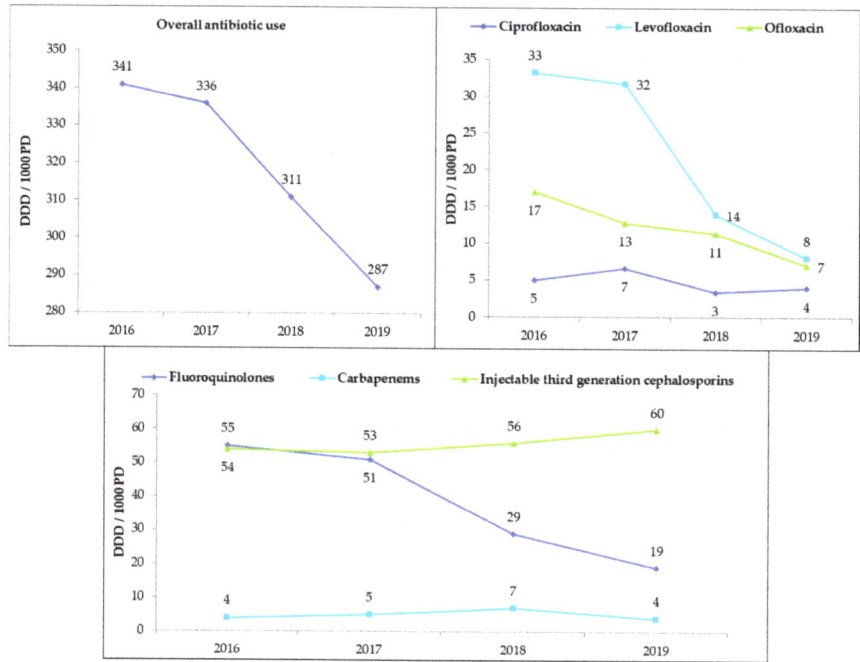

Figure 5. Evolution over time of antibiotic consumption in secondary care hospital of Bassin de Thau. Data are presented as defined daily dose of antibiotics per 1000 patient-days (DDD$_{1000PD}$).

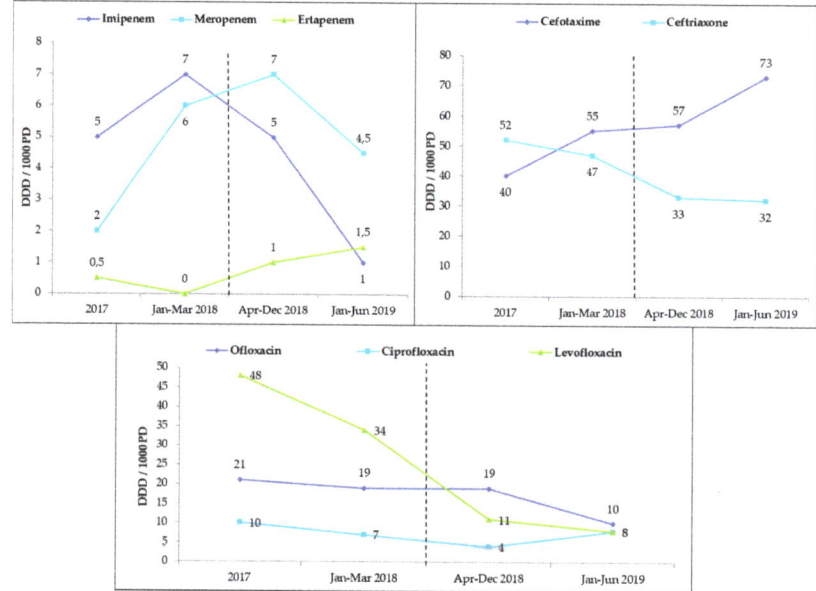

Figure 6. Evolution over time of antibiotic consumption in the eight units that tested the prospective audit and feedback intervention (antibiotics prescription review). Dotted lines represent initiation of critical antibiotics review in association with pharmacy unit members. Data are presented as defined daily dose of antibiotics per 1000 patient-days.

2.4. User Experience Assessment: Satisfaction Survey

Ninety-five physicians that participated in the ASP were surveyed for satisfaction, of which 49 responded. All physicians were satisfied with the dedicated phone line provided and wanted on-request IDSCS to be continued, as well as LAB-M interventions. Regarding PAF actions, only 2/32 physicians were not satisfied with this kind of intervention and did not wish for it to be carried on. All results are summarized in Supplementary Table S1.

3. Discussion

We demonstrated that implementation of a whole ASP combining solicited and unsolicited interventions is possible and that the different modes of intervention are complementary. The multimodal ASP implemented in the hospital of Bassin de Thau (HBT) led to a decrease of antibiotic use, especially fluoroquinolones, without impacting deep infection mortality. We also observed a slightly decreased trend in the length of hospital stay in these patients.

Many ASP strategies have already shown their efficacy; for example, development and implementation of facility-specific clinical practice guidelines for common infectious diseases syndromes, IDS systematic referral for *Staphylococcus aureus* bacteremia clinical cases, PAF, preprescription authorization for certain antibiotics, specific interventions depending on infection type or clinical department, microbiological laboratory interventions, and so on [10,11,24,28,29]. To the best of our knowledge, our study is the first to evaluate the potential synergy between different kinds of actions. Our main contribution is to demonstrate that multimodal interventions are synergic. Indeed, opposite to former studies evaluating the impact of specific different antibiotic stewardship interventions, our global approach highlighted the complementarity of each intervention in the success of the holistic ASP. It is noteworthy that this study was set up in the French healthcare system where interfering methods are not developed [19]. Thanks to the progressive implementation of this system, we were able to highlight the complementarity of the interventions. Indeed, the on-request IDSCS, LAB-M, and ICU-M interventions number was stable overtime, even after implementation of PAF strategies, i.e., PHARM-cATB and PHARM-7d review. This highlights a cumulative effect between the different modes of intervention, suggesting that each kind of intervention responded to a specific type of problem. Indeed, on-request IDSCS led to escalation or lengthening of antibiotic therapy in more than 50% of cases, while PHARM-cATB resulted in escalation or lengthening in only 14%. Conversely, PHARM-cATB reviews resulted in de-escalation, stopping, or shortening of antibiotic therapy in 60% of cases. This proportion was even higher within PHARM-7d review. Thus, the different modes of intervention were complementary, both qualitatively and quantitatively.

Antibiotic use analysis also revealed the same pattern. Interestingly, the decreased consumption accelerated after implementation of PAF methods, suggesting a stronger impact of interfering methods on overall antibiotic use. Similar results were found by Tamma et al., whose study highlighted the effectiveness of this method and its major impact on antibiotic use in a cross-over trial [30]. According to these results, a recent retrospective study analyzed the impact of interventionist strategies as PAF or preprescription authorization on fluoroquinolone consumption in 48 U.S. hospitals [31]. Fluoroquinolone use was significantly decreased by 26% over two years between establishment with ASP targeting fluoroquinolone and those with no ASP.

We did not find evidence of any statistically significant differences on mean LOS, 30-DRR, or mortality between the two periods. However, we observed a downward trend in the mean LOS with a decrease of 0.6 days of hospitalization per stay. Indeed, the reduction in antibiotic consumption, particularly intravenous antibiotics, might lead to a reduction in adverse effects and an earlier discharge of patients. The absence of statistical significance might be because of a lack of power for this criteria; however, it was not the primary endpoint of this study. In the literature, some arguments tend to confirm this hypothesis: Sasikumar et al. showed a significant impact of IDS interventions on mortality and medical stay costs, especially for ICU stays [32]. Although there was no significant positive impact on mortality, 30-DRR, and mean LOS in our study, we did not observe any negative impact on patients' clinical outcomes. Moreover, the high prevalence of patients with chronic respiratory failure, end-stages renal diseases, immunosuppression, and diabetes in the second analysis period could lead to an underestimation of the potential positive impact of our ASP on these outcomes.

These data highlight the importance of using a multimodal strategy when setting up an ASP, keeping in mind that different interventions would respond to different needs. The 2016 IDSA guidelines emphasized PAF and preprescription authorization methods, while underlining the potential for better acceptance of PAF as prescriber autonomy is maintained [24]. In our study, the acceptance rate of PAF intervention was high (79%), despite the fact that unsolicited specialist consulting is not culturally ingrained into the French medical community. Most physicians interviewed in the satisfaction survey agreed that on-request IDSCS and LAB-M actions were improving clinical outcomes and should be continued, whereas only two physicians viewed unsolicited interventions as intrusive to their practice and were reluctant to maintain these methods. PAF acceptance was probably better than expected thanks to its implementation over a second phase of the program, whereas more conventional methods, i.e., on-request IDSCS and LAB-M, were already set up. So, sequential implementation can be identified as a facilitator regarding acceptance of interventionist methods. These results reinforce IDSA recommendations to develop and promote PAF strategies.

We show that they may be implemented within French hospitals considering their efficiency and their complementarity to other methods. It is important to note that, without an EMR, it is challenging to set up such a program with unsolicited interventions.

Nevertheless, this kind of program is time-consuming and labor-intensive; indeed, PAF interventions represented 10 h of work per week for one IDS and one pharmacist, while LAB-M interventions counted for 5 h of work, without including intervention retranscription in the electronic patient record (about 30 min for each intervention, i.e., 25 h weekly). This organization requires dedicated medical time for this activity, as recommended by European Society of Clinical Microbiology and Infectious Diseases (ESCMID) [26].

There are limitations to our study. The impact on antibiotic resistance was not assessed because of the short-term study design. This key outcome will be analyzed after several years of operating under the program in order to compare antimicrobial resistance before and after implementation of this system. Our study did not include medico-economic analysis. Nevertheless, the 0.6 days of stay decrease for inpatients with ID diagnosis would allow some healthcare cost saving, despite this result not being statistically significant. We were also not able to set up, in parallel to our ASP, an educational program that could lead to improved practitioner adherence as well as antibiotics prescribing over the long term [33]. Indeed, in a recent Spanish study, the quality of antimicrobial prescribing improved markedly, and the inappropriate treatment rate was significantly lower over 3 years thanks to regular educational interviews [34]. In addition, we could not evaluate antibiotic prescription at the discharge because of the lack of computerization. Indeed, Vaughn et al. recently highlight that hospital-based stewardship interventions did not affect antibiotic prescription at the discharge [31]. In this study, 14/48 hospitals reported using pre-prescription approval and/or PAF to target fluoroquinolone prescriptions, but hospitals with fluoroquinolone stewardship had twice as many new fluoroquinolone starts after discharge as hospitals without. Weber et al. analyzed discharge prescriptions in a 576-bed academic hospital in Portland. Among 6701 discharges, 22.9% were prescribed antibiotics upon discharge [35]. To complete these data, Scarpato et al. analyzed the appropriateness of antimicrobial agents prescribed on discharge [36]. They found that 70% of discharge antibiotics were inappropriate in antibiotic drug choice, dose, or duration. Analysis of discharge prescriptions should be the next step of our ASP with the implementation of an educational program to improve the prescription of discharge antibiotics. Moreover, there are biases inherent to the design of our study. Indeed, as for many "before–after" studies, the two groups we compared are heterogeneous. However, we found more pre-existing medical conditions for patients in the period after implementation of our ASP; therefore, this might lead to underestimation of the impact on the mean LOS downward trend we observed.

Finally, there was a center's effect limiting the extrapolation of our results as our study took place in a small hospital with less than 300 beds for the medicine, surgery, and obstetrics departments. The small hospital size likely facilitated the rapid establishment of this multidisciplinary system. One of the reasons of our success is probably the direct and confident relationship established between the IDS, the pharmacist, the microbiologist, and the prescribers, which may not be possible to install in other settings. Additional multicentric studies are needed to confirm our results and go further.

4. Materials and Methods

4.1. Study Setting and Interventions

Two hospitals (secondary care hospital of Bassin de Thau (HBT) and university hospital of Montpellier (UHM)) created a shared infectious disease specialist (IDS) position to sequentially implement an innovative multimodal ASP within HBT. The HBT is a 938-bed hospital with establishments providing care for dependent elderly people (376 beds); psychiatric unit (57 beds); geriatric and follow-up care and rehabilitation unit (167 beds); and acute care unit, medicine, surgery, and obstetrics unit (274 beds). On the whole, 406 beds are provided with an electronic medical record (EMR).

The infectious disease EMR pattern was duplicated from UHM to HBT to allow IDS response in real time with a complete traceability in the patient EMR for each intervention [37].

Several interventions centralized by the same IDS were progressively implemented:

January 2018: Simultaneous implementation of (i) a dedicated phone line for the infectious diseases specialist consulting service (IDSCS), (ii) weekly intensive care unit multidisciplinary clinical team meetings (ICU-M), and (iii) IDS intervention triggered by a bi-weekly microbiological laboratory meeting (LAB-M) for the revision of antibiotics based on microbiological data (blood cultures, per-operative samples, lumbar, pleural, and joint punctures). In addition, monthly educational training on antibiotic use was proposed to all residents of the hospital.

April to December 2018: Establishment of PAF interventions in association with pharmacy unit members. Initiation of critical antibiotics prescription review (PHARM-cATB) in April 2018. This consists of a systematized analysis of critical antibiotics prescription (injectable third-generation cephalosporins, fluoroquinolones (FQ), and carbapenems) performed twice a week within the eight wards with the greatest antibiotics use, with feedback to the prescriber.

Initiation of longer than 7 days antibiotics prescription review (PHARM-7d) in December 2018. A systematized analysis was performed on the whole hospital with feedback to the prescriber.

Each intervention was noted in the EMR in real time and was analyzed to evaluate intervention acceptance. An intervention was defined as having been followed if the proposed antibiotic type, duration, and dosage were accepted by the prescribing physician. The whole system organization is summarized in Figure 7.

4.2. Outcomes

The complementarity of the different actions was assessed by the quantitative and qualitative analysis of all interventions traced in the EMR (number of different types of interventions over time, analysis of proposal for each intervention, and impact of interventions on antibiotic use). Antibiotic consumption, defined in daily dose of antibiotics per 1000 patient-days (DDD_{1000PD}), was calculated with ConsoRes® software [38] for the years 2016–2019 in the whole hospital. The impact on mean LOS, 30-DRR, and in-hospital mortality was assessed on patients with deep infections from the eight wards (medicine, surgery, and intensive care unit) representing 274 acute care beds that benefited from all the interventions of ASP by comparing two groups of patients over two periods of 18 months: January 2016–May 2017 versus January 2018–May 2019. All patients who were diagnosed with deep infections based on the International Classification of Diseases, Information System Medicalization Program were included in this comparison.

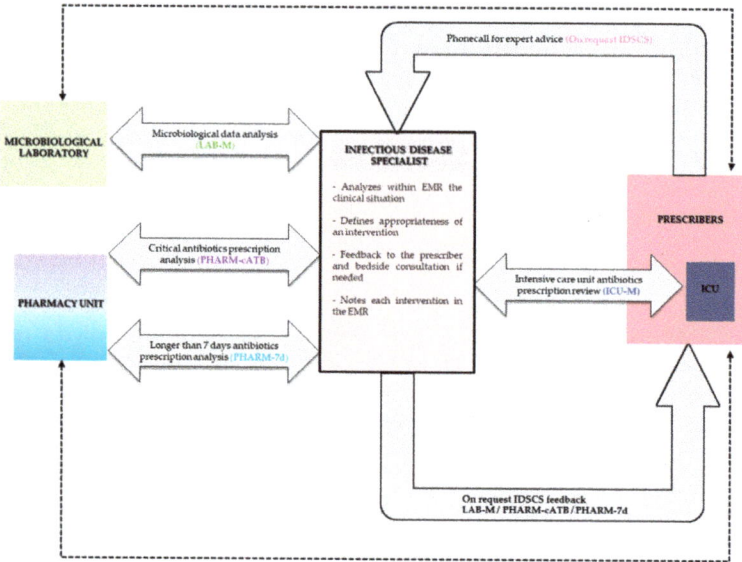

Figure 7. Antibiotic stewardship program organization in the studied hospital when fully established in December 2018. Dotted lines represent pre-existent relationship before implementation of the antibiotic stewardship program. On request IDSCS: on request infectious diseases specialist consulting service via a dedicated phone line. ICU-M: intensive care unit multidisciplinary clinical team meetings for weekly antibiotics prescription review in the ward. LAB-M: microbiological laboratory meetings for bi-weekly analysis of microbiological samples with microbiologists and infectious diseases specialist. PHARM-cATB: critical antibiotics prescription review twice a week with pharmacist and infectious diseases specialist. PHARM-7d: longer than 7 days antibiotic prescriptions review twice a week with pharmacist and infectious diseases specialist. EMR: electronic medical records. ICU: intensive care unit.

4.3. User Experience Assessment

An anonymous satisfaction survey was sent after 12 months of implementation of the system to all clinicians, followed by two reminder letters.

4.4. Statistical Approach

Comparisons between the two periods were made using a χ^2 test for qualitative variables. Comparisons between the two periods were performed using a χ^2 test for mortality and readmission rate, a Mann–Whitney U test for the mean LOS, and a linear regression test to analyze antibiotic consumption.

4.5. Ethics

This study was conducted according to the principles of the declaration of Helsinki and in compliance with International Conference on Harmonization/Good Clinical Practice regulations. According to the French law, the study was in accordance with the recommendations of the local ethics committee, without the need for consent.

5. Conclusions

This study is among the first to analyze the complementarity and impact of combining different strategies, especially interventionist methods, developed within ASPs. This system set up with reasonable human resources could easily be transposable to size-equivalent hospitals. A good acceptance rate of PAF interventions and clear complementarity of the different types of actions, leading to a major decrease in fluoroquinolones use and overall antibiotic use, without a negative impact on mortality or 30-DRR, are key points of this study.

Further studies are needed to strengthen the scope of our results, including multidisciplinary and educational programs; long-stay healthcare structures; analysis of discharge prescriptions; and giving a more important role to PAF interventions, which currently are likely not sufficiently developed [39,40]. As this type of system is probably cost-effective, the economic aspect should not be an obstacle to its implementation.

Supplementary Materials: The following are available online at http://www.mdpi.com/2079-6382/9/12/848/s1, Table S1: Satisfaction survey regarding the antibiotic stewardship program in a tertiary hospital.

Author Contributions: Conceptualization, F.B., D.D., L.G., and D.M.; methodology, F.B., L.G., A.L., and D.M.; software, F.C., D.D., and A.L.; writing—original draft preparation, F.B.; writing—review and editing, V.L.M. and D.M.; supervision, V.L.M. and J.R. All authors have read and agreed to the published version of the manuscript.

Funding: This research received no external funding.

Conflicts of Interest: The authors declare no conflict of interest.

References

1. Cassini, A.; Högberg, L.D.; Plachouras, D.; Quattrocchi, A.; Hoxha, A.; Simonsen, G.S.; Colomb-Cotinat, M.; Kretzschmar, M.E.; Devleesschauwer, B.; Cecchini, M.; et al. Attributable deaths and disability-adjusted life-years caused by infections with antibiotic-resistant bacteria in the EU and the European Economic Area in 2015: A population-level modelling analysis. *Lancet Infect. Dis.* **2019**, *19*, 56–66. [CrossRef]
2. Publications|AMR Review. Available online: https://amr-review.org/Publications.html (accessed on 29 August 2019).
3. Laxminarayan, R.; Duse, A.; Wattal, C.; Zaidi, A.K.M.; Wertheim, H.F.L.; Sumpradit, N.; Vlieghe, E.; Hara, G.L.; Gould, I.M.; Goossens, H.; et al. Antibiotic resistance-the need for global solutions. *Lancet Infect. Dis.* **2013**, *13*, 1057–1098. [CrossRef]
4. Rieg, S.; Küpper, M.F. Infectious diseases consultations can make the difference: A brief review and a plea for more infectious diseases specialists in Germany. *Infection* **2016**, *44*, 159–166. [CrossRef] [PubMed]
5. Carling, P.; Fung, T.; Killion, A.; Terrin, N.; Barza, M. Favorable impact of a multidisciplinary antibiotic management program conducted during 7 years. *Infect. Control. Hosp. Epidemiol.* **2003**, *24*, 699–706. [CrossRef]
6. DiazGranados, C.A. Prospective audit for antimicrobial stewardship in intensive care: Impact on resistance and clinical outcomes. *Am. J. Infect. Control.* **2012**, *40*, 526–529. [CrossRef]
7. Karanika, S.; Paudel, S.; Grigoras, C.; Kalbasi, A.; Mylonakis, E. Systematic Review and Meta-analysis of Clinical and Economic Outcomes from the Implementation of Hospital-Based Antimicrobial Stewardship Programs. *Antimicrob. Agents Chemother.* **2016**, *60*, 4840–4852. [CrossRef]
8. Baur, D.; Gladstone, B.P.; Burkert, F.; Carrara, E.; Foschi, F.; Döbele, S.; Tacconelli, E. Effect of antibiotic stewardship on the incidence of infection and colonisation with antibiotic-resistant bacteria and Clostridium difficile infection: A systematic review and meta-analysis. *Lancet Infect. Dis.* **2017**, *17*, 990–1001. [CrossRef]
9. Kim, J.; Joo, E.-J.; Ha, Y.E.; Park, S.Y.; Kang, C.-I.; Chung, D.R.; Song, J.-H.; Peck, K.R. Impact of a computerized alert system for bacteremia notification on the appropriate antibiotic treatment of Staphylococcus aureus bloodstream infections. *Eur. J. Clin. Microbiol. Infect. Dis.* **2013**, *32*, 937–945. [CrossRef]
10. Bai, A.D.; Showler, A.; Burry, L.; Steinberg, M.; Ricciuto, D.R.; Fernandes, T.; Chiu, A.; Raybardhan, S.; Science, M.; Fernando, E.; et al. Impact of Infectious Disease Consultation on Quality of Care, Mortality, and Length of Stay in Staphylococcus aureus Bacteremia: Results From a Large Multicenter Cohort Study. *Clin. Infect. Dis.* **2015**, *60*, 1451–1461. [CrossRef]
11. Schmitt, S.; McQuillen, D.P.; Nahass, R.; Martinelli, L.; Rubin, M.; Schwebke, K.; Petrak, R.; Ritter, J.T.; Chansolme, D.; Slama, T.; et al. Infectious diseases specialty intervention is associated with decreased mortality and lower healthcare costs. *Clin. Infect. Dis.* **2014**, *58*, 22–28. [CrossRef]
12. Cunha, C.B. The Pharmacoeconomic Aspects of Antibiotic Stewardship Programs. *Med. Clin. North Am.* **2018**, *102*, 937–946. [CrossRef]

13. Abbara, S.; Pitsch, A.; Jochmans, S.; Hodjat, K.; Cherrier, P.; Monchi, M.; Vinsonneau, C.; Diamantis, S. Impact of a multimodal strategy combining a new standard of care and restriction of carbapenems, fluoroquinolones and cephalosporins on antibiotic consumption and resistance of Pseudomonas aeruginosa in a French intensive care unit. *Int. J. Antimicrob. Agents* **2019**, *53*, 416–422. [CrossRef]
14. Dyar, O.J.; Tebano, G.; Pulcini, C.; ESGAP (ESCMID Study Group for Antimicrobial StewardshiP). Managing responsible antimicrobial use: Perspectives across the healthcare system. *Clin. Microbiol. Infect.* **2017**, *23*, 441–447. [CrossRef] [PubMed]
15. Parente, D.M.; Morton, J. Role of the Pharmacist in Antimicrobial Stewardship. *Med. Clin. North Am.* **2018**, *102*, 929–936. [CrossRef] [PubMed]
16. Carlet, J.; Le Coz, P. *Proposals of the Special Working Group for Keeping Antibiotics Effective*; ESCMID: Basel, Switzerland, 2015; 150p.
17. Pulcini, C.; Morel, C.M.; Tacconelli, E.; Beovic, B.; de With, K.; Goossens, H.; Harbarth, S.; Holmes, A.; Howard, P.; Morris, A.M.; et al. Human resources estimates and funding for antibiotic stewardship teams are urgently needed. *Clin. Microbiol. Infect.* **2017**, *23*, 785–787. [CrossRef] [PubMed]
18. Amann, S.; Neef, K.; Kohl, S. Antimicrobial resistance (AMR). *Eur. J. Hosp. Pharm. Sci. Prac.* **2019**, *26*, 175–177. [CrossRef] [PubMed]
19. Binda, F.; Tebano, G.; Kallen, M.C.; Ten Oever, J.; Hulscher, M.E.; Schouten, J.A.; Pulcini, C. Nationwide survey of hospital antibiotic stewardship programs in France. *Med. Mal. Infect.* **2020**, *50*, 414–422. [CrossRef] [PubMed]
20. Dyar, O.J.; Nathwani, D.; Monnet, D.L.; Gyssens, I.C.; Stålsby Lundborg, C.; Pulcini, C.; ESGAP Student-PREPARE Working Group. Do medical students feel prepared to prescribe antibiotics responsibly? Results from a cross-sectional survey in 29 European countries. *J. Antimicrob. Chemother.* **2018**, *73*, 2236–2242. [CrossRef]
21. Mehta, J.M.; Haynes, K.; Wileyto, E.P.; Gerber, J.S.; Timko, D.R.; Morgan, S.C.; Binkley, S.; Fishman, N.O.; Lautenbach, E.; Zaoutis, T.; et al. Comparison of prior authorization and prospective audit with feedback for antimicrobial stewardship. *Infect. Control. Hosp. Epidemiol.* **2014**, *35*, 1092–1099. [CrossRef]
22. Cosgrove, S.E.; Seo, S.K.; Bolon, M.K.; Sepkowitz, K.A.; Climo, M.W.; Diekema, D.J.; Speck, K.; Gunaseelan, V.; Noskin, G.A.; Herwaldt, L.A.; et al. Evaluation of postprescription review and feedback as a method of promoting rational antimicrobial use: A multicenter intervention. *Infect. Control. Hosp. Epidemiol.* **2012**, *33*, 374–380. [CrossRef]
23. Davey, P.; Marwick, C.A.; Scott, C.L.; Charani, E.; McNeil, K.; Brown, E.; Gould, I.M.; Ramsay, C.R.; Michie, S. Interventions to improve antibiotic prescribing practices for hospital inpatients. *Cochrane Database Syst. Rev.* **2017**, *2017*. [CrossRef] [PubMed]
24. Barlam, T.F.; Cosgrove, S.E.; Abbo, L.M.; MacDougall, C.; Schuetz, A.N.; Septimus, E.J.; Srinivasan, A.; Dellit, T.H.; Falck-Ytter, Y.T.; Fishman, N.O.; et al. Implementing an Antibiotic Stewardship Program: Guidelines by the Infectious Diseases Society of America and the Society for Healthcare Epidemiology of America. *Clin. Infect. Dis.* **2016**, *62*, e51–e77. [CrossRef] [PubMed]
25. Pollack, L.A.; Srinivasan, A. Core elements of hospital antibiotic stewardship programs from the Centers for Disease Control and Prevention. *Clin. Infect. Dis.* **2014**, *59* (Suppl. 3), S97–S100. [CrossRef] [PubMed]
26. Pulcini, C.; Binda, F.; Lamkang, A.S.; Trett, A.; Charani, E.; Goff, D.A.; Harbarth, S.; Hinrichsen, S.L.; Levy-Hara, G.; Mendelson, M.; et al. Developing core elements and checklist items for global hospital antimicrobial stewardship programmes: A consensus approach. *Clin. Microbiol. Infect.* **2019**, *25*, 20–25. [CrossRef] [PubMed]
27. Buckel, W.R.; Veillette, J.J.; Vento, T.J.; Stenehjem, E. Antimicrobial Stewardship in Community Hospitals. *Med. Clin. N. Am.* **2018**, *102*, 913–928. [CrossRef] [PubMed]
28. Bishop, B.M. Antimicrobial Stewardship in the Emergency Department: Challenges, Opportunities, and a Call to Action for Pharmacists. *J. Pharm. Prac.* **2016**, *29*, 556–563. [CrossRef] [PubMed]
29. Morrill, H.J.; Gaitanis, M.M.; LaPlante, K.L. Antimicrobial stewardship program prompts increased and earlier infectious diseases consultation. *Antimicrob. Resist. Infect. Control.* **2014**, *3*, 12. [CrossRef]
30. Tamma, P.D.; Avdic, E.; Keenan, J.F.; Zhao, Y.; Anand, G.; Cooper, J.; Dezube, R.; Hsu, S.; Cosgrove, S.E. What is the More Effective Antibiotic Stewardship Intervention: Preprescription Authorization or Postprescription Review with Feedback? *Clin. Infect. Dis.* **2017**, *64*, 537–543. [CrossRef]

31. Vaughn, V.M.; Gandhi, T.; Conlon, A.; Chopra, V.; Malani, A.N.; Flanders, S.A. The Association of Antibiotic Stewardship With Fluoroquinolone Prescribing in Michigan Hospitals: A Multi-hospital Cohort Study. *Clin. Infect. Dis.* **2019**, *69*, 1269–1277. [CrossRef]
32. Sasikumar, M.; Boyer, S.; Remacle-Bonnet, A.; Ventelou, B.; Brouqui, P. The value of specialist care-infectious disease specialist referrals-why and for whom? A retrospective cohort study in a French tertiary hospital. *Eur. J. Clin. Microbiol. Infect. Dis.* **2017**, *36*, 625–633. [CrossRef]
33. Pulcini, C.; Gyssens, I.C. How to educate prescribers in antimicrobial stewardship practices. *Virulence* **2013**, *4*, 192–202. [CrossRef] [PubMed]
34. Rodríguez-Baño, J.; Pérez-Moreno, M.A.; Peñalva, G.; Garnacho-Montero, J.; Pinto, C.; Salcedo, I.; Fernández-Urrusuno, R.; Neth, O.; Gil-Navarro, M.V.; Pérez-Milena, A.; et al. Outcomes of the PIRASOA programme, an antimicrobial stewardship programme implemented in hospitals of the Public Health System of Andalusia, Spain: An ecologic study of time-trend analysis. *Clin. Microbiol. Infect.* **2020**, *26*, 358–365. [CrossRef] [PubMed]
35. Weber, B.R.; Noble, B.N.; Bearden, D.T.; Crnich, C.J.; Ellingson, K.D.; McGregor, J.C.; Furuno, J.P. Antibiotic Prescribing upon Discharge from the Hospital to Long-Term Care Facilities: Implications for Antimicrobial Stewardship Requirements in Post-Acute Settings. *Infect. Control. Hosp. Epidemiol.* **2019**, *40*. [CrossRef]
36. Scarpato, S.J.; Timko, D.R.; Cluzet, V.C.; Dougherty, J.P.; Nunez, J.J.; Fishman, N.O.; Hamilton, K.W.; CDC Prevention Epicenters Program. An Evaluation of Antibiotic Prescribing Practices upon Hospital Discharge. *Infect. Control. Hosp. Epidemiol.* **2017**, *38*, 353–355. [CrossRef]
37. Morquin, D.; Ologeanu-Taddei, R.; Koumar, Y.; Reynes, J. Tele-Expertise System Based on the Use of the Electronic Patient Record to Support Real-Time Antimicrobial Use. *Int. J. Technol. Assess. Health Care* **2018**, *34*, 156–162. [CrossRef]
38. Boussat, S.; Demoré, B.; Lozniewski, A.; Aissa, N.; Rabaud, C. How to improve the collection and analysis of hospital antibiotic consumption: Preliminary results of the ConsoRes software experimental implementation. *Med. Mal. Infect.* **2012**, *42*, 154–160. [CrossRef]
39. Howard, P.; Pulcini, C.; Levy Hara, G.; West, R.M.; Gould, I.M.; Harbarth, S.; Nathwani, D.; ESCMID Study Group for Antimicrobial Policies (ESGAP); ISC Group on Antimicrobial Stewardship. An international cross-sectional survey of antimicrobial stewardship programmes in hospitals. *J. Antimicrob. Chemother.* **2015**, *70*, 1245–1255. [CrossRef]
40. Perozziello, A.; Lescure, F.X.; Truel, A.; Routelous, C.; Vaillant, L.; Yazdanpanah, Y.; Lucet, J.C.; CEFECA Study Group. Prescribers' experience and opinions on antimicrobial stewardship programmes in hospitals: A French nationwide survey. *J. Antimicrob. Chemother.* **2019**, *74*, 2451–2458. [CrossRef]

Publisher's Note: MDPI stays neutral with regard to jurisdictional claims in published maps and institutional affiliations.

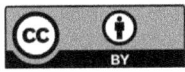

© 2020 by the authors. Licensee MDPI, Basel, Switzerland. This article is an open access article distributed under the terms and conditions of the Creative Commons Attribution (CC BY) license (http://creativecommons.org/licenses/by/4.0/).

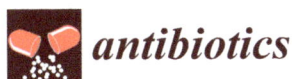

Article

Impact of a Rapid Diagnostic Meningitis/Encephalitis Panel on Antimicrobial Use and Clinical Outcomes in Children

Danielle McDonald [1], Christina Gagliardo [2,3], Stephanie Chiu [4] and M. Cecilia Di Pentima [2,3,5,*]

1. Department of Pharmacy, Cooper University Health Care, Camden, NJ 08103, USA; danimcd2@gmail.com
2. Department of Pediatrics, Goryeb Children's Hospital, Atlantic Health System, Morristown, NJ 07960, USA; Christina.Gagliardo@atlantichealth.org
3. Department of Pediatrics, Sidney Kimmel Medical College at Thomas Jefferson University, Philadelphia, PA 19107, USA
4. Atlantic Center for Research, Atlantic Health System, Morristown, NJ 07960, USA; Stephanie.Chiu@atlantichealth.org
5. Department of Pediatrics, Infectious Diseases Division, Atlantic Health System, Thomas Jefferson University, Morristown, NJ 07960, USA
* Correspondence: mariacecilia.dipentima@Atlantichealth.org

Received: 9 October 2020; Accepted: 13 November 2020; Published: 18 November 2020

Abstract: Rapid molecular diagnostic assays are increasingly used to guide effective antimicrobial therapy. Data on their effectiveness to decrease antimicrobial use in children have been limited and varied. We aimed to assess the impact of the implementation of the FilmArray Meningitis Encephalitis Panel (MEP) on antimicrobial use and outcomes in children. In an observational retrospective study performed at Atlantic Health System (NJ), we sought to evaluate the duration of intravenous antibiotic treatment (days of therapy (DoT)) for patients <21 years of age hospitalized and evaluated for presumptive meningitis or encephalitis before and after the introduction of the MEP. A secondary analysis was performed to determine if recovery of a respiratory pathogen influenced DoT. The median duration of antibiotic therapy prior to the implementation of the MEP was 5 DoT (interquartile range (IQR): 3–6) versus 3 DoT (IQR: 1–5) ($p < 0.001$) when MEP was performed. The impact was greatest on intravenous third-generation cephalosporin and ampicillin use. We found a reduction in the number of inpatient days associated with the MEP. In the regression analysis, a positive respiratory pathogen panel (RPP) was not a significant predictor of DoT ($p = 0.08$). Furthermore, we found no significant difference between DoT among patients with negative and positive RPP ($p = 0.12$). Our study supports the implementation of rapid diagnostics to decrease the utilization of antibiotic therapy among pediatric patients admitted with concerns related to meningitis or encephalitis.

Keywords: meningitis; encephalitis; FilmArray; multiplex PCR; antimicrobial; rapid diagnostic technology; stewardship; children; adolescents; outcomes

1. Introduction

With the aid of rapid molecular diagnostics and the introduction of effective vaccines against *Haemophilus influenzae* type b, *Streptococcus pneumoniae*, and most recently *Neisseria meningitides*, the epidemiology of meningitis and encephalitis remains a rapidly evolving field [1]. The impact of vaccines has mainly affected children in developed countries, with an over 60% reduction in the incidence of bacterial meningitis in this patient population [2]. In a study performed in the United States in 2006, roughly 72,000 adult hospitalizations were related to meningitis [3]. While the majority of these were due to viral etiologies (54.6%), the estimated healthcare cost reached USD 1.2 billion [3]. More recent data show that the global incidence of meningitis increased from 2.5 million cases in 1990 to 2.82 million cases in 2016, with the highest rates found in sub-Saharan African countries, also known as the meningitis belt [4]. Kwambana-Adams et al. published the prevalence of bacterial, viral and parasitic infection in children younger than 5 years of age in West Africa following the rollout of conjugate vaccines against pneumococcus (PVC), meningococcus (MenAfriVac) and *Haemophilus influenzae* [5]. *Escherichia coli* (4.8%), followed by *S. pneumoniae* (3.5%) and *Plasmodium* (3.5%), were the most prevalent etiologies of meningitis in this age group. Because serotyping for pneumococcal isolates was not reported, the impact of PVC could not be determined. Gram negative rods, particularly *Escherichia coli* and *Klebsiella pneumoniae*, were more commonly identified in newborns.

The initial clinical manifestations of central nervous system (CNS) infections in neonates and children can be non-specific, difficult to diagnose and devastating if not treated correctly. The implementation of diagnostic stewardship entails optimization of clinical care and antimicrobial therapy guided by timely and personalized effective testing [6,7]. Rapid diagnostics have been shown to improve clinical outcomes in patients with bacteremia and infections with multidrug-resistant organisms when the introduction of these tests are linked to effective antibiotic stewardship strategies [7,8]. Data on the performance and impact of the FilmArray Meningitis Encephalitis Panel (MEP) in children are limited [9]. The MEP is a rapid multiplex polymerase chain reaction (PCR) assay designed to detect 14 pathogens in the cerebrospinal fluid (CSF). These pathogens include six bacteria, seven viruses, and one yeast group. In the cases of meningitis or encephalitis, quick pathogen identification aids in the initiation/continuation of appropriate targeted therapy as well as discontinuation of unnecessary empiric antimicrobials. Timely diagnosis directly impacts patient outcomes and healthcare costs.

Prior to Food and Drug Administration (FDA) approval of the MEP, a large, prospective, multicenter study of 1560 CSF specimens was conducted to compare the MEP to standard diagnostics, bacterial culture and viral PCR [10]. In this study, the MEP yielded a percent positive agreement (PPA) of 100% for 9 of 14 analytes. Enterovirus yielded a 95.7% PPA, and human herpes virus type 6 had an agreement of 85.7%. *Streptococcus agalactiae* had one false-positive and one false-negative result. *Listeria monocytogenes* and *Neisseria meningitides* were not evaluated.

Additional studies augmented the results and strengthened the findings of this initial study. Liesman et al. evaluated 291 CSF specimens and found a PPA of 85.6% [11]. When results for *Cryptococcus neoformans/gattii* were excluded, the PPA increased to 92.5%. Naccache et al. evaluated 251 samples and showed a low false positivity rate [12]. Piccirilli et al. demonstrated 90.9% concordance between the FilmArray MEP and conventional microbiological procedures in 77 CSF samples studied [13]. Additionally, two published reviews had a pediatric focus. Graf et al. used 67 retrospective viral PCR or bacterial culture-positive samples and identified 92.5% that were positive for the same target on the panel [14]. Messacar et al. tested 138 CSF samples and concluded an overall agreement of 96% as compared to conventional diagnostic methods in children with CNS infections [15]. In a recently published meta-analysis by Tansarli and Chapin, and as previously reported by Liesman et al., the MEP was found to have higher rates of false-negative results for herpes simplex virus 1 and 2 and enterovirus when compared with standard PCR assays [11,16].

More recently, several studies demonstrated cost savings and reductions in antibiotic days of therapy (DoT) with implementation of the MEP [17–21]. Nabower et al. demonstrated decreased length of stay (LOS) and fewer acyclovir doses administered, while Weber et al. demonstrated hospital cost savings in a military treatment facility [17,18]. Posnakoglou et al. supplemented these findings, demonstrating decreased LOS, a reduction in antimicrobial use, and a decrease in total cost [19]. Similarly, Hagen et al. noted a decreased duration of empiric therapy, with the largest effect documented in infants [20]. Messacar et al. focused on herpes simplex virus in patients >60 days of age and observed a doubling of herpes simplex virus testing with a reduction in acyclovir duration of therapy [21]. These studies begin to validate the clinical utility of the MEP in pediatric patients with results that support opportunities for antimicrobial stewardship.

The purpose of this study was to evaluate the impact of the implementation of the FilmArray MEP in pediatric patients receiving empiric therapy for meningitis and/or encephalitis. The potential confounding role of respiratory pathogens was examined in a secondary analysis.

2. Methods

In an observational retrospective study performed at Atlantic Health System (AHS), we reviewed 297 medical records of patients <21 years of age evaluated for meningitis and/or encephalitis between January 2015 and September 2018. AHS is a not-for-profit private healthcare corporation operating five hospitals in northern New Jersey. Subjects evaluated at two AHS hospitals were included in the study: Goryeb Children's Hospital in Morristown and Goryeb Children's Center at Overlook Medical Center in Summit.

Admitted patients evaluated for meningitis by lumbar puncture prior to MEP incorporation were categorized and analyzed as "pre-implementation" subjects (January 2015–October 2016), whereas admissions on or after incorporation were categorized as "post-implementation" subjects (November 2017–September 2018). In order to only assess duration of empiric therapy, patients with confirmed bacterial infections and patients with herpes simplex meningoencephalitis were excluded from the study. Confirmation was based on positive MEP and CSF, blood cultures, and urine cultures. Hematology–oncology and neurosurgery patients were also excluded. A total of 247 patients were included in the final analysis.

The FilmArray MEP (BioFire Diagnostics, Salt Lake City, UT, USA) was incorporated at AHS on November 1, 2016. Analytes on the MEP include *Escherichia coli* (K1 capsular type), *Haemophilus influenzae*, *Listeria monocytogenes*, *Neisseria meningitides*, *Streptococcus agalactiae*, *Streptococcus pneumoniae*, *Cytomegalovirus*, *Enterovirus*, *Epstein-Barr virus*, *Herpes simplex viruses 1 and 2*, *Human Herpes virus 6*, *Varicella zoster*, *Human parechovirus*, and *Cryptococcus neoformans/gattii*. The sample size required is 200 microliters (µL), and the turnaround time for reporting the MEP at AHS is approximately 2 h. FilmArray Respiratory Pathogen panel (RPP; BioFire Diagnostics, Salt Lake City, UT, USA) was incorporated in 2011. Analytes of the RPP include Adenovirus, Coronaviruses (HKU1, NL63, 229E, OC43), Human metapneumovirus, Human rhinovirus/Enterovirus, Influenza A (A/H1, A/H#, A/H1-2009) and Influenza B viruses, Parainfluenza (1–4) viruses, Respiratory Syncytial Virus, *Bordetella pertussis*, *Bordetella parapertussis*, *Chlamydia pneumonia*, and *Mycoplasma pneumoniae*.

Data collected included patient age, gender, admission date, event date, CSF studies, diagnosis, antimicrobial therapy, RPP if performed, mortality and 30-day readmission.

The primary outcome of the study was to evaluate the duration of empiric antimicrobial therapy measured as DoT before and after incorporation of the MEP. Secondary outcomes included length of stay (LOS), all-cause mortality and 30-day readmission rates. Patient outcomes were compared pre- and post-implementation.

3. Statistical Analysis

Patient characteristics were summarized using medians and interquartile range (IQR) for continuous variables and proportions for categorical data. Total DoT and LOS failed normality tests, so non-parametric comparative analyses, Mann–Whitney, were performed to assess the data between the two groups. Binomial variables were compared using 2 proportions, and binary regression analyses were used to determine significant predictor variables. Categorical variables were evaluated using a chi-square test. All tests were 2-tailed at a level of significance of less than 0.05.

The AHS institutional review board approved this study (Protocol Number: 1107015-1).

4. Results

Two-hundred and forty-seven children with suspected meningitis or encephalitis who received empiric antimicrobial therapy were included in the study analysis. Of these, 186 patients were part of the pre-implementation period while 61 patients had an MEP performed during the post-implementation period. Patient characteristics for each group are depicted in Table 1. Age and gender were similar in both groups. The median age for all patients was less than 1 year of age. A total of 113 (60%) and 37 (64%) patients were males before and after the implementation of the MEP, respectively. Even when a higher proportion of patients was admitted to intensive care units during the pre-implementation phase, this difference was not statistically significant ($p = 0.16$). Patients were more likely to have a positive RPP prior to the implementation of the MEP ($p < 0.01$).

Table 1. Patient Characteristics.

Characteristics	Pre-MEP (N:186)	Post-MEP (N:61)	p-Value
Age in years, median (IQR)	0 (0–3.5)	0 (0–4)	0.24 †
Male patients, n (%)	113 (59.8)	37 (63.7)	0.59 *
NICU/PICU care, n (%)	43 (23)	20 (32)	0.16 *
CSF WBC, median (IQR)	4 (1–22.3) cells/mm^3	3 (1–13.5) cells/mm^3	0.71 †
Respiratory pathogen panel positive n (%)	105/109 (96.3)	17/40 (42.5)	<0.01 *

† Mann–Whitney, * chi-square test, IQR: interquartile range, NICU: neonatal intensive care unit, PICU: pediatric intensive care unit, CSF: cerebrospinal fluid, WBC: white blood cells.

The median duration of antibiotic therapy in the pre-implementation group was five DoT (IQR: 3–6) versus three DoT (IQR: 1–5) ($p < 0.001$) post–implementation. Figure 1 illustrates antibiotic utilization before and after the MEP was introduced into clinical practice in our study population.

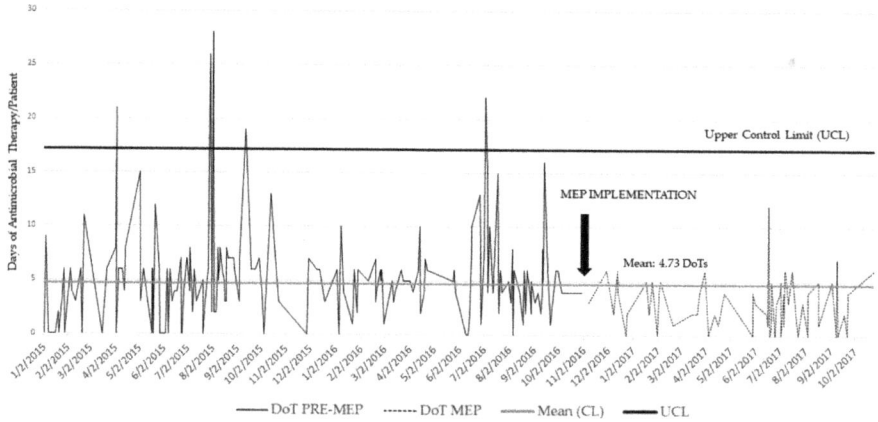

Figure 1. Patient-specific empiric antimicrobial utilization.

During the pre-implementation period, the median DoT for individual antibiotics was 3 DoT (IQR: 1) for third-generation cephalosporins, including ceftriaxone and cefotaxime (n:23), 3 DoT (IQR: 3) for ampicillin (n:113) and 2 DoT (IQR: 2–3) for vancomycin (n:40). Ceftazidime was not used in either cohort.

The median duration of empiric antibiotic therapy in patients with suspected meningitis or encephalitis during the post-implementation period was 2 DoT (IQR: 2–3) for third-generation cephalosporins (n:31) ($p = 0.02$), 2 DoT (IQR: 2–3) for ampicillin (n:22) ($p = 0.017$) and 2 DoT (IQR: 2–3) for vancomycin (n:7) ($p = 0.2$). Gentamicin was used in 65 and 17 subjects, before and after the implementation of the MEP with a median duration of 2 DoT for both patient groups ($p = 0.13$). We found no statistical differences in the median duration of cefepime ($p = 0.70$), doxycycline ($p = 0.9$) or piperacillin-tazobactam ($p = 0.95$) between the two cohorts.

Few patients received acyclovir before (n:32) and after implementation of the MEP (n:9). Median utilization of acyclovir was 3 DoT (IQR: 3–4) and 2 DoT (IQR: 2–3), respectively ($p = 0.76$).

In the regression analysis, in patients evaluated for meningitis or encephalitis, a positive RPP was not a significant predictor of duration of antibiotic therapy (Odds Ratio: 1.15; 95% Confident Interval: 0.1–1.34). Furthermore, we found no significant differences between DoT among patients with negative (median: 4 DoT; range 0–6) and positive (median: 4 DoT; range 0–21) RPP ($p = 0.12$).

Secondary outcomes are summarized in Table 2. We found a statistically significant reduction in the median number of inpatient days after the implementation of the MEP ($p < 0.01$). All-cause readmission was higher in the pre-implementation group but did not reach statistical significance ($p = 0.24$). No deaths occurred in either cohort.

Table 2. Patient Outcomes.

Outcomes	Pre-MEP (N:186)	Post-MEP (N:61)	p-Value
LOS, median (IQR)	4 (1–3)	3 (0–4)	<0.001 [†]
All-cause 30 day-readmission (%)	4 (2.2%)	0	0.24 [*]
All-cause mortality	0	0	

[†] Mann–Whitney, [*] chi-square test.

5. Discussion

In our experience, implementation of the MEP decreased antimicrobial use and LOS among hospitalized children evaluated for presumptive meningitis or encephalitis, without having a negative impact on readmissions or mortality.

Performing a lumbar puncture in young infants and children can be challenging, limiting the ability to obtain large volumes of CSF to submit for multiple tests, especially when standard antigen, PCR and/or antibody testing must be performed at different reference laboratories. The MEP uses only 200 µL of CSF. Reference laboratories usually request a minimum of 500 µL of CSF to perform individual pathogen testing such as *Cryptococcus* antigen, HSV or enterovirus PCRs. CSF culture, although still the gold standard for diagnosis, takes a longer time to result. Standard microbiological methods for recovery and identification of an organism can take up to 48–72 h to report, and turnaround times for reference laboratories mean that it can take days to deliver results. At our institution, the MEP is reported within 2 h of obtaining the CSF sample. Furthermore, culture results can be difficult to interpret in patients who previously received antibiotic treatment. In a small study of 62 CSF samples from young infants with suspected meningitis, seven samples were positive on the PCR panel with no culture growth [22]. These seven samples were obtained from infants who had been pretreated with antibiotics. While false-positive and false-negative results from the MEP are possible, and results need to be interpreted in the context of the patient's clinical condition, the MEP may increase the ability to recover a clinically significant organism in children who have been pretreated with antimicrobials.

We noted that impact on antibiotic utilization mainly affected intravenous ampicillin, commonly used in newborns with suspected early or late onset sepsis and/or meningitis when *Streptococcus agalactiae*, *Listeria monocytogenes*, *E. coli*, and other Gram-negative pathogens are a consideration. With rates of ampicillin-resistant *E. coli* surpassing 50%, early identification of a potential etiology can guide appropriate antibiotic therapy. Similar impact was noted on third-generation cephalosporins, the antibiotics of choice for empiric therapy for infants and children with suspected CNS infections. Despite the intermittent shortages and eventual discontinuation of cefotaxime, and the age limitations for the use of ceftriaxone during the newborn period, we did not find a statistically significant change in the use of cefepime. Ceftazidime, an alternative to cefotaxime recommended by the American Academy of Pediatrics for infants under 2 months of age with suspected meningitis, was not used in our patient population. While the duration of empiric gentamicin use did not change with the rollout of the MEP, fewer patients were started on this antibiotic after the MEP was implemented.

The impact found on antibiotic utilization was independent of patients diagnosed with a respiratory viral pathogen. Furthermore, a positive RPP was not associated with a shorter duration of antibiotic therapy, implying that diagnosis of a viral respiratory infection did not drive antibiotic management in this patient population. Studies assessing the impact of rapid diagnostics in children with acute respiratory tract infections found that these assays reduce LOS and empiric antibiotic utilization [23]. To the best of our knowledge, prior studies assessing the impact of RPP in children admitted with possible CNS infection has not been published. Our data suggest that rapid syndromic molecular testing has a more meaningful impact when aimed at the diagnosis of concern rather than in combination.

Herpes simplex virus can be a devastating CNS infection in newborns. Although rare, with rates in the United States ranging between 1 in 2000 to 1 in 13,000 live births, early diagnosis and treatment remain critical to impact mortality and neurologic outcomes in this patient population [24]. In our institution, prior to the implementation of the MEP, CSF herpes simplex virus DNA testing was sent out to an outside laboratory, delaying turnaround time by several days. Though acyclovir use decreased after the implementation of the MEP, the small sample size made it difficult to assess the statistical impact on acyclovir DoT. However, rapid negative herpes simplex virus results from the MEP reduced the number of patients receiving empiric acyclovir therapy for several days pending results, as was seen in the pre-implementation period. These findings are critically important in the phase of recurrent shortages of intravenous acyclovir. Acyclovir shortages trigger the need to use alternative therapies such as IV ganciclovir or high-dose oral valacyclovir [25]. Of particular concern is the potentially negative economic and clinical impact associated with drug shortages described in the literature [26]. As of 22 September 2020, acyclovir remains in the drug shortage list kept by the American Society of Health-Systems Pharmacists [27]. The COVID-19 pandemic has generated an additional challenge to the chronic problem of antimicrobial shortages by creating an imbalance between supply and demand [28]. Furthermore, it is estimated that the global public health crisis generated by the severe acute respiratory syndrome COVID-19 resulted in an increased use of antimicrobials and could amplify the threat of antimicrobial resistance [29].

There are limitations to this study. We excluded hematology, oncology and neurosurgery patients. However, we purposely excluded these populations, in whom empiric antibiotic therapy might be guided based on risks associated with their underlying conditions. We also excluded hospitalized patients with documented infections to assess only the duration of empiric antimicrobial therapy. Our patient population represents a single institution, and the results might not be generalizable to all centers caring for children. Our study did not include an economic analysis. Duff et al. evaluated the financial outcome of the implementation of the BioFire® MEP in adult and pediatric populations at a single institution [30,31]. Greater savings were found when testing was performed in all suspected cases rather than in those with abnormal CSF findings for both pediatric (USD 3481/case) and adult (USD 2213/case) patients [30,31]. While antibiotic use is known to be associated with the emergence of antibiotic resistance, the direct impact of a single rapid diagnostic test is difficult to discern. To the best of our knowledge, studies evaluating the potential impact of the MEP on antibiotic resistance has not been published.

The World Health Organization is committed to decreasing the scourge of bacterial meningitis, especially for pathogens affecting young children, such as *Streptococcus agalactiae*, *Neisseria meningitidis*, *Streptococcus pneumoniae*, and *Haemophilus influenzae* [32]. The "Defeating meningitis by 2030" global roadmap is a multi-organization partnership that calls for the development and wide implementation of molecular-based multiplex meningitis rapid diagnostic assays at the point of care [32]. Newer generation meningitis assays will be needed to accomplish these goals worldwide [33]. Despite all the benefits described, rapid diagnostic tests should not replace routine bacterial and fungal cultures. Moreover, diagnostic testing should be interpreted in the context of the patient's clinical manifestations, and the possibility of either a false-positive or false-negative result should be considered based on the index of clinical and laboratory suspicion.

6. Conclusions

Meningitis remains a prevalent and devastating disease worldwide. While the timely administration of antimicrobial therapy is critical to optimizing the outcomes of children with CNS infections, unnecessary treatments and prolonged hospitalizations represent a burden on our healthcare system and contribute to antimicrobial shortages and resistance. In our experience, the implementation of rapid CSF multiplex PCR assays aided in antimicrobial stewardship initiatives and shortened the duration of hospital stays in children with suspected meningitis and encephalitis.

Author Contributions: Conceptualization, M.C.D.P.; formal analysis, S.C.; investigation, D.M., C.G. and M.C.D.P.; writing—original draft, D.M. and M.C.D.P.; writing—review and editing, C.G. All authors have read and agreed to the published version of the manuscript.

Funding: This research received no external funding.

Conflicts of Interest: The authors have no conflicts of interest or financial relationships relevant to this article to disclose.

References

1. Thigpen, M.C.; Whitney, C.G.; Messonnier, N.E.; Zell, E.R.; Lynfield, R.; Hadler, J.L.; Harrison, L.H.; Farley, M.M.; Reingold, A.; Bennett, N.M.; et al. Bacterial meningitis in the United States, 1998–2007. *N. Engl. J. Med.* **2011**, *364*, 2016–2025. [CrossRef]
2. Castelblanco, R.L.; Lee, M.; Hasbun, R. Epidemiology of bacterial meningitis in the USA from 1997 to 2010: A population-based observational study. *Lancet Infect. Dis.* **2014**, *14*, 813–819. [CrossRef]
3. Holmquist, L.; Russo, C.A.; Elixhauser, A. Meningitis-Related Hospitalizations in the United States, 2006: Statistical Brief #57. In *Healthcare Cost and Utilization Project (HCUP) Statistical Briefs*; Agency for Healthcare Research and Quality: Rockville, MD, USA, 2006.
4. Collaborators, G.B.D.M. Global, regional, and national burden of meningitis, 1990–2016: A systematic analysis for the Global Burden of Disease Study 2016. *Lancet Neurol.* **2018**, *17*, 1061–1082. [CrossRef]
5. Kwambana-Adams, B.A.; Liu, J.; Okoi, C.; Mwenda, J.M.; Mohammed, N.I.; Tsolenyanu, E.; Renner, L.A.; Ansong, D.; Tagbo, B.N.; Bashir, M.F.; et al. Etiology of Pediatric Meningitis in West Africa Using Molecular Methods in the Era of Conjugate Vaccines against Pneumococcus, Meningococcus, and *Haemophilus influenzae* Type b. *Am. J. Trop. Med. Hyg.* **2020**, *103*, 696–703. [CrossRef]
6. Messacar, K.; Parker, S.K.; Todd, J.K.; Dominguez, S.R. Implementation of Rapid Molecular Infectious Disease Diagnostics: The Role of Diagnostic and Antimicrobial Stewardship. *J. Clin. Microbiol.* **2017**, *55*, 715–723. [CrossRef]
7. Patel, R.; Fang, F.C. Diagnostic Stewardship: Opportunity for a Laboratory-Infectious Diseases Partnership. *Clin. Infect. Dis.* **2018**, *67*, 799–801. [CrossRef]
8. Bauer, K.A.; Perez, K.K.; Forrest, G.N.; Goff, D.A. Review of rapid diagnostic tests used by antimicrobial stewardship programs. *Clin. Infect. Dis.* **2014**, *59*, 134–145. [CrossRef]
9. Broadhurst, M.J.; Dujari, S.; Budvytiene, I.; Pinsky, B.A.; Gold, C.A.; Banaei, N. Utilization, Yield, and Accuracy of the FilmArray Meningitis/Encephalitis Panel with Diagnostic Stewardship and Testing Algorithm. *J. Clin. Microbiol.* **2020**, *58*. [CrossRef]
10. Leber, A.L.; Everhart, K.; Balada-Llasat, J.M.; Cullison, J.; Daly, J.; Holt, S.; Lephart, P.; Salimnia, H.; Schreckenberger, P.C.; DesJarlais, S.; et al. Multicenter Evaluation of BioFire FilmArray Meningitis/Encephalitis Panel for Detection of Bacteria, Viruses, and Yeast in Cerebrospinal Fluid Specimens. *J. Clin. Microbiol.* **2016**, *54*, 2251–2261. [CrossRef]
11. Liesman, R.M.; Strasburg, A.P.; Heitman, A.K.; Theel, E.S.; Patel, R.; Binnicker, M.J. Evaluation of a Commercial Multiplex Molecular Panel for Diagnosis of Infectious Meningitis and Encephalitis. *J. Clin. Microbiol.* **2018**, *56*. [CrossRef]
12. Naccache, S.N.; Lustestica, M.; Fahit, M.; Mestas, J.; Dien Bard, J. One Year in the Life of a Rapid Syndromic Panel for Meningitis/Encephalitis: A Pediatric Tertiary Care Facility's Experience. *J. Clin. Microbiol.* **2018**, *56*. [CrossRef]

13. Piccirilli, G.; Chiereghin, A.; Gabrielli, L.; Giannella, M.; Squarzoni, D.; Turello, G.; Felici, S.; Vocale, C.; Zuntini, R.; Gibertoni, D.; et al. Infectious meningitis/encephalitis: Evaluation of a rapid and fully automated multiplex PCR in the microbiological diagnostic workup. *New Microbiol.* **2018**, *41*, 118–125. [PubMed]
14. Graf, E.H.; Farquharson, M.V.; Cardenas, A.M. Comparative evaluation of the FilmArray meningitis/encephalitis molecular panel in a pediatric population. *Diagn. Microbiol. Infect. Dis.* **2017**, *87*, 92–94. [CrossRef]
15. Messacar, K.; Breazeale, G.; Robinson, C.C.; Dominguez, S.R. Potential clinical impact of the film array meningitis encephalitis panel in children with suspected central nervous system infections. *Diagn. Microbiol. Infect. Dis.* **2016**, *86*, 118–120. [CrossRef]
16. Tansarli, G.S.; Chapin, K.C. Diagnostic test accuracy of the BioFire(R) FilmArray(R) meningitis/encephalitis panel: A systematic review and meta-analysis. *Clin. Microbiol. Infect.* **2020**, *26*, 281–290. [CrossRef] [PubMed]
17. Nabower, A.M.; Miller, S.; Biewen, B.; Lyden, E.; Goodrich, N.; Miller, A.; Gollehon, N.; Skar, G.; Snowden, J. Association of the FilmArray Meningitis/Encephalitis Panel with Clinical Management. *Hosp. Pediatr.* **2019**, *9*, 763–769. [CrossRef]
18. Weber, Z.; Sutter, D.; Baltensperger, A.; Carr, N. Economic Evaluation: Onsite HSV PCR Capabilities for Pediatric Care. *Pediatr. Qual. Saf.* **2020**, *5*, 266. [CrossRef]
19. Posnakoglou, L.; Siahanidou, T.; Syriopoulou, V.; Michos, A. Impact of cerebrospinal fluid syndromic testing in the management of children with suspected central nervous system infection. *Eur. J. Clin. Microbiol. Infect. Dis.* **2020**. [CrossRef]
20. Hagen, A.; Eichinger, A.; Meyer-Buehn, M.; Schober, T.; Huebner, J. Comparison of antibiotic and acyclovir usage before and after the implementation of an on-site FilmArray meningitis/encephalitis panel in an academic tertiary pediatric hospital: A retrospective observational study. *BMC Pediatr.* **2020**, *20*, 56. [CrossRef]
21. Messacar, K.; Gaensbauer, J.T.; Birkholz, M.; Palmer, C.; Todd, J.K.; Tyler, K.L.; Dominguez, S.R. Impact of FilmArray meningitis encephalitis panel on HSV testing and empiric acyclovir use in children beyond the neonatal period. *Diagn. Microbiol. Infect. Dis.* **2020**, *97*, 115085. [CrossRef]
22. Arora, H.S.; Asmar, B.I.; Salimnia, H.; Agarwal, P.; Chawla, S.; Abdel-Haq, N. Enhanced Identification of Group B Streptococcus and Escherichia Coli in Young Infants with Meningitis Using the Biofire Filmarray Meningitis/Encephalitis Panel. *Pediatr. Infect. Dis. J.* **2017**, *36*, 685–687. [CrossRef]
23. Lee, B.R.; Hassan, F.; Jackson, M.A.; Selvarangan, R. Impact of multiplex molecular assay turn-around-time on antibiotic utilization and clinical management of hospitalized children with acute respiratory tract infections. *J. Clin. Virol.* **2019**, *110*, 11–16. [CrossRef] [PubMed]
24. Muller, W.J.; Zheng, X. Laboratory Diagnosis of Neonatal Herpes Simplex Virus Infections. *J. Clin. Microbiol.* **2019**, *57*. [CrossRef] [PubMed]
25. McLaughlin, M.M.; Sutton, S.H.; Jensen, A.O.; Esterly, J.S. Use of High-Dose Oral Valacyclovir during an Intravenous Acyclovir Shortage: A Retrospective Analysis of Tolerability and Drug Shortage Management. *Infect. Dis.* **2017**, *6*, 259–264. [CrossRef]
26. Phuong, J.M.; Penm, J.; Chaar, B.; Oldfield, L.D.; Moles, R. The impacts of medication shortages on patient outcomes: A scoping review. *PLoS ONE* **2019**, *14*, e0215837. [CrossRef] [PubMed]
27. ASHP. Current Drug Shortages. Available online: https://www.ashp.org/drug-shortages/current-shortages/drug-shortages-list?page=CurrentShortages (accessed on 10 October 2020).
28. Choo, E.K.; Rajkumar, S.V. Medication Shortages During the COVID-19 Crisis: What We Must Do. *Mayo Clin. Proc.* **2020**, *95*, 1112–1115. [CrossRef]
29. Murray, A.K. The Novel Coronavirus COVID-19 Outbreak: Global Implications for Antimicrobial Resistance. *Front. Microbiol.* **2020**, *11*, 1020. [CrossRef]
30. Duff, S.; Hasbun, R.; Balada-Llasat, J.M.; Zimmer, L.; Bozzette, S.A.; Ginocchio, C.C. Economic analysis of rapid multiplex polymerase chain reaction testing for meningitis/encephalitis in adult patients. *Infection* **2019**, *47*, 945–953. [CrossRef]
31. Duff, S.; Hasbun, R.; Ginocchio, C.C.; Balada-Llasat, J.M.; Zimmer, L.; Bozzette, S.A. Economic analysis of rapid multiplex polymerase chain reaction testing for meningitis/encephalitis in pediatric patients. *Future Microbiol.* **2018**, *13*, 617–629. [CrossRef]

32. WHO. Defeating Meningitis by 2030: A Global Road Map. Available online: https://www.who.int/immunization/research/development/DefeatingMeningitisRoadmap.pdf (accessed on 17 November 2020).
33. Feagins, A.R.; Ronveaux, O.; Taha, M.K.; Caugant, D.A.; Smith, V.; Fernandez, K.; Glennie, L.; Fox, L.M.; Wang, X. Next generation rapid diagnostic tests for meningitis diagnosis. *J. Infect.* **2020**. [CrossRef]

Publisher's Note: MDPI stays neutral with regard to jurisdictional claims in published maps and institutional affiliations.

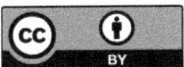

© 2020 by the authors. Licensee MDPI, Basel, Switzerland. This article is an open access article distributed under the terms and conditions of the Creative Commons Attribution (CC BY) license (http://creativecommons.org/licenses/by/4.0/).

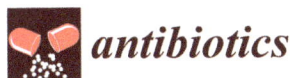

Article

Implementation of a Delayed Prescribing Model to Reduce Antibiotic Prescribing for Suspected Upper Respiratory Tract Infections in a Hospital Outpatient Department, Ghana

Sam Ghebrehewet [1,*], Wendi Shepherd [1,2], Edwin Panford-Quainoo [2], Saran Shantikumar [3], Valerie Decraene [4], Rajesh Rajendran [5], Menaal Kaushal [6], Afua Akuffo [6], Dinah Ayerh [6] and George Amofah [6]

1. Public Health England North West Health Protection Team, Liverpool L3 1JR, UK; wendi.shepherd@phe.gov.uk
2. Liverpool School of Tropical Medicine, Liverpool L3 5QA, UK; 248964@lstmed.ac.uk
3. Warwick Medical School, University of Warwick, Coventry CV4 7HL, UK; Saran.Shantikumar@warwick.ac.uk
4. Public Health England National Infection Service, Liverpool L3 1JR, UK; Valerie.decraene@phe.gov.uk
5. Mid Cheshire NHS Foundation Trust, Crewe CW1 4QJ, UK; rajeshrajendran@nhs.net
6. LEKMA Hospital, Accra, Ghana; menaal.kaushal@gmail.com (M.K.); afuaakuffo@yahoo.com (A.A.); dinash51@yahoo.com (D.A.); george.amofah@ghsmail.org (G.A.)
* Correspondence: sam.ghebrehewet@phe.gov.uk; Tel.: +44-344-225-0562

Received: 31 August 2020; Accepted: 31 October 2020; Published: 4 November 2020

Abstract: *Background*: High levels of antimicrobial resistance (AMR) in Ghana require the exploration of new approaches to optimise antimicrobial prescribing. This study aims to establish the feasibility of implementation of different delayed/back-up prescribing models on antimicrobial prescribing for upper respiratory tract infections (URTIs). *Methods*: This study was part of a quality improvement project at LEKMA Hospital, Ghana, (Dec 2019–Feb 2020). Patients meeting inclusion criteria were assigned to one of four groups (Group 0: No prescription given; Group 1; Patient received post-dated antibiotic prescription; Group 2: Offer of a rapid reassessment of patient by a nurse practitioner after 3 days; and Group 3: Post-dated prescription forwarded to hospital pharmacy). Patients were contacted 10 days afterwards to ascertain wellbeing and actions taken, and patients were asked rate the service on a Likert scale. Post-study informal discussions were conducted with hospital staff. *Results*: In total, 142 patients met inclusion criteria. Groups 0, 1, 2 and 3 had 61, 16, 44 and 21 patients, respectively. Common diagnosis was sore throat (73%). Only one patient took antibiotics after 3 days. Nearly all (141/142) patients were successfully contacted on day 10, and of these, 102 (72%) rated their experiences as good or very good. Informal discussions with staff revealed improved knowledge of AMR. *Conclusions*: Delayed/back-up prescribing can reduce antibiotic consumption amongst outpatient department patients with suspected URTIs. Delayed/back-up prescribing can be implemented safely in low and middle-income countries (LMICs).

Keywords: antimicrobial resistance (AMR); antimicrobial stewardship (AMS); delayed/back-up prescribing; upper respiratory tract infections; developing countries; LMICs; Ghana

1. Introduction

Resistance to antimicrobials poses a substantial threat to individual and public health. Antimicrobial resistance (AMR) is responsible for around 700,000 deaths globally per annum—this figure is predicted to rise to 10 million by 2050 if current trends continue unabated [1] with a disproportionately heavier burden in developing countries [2]. Antimicrobial stewardship (AMS) as an organisational, healthcare system-wide approach to promoting and monitoring judicious use of antimicrobials to preserve their future effectiveness has a critical role in reversing these trends [3].

Upper respiratory tract infections (URTIs) antibiotic prescriptions account for the vast majority of antibiotic prescribing—usually in primary care [4]—where they are frequently prescribed for conditions where there is limited evidence of benefit, including acute otitis media and pharyngitis, and where there is no evidence of benefit, such as the common cold [5–7]. Delayed/back-up prescribing (where antibiotics can be accessed at a later time after the initial consultation) [8] is one strategy that can be implemented to reduce antibiotic prescribing.

Current British National Institute for Clinical Excellence (NICE) guidance suggests that a delayed antibiotic prescribing strategy "encourages self-management ... but allows a person to access antimicrobials without another appointment if their condition gets worse" [9]. Delayed/back-up prescribing should not be used where there is evidence of serious illness or complications, or where the patient is in a clinical risk group [10].

A Cochrane systematic review identified 10 randomised clinical trials that investigated the effectiveness of delayed and no prescriptions strategies for respiratory tract infections [11]. The review found that there was no difference for adverse effects or results favoured delayed antibiotics over immediate antibiotic prescribing; significant reduction in antibiotic use compared to immediate prescription; patient satisfaction favoured delayed prescribing over no antibiotics and there was no difference in patient satisfaction.

Delayed/back-up prescribing can be implemented in a wide variety of ways. An English Ipsos-MORI survey of 1625 participants in 2015 showed that 15% of participants that were prescribed an antibiotics received a delayed prescription [12]. The same study showed a lack of awareness by the public of what the term "delayed prescription" means—after explanation, just 30% of respondents were opposed to General Practitioners (GPs) using this prescribing method for throat, urinary tract, ear, or chest infections. Furthermore, another study [13] reported that delayed prescribing is acceptable no matter how the delay is operationalised, but explanation of the rationale is needed and care taken to minimise mixed messages about the severity of illnesses and causation by viruses or bacteria. A Randomised Control Trial (RCT) considering delayed antibiotic prescribing for uncomplicated acute respiratory tract infections surmised that the practice of delayed prescribing was "associated with slightly greater but clinically similar symptom burden and duration and also with substantially reduced antibiotic use when compared with an immediate strategy" [14].

Delayed/back-up prescribing can be undertaken or approached in different ways. For example, practitioner-centred (when the health professional is responsible for completing the delayed prescription process) or patient-centred, where the patient has responsibility. An advantage of delayed/back-up prescribing is that it provides clinicians and patients with a safety net should an infection deteriorate or fail to improve. Other options may include a systems approach (if diagnosis is clearly identified) whereby local prescribing only allows for delayed prescription—however this may have significant limitations as it does not include the opportunity to review the patient's condition and consider appropriateness of delayed prescribing. Different approaches may be more appropriate for separate patient groups, practitioners, health facilities, or health systems. A typography of approaches is shown in Figure S1.

Ghana has high levels of AMR, with one study showing multidrug resistance rates of over 75% for some organisms [15]. This demonstrates an urgent need to introduce models of care that optimise antibiotic prescribing within a Ghanaian setting [16].

In 2019, a health partnership between the UK Faculty of Public Health (Africa Special Interest Group) and Ghana Public Health Association secured a global volunteering grant from the Fleming Fund's Commonwealth Partnerships for Antimicrobial Stewardship (CwPAMS), supported by Tropical Health and Education Trust (THET) and Commonwealth Pharmacists Association (CPA) to undertake a series of stewardship programmes at LEKMA hospital in Ghana. It was felt that there was an opportunity to try different models of antibiotic prescribing within a Ghana healthcare setting to understand what the barriers would be for implementation of a change to existing antibiotic prescribing practices in a low to middle-income country (LMIC) context. Theoretical work to understand challenges to tackling AMR in LMICs has demonstrated that a broad range of factors such as weak governance and poor regulatory measures, compounded by low public awareness of AMR and technological limitations to adequate surveillance, may present complexities not present in non-LMIC settings [2].

The main aim of this study was to explore the feasibility and practical application of different delayed/back-up prescribing models of antibiotics for the management of URTI within a large outpatient facility in a LMIC. This study also aimed to determine if delayed prescribing was safe within this setting, and to test the model's acceptability to both patients and clinicians.

2. Results

2.1. Quantitative Results

Over a 3-month period from December 2019 to February 2020, 142 patients who attended LEKMA hospital outpatient's department and were cared for by one of three medical doctors were eligible for delayed/back-up prescribing. Of these, 86 (61%) were female, 53 (37%) were male; and 3 (2%) did not specify gender (Table 1).

Table 1. Group description and characteristics of participants.

Characteristics			Group			
			0	1	2	3
	Description		Not considered in need of a back-up prescription. However, they were given a leaflet that outlines the reasons for the clinical decision	Post-dated prescription (given to patient)	Rapid reassessment by nurse at 3-days post initial presentation	Post-date prescription forwarded to hospital pharmacy
Participants (n = 142)	(% of total)		61 (43%)	16 (11%)	44 (31%)	21 (15%)
Sex	(n, % of group)	Females	40 (66%)	9 (56%)	24 (55%)	13 (62%)
Age distribution	(median, IQR in years)		22.5 (2–49)	19 (4–63)	17 (4–30.5)	24 (5–46)

With regard to the different models of delayed/back-up prescribing, 61 (43%) patients were managed conservatively without a back-up prescription or reassessment option (Group 0), 16 (11%) had a post-dated prescription issued (Group 1), 44 (31%) were offered a follow-up appointment for reassessment with a nurse in 3-days if required (Group 2), and 21 (15%) had a prescription left for collection at the hospital pharmacy (Group 3) (Table 1).

As shown in Table 2, nearly half the participants (67, 47%) were working age adults, followed by children under 10 years of age (52, 36%).

Table 2. Age Profile of Participants.

Age Band	Number (n = 142)	%	Cumulative Age Band	%
0–10 years	52	6%	0–10 years	37%
1–10 years	43	30%		
11–19 years	11	8%		47%
20–45 years	37	26%	11–65 years	
46–65 years	19	13%		
≥66 years	13	9%	≥66 years	9%
Not recorded	10	7%	Not recorded	7%

The most common clinical diagnoses were sore throat (72%; n = 102), common cold (15%; n = 22) and acute sinusitis (5%; n = 10) with a similar distribution across the four groups (Table 3). Clinical diagnosis was not recorded for three participants. All participants were successfully contacted at day 10 to record outcome data. In all, only 12 (9%) patients remained mildly symptomatic at day 10, although they all indicated they were feeling better and none had sought further healthcare advice. A lower proportion of those in Group 0 had symptoms at day 10, compared with the other groups. Only one individual in the entire eligible patient population (from Group 3) took antibiotics based on worsening symptoms after 3 days. This patient was diagnosed with sore throat, which had subsided when contacted at day 10 and they had completed course of antibiotics.

Table 3. Characteristics and outcomes of participants by group where recorded.

Characteristics			Group			
			0	1	2	3
Diagnosis	(n, % of group)	Sore throat	46 (75%)	10 (63%)	33 (75%)	13 (62%)
		Common cold	9 (15%)	3 (19%)	7 (16%)	3 (14%)
		Sinusitis	3 (5%)	1 (6%)	4 (9%)	2 (10%)
		Other	2 (3%)	1 (6%)	0 (0%)	2 (10%)
		Not specified	1 (2%)	1 (6%)	0 (0%)	1 (5%)
Symptoms at day 10	(n, % of group)		1 (2%)	4 (25%)	3 (7%)	4 (19%)
Antibiotics taken	(n, % of group)		0 (0%)	0 (0%)	0 (0%)	1 (5%)
Experience reported as good/very good	(proportion of respondents, %)		57/57 (100%)	5/5 (100%)	30/34 (88%)	10/11 (91%)

A Likert Scale of 1–5 was used which has been found to have the most reliability and validity of available Likert Scale methodologies [17]. It should be noted that gaps in the dataset exist where patients were contacted for follow-up but either did not answer questions or the answers were not recorded. Most patients [102 (72%)] rated their experience as good or very good. No patients rated the care they received as poor. When considered by group, the group not given a back-up prescription or an appointment for reassessment (Group 0) were most satisfied with their experience (Table 3).

No adverse events or serious deterioration of illness were reported as a result of the delayed/back-up prescribing model during the 10-day follow-up period for all participants.

2.2. Informal Discussions

Following the period of data collection, informal/unstructured discussions were held with LEKMA Hospital staff (doctors, nurse practitioners and pharmacists) involved in the project. This approach, rather than structured interviews, was adopted to give the LEKMA healthcare workers the flexibility to discuss the key components of the pilot from their perspective and important considerations for their patients. These conversations were based on the rapport that had been built between the researchers and the staff at the hospital during the study. This approach, however, meant that each discussion was unique. From these discussions, we were able to ascertain both areas for development as well as successes to inform future delayed/back-up prescribing projects in LMICs.

The main areas for consideration all appear to stem from the lack of visible senior clinical leadership from project implementation. The senior team at LEKMA Hospital were all very supportive of the project from the outset, but the promotion of the project in the outpatients' department was delegated to the project/study staff. This resulted in misunderstanding by staff about the project aims and the role of clinical staff in delivery of the project. Inevitably, this comprehension impacted on the recruitment of participants to the project as clinical staff did not wish to engage. These issues were addressed once dedicated training had been delivered to the outpatients' department clinical staff, together with the active promotion of the project by senior leadership.

In-depth understanding of some of the root-causes for AMR and the potential solutions are not commonly/widely shared in Ghana—either by clinicians or by patients. The project provided an opportunity to raise awareness and educate both groups on the importance of the issue via face-to-face discussion with patients and regular AMR training sessions for staff in the outpatients' department. Furthermore, dedicated nurse practitioners input to the project provided opportunities for nurse practitioners to discuss other aspects of health and healthy living with the patients—this was particularly important as there is a low level of literacy in Ghana [16], and therefore traditional health messages via printed media may be missed.

3. Discussion

Our project setting was LEKMA, Greater Accra (Ghana), which has a population of 263,631 representing approximately 5.7% and 0.92% of the Greater Accra and Ghanaian populations, respectively. The population is young, 52% female, with a broad-based population pyramid which tapers towards the top, with very few individuals aged over 65. The catchment area population for LEKMA district general hospital is like that of most hospitals in LMICs, especially in Africa. Therefore, considering some of the cultural and socioeconomic factors, we believe the findings of this study are likely to be applicable to most LMICs, especially African countries.

There was an initial cost to this project (nurse practitioners' time) which, if the model was to be implemented on a long-term basis, would need investment. Depending on the funding arrangements within the setting of application, this could be viewed as a long-term investment initiative through the reduction of antibiotic prescribing and associated reduction in AMR which will offset the on-going staff support costs. The provision of nursing support did not affect the patient experience or clinical outcome—rather this reassured medical colleagues about the safety of the model—so delayed/back-up prescribing within an LMIC setting for URTIs could be a cost-neutral endeavour if medical support for the model is in place from the outset. More detailed work on the financial aspects of delayed prescribing in LMICs is required to determine the specific cost-benefit of the strategy, but this is likely to be dependent on the specific funding structures for healthcare in local settings.

The primary message from this project is the practical demonstration and evidence that delayed prescribing models for URTIs can be safely utilised in primary care in the Ghanaian healthcare setting—albeit with some areas which require further redress for sustainability and professional acceptance.

3.1. Safety and Patient Outcomes

This study demonstrates that all the models of delayed prescribing, including the group given no further follow-up options (Group 0), were acceptable to both staff and patients. With the exception of one patient, all other patients involved in the project reported no deterioration of symptoms as a result of participation. Indeed, there were no adverse events related to the patients' presenting symptoms during the project and follow-up period (10 days post presentation).

Most patients (91%) who participated in the study had indicated presenting symptoms had resolved by day 10. This reinforces the findings and conclusions from several studies which have demonstrated no differences in antibiotic prescription rates or clinical outcomes between immediate and delayed prescription and, in the short term, there is also little difference in symptom control between delayed prescription, no prescription, or immediate prescription. Delayed/back-up antibiotic prescription resulted in the minority of patients using antibiotics, and any strategy of delayed prescribing is likely to result in fewer than 40% of patients using antibiotics [17]. In this project, a significantly lower proportion of those in Group 0 (2%) had symptoms, albeit milder, at day 10 compared with the other groups. There is a possibility that these patients were generally less unwell at time of presentation, so clinicians felt more comfortable in not providing any treatment or delayed/back-up prescribing options.

It has been found that patients who had been prescribed an antibiotic for cough in the previous two years were over twice as likely to consult for a similar illness, and that a delayed antibiotic prescription strategy reduced re-consultation by 78% in this group [11]. Another study into paediatric antibiotic use also found that "delayed (rather than immediate) antibiotics reduced re-consultations for deterioration for children with URTI in RCT" [18]—a view supported by other studies into antimicrobial prescribing strategies [18,19]. Although the follow-up period in this project was short (10 days), none of the participants sought further heath advice or took antibiotics from any other source. There was also no need for re-consultation in the follow-up period. A longer period of follow-up, however, is required to confirm that there was no further deterioration or need for clinical re-assessment after the 10-day period, as well as the long-term impact on repeat antibiotic usage in the project population.

The research team had expected that there may be some logistical barriers to uptake of different models within the project, such as travel time and expense to return if symptoms did not spontaneously resolve or if clinical condition deteriorated, which may result in poorer clinical outcomes. It is acknowledged that we did not have a complete response to these questions from all participants (39/82 in Groups 1–3), but 37/38 (97.4%) of those who did respond stated that these factors were not an issue meaning that these factors were not a primary concern for patients in the LEKMA project. Although care should be taken in interpreting these results as they are based on a small number of responses, it is not unreasonable to suggest these results are likely to generalisable to the wider catchment area of LEKMA Hospital and beyond in Ghana, i.e., given the similar geographic or population economic circumstances.

3.2. Reduction in Antibiotic Prescribing

Over the course of the project, there was a reduction of at least 141 antibiotic prescriptions (one prescription per individual but some individuals may have received multiple prescriptions to treat the same infection). It is reasonable to extrapolate the potential number of antibiotic prescriptions that could be saved over a year if this service improvement project is extended to all clinical staff. Based on surveillance data from LEKMA Hospital, and assuming that all patients presenting with URTI will be prescribed antibiotics [personal communication with LEKMA hospital doctors] we estimated that at least, well over 2000 antibiotic prescriptions can be avoided for just two of the commonest URTIs in LEKMA hospital (common cold and sore throat) in the peak URTI season (October to December), i.e., if all LEKMA hospital outpatient clinicians were involved in the implementation of delayed/back-up prescribing. This figure could be at least 3× higher (>6000 antibiotic prescriptions) if delayed/back-up prescribing is implemented for a full 12-month period for all URTI and by all out-patient department clinicians (Figure 1).

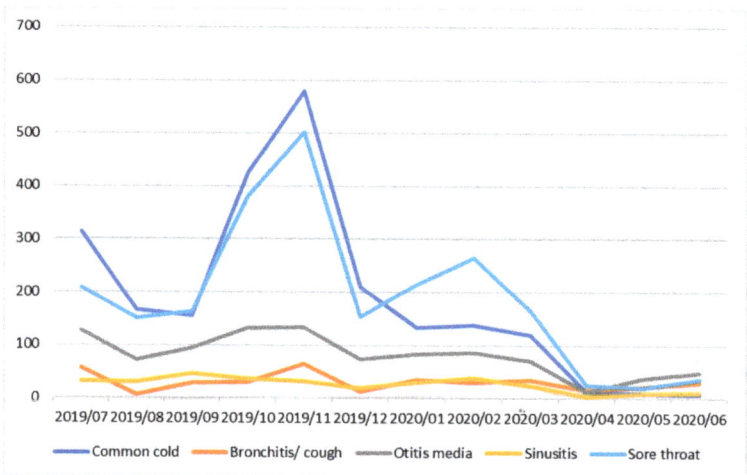

Figure 1. Attendance of Patients with upper respiratory tract infections (URTIs) at LEKMA Hospital, July 2019–June 2020.

3.3. Behaviour Change and Acceptability

The delayed prescribing model was rated as good or very good by 95% of patients. After initial trepidation about the model by clinicians, staff awareness sessions and visible senior clinical leadership were successful methods of ensuring clinician buy-in to the delayed/back-up prescribing model.

Contrary to the perceptions of some local clinicians, Group 0 were the most satisfied with their experience. LEKMA clinicians felt that a potential barrier to the project was that individuals would not wish to leave the outpatient department without a prescription of some nature. This mirrors research considering the issue of increasing antimicrobial resistance, where the authors concluded that "where clinicians feel it is safe not to prescribe antibiotics immediately for people with respiratory infections, no antibiotics with advice to return if symptoms do not resolve is likely to result in the least antibiotic use while maintaining similar patient satisfaction and clinical outcomes to delaying prescription of antibiotics. Where clinicians are not confident in using a no antibiotic strategy, a delayed antibiotics strategy may be an acceptable compromise in place of immediate prescribing to significantly reduce unnecessary antibiotic use for URTIs, and thereby reduce antibiotic resistance, while maintaining patient safety and satisfaction levels" [1].

Our findings demonstrate that, not only was the use of no prescribing (delayed/back-up) acceptable to patients, it was also safe. In addition, the delayed/back-up strategy meant that medical staff were reassured that patients had a point of contact in the nursing team if their condition did not improve/deteriorated, so that they could access further advice and treatment—even if they had been assigned to the Group 0. We hope that these findings can contribute to changing the behaviour of healthcare professionals when considering whether or not to prescribe antibiotics for URTIs.

The experiences of staff during the project, while positive overall, indicate the complexities of the healthcare system in Ghana, the need for complete transparency as to the rationale for such a programme, and the importance of visible senior leadership from the outset. The need for dedicated training and awareness raising of the scheme and the rationale prior to commencement of the project, in addition to senior clinical leadership, cannot be overemphasised.

3.4. Strengths of Project

This project contributes to the evidence base around the use of delayed prescribing as a strategy to reduce antibiotic usage within outpatient settings in LMICs. We have found no previous studies that have examined or implemented the strategy of delayed/back-up prescribing in LMICs in our extensive literature searches on Medline, CINAHL, or Global Health databases until July 2020.

The real-life setting of this project provides evidence for the applicability of delayed/back-up prescribing models in similar settings. Through implementation of the project in a functioning and very busy outpatient department, we were able to confirm theoretical principles into practice. Furthermore, the use of different grouping to test all the current suggested delayed prescribing models, including an information only option (Group 0), demonstrates that there was no major difference in outcomes based on the model used.

The use of Group 0 also removes doubt regarding the possibility that delayed/back-up prescriptions may have been used on those who did not require them. Coupled with proactive efforts to reduce private antibiotic sales from local community pharmacies, we can be confident that the results outlined above are an accurate reflection of the treatment each participant received for their condition.

Use of a 10-day follow-up period within the project increased patient safety as it ensured that all patients had a point of rapid access in case of lack of improvement in their condition. Provision of a call to the patient at the end of the follow-up period allowed documentation of clinical outcome.

Finally, the project had an excellent response rate from participants—both on enrolment and at the end of the follow-up period—which provides assurance as to the accuracy of the findings.

3.5. Limitations of Project

This service improvement project had some limitations which require discussion to build on our experiences for future delayed/back-up prescribing projects in similar settings.

This initiative had a relatively small number of eligible participants. In part, this may be due to buy-in and understanding of the project from clinicians within LEKMA outpatients' department in the early period of the project. Although training was offered, it did not reach all outpatients' department doctors, and this may have contributed to the lack of engagement from all the doctors who worked at LEKMA outpatients' department at the time. We did not interview clinicians who were not involved in the project to see what factors may have been responsible for the low take-up of the model by prescribing staff.

Although we have one year's data, we do not know the true trend of URTIs at LEKMA Hospital. Further analysis on general rates of URTIs over the project period may also yield information about whether there was simply a lower burden of URTIs than expected compared with previous years. It was not possible to run the project over all outpatient clinics throughout the week due to project resources only being available on weekdays, so we do not have information on weekend and out of hours attendance for URTIs. We did not collect information on patient's medical history or existing comorbidities, and these may have impacted on patient outcomes, i.e., persistence of illness or need for antibiotics. In addition, outcomes were self-reported and not validated by clinical examination.

More extensive qualitative and quantitative research throughout the project would have been beneficial to understand other reasons for low take-up—for example, we do not have information on number of potential participants approached who did not consent to being in the project, the number of patients with an URTI who came to the clinic who were not included in the study who may have been given antibiotic treatment. We also do not have information on the exact impact of COVID-19 on potential participant attendance at the outpatients' department, especially in February 2020. These low numbers of participants, and the single site setting, may limit the generalisability of these findings and inference to other settings in Ghana and other LMICs. This is compounded by this not being an RCT design, and therefore a comparative, standardised study design was not undertaken.

Data quality and data completeness have affected the comprehensiveness of the findings, as there are significant gaps in participant responses—particularly towards the end of the project period when staff were undertaking additional duties to assist with the COVID-19 efforts. Counter to this, at the start of the project, participants were not sequentially allocated to a group, which may have led to some bias. Staff involved in the project have commented that they were not aware of the importance of sequential allocation initially. It was also not possible to blind the study due to the service nature of the project, which may have affected our outcomes. Additional training of project staff in service improvement methodology prior to the commencement of the project may have increased local ownership and understanding of the rationale behind the data collection tools which may have improved data quality. This would have the added benefit of allowing local adaptation of tools to fit local circumstance based on local knowledge.

We recommend that further studies are conducted to address some of these issues in other settings.

4. Materials and Methods

The service improvement pilot ran from December 2019 to February 2020 within the outpatients' department of LEKMA Hospital, Accra, Ghana. Inclusion criteria were all patients who presented at the setting with URTI symptoms during the project period and were deemed to be eligible for the study by the examining clinician. Exclusion criteria were any patient who is diagnosed with URTI but clinician considered that delayed antibiotic prescription was inappropriate or any patient that did not verbally consent to take part. As this was not clinical research, the quality improvement project was discussed with LEKMA Hospital management, and all available evidence regarding back-up/delayed prescribing was presented. The consensus by LEKMA management was that this is evidence-based good practice that would be a key component of quality improvement for the hospital and would not alter patient choices and opportunities; therefore, no ethics approval was required.

There were four different models of delayed/back-up prescribing—no prescription given (only information leaflet); post-dated prescriptions being given to patients at time of first clinical appointment to use if no symptom resolution 3 days after clinic visit; rapid access to a nurse-led clinic for re-assessment after three days, i.e., if symptoms did not improve/patient's condition deteriorate; and prescription forwarded to the hospital pharmacy and clinician/nurse practitioner asking patient to visit the hospital pharmacy to collect a pre-written antibiotic prescription if symptoms did not improve within 3 days. Delayed/back-up antibiotic prescribing was only to take place when it was deemed clinically appropriate to do so—this decision was at the sole discretion of the clinician responsible for the patients' care. The clinical pathways are available in Figure S2.

Two experienced nurses were recruited from the hospital staff to provide support to the project on a full-time basis for the project duration, although their time was diverted to COVID-19 response towards the end of the project. A data collection tool was developed using Microsoft Excel to ensure contemporaneous data capture by these nurses and provide a database of clinical presentation, clinical outcome at the end of follow-up period, and general evaluation information. Patient information leaflets were prepared for different groups. All project materials are available in the Supplementary Information.

Participants were allocated to one of the four groups on a sequential basis by the nursing team. The study was designed so that there was sequential randomisation of participants but, in reality, this was initially more ad-hoc than was planned which resulted in unequal sized groups between the different interventions and may have introduced bias into the study.

Dedicated face-to-face training to medical, nursing, and administrative staff in the outpatients' department and pharmacy was provided by the UK partnership staff in advance of the project to advise them of the project aims and objectives. Further training was provided in January 2020 by senior medical staff at LEKMA Hospital.

Community pharmacists in the area surrounding LEKMA Hospital were visited by the project team to try to minimise non-prescribed antibiotic purchases direct from pharmacists.

All patients were contacted via telephone 10-days after their initial presentation to ascertain if they were still symptomatic; if they had consulted other medical professionals over the 10-day period; antibiotics taken in previous 10-days (and source); and their experience of the care they received using a Likert scale.

Informal discussions with LEKMA staff members actively involved in the project were undertaken, and their transcripts were analysed to understand how the field experience at the local level in Ghana related to the potential barriers outlined in other work on antimicrobial prescribing in LMICs [2].

5. Conclusions

Despite good evidence for a delayed prescribing approach in other regions (mainly high-income countries), there is sparse published evidence for the use of delayed/back-up prescribing in LMICs—particularly in Africa, where alternative methods of gaining antibiotics may exist (such as direct illicit purchase from community pharmacists, as can occur in Ghana). Furthermore, in LMIC hospital outpatient departments, which see new clinical presentations of illness (much like in primary care), the proportion of antibiotic prescriptions that are written for URTIs is unknown, and inappropriate antibiotic prescribing is likely to be high.

The results from this service improvement project show support from both clinicians and patients for more dedicated interventions to reduce inappropriate prescribing of antibiotics in LMICs with little preference for which model of delay/back-up prescribing used. The success of the models is reflected through a significant reduction in antibiotic use for URTIs in LEKMA outpatients during the project with no serious illness or adverse events recorded over the 10-day follow-up period. Furthermore, upscaling implementation delayed/back-up prescribing in LMICs could contribute to improvement in clinicians' confidence, optimise antibiotic prescribing and reduce antimicrobial resistance.

Further in-depth exploration of clinicians' and patients' experiences and perceptions need to be captured to help optimise delayed/back-up prescribing implementation. Extended project schemes along the same model should be used in different settings and with larger cohorts of patients to prove the clinical applicability of the model to other LMIC settings using a bigger data set.

Supplementary Materials: The following are available online at http://www.mdpi.com/2079-6382/9/11/773/s1, Figure S1: Typography of approaches to delayed antibiotic prescription, Figure S2: Patient pathways for project of delayed prescribing in LEKMA Hospital outpatients' department, Ghana.

Author Contributions: S.G., W.S., E.P.-Q., and S.S. drafted the paper and contributed to the project idea, conceptualisation, design and implementation of the study. V.D., G.A., M.K., A.A., D.A. and R.R. contributed to the design and implementation of the study and commented on the manuscript. All authors have read and agreed to the published version of the manuscript.

Funding: This project was funded as part of the Commonwealth Partnerships for Antimicrobial Stewardship Scheme (CwPAMS) supported by Tropical Health and Education Trust (THET) and Commonwealth Pharmacists Association (CPA) using Official Development Assistance (ODA) funding, through the Department of Health and Social Care's Fleming Fund. The views expressed in this publication are those of the author(s) and not necessarily those of the NHS, PHE, the Fleming Fund, the Department of Health and Social Care, THET or CPA.

Acknowledgments: On behalf of the UK Faculty of Public Health (Africa Special Interest Group), and Ghana Public Health Association, we would like to thank all the UK FPH and GPHA partnership members for their invaluable input and support in the implementation of this projects. The partnership members are: Col. Edwin Afari (Rtd.), President of the GPHA; Perdita Hilary Lopes, Financial Secretary & Deputy Project Coordinator; Michael Adjabeng, GPHA Secretary; Amoah James McKeown, Public Relations Officer, GPHA; Samantha Walker, Lead Nurse—Infection Prevention and Control, Countess of Chester Hospital NHS Foundation Trust; Indu Das, Antimicrobial Specialist Pharmacist, East Cheshire NHS Trust. We are also grateful for LEKMA Hospital Senior Management, especially Juliana Ameh, Medical Superintendent (during the project period), for hercommitment to support the project with 2 full-time nurse practitioners. In addition, we would like to thank the following members of LEKMA Hospital staff for providing information, and support in coordination and implementation of the project: Akua Gyimah-Asante, Medical Superintendent; Stella Siriboe, Director of Nursing; Anthonia Aba Bannerman-Quist, Chief Pharmacist; Paul Beson, Infection Prevention & Control (IPC), Focal Lead; Abdul Razak Amari, Head of Laboratory; and Doreen Atta-Fynn. Finally, we would like to thank Merav Kliner and Peter MacPherson for their initial work in 2015 on the evidence base for delayed prescribing models within the UK.

Conflicts of Interest: The authors declare no conflict of interest.

References

1. Villegas, M.V.; Lyon, S. Gram-Negative Infections: Evolving Treatments with Expanding Options. *Futur. Sci. OA* **2018**, *4*, 2–5. [CrossRef] [PubMed]
2. Pokharel, S.; Raut, S.; Adhikari, B. Tackling Antimicrobial Resistance in Low-Income and Middle-Income Countries. *BMJ Glob. Health* **2019**, *4*, 4–6. [CrossRef] [PubMed]
3. Dyar, O.J.; Huttner, B.; Schouten, J.; Pulcini, C. What Is Antimicrobial Stewardship? *Clin. Microbiol. Infect.* **2017**, *23*, 793–798. [CrossRef] [PubMed]
4. Public Health England. English Surveillance Programme for Antimicrobial Utilisation and Resistance (ESPAUR). 2016. Available online: https://improvement.nhs.uk/resources/english-surveillance-programme-antimicrobial-utilisation-and-resistance-espaur/ (accessed on 1 August 2020).
5. Venekamp, R.P.; Sanders, S.L.; Glasziou, P.P.; Del Mar, C.B.; Rovers, M.M. Antibiotics for Acute Otitis Media in Children. *Cochrane Database Syst. Rev.* **2015**, *2015*, CD000219. [CrossRef] [PubMed]
6. Spinks, A.; Glasziou, P.; Del Mar, C. Antibiotics for Sore Throat. *Cochrane Database Syst. Rev.* **2013**, *2013*, CD000023. [CrossRef] [PubMed]
7. Kenealy, T.; Arroll, B. Antibiotics for the Common Cold and Acute Purulent Rhinitis. *Cochrane Database Syst. Rev.* **2013**, *2013*, CD000247. [CrossRef] [PubMed]
8. Public Health England. Tackling Antimicrobial Resistance 2019–2024: UK 5-Year Action Plan. 2019. Available online: https://www.gov.uk/government/publications/uk-5-year-action-plan-for-antimicrobial-resistance-2019-to-2024 (accessed on 1 August 2020).
9. NICE. *Antimicrobial Stewardship: Quality Statement 2*; National Institute for Health and Care Excellence: London, UK, 2016.

10. NICE. *Antimicrobial Stewardship: Systems and Processes for Effective Antimicrobial Medicine Use*; National Institute for Health and Care Excellence: London, UK, 2015.
11. Spurling, G.; Del Mar, C.; Dooley, L.; Foxlee, R.; Farley, R. Delayed Antibiotic Prescriptions for Respiratory Infections (Review). *Cochrane Database Syst. Rev.* **2019**, *9*, CD004417. [CrossRef]
12. McNulty, C.A.M.; Lecky, D.M.; Hawking, M.K.D.; Quigley, A.; Butler, C.C. Delayed/Back up Antibiotic Prescriptions: What Do the Public Think? *BMJ Open* **2015**, *5*, e009748. [CrossRef]
13. McDermott, L.; Leydon, G.M.; Halls, A.; Kelly, J.; Nagle, A.; White, J.; Little, P. Qualitative Interview Study of Antibiotics and Self-Management Strategies for Respiratory Infections in Primary Care. *BMJ Open* **2017**, *7*, 1–7. [CrossRef]
14. De La Poza Abad, M.; Dalmau, G.M.; Bakedano, M.M.; González, A.I.G.; Criado, Y.C.; Anadón, S.H.; Del Campo, R.R.; Monserrat, P.T.; Palma, A.N.; Ortiz, L.M.; et al. Prescription Strategies in Acute Uncomplicated Respiratory Infections a Randomized Clinical Trial. *JAMA Intern. Med.* **2016**, *176*, 21–29. [CrossRef]
15. Little, P.; Stuart, B.; Smith, S.; Thompson, M.J.; Knox, K.; Van Den Bruel, A.; Lown, M.; Moore, M.; Mant, D. Antibiotic Prescription Strategies and Adverse Outcome for Uncomplicated Lower Respiratory Tract Infections: Prospective Cough Complication Cohort (3C) Study. *BMJ* **2017**, *357*, j2148. [CrossRef] [PubMed]
16. Little, P.; Moore, M.; Kelly, J.; Williamson, I.; Leydon, G.; McDermott, L.; Mullee, M.; Stuart, B. Delayed Antibiotic Prescribing Strategies for Respiratory Tract Infections in Primary Care: Pragmatic, Factorial, Randomised Controlled Trial. *BMJ* **2014**, *348*, 1–8. [CrossRef]
17. Louangrath, P.I.; Sutanapong, C. Validity and Reliability of Survey Scales. *Int. J. Res. Methodol. Soc. Sci.* **2018**, *4*, 99–115. [CrossRef]
18. Redmond, N.M.; Turnbull, S.; Stuart, B.; Thornton, H.V.; Christensen, H.; Blair, P.S.; Delaney, B.C.; Thompson, M.; Peters, T.J.; Hay, A.D.; et al. Impact of Antibiotics for Children Presenting to General Practice with Cough on Adverse Outcomes: Secondary Analysis from a Multicentre Prospective Cohort Study. *Br. J. Gen. Pract.* **2018**, *68*, e682–e693. [CrossRef] [PubMed]
19. Literacy Rate, Adult Total (% of People Ages 15 and Above)—Ghana. Available online: https://data.worldbank.org/indicator/SE.ADT.LITR.ZS?locations=GH (accessed on 12 August 2020).

Publisher's Note: MDPI stays neutral with regard to jurisdictional claims in published maps and institutional affiliations.

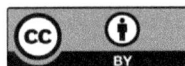

© 2020 by the authors. Licensee MDPI, Basel, Switzerland. This article is an open access article distributed under the terms and conditions of the Creative Commons Attribution (CC BY) license (http://creativecommons.org/licenses/by/4.0/).

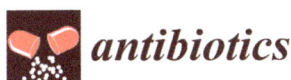

Article

Is Antimicrobial Dosing Adjustment Associated with Better Outcomes in Patients with Severe Obesity and Bloodstream Infections? An Exploratory Study

Stéphanie Sirard [1], Claire Nour Abou Chakra [1], Marie-France Langlois [2], Julie Perron [3], Alex Carignan [1] and Louis Valiquette [1,*]

1. Department of Microbiology and Infectious Diseases, Université de Sherbrooke, Sherbrooke, QC J1H 5N4, Canada; stephanie.sirard@USherbrooke.ca (S.S.); claire.nour.abou.chakra@usherbrooke.ca (C.N.A.C.); alex.carignan@usherbrooke.ca (A.C.)
2. Department of Medicine, Division of Endocrinology, Université de Sherbrooke, Sherbrooke, QC J1H 5N4, Canada; marie-france.langlois@usherbrooke.ca
3. Department of Pharmacy, Centre Intégré Universitaire de Santé et de Services Sociaux de l'Estrie-Centre Hospitalier Universitaire de Sherbrooke, Granby, QC J2G 1T7, Canada; julie.perron2@usherbrooke.ca
* Correspondence: louis.valiquette@USherbrooke.ca; Tel.: +1-819-821-8000 (ext. 72568)

Received: 8 September 2020; Accepted: 14 October 2020; Published: 16 October 2020

Abstract: The impact of adjusted treatment on clinical outcomes in patients with severe obesity is unclear. This study included adults with severe obesity admitted for bloodstream infections between 2005 and 2015. The patients were grouped according to the percentage of the appropriateness of the dosage of their antimicrobial treatment: 80–100% = good, 20–79% = moderate, and 0–19% = poor. The association between antimicrobial adjustment and a composite of unfavourable outcomes [intensive care unit stay ≥72 h, duration of sepsis >3 days, length of stay ≥7 days or all-cause 30-day mortality] was assessed using logistic regression. Of 110 included episodes, the adjustment was rated good in 47 (43%) episodes, moderate in 31 (28%), and poor in 32 (29%). Older age, Pitt bacteremia score ≥2, sepsis on day 1, and infection site were independent risk factors for unfavourable outcomes. The level of appropriateness was not associated with unfavourable outcomes. The number of antimicrobials, consultation with an infectious disease specialist, blood urea nitrogen 7–10.9 mmol/L, and hemodialysis were significantly associated with adjusted antimicrobial dosing. While the severity of the infection had a substantial impact on the measured outcomes, we did not find an association between dosing optimization and better outcomes.

Keywords: obesity; bloodstream infection; antimicrobials; prescription

1. Introduction

In the last 40 years, the prevalence of obesity has doubled in more than 70 countries, accounting for over 2 million deaths worldwide [1]. Aside from comorbidities such as type 2 diabetes, hypertension, and cardiovascular diseases, obesity is associated with a high risk of infections [2,3]. Physiologic alterations in patients with obesity influence the pharmacokinetics (PK) and pharmacodynamics (PD) of many drugs, including antimicrobials [4,5]. Underdosing of antimicrobials in patients with obesity could lead to sub-inhibitory concentrations, which, in turn, could impair treatment and lead to clinical failure [6–9]. For example, in patients with severe obesity and cellulitis, a low antimicrobial dose upon hospital discharge was associated with either recurrence, emergency room visit, rehospitalization, or 30-day attributable death (odds ratio [OR] 3.6 95% CI 1.4–9.4) [7]. In a cohort of critically ill patients with complicated intra-abdominal and skin and soft tissue infections, high doses of tigecycline resulted in a significant reduction in mortality, intensive care unit (ICU) length of stay (LOS), and occurrence of bacteremia and septic shock [10].

Bloodstream infections (BSI) are severe infections and one of the leading causes of death in North America and Europe [11]. In one study, the risk of BSI was higher in patients with obesity than in normal-weight patients (31% for body mass index (BMI) of 30–34.9, 87% for BMI of 35–39.9, and 210% for BMI of ≥40) [12]. While obesity had no association with short-term all-cause mortality and clinical outcomes in patients with BSIs [13], another study found that high BMI was associated with organ failure and all-cause hospital mortality in patients with BSIs due to Gram-negative bacteria [14].

Although some studies have investigated the link between obesity and unfavourable outcomes associated with BSI, to our knowledge, none has focused on the impact of antimicrobial dose adjustment in BSI patients with class III obesity [12–16].

In this article, we describe a retrospective cohort of adults with class III obesity hospitalized for BSI, where we assessed factors associated with adjustment of antimicrobial dosing and compared clinical outcomes according to the appropriateness of antimicrobial dose adjustments.

2. Materials and Methods

2.1. Population and Study Design

This retrospective study was conducted at the Centre intégré universitaire de santé et de services sociaux de l'Estrie-Centre hospitalier universitaire de Sherbrooke (CIUSSSE-CHUS), a 677-bed academic centre in the Province of Quebec, Canada. Approval was obtained from CIUSSSE-CHUS institutional review board (#12–187). Subjects were identified through a clinical data warehouse. All adult patients with documented class III obesity (BMI ≥ 40 kg/m^2) hospitalized between 1 August 2005 and 31 August 2015 for BSI were included.

BSI was defined by the presence of a pathogen in one blood culture or the presence of a skin flora microorganism (coagulase-negative staphylococci, alpha-hemolytic streptococci, *Micrococcus* species, *Propionibacterium/Cutibacterium* species, *Corynebacterium* species, and *Bacillus* species) in at least two consecutive blood cultures (from two different sites).

Specific populations for whom the BMI was not reliable, such as pregnant women, patients with dwarfism, those with above-the-knee bilateral amputation, or those with a history of bariatric surgery were excluded. Other exclusion criteria were: presence of fungemia, transfer from another hospital after ≥48 h, receiving palliative care, presence of more than one bacterial infection, or two or more distinct episodes during hospitalization. We excluded patients who were treated for the whole or the majority of the treatment (>80%) with an antimicrobial requiring no adjustment for obesity (cefixime, moxifloxacin, ertapenem, fosfomycin, and tigecycline) and those treated with vancomycin or aminoglycosides only, especially cases where it was the only effective antimicrobial. In addition, patients who died or did not received an antimicrobial within the first 48 h after the initial positive blood culture, or had inadequate antimicrobial coverage for >48 h were excluded.

2.2. Data Collection

A standardized form was used to collect data on clinical variables from computerized medical charts. Pathogens isolated from blood samples were noted along with antimicrobial susceptibility test results. Immunosuppression was defined as the presence of leukaemia, lymphoma, HIV infection, neutropenia (neutrophils < 1800/µL), organ transplantation, and connective tissue disease or use of immunosuppressive drugs for over one month within the previous six months. To evaluate the severity of illness, the Pitt bacteremia score (PBS) (ranging from 0 to 18) was documented on the day of the positive blood culture and up to 48 h prior [17,18]. The time to effective antimicrobial was determined by the time between admission and the administration of the first effective antimicrobial related to the infection. All antimicrobial prescriptions relevant to the treatment of BSI were reviewed for the route of administration, dose, and dosing interval and were compared to the local guidelines for adults with class III obesity based on the current literature (see Table 1) [5,19,20].

Table 1. Dosing regimens for the most frequently prescribed antimicrobials.

Antimicrobial	Creatinine Clearance *			
	>50 mL/min	30–50 mL/min	10–30 mL/min	<10 mL/min
Penicillins				
ampicillin	2000 mg q4h	2000 mg q6h	2000 mg q6h	2000 mg q6h
penicillin (IV)	4 million units q4h	3 million units q4h	3 million units q4h	2 million units q4h
(PO)	600 mg q6h	600 mg q6h	600 mg q6h	600 mg q8h
piperacillin/tazobactam	(CrCl > 40 mL/min) 3000 mg q4h or 4000 mg q6h	(CrCl 20–40 mL/min) 3000 mg q6h	(CrCl 0–20 mL/min) 2000 mg q6h	(CrCl 0–20 mL/min) 2000 mg q6h
Cephalosporins				
cefazolin	2000 mg q4h	(CrCl 35–50mL/min) 2000 mg q8h	(CrCl 10–35 mL/min) 2000 mg q12h	2000 mg q24h
ceftriaxone	2000 mg q12h	2000 mg q12h	2000 mg q12h	2000 mg q12h
Quinolones				
ciprofloxacin (IV)	400 mg q8h	400 mg q12h	400 mg q24h	400 mg q24h
(PO)	750 mg q12h	500 mg q12h	500 mg q24h	500 mg q24h
Aminoglycosides				
gentamicin	1 mg/kg q8h	1 mg/kg q12h	1 mg/kg q24h	1 mg/kg q48h

Abbreviations: CrCl: creatinine clearance, IV: intravenous, PO: oral administration. * estimated with the Cockcroft-Gault equation with adjusted body weight.

Cockcroft-Gault equation with adjusted body weight was used to estimate creatinine clearance (CrCl) at the beginning of all prescriptions and for every significant change in creatinine values [21]. A prescription was deemed inadequate if either the dose and/or the dosing intervals were lower than expected for class III obesity. When multiple antimicrobials were administered at the same time, we considered the whole prescription adequate if at least one antimicrobial dosing and the spectrum were adequate. The first prescription was also carefully reviewed. The percentage of the appropriateness of the dose and dosing intervals was calculated by dividing the number of days of adequate treatment by the total number of days of treatment and was considered good (80–100%), moderate (20–79%), or poor (0–19%). This classification has been selected after discussion with infectious disease experts, locally.

2.3. Outcomes

To reflect unfavourable outcomes potentially associated with unadjusted antimicrobial dosing and because of the low frequency of each component, we constructed a composite primary endpoint including clinically relevant components: ICU stay ≥72 h, duration of sepsis >3 days, LOS ≥7 days, or all-cause 30-day mortality. Other secondary endpoints collected per hospitalization were time to defervescence, time to white blood cells (WBC) normalization, time to sepsis normalization, ICU LOS, need for and duration of mechanical ventilation, and hospital LOS. Fever was defined as an increase in body temperature above 37.5 °C orally, 38 °C rectally and centrally, or 37.3 °C axillary. Time to defervescence was the time between the first abnormal value and the first normal value that remained within normal values for at least 48 h. Only the first febrile episode within 48 h of the first positive blood culture was considered in this calculation. WBC normalization associated with the first positive blood culture was defined as a stable return within the normal range during hospitalization. We could not calculate this variable in patients for whom WBC counts were within or below normal range during the entire study period. To define sepsis, we used a modified sequential organ failure assessment (mSOFA) to overcome the limitations due to missing values [22,23]. A serial mSOFA was calculated on days 1, 3, 5, and 7 with the most abnormal values in the 24-h period. Missing values were imputed with normal values, and the corresponding parameter of mSOFA was attributed a score of 0. Sepsis was defined as an mSOFA score of ≥2. All-cause readmission within 30 days of hospital discharge was assessed, and relapse was considered when patients were hospitalized for the initial infection or a complication.

2.4. Statistical Analysis

Data were analyzed using IBM SPSS Statistics for Windows, version 25 (IBM Corp., Armonk, NY, USA). Groups of patients were compared on the basis of the appropriateness of the antimicrobial dosage. To account for potential changes linked to the impact of an antimicrobial stewardship program based on a decision support system (APSS, Lumed Inc., Canada) implemented in August 2010, we divided the study period into three segments: pre-APSS (2005–July 2010), early-APSS (August 2010–2012), and late-APSS (2013–2015). The Antimicrobial Prescription Surveillance System (APSS) is an asynchronous system that generates alerts for potentially inappropriate antimicrobial prescriptions based on published recommendations and expert opinions. These alerts are reviewed by pharmacists who are part of the antimicrobial stewardship program team and recommendations are made to physicians. Special rules were developed for patients with class III obesity [24].

Descriptive statistics were used to characterize baseline demographic characteristics, comorbidities, and outcomes, stratified by the level of appropriateness. Descriptive analyses are presented using three groups based on the level of appropriateness (good, moderate and poor). For some comparisons, we combined the moderate and poor groups and compared to the most optimal group (good). Categorical variables were reported as number and percentage for each group and were compared using the χ^2 test or binary logistic regression, when appropriate. Continuous variables were reported as median values with their interquartile range (IQR) and were compared with the Wilcoxon test. Logistic regression was used to assess the association between adjusted antimicrobial dosing and unfavourable outcomes and to identify factors associated with adjusted antimicrobial therapy (0–19% poor compared to 20–100%). Selected variables and variables identified in univariable analysis were included in a multivariable model in order of the lowest *P*-value and results of the likelihood ratio test. The results are presented as unadjusted or adjusted OR (aOR) with 95% confidence interval (CI).

3. Results

During the study period, 160 clinical episodes of positive blood cultures in adults with class III obesity were identified in our centre, and 110 episodes occurring in 96 patients met the eligibility criteria (Supplementary Data, Figure S1). The excluded patients were similar to the study population, except for higher rates of intra-abdominal (16% vs. 5%, $p = 0.04$) and catheter (16% vs. 4%, $p = 0.009$) infections. Patients' characteristics and comorbidities are presented in Table 2. Antimicrobial treatment was classified as 80–100% adequate (good) in 47, 20–79% adequate (moderate) in 31, and 0–19% adequate (poor) in 32 patients.

Overall, the median BMI was 44.9 kg/m^2 (IQR 42–49), 20% ($n = 22$) of the patients had a BMI over 50 kg/m^2, and 85% ($n = 94$) had at least one chronic underlying illness. The most frequent comorbidities were diabetes (69%, $n = 76$), coronary artery disease (32%, $n = 35$), and chronic obstructive pulmonary disease (25%, $n = 27$). One in five patients (21%, $n = 23$) had renal failure and 15% ($n = 17$) were immunocompromised. Apart from a significantly greater proportion of hemodialysis patients in the group with good adjustment, all other demographic variables and comorbidities were similar between groups.

The most common source of BSI was urinary tract infections (34%), followed by skin and soft tissue infections (25%). Infections in patients who had good antimicrobial adjustment were more severe, with a lower proportion of urinary tract infections (21% vs. 43%, $p = 0.018$), and a greater proportion of patients with a Pitt bacteremia score (PBS) ≥ 2 (68% vs. 40%, $p = 0.003$); there was a significantly higher frequency of sepsis in this group than in those with moderate or poor levels of adjustment (79% vs. 59%, $p = 0.027$). *Escherichia coli* was the most frequently isolated pathogen (28% of episodes). Enterobacteriaceae were recovered less often from patients with a good adjustment than from patients in the other groups (28% vs. 51%, $p = 0.015$).

Table 2. Patient demographics and medical conditions stratified by the level of appropriateness.

Characteristics	Good (80–100%) n = 47	Moderate (20–79%) n = 31	Poor (0–19%) n = 32	Total Cohort N = 110
Female sex	25 (53)	17 (55)	17 (53)	59 (54)
Age (years), median (IQR)	59 (54–66)	66 (51–76)	62 (57–65)	62 (54–67)
BMI (kg/m^2), median (IQR)	45.3 (41.8–50.2)	43.7 (42.2–47.3)	45.0 (42.3–49.2)	44.9 (42.1–48.9)
Weight (kg), median (IQR)	127.0 (113.0–145.0)	121.0 (107.5–136.9)	122.0 (108.4–147.9)	124.6 (111.2–142.8)
Comorbidities				
Immunosuppression	11 (23)	3 (10)	3 (9)	17 (15)
Coronary artery disease	15 (32)	8 (26)	12 (38)	35 (32)
Diabetes	32 (68)	19 (61)	25 (78)	76 (69)
COPD	10 (21)	9 (29)	8 (25)	27 (25)
Chronic kidney failure	11 (23)	5 (16)	7 (22)	23 (21)
Charlson comorbidity index				
0–3	17 (36)	13 (42)	15 (47)	45 (41)
4–6	26 (55)	9 (29)	9 (28)	44 (40)
≥7	4 (9)	9 (29)	8 (25)	21 (19)
Infection site				
Urinary tract	10 (21)	11 (36)	16 (50)	37 (34)
Skin and soft tissue	11 (23)	9 (29)	7 (22)	27 (25)
Pulmonary	8 (17)	4 (13)	1 (3)	13 (12)
Intra-abdominal	2 (4)	3 (10)	1 (3)	6 (5)
Others [a]	16 (34)	4 (13)	7 (22)	27 (25)
Severity				
PBS, median (IQR)	2 (1–4)	1 (0–2)	1 (0–3)	2 (1–3)
PBS ≥ 2	32 (68)	11 (36)	14 (44)	57 (52)
Sepsis on day 1 [b]	37 (79)	21 (68)	16 (50)	74 (67)
Pathogens isolated				
Gram-positive				
S. aureus	8 (17)	3 (10)	3 (9)	14 (13)
S. pneumoniae	9 (19)	2 (7)	1 (3)	12 (11)
Others [c]	12 (26)	9 (29)	8 (25)	29 (26)
Gram-negative				
Enterobacteriaceae [d]	13 (28)	13 (42)	19 (59)	45 (41)
Other [e]	7 (15)	4 (13)	2 (6)	13 (12)
Polymicrobial infection	5 (11)	3 (10)	2 (6)	10 (9)
Others				
Consultation with an infectious disease specialist	31 (66)	13 (42)	10 (31)	54 (49)

Results are reported as number (%) or median (IQR). Abbreviations: IQR: interquartile range, BMI: body mass index, COPD: chronic obstructive pulmonary disease, PBS: Pitt bacteremia score. [a] Bones and joints (6), cardiovascular (5), hepatic/biliary (5), catheter (4), undetermined (3), thoracic (2), central nervous system (1), vascular system (1). [b] Since it was present upon arrival or occurred early after initiation of antimicrobial treatment, sepsis at day 1 was considered a severity factor rather than a clinical outcome. [c] β-hemolytic (groups A, B, C and G) (27) and non-hemolytic streptococci (S. gallolyticus, S. mitis) (2). [d] Escherichia coli (31), Klebsiella pneumoniae (10), Serratia marcescens (3), Citrobacter freundii (2), Enterobacter cloacae (2), Proteus mirabilis (2), Morganella morganii (1), Klebsiella oxytoca (1). [e] Enterococcus faecalis (3), Haemophilus influenzae (2), Aerococcus urinae (1), Bacteroides thetaiotaomicron (1), Bilophila wadsworthia (1), Clostridium septicum (1), Clostridium ramosum (1), Pasteurella multocida (1), Prevotella loescheii (1), Pseudomonas aeruginosa (1).

During hospitalization, patients received an average of 3.1 ± 1.2 antimicrobials for their infection, of which 1.8 ± 0.9 had inadequate posology. The first prescription was unadjusted for the dose and/or the interval in 60% of patients ($n = 66$), and the dose was insufficient in 68% of the cases. Piperacillin-tazobactam (25%), ciprofloxacin (20%), and ceftriaxone (10%) were the most frequently non-adjusted antimicrobials.

More than half of the episodes (54%, $n = 59$) occurred after the implementation of APSS. There was a significant increase in the median appropriateness percentage of the treatment in the late-APSS period (84% [IQR 35–100], $p = 0.031$) compared with the other periods (pre-APSS: 27% [IQR 12–86]; early-APSS: 60% [IQR 9–97]) (Suppl. Data, Table S1). The proportion of inadequate prescriptions upon discharge was significantly lower (44% vs. 75% $p = 0.02$) in the late-APSS than in the pre-APSS period. Further, consultation with an infectious disease specialist was more frequent among patients with a good level of appropriateness than in the other categories (66% vs. 37%, $p = 0.002$).

3.1. Outcomes

The clinical outcomes (hospital outcomes and 30-day outcomes) are presented in Table 3. Overall, 53% ($n = 58$) of patients were admitted to the ICU and the median time to ICU admission was 7.4 h (IQR 4.0–14.9). Patients in the good appropriateness category tended to be admitted sooner (5.6 h IQR 3.7–10.4, $p = 0.25$) compared with the other groups (9.4 h [IQR 5.0–25.4]; 8.0 h [IQR 4.0–21.8]). Time from admission to first effective antimicrobial did not differ between groups ($p = 0.84$). The first antimicrobial was administered before ICU admission in most patients (89%, $n = 98$), but half of the patients who received their first antimicrobial in the ICU were in the good level of appropriateness. The patients in this group experienced more sepsis on days three and five and required more mechanical ventilation.

Table 3. Clinical outcomes stratified by the level of appropriateness.

Outcomes	Good (80–100%) $n = 47$	Moderate (20–79%) $n = 31$	Poor (0–19%) $n = 32$	Total Cohort N = 110
Hospital outcomes				
Time to defervescence (hours), median (IQR)	40.4 (71.9–84.5)	45.2 (17.9–84.5)	53.7 (26.2–90.3)	45 (15.4–87.6)
WBC time to normalization, (hours), median (IQR)	60.6 (24.4–144.8)	70.6 (35.1–111.0)	62.1 (43.8–109.9)	68.3 (32.2–114.0)
Sepsis [a]	38 (81)	23 (74)	17 (53) *	78 (71)
Day 3	23/46 (50)	16/31 (52)	7/31 (23) *	46/108 (43)
Day 5	17/39 (44)	5/26 (19) *	7/23 (30)	29/88 (33)
Mechanical ventilation	17 (36)	9 (29)	4 (13) *	30 (27)
Duration of mechanical ventilation (days), median (IQR)	4 (2–6)	3 (1–6)	2 (1–7)	3 (2–6)
ICU LOS (hours), median (IQR)	117.6 (67.8–204.7)	107.9 (67.8–141.9)	39.0 (27.4–109.3)	99.7 (43.6–174.5)
LOS (hours), median (IQR)	258.1 (126.7–496.0)	171.9 (117.9–293.3) *	174.6 (98.8–289.1) *	194.5 (114.8–417.4)
30-day outcomes				
Readmission				
All-causes	4/41 (10)	5/28 (18)	2/32 (6)	11/101 (11)
Relapse	1/41 (2)	3/28 (11)	1/32 (6)	5/101 (5)
Time to readmission (days), median (IQR) [b]	13 (3–21)	11 (5–19)	-	11 (7–18)
All-cause 30-day mortality	6 (13)	3 (10)	0	9 (8)

Results are reported as number (%) or median (IQR). Abbreviations: IQR: interquartile range, WBC: white blood cells, ICU: intensive care unit, LOS: length of stay. [a] At least one day with mSOFA ≥ 2, on days 1, 3, 5, 7. [b] In cases with poor appropriateness, only 2 patients were readmitted with time to readmission of 9 and 18 days. * Statistically significant difference (p value < 0.05), reference category: good (80–100%).

Although more patients from the good and moderate appropriateness groups were readmitted within 30 days from discharge and had high mortality rates, these differences did not reach statistical significance.

3.2. Factors Associated with Adjusted Antimicrobial Therapy

Factors associated with antimicrobial dosing adjusted for obesity are presented in Table 4. In the adjusted model, the number of antimicrobials (aOR 2.2, 95% CI 1.4–3.4,), consultation with an infectious disease specialist (aOR 3.3, 95% CI 1.3–8.6), blood urea nitrogen (BUN) 7–10.9 mmol/L (aOR 7.3, 95% CI 1.8–29.5), and hemodialysis (aOR 10.30, 95% CI 1.62–65.56) were significantly associated with high appropriateness. BMI >50 or weight >120 kg was not associated with adjusted antimicrobial dosing.

Table 4. Factors associated with adjusted antimicrobial therapy.

Factors	No. Adjusted Therapy/ Total (%)	Univariable OR (95% IC)	p Value	Multivariable OR (95% IC)	p Value
Number of antimicrobials	-	2.19 (1.43–3.14)	<0.001	2.17 (1.40–3.37)	<0.001
Consultation with an infectious disease specialist					
No	16/56 (29)	reference		reference	
Yes	31/54 (57)	3.37 (1.53–7.44)	0.003	3.33 (1.29–8.58)	0.013
Sepsis on day 1					
No	10/36 (28)	reference			
Yes	37/74 (50)	2.60 (1.10–6.14)	0.03		
BUN (mmol/L)					
<7	7/32 (22)	reference		reference	
7–10.9	14/22 (64)	6.25 (1.87–20.90)	0.003	7.34 (1.83–29.48)	0.005
≥11	25/52 (48)	3.31 (1.22–8.98)	0.02	2.51 (0.74–8.46)	0.14
missing	1/4 (25)	1.190 (0.11–13.30)	0.89	0.51 (0.03–8.49)	0.6
APSS					
No	17/51 (33)	reference			
Yes	30/59 (51)	2.07 (0.95–4.49)	0.066		
Immunosuppression					
No	36/93 (39)	reference			
Yes	11/17 (65)	2.90 (0.99–8.54)	0.05		
Hemodialysis					
No	39/100 (39)	reference		reference	
Yes	8/10 (80)	6.26 (1.26–31.01)	0.03	10.30 (1.62–65.56)	0.014
Charlson comorbidity index					
0–3	17/45 (38)	reference			
4–6	26/44 (59)	2.38 (1.02–5.57)	0.05		
≥7	4/21 (19)	0.388 (0.11–1.35)	0.14		
PBS					
0–1	15/53 (28)	reference			
≥2	32/57 (56)	3.24 (1.47–7.18)	0.004		
Infection site					
Urinary	10/37 (27)	reference			
Pulmonary	8/13 (62)	4.32 (1.14–16.37)	0.03		
Skin and soft tissue	11/27 (41)	1.86 (0.65–5.34)	0.25		
Other	18/33 (55)	3.24 (1.19–8.79)	0.02		

Reference category: 0–19% poor (vs. 20–100%). Abbreviations: BUN: blood urea nitrogen, APSS: Antimicrobial Prescription Surveillance System, PBS: Pitt bacteremia score.

3.3. Factors Associated with Unfavourable Outcomes

Overall, 55% ($n = 60$) of the patients had at least one of the following components of a composite outcome: ICU stay ≥72 h (33%, $n = 36$), duration of sepsis >3 days (34%, $n = 37$), LOS ≥7 days (55%, $n = 61$), and 30-day mortality (8%, $n = 9$). Risk factors for unfavourable outcomes are shown in Table 5. In multivariable analysis, age (aOR 1.07, 95% CI 1.02–1.12, $p = 0.009$), PBS ≥2 (aOR 7.30, 95% CI 2.09–25.52, $p = 0.002$), sepsis on day 1 (aOR 16.78, 95% CI 3.93–71.63, $p < 0.001$), and infection site (pulmonary aOR 7.52, 95% CI 1.20–47.15, $p = 0.031$, skin and soft tissue aOR 7.79, 95% CI 1.67–36.41, $p = 0.009$, others aOR 9.47, 95% CI 1.99–45.10, $p = 0.005$) were significantly associated with unfavourable outcomes. After adjustment, no measure of treatment appropriateness (first adjusted prescription, adjusted prescription within the first 72 h, and level of appropriateness) was associated with unfavourable outcomes.

Table 5. Factors associated with unfavourable outcomes.

Factors	No. Unfavourable Outcomes/ Total (%)	Univariable OR (95% CI)	p Value	Multivariable OR (95% CI)	p Value
Age (years)	-	1.05 (1.01–1.08)	0.01	1.07 (1.02–1.12)	0.009
BMI (kg/m^2)	-	1.02 (0.95–1.08)	0.64		
Charlson comorbidity index	-	1.19 (1.02–1.38)	0.02		
Hemodialysis					
No	58/100 (58)	reference			
Yes	2/10 (20)	0.18 (0.04–0.90)	0.04		
PBS ≥ 2					
No	15/53 (28)	reference		reference	
Yes	45/57 (79)	9.50 (3.97–22.75)	<0.001	7.30 (2.09–25.52)	0.002
Sepsis on day 1					
No	4/36 (11)	reference		reference	
Yes	56/74 (76)	24.89 (7.75–79.97)	<0.001	16.78 (3.93–71.63)	<0.001
Infection site					
Urinary	11/37 (30)	reference		reference	
Pulmonary	10/13 (77)	7.88 (1.81–34.28)	0.01	7.52 (1.20–47.15)	0.031
Skin and soft tissue	20/27 (74)	6.75 (2.22–20.55)	0.001	7.79 (1.67–36.41)	0.009
Other	19/33 (58)	3.21 (1.20–8.60)	0.02	9.47 (1.99–45.10)	0.005
BUN (mmol/L)					
<7	9/32 (28)	reference			
7–10.9	16/22 (73)	6.82 (2.02–22.95)	0.002		
≥11	35/52 (67)	5.26 (2.01–13.80)	0.001		
missing	0/4 (0)	-			
Appropriateness category					
Good (80–100%)	30/47 (64)	2.94 (1.16–7.46)	0.02		
Moderate (20–79%)	18/31 (58)	2.31 (0.84–6.34)	0.11		
Poor (0–19%)	12/32 (38)	reference			
Number of antimicrobials	-	1.98 (1.34–2.93)	0.001		
Type of antimicrobial (based on PD)					
Concentration-dependent	1/11 (9)	reference			
Time-dependent	25/38 (66)	19.23 (2.21–167.11)	0.007		
Mixed	34/61 (56)	12.59 (1.52–104.58)	0.02		

Abbreviations: BMI: body mass index, PBS: Pitt bacteremia score, BUN: blood urea nitrogen, PD: pharmacodynamics.

4. Discussion

Since the prevalence of obesity continues to rise, and as individuals with obesity are likely to receive a high number of antimicrobials [25,26] and complex antimicrobial treatment [27], a better understanding of the impact of optimal dosing adjustment in patients with obesity is needed. In this study, we retrospectively assessed the impact of the appropriateness of antimicrobial dosing in patients with severe obesity hospitalized for BSI.

We observed low adherence to our local guidelines on the adjustment of doses for patients with severe obesity, with the first prescription being adequate in 40% of the episodes and the treatment being fully adequate in only 24% of the cases. These findings are consistent with those of previous studies, where recommendations (published or local guidelines) were rarely followed [28–31]. For instance, in patients with class III obesity, initial doses of vancomycin [28], ciprofloxacin, cefazolin, and cefepime [31] were adequate in only 0%, 1.2%, 3%, and 8% of the cases, respectively. However, in our centre, a computerized clinical decision support system designed to assist the antimicrobial stewardship program team [24] had an impact on the prescriptions for patients with obesity, as shown by a three-fold increase in the median appropriateness of the antimicrobial treatment from the pre-APSS to the late-APSS period. In addition, patients who benefited from a consultation in infectious diseases had a higher likelihood of receiving a dosage adjusted for severe obesity than those who did not. Other factors associated with a high likelihood of adjustment were the number of antimicrobials, BUN between 7 and 10.9 mmol/L, and hemodialysis.

In the univariable analysis, we initially found a significant association between good prescription adjustment (>80%) and the occurrence of unfavourable outcomes. This association is counterintuitive as it implies that optimized dosage leads to negative outcomes. However, the association ceased to exist after adjustment for disease severity and the presence of sepsis on day one. It is common practice to increase antimicrobial dosage in the sickest patients, given their altered antimicrobial pharmacokinetics [32,33]. The presence of severe obesity in these patients is an additional reason to adjust the dosage upwards [5,19]. Finally, the wide therapeutic index of most antimicrobials used in this setting favours adjustments towards higher doses, given the imbalance between the severity of their condition and the low risk of adverse effects associated with overdosing with most antimicrobials. The same pattern was observed when we used adjustment of the first dose or adjustment within the first 72 h of treatment to measure the level of dosage optimization. Interestingly, we found a negative association between secondary outcomes and level of adjustment, but it did not reach statistical significance.

The literature on the impact of dose adjustment on clinical outcomes in patients with severe obesity treated for infection is scarce. In one study, high doses of tigecycline (100 mg every 12 h) administered to patients with obesity significantly improved clinical outcomes by reducing mortality, ICU stay, recurrent infections, and septic shock events [10]. However, this retrospective cohort study was limited by the small sample (only 11 patients with obesity), and the authors did not adjust for potential confounding factors. In another study, in a subgroup analysis of patients with severe obesity hospitalized for cellulitis, a low antimicrobial dose (TMP-SMX 1 DS PO twice a day or clindamycin 150–300 mg PO every 6–8 h) was associated with a high rate of clinical failure after discharge [7]. Again, this study was limited by its small sample (46 patients with severe obesity) and by the selection of unusual agents for cellulitis treatment [34]. Finally, inadequate dosing but neither weight nor obesity was associated with clinical failure in another study, and patients weighing ≥120 kg were more likely to receive adequate doses of TMP-SMX upon discharge [35]. Time-dependent killing antimicrobials were also associated with worse outcomes but this association did not remain significant after adjustment for covariates. Most patients in our study ($n = 60$, 55%) received both time-dependent and concentration-dependent killing antimicrobials. Since 2010, β-lactams, especially piperacillin-tazobactam have generally been administered as prolonged infusions in the ICU of our center to improve drug exposures. Prolonged perfusion is an important strategy to optimize PD parameters in β-lactams (increasing the time that concentrations remain above the minimum inhibitory concentration (MIC)), rather than only increasing the dose [36,37]. Besides, MIC values and organisms must be considered when assessing effectiveness and outcomes. In our cohort, the impact of bacterial resistance was limited because we excluded episodes where the pathogen was resistant to the antimicrobial received for more than 48 h.

The PBS was chosen to determine the severity of BSI, because it is simple to calculate, and has been described to better predict outcomes in patients with sepsis (which represented 71% of our cohort) than the Acute Physiology and Chronic Health Evaluation II (APACHE II) [17]. Moreover, in retrospective studies, complex scores such as APACHE II or SOFA are likely to be unhelpful due to missing values. We used the modified SOFA (mSOFA) score to limit the impact on missing variables, due to the retrospective nature of our study [22,23].

This study has several limitations. First, the study is subject to biases and missing data due to its retrospective design. Therefore, serum concentrations were not standardized, and it was impossible to perform pharmacokinetic calculations and measure concentrations to assess the appropriateness of the patients' regimens. Consequently, we decided not to include vancomycin. However, our local guidelines related to adjustments are based on published studies in which PK/PD data were available. We could not assess microbiologic clearance or the duration of BSI because blood samples are not routinely collected after the onset of BSI or they are but at various intervals. To our knowledge, no validated criteria exist to quantify the level of appropriateness. Our classification is subjective, but has been reviewed by two infectious disease specialists (A.C. and L.V.) for its clinical relevance. This classification, although far from being perfect, provides the reader with an order of magnitude regarding adjustment, but further research on this topic is needed. Finally, a posteriori, the study was limited by its small sample size, and it had 38% power to detect a difference of 15% in unfavourable outcomes between patients with and without dose adjustment, coming from a single centre. The small sample size could be explained by the limited proportion of patients hospitalized in our centre with severe obesity and infection treated with antimicrobials requiring adjustment.

However, despite these limitations, this study is the first to evaluate the association between adjustment for obesity and outcomes in patients with severe obesity and BSIs, such as urinary tract infection, pneumonia, cholangitis, and skin and tissue infections. We could assess short- and medium-term outcomes in several types of infections from various sites and of various severities, from mild symptoms to septic shock, thus providing an overview on the need for and impact of dose adjustment for patients with obesity. Most importantly, each prescription was evaluated considering renal function, which may have changed during hospitalization.

5. Conclusions

In conclusion, after adjustment for confounding factors, we did not find an association between dosing optimization and better outcomes in this cohort of patients with severe obesity and BSIs. However, in the absence of measured concentrations of antimicrobials, links between adjusted doses and outcomes can hardly be made. This study was exploratory and ideally a prospective study with the dosage of antimicrobials would be needed. This would maybe allow identifying a link between the adjustment and the outcomes, which we were unable to demonstrate. We did not find any study investigating the link between antimicrobial adjustment and outcomes like we did, in patients with class III obesity hospitalized for a bloodstream infection. Our study is intended as a first step in a field where knowledge remains extremely limited. Yet, given the wide therapeutic index of most antimicrobials and the trend of their effect on secondary outcomes, mortality, and morbidity associated with BSIs, and PK/PD data, it would be wise to continue to adjust antimicrobials upwards in patients with severe obesity and BSIs, while we wait for further evidence. Prolonged infusions also remain important strategies in optimizing PD as they may have a greater influence than dose increment. Finally, we have shown the positive impact of consultations with infectious disease specialists and an antimicrobial stewardship program based on an expert system in increasing the adherence to antimicrobial dosing adapted to patients with obesity.

Supplementary Materials: The following are available online at http://www.mdpi.com/2079-6382/9/10/707/s1, Figure S1: Flowchart of included and excluded episodes of bloodstream infections, Table S1: Variables related to the appropriateness according to the period of admission.

Author Contributions: Conceptualization, S.S., C.N.A.C., M.-F.L., J.P., A.C. and L.V.; methodology, S.S., C.N.A.C., M.-F.L., J.P. and L.V.; formal analysis, S.S., C.N.A.C. and L.V.; investigation, S.S.; writing—original draft preparation, S.S.; writing—review and editing, S.S., C.N.A.C., J.P., M.-F.L., A.C., L.V.; supervision, M.-F.L. and L.V.; funding acquisition, L.V. All authors have read and agreed to the published version of the manuscript.

Funding: This work was supported by The Canadian Medical Protective Association (CMP2519).

Conflicts of Interest: L.V. is a shareholder and medical advisor to Lumed Inc. All other authors: none to declare.

References

1. The GBD 2015 Obesity Collaborators; Afshin, A.; Forouzanfar, M.H.; Reitsma, M.B.; Sur, P.; Estep, K.; Lee, A.; Marczak, L.; Mokdad, A.H.; Moradi-Lakeh, M.; et al. Health effects of overweight and obesity in 195 countries over 25 years. *N. Engl. J. Med.* **2017**, *377*, 13–27. [CrossRef] [PubMed]
2. Falagas, M.E.; Kompoti, M. Obesity and infection. *Lancet Infect. Dis.* **2006**, *6*, 438–446. [CrossRef]
3. Huttunen, R.; Syrjänen, J. Obesity and the risk and outcome of infection. *Int. J. Obes. (Lond.)* **2013**, *37*, 333–340. [CrossRef] [PubMed]
4. Hanley, M.; Abernethy, D.R.; Greenblatt, D.J. Effect of obesity on the pharmacokinetics of drugs in humans. *Clin. Pharmacokinet.* **2010**, *49*, 71–87. [CrossRef] [PubMed]
5. Alobaid, A.S.; Hites, M.; Lipman, J.; Taccone, F.S.; Roberts, J.A. Effect of obesity on the pharmacokinetics of antimicrobials in critically ill patients: A structured review. *Int. J. Antimicrob. Agents* **2016**, *47*, 259–268. [CrossRef] [PubMed]
6. Abdullahi, M.; Annibale, B.; Capoccia, D.; Tari, R.; Lahner, E.; Osborn, J.; Leonetti, F.; Severi, C. The eradication of *Helicobacter pylori* is affected by body mass index (BMI). *Obes. Surg.* **2008**, *18*, 1450–1454. [CrossRef]
7. Halilovic, J.; Heintz, B.H.; Brown, J. Risk factors for clinical failure in patients hospitalized with cellulitis and cutaneous abscess. *J. Infect.* **2012**, *65*, 128–134. [CrossRef]
8. Longo, C.; Bartlett, G.; Macgibbon, B.; Mayo, N.; Rosenberg, E.; Nadeau, L.; Daskalopoulou, S.S. The effect of obesity on antibiotic treatment failure: A historical cohort study. *Pharmacoepidemiol. Drug Saf.* **2013**, *22*, 970–976. [CrossRef]
9. Theofiles, M.; Maxson, J.; Herges, L.; Marcelin, A.; Angstman, K.B. Cellulitis in obesity: Adverse outcomes affected by increases in body mass index. *J. Prim. Care Community Health* **2015**, *6*, 233–238. [CrossRef]
10. Ibrahim, M.M.; Abuelmatty, A.M.; Mohamed, G.H.; Nasr, M.A.; Hussein, A.K.; El Deen Ebaed, M.; Sarhan, H.A. Best tigecycline dosing for treatment of infections caused by multidrug-resistant pathogens in critically ill patients with different body weights. *Drug Des. Dev. Ther.* **2018**, *12*, 4171–4179. [CrossRef]
11. Goto, M.; Al-Hasan, M.N. Overall burden of bloodstream infection and nosocomial bloodstream infection in North America and Europe. *Clin. Microbiol. Infect.* **2013**, *19*, 501–509. [CrossRef]
12. Paulsen, J.; Askim, Å.; Mohus, R.M.; Mehl, A.; Dewan, A.; Solligård, E.; Damås, J.K.; Åsvold, B.O. Associations of obesity and lifestyle with the risk and mortality of bloodstream infection in a general population: A 15-year follow-up of 64 027 individuals in the HUNT Study. *Int. J. Epidemiol.* **2017**, *46*, 1573–1581. [CrossRef]
13. Atamna, A.; Elis, A.; Gilady, E.; Gitter-Azulay, L.; Bishara, J. How obesity impacts outcomes of infectious diseases. *Eur. J. Clin. Microbiol. Infect. Dis.* **2017**, *36*, 585–591. [CrossRef]
14. Lizza, B.D.; Rhodes, N.J.; Esterly, J.S.; Toy, C.; Lopez, J.; Scheetz, M.H. Impact of body mass index on clinical outcomes in patients with gram-negative bacteria bloodstream infections. *J. Infect. Chemother.* **2016**, *22*, 671–676. [CrossRef] [PubMed]
15. Lam, S.W.; Athans, V. Clinical and microbiological outcomes in obese patients receiving colistin for carbapenem-resistant gram-negative bloodstream infection. *Antimicrob. Agents Chemother.* **2019**, *63*, e00531-19. [CrossRef] [PubMed]
16. Lines, J.; Yang, Z.; Bookstaver, P.B.; Catchings, E.; Justo, J.A.; Kohn, J.; Albrecht, H.; Al-Hasan, M.N.; Palmetto Health Antimicrobial Stewardship and Support Team. Association between body mass index and mortality in patients with gram-negative bloodstream infections. *Infect. Dis. Clin. Pract.* **2019**, *27*, 90–95. [CrossRef]
17. Rhee, J.Y.; Kwon, K.T.; Ki, H.K.; Shin, S.Y.; Jung, D.S.; Chung, D.R.; Ha, B.C.; Peck, K.R.; Song, J.H. Scoring systems for prediction of mortality in patients with intensive care unit-acquired sepsis: A comparison of the Pitt bacteremia score and the Acute Physiology and Chronic Health Evaluation II scoring systems. *Shock* **2009**, *31*, 146–150. [CrossRef]
18. Paterson, D.L.; Ko, W.C.; Von Gottberg, A.; Mohapatra, S.; Casellas, J.M.; Goossens, H.; Mulazimoglu, L.; Trenholme, G.; Klugman, K.P.; Bonomo, R.A.; et al. International prospective study of *Klebsiella pneumoniae* bacteremia: Implications of extended-spectrum beta-lactamase production in nosocomial infections. *Ann. Intern. Med.* **2004**, *140*, 26–32. [CrossRef] [PubMed]
19. Meng, L.; Mui, E.; Holubar, M.K.; Deresinski, S.C. Comprehensive guidance for antibiotic dosing in obese adults. *Pharmacotherapy* **2017**, *37*, 1415–1431. [CrossRef]
20. Srinivas, N.R. Influence of morbid obesity on the clinical pharmacokinetics of various anti-infective drugs: Reappraisal using recent case studies-issues, dosing implications, and considerations. *Am. J. Ther.* **2018**, *25*, e224–e246. [CrossRef]

21. Winter, M.A.; Guhr, K.N.; Berg, G.M. Impact of various body weights and serum creatinine concentrations on the bias and accuracy of the Cockcroft-Gault equation. *Pharmacotherapy* **2012**, *32*, 604–612. [CrossRef] [PubMed]
22. Grissom, C.K.; Brown, S.M.; Kuttler, K.G.; Boltax, J.P.; Jones, J.; Jephson, A.R.; Orme, J.F., Jr. A modified sequential organ failure assessment score for critical care triage. *Disaster Med. Public Health Prep.* **2010**, *4*, 277–284. [CrossRef] [PubMed]
23. Rahmatinejad, Z.; Reihani, H.; Tohidinezhad, F.; Rahmatinejad, F.; Peyravi, S.; Pourmand, A.; Abu-Hanna, A.; Eslami, S. Predictive performance of the SOFA and mSOFA scoring systems for predicting in-hospital mortality in the emergency department. *Am. J. Emerg. Med.* **2019**, *37*, 1237–1241. [CrossRef] [PubMed]
24. Nault, V.; Pepin, J.; Beaudoin, M.; Perron, J.; Moutquin, J.M.; Valiquette, L. Sustained impact of a computer-assisted antimicrobial stewardship intervention on antimicrobial use and length of stay. *J. Antimicrob. Chemother.* **2017**, *72*, 933–940. [CrossRef] [PubMed]
25. Counterweight Project Team. The impact of obesity on drug prescribing in primary care. *Br. J. Gen. Pract.* **2005**, *55*, 743–749.
26. Papadimitriou-Olivgeris, M.; Aretha, D.; Zotou, A.; Koutsileou, K.; Aikaterini, Z.; Aikaterini, L.; Sklavou, C.; Marangos, M.; Fligou, F. The role of obesity in sepsis outcome among critically ill patients: A retrospective cohort analysis. *Biomed. Res. Int.* **2016**, *2016*, 5941279. [CrossRef]
27. Charani, E.; Gharbi, M.; Frost, G.; Drumright, L.; Holmes, A. Antimicrobial therapy in obesity: A multicentre cross-sectional study. *J. Antimicrob. Chemother.* **2015**, *70*, 2906–2912. [CrossRef]
28. Hall, R.G.; Payne, K.D.; Bain, A.M.; Rahman, A.P.; Nguyen, S.T.; Eaton, S.A.; Busti, A.J.; Vu, S.L.; Bedimo, R. Multicenter evaluation of vancomycin dosing: Emphasis on obesity. *Am. J. Med.* **2008**, *121*, 515–518. [CrossRef]
29. Davis, S.L.; Scheetz, M.H.; Bosso, J.A.; Goff, D.A.; Rybak, M.J. Adherence to the 2009 consensus guidelines for vancomycin dosing and monitoring practices: A cross-sectional survey of U.S. hospitals. *Pharmacotherapy* **2013**, *33*, 1256–1263. [CrossRef]
30. Rosini, J.M.; Grovola, M.R.; Levine, B.J.; Jasani, N.B. Prescribing habits of vancomycin in the Emergency Department: Are we dosing appropriately? *J. Emerg. Med.* **2013**, *44*, 979–984. [CrossRef]
31. Roe, J.L.; Fuentes, J.M.; Mullins, M.E. Underdosing of common antibiotics for obese patients in the ED. *Am. J. Emerg. Med.* **2012**, *30*, 1212–1214. [CrossRef] [PubMed]
32. Liang, S.Y.; Kumar, A. Empiric antimicrobial therapy in severe sepsis and septic shock: Optimizing pathogen clearance. *Curr. Infect. Dis. Rep.* **2015**, *17*, 493. [CrossRef] [PubMed]
33. Rhodes, A.; Evans, L.E.; Alhazzani, W.; Levy, M.M.; Antonelli, M.; Ferrer, R.; Kumar, A.; Sevransky, J.E.; Sprung, C.L.; Nunnally, M.E.; et al. Surviving Sepsis Campaign: International Guidelines for Management of Sepsis and Septic Shock: 2016. *Intensive Care Med.* **2017**, *43*, 304–377. [CrossRef]
34. Stevens, D.L.; Bisno, A.L.; Chambers, H.F.; Dellinger, E.P.; Goldstein, E.J.C.; Gorbach, S.L.; Hirschmann, J.V.; Kaplan, S.L.; Montoya, J.G.; Wade, J.C. Practice guidelines for the diagnosis and management of skin and soft tissue infections: 2014 update by the Infectious Diseases Society of America. *Clin. Infect. Dis.* **2014**, *59*, e10–e52. [CrossRef] [PubMed]
35. Cox, K.K.; Alexander, B.; Livorsi, D.J.; Heintz, B.H. Clinical outcomes in patients hospitalized with cellulitis treated with oral clindamycin and trimethoprim-sulfamethoxazole: The role of weight-based dosing. *J. Infect.* **2017**, *75*, 486–492. [CrossRef]
36. Cheatham, S.C.; Fleming, M.R.; Healy, D.P.; Chung, C.E.K.; Shea, K.M.; Humphrey, M.L.; Kays, M.B. Steady state pharmacokinetics and pharmacodynamics of piperacillin and tazobactam administered by prolonged infusion in obese patients. *Int. J. Antimicrob. Agents* **2013**, *41*, 52–56. [CrossRef] [PubMed]
37. Chung, E.K.; Cheatham, S.C.; Fleming, M.R.; Healy, D.P.; Shea, K.M.; Kays, M.B. Population pharmacokinetics and pharmacodynamics of piperacillin and tazobactam administered by prolonged infusion in obese and nonobese patients. *J. Clin. Pharmacol.* **2015**, *55*, 899–908. [CrossRef] [PubMed]

Publisher's Note: MDPI stays neutral with regard to jurisdictional claims in published maps and institutional affiliations.

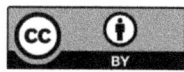

© 2020 by the authors. Licensee MDPI, Basel, Switzerland. This article is an open access article distributed under the terms and conditions of the Creative Commons Attribution (CC BY) license (http://creativecommons.org/licenses/by/4.0/).

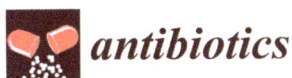

Article

Effective Treatment for Uncomplicated Urinary Tract Infections with Oral Fosfomycin, Single Center Four Year Retrospective Study

Miroslav Fajfr [1,2], Michal Balik [2,3], Eva Cermakova [4] and Pavel Bostik [1,2,5,*]

1. Institute of Clinical Microbiology, University Hospital, Sokolska 581, 500 05 Hradec Kralove, Czech Republic; miroslav.fajfr@fnhk.cz
2. Faculty of Medicine in Hradec Kralove, Charles University in Prague, Simkova 870, 500 38 Hradec Kralove, Czech Republic; michal.balik@fnhk.cz
3. Department of Urology, University Hospital, Sokolska 581, 500 05 Hradec Kralove, Czech Republic
4. Faculty of Medicine in Hradec Kralove, Department of Medical Biophysics, Charles University in Prague, Simkova 870, 500 38 Hradec Kralove, Czech Republic; cermakovae@lfhk.cuni.cz
5. Faculty of Military Health Sciences, University of Defence, Trebesska 1575, 500 01 Hradec Kralove, Czech Republic
* Correspondence: pavel.bostik@unob.cz; Tel.: +420-724-692-609

Received: 16 July 2020; Accepted: 11 August 2020; Published: 13 August 2020

Abstract: Fosfomycin represents a relatively old antibiotic, but it is experiencing a comeback in recent years. According to some studies, the increasing therapeutic use of this drug led to a rapid increase in the levels of resistance in bacteria causing urinary tract infection. In the presented study, levels of resistance to fosfomycin in more than 3500 bacterial isolates before and after fosfomycin introduction into therapeutic use in the Czech Republic and the clinical efficacy of treatment in 300 patients using this drug were assessed. The results show that the resistance levels to fosfomycin in *Escherichia coli* isolates before and after the drug registration were not significantly different (3.4% and 4.4%, respectively). In some other Gram-negative rods, such as otherwise susceptible *Enterobacter*, resistance to fosfomycin increased significantly from 45.6% to 76.6%. Fosfomycin treatment of urinary tract infections showed an excellent seven-day clinical efficacy (79.7%). However, when used to treat recurrent or complicated urinary tract infections, fosfomycin treatment was associated with high levels of infection relapse, leading to relapse in a total of 20.4% of patients during the first two months. This indicates that fosfomycin exhibits good efficacy only for the treatment of uncomplicated urinary tract infections

Keywords: fosfomycin; urinary infection; resistance

1. Introduction

Fosfomycin was introduced for the first time in 1969 as a product of *Streptomyces fradiae*, and it was also isolated from some members of the *Pseudomonas* species [1]. This drug was used for a long time in the treatment of urinary tract infections (UTIs), but the development of newer antibiotics led to a gradual decrease in its use. However, with the development of bacterial resistance to many antibiotics (i.e., β-lactam antibiotics, quinolones, aminglycosides) worldwide, fosfomycin is coming back as a viable alternative. Many countries adopted fosfomycin trometamol in their guidelines for urinary tract infection management not only for uncomplicated infections, but also for infections caused by multidrug-resistant bacteria [2,3]. However, this was associated, in turn, with a rapid increase in the resistance level of bacteria to fosfomycin, according to data from several countries. Data from Spain show an increase in Fosfomycin-resistant *Escherichia coli* extended-spectrum beta-lactamase (ESBL)-producing isolates from 4.4% in 2005 to 11.4% in 2009. However, the overall resistance level of all

Escherichia coli isolates (ESBL producers and ESBL non-producers) to fosfomycin in this study remained low at 2.9% in 2019. Another study from China showed that a high percentage of carbapenemase (KPC)-producing *Klebsiella pneumoniae* isolates harbor FosA3 (34%), which would suggest the loss of effectiveness of fosfomycin and the multidrug resistance (MDR) of these bacteria. Data from Poland show the overall susceptibility of *E. coli* isolates to fosfomycin to be 62.2% in complicated UTIs and 77.6% in uncomplicated UTIs [4–6]. These data, thus, indicate a potential problem in the use of fosfomycin in the treatment of nosocomial acquired urinary tract infections (UTIs).

In the Czech Republic, fosfomycin trometamol was not licensed for clinical use until October 2014. The resistance of bacteria was, therefore, very low, as described in our previous work and as also reported from other countries [7,8]. In 2015, oral fosfomycin trometamol was implemented into the Czech national UTI treatment guidelines as a drug of second choice for uncomplicated infections of the lower urinary tract. Here, we describe a study of the clinical effects of fosfomycin trometamol use in the University Hospital in Hradec Kralove, Czech Republic, and we evaluate trends in bacterial susceptibility to fosfomycin during the first four years of its use for the treatment of UTIs.

2. Results

2.1. Susceptibility of Bacteria Causing UTI to Fosfomycin

The prevalence of individual bacterial strains isolated from urine samples was similar when comparing samples from two patient cohorts before (Cohort 1) and after (Cohort 2) the introduction of fosfomycin into the treatment of UTIs. The most frequent bacterium isolated was *Escherichia coli*, with levels of 46.1% and 49.7%, respectively. Other bacteria isolated more frequently than in 10% of samples were *Enterococcus faecalis* and *Klebsiella* species. The similar bacterial stratification allowed for a comparison of both cohorts in the next step. The entire spectrum of bacteria isolated is shown in Figure 1.

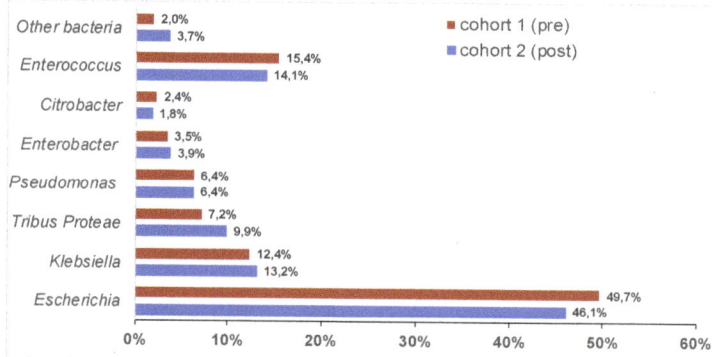

Figure 1. Proportional representation of bacteria isolated from urine samples in Cohort 1 (before fosfomycin registration) and Cohort 2 (after fosfomycin registration). Bacteria were stratified by families; Tribus *Proteae* includes *Proteus* spp., *Morganella* spp., and *Providentia* spp.

The general level of resistance (beta-lactamase production, resistance to fluoroquinolones, and multidrug resistance) of Gram-negative bacteria showed a notable increase over time when analyzed in the older (Cohort1) and more recent (Cohort 2) samples (Table 1). Thus, the number of high-risk beta-lactamase-positive (ESBL, AmpC, and K1) bacterial strains rose from 11.7% to 19.8%, and the number of fluoroquinolone-resistant ones rose from 25.9% to 33.8%. *Escherichia* species isolates generally showed lower levels of resistance to antibiotics with no significant increase over time ($p = 0.23304$). The highest level of resistance was detected in *Klebsiella* species isolates, but there was also no significant increase when comparing the two cohorts ($p = 0.53870$). On the contrary, multidrug-resistant (MDR) *Pseudomonas* isolates (defined as resistant to beta-lactams, carbapenems, and fluoroquinolones) showed a markable and statistically significant increase over time from 5.6% to 13.3% ($p = 0.00026$).

Table 1. Resistance levels of the most frequent pathogenic bacteria from urine samples before (Cohort 1) and after (Cohort 2) fosfomycin registration. Brackets indicate statistically significant differences ($p < 0.05$) between Cohort 1 and Cohort 2.

Bacteria	Cohort 1													Cohort 2												
	BL (ESBL, AmpC, K1)		iAmpC		FQR		MDR		NO RES		BL (ESBL, AmpC, K1)		iAmpC		FQR		MDR		NO RES	
	%	No.	%	No.	%	No.	%	No.	%	No.	%	No.	%	No.	%	No.	%	No.	%	No.
Citrobacter spp.	12.1	4	(0.0)	0	9.1	3	0.0	0	(78.8)	26	10.5	10	(25.3)	24	12.6	12	0.0	0	(51.6)	49
Enterobacter spp.	19.2	10	(0.0)	0	19.2	10	0.0	0	(61.6)	32	26.9	56	(24.5)	51	14.9	31	0.0	0	(33.7)	70
Escherichia coli	5.4	37	0.0	0	17.0	116	0.0	0	77.6	530	7.3	166	0.2	4	17.2	392	0.0	0	75.3	1714
Klebsiella spp.	29.0	64	0.0	0	37.5	83	0.0	0	33.5	74	30.8	252	0.4	3	33.2	272	0.0	0	35.6	291
Pseudomonas spp.	0.0	0	0.0	0	(42.7)	38	(5.6)	5	51.7	46	0.0	0	0.0	0	(21.9)	66	(13.3)	40	64.8	195
Tribus *Proteae*	2.1	2	(0.0)	0	27.8	27	0.0	0	(70.1)	68	4.3	21	(11.6)	57	32.4	159	0.0	0	(51.7)	254

BL—high-risk beta-lactamases (ESBL, AmpC, K1); iAmpC—inducibile AmpC beta-lactamases; FQR—fluoroquinolone resistance; MDR—multidrug resistance; NO RES—no resistance; Tribus *Proteae*—*Proteus* spp., *Morganella* spp., and *Providentia* spp.

The analysis of resistance of the three most common Gram-negative rods to fosfomycin and its development over time is shown in Table 2. Eesistance to fosfomycin was generally low in all *Escherichia* isolates, with no statistically significant differences before and after the fosfomycin registration, with levels of 4.4% and 3.4%, respectively. However, both *Klebsiella* and *Enterobacter* isolates showed statistically significant increases in resistance after the introduction of fosfomycin. Thus, in the high-risk beta-lactamase-producing *Klebsiella* isolates, the resistance to fosfomycin increased from 87% to 95.2% ($p = 0.0467$). In the *Enterobacter* isolates with no other resistance detected, fosfomycin resistance increased dramatically from 45.6% to 76.6% ($p = 0.0105$). However, the overall increase in fosfomycin resistance in all *Enterobacter* isolates was also high and statistically significant (55.2% vs. 74.4%; $p = 0.0468$). Taken together, of the more prevalent bacterial isolates from the UTIs that showed other drug resistances (high-risk beta-lactamases production or resistance to fluroquinolones), only the *E. coli* isolates were sufficiently susceptible to fosfomycin both before and after its introduction into the treatment regimes.

Table 2. Resistance levels of the most frequent Gram-negative bacteria from urine samples to fosfomycin before (Cohort 1) and after (Cohort 2) fosfomycin registration. Brackets indicate statistically significant differences ($p < 0.05$) between Cohort 1 and Cohort 2.

Bacteria		Cohort 1		Cohort 2	
	Resistance	Fosfomycin Resistant (%)	Total	Fosfomycin Resistant (%)	Total
Escherichia coli	BL	16.0	25	8.7	161
	FQR	0.0	43	3.8	262
	NO	4.0	273	2.8	1702
Escherichia coli in total	ALL	4.4		3.4	
Klebsiella species	BL	(87.0)	54	(95.2)	165
	FQR	83.3	12	90.6	32
	NO	74.5	47	79.6	147
Klebsiella species in total	ALL	81.4		88.1	
Enterobacter species	BL	85.7	7	81.0	21
	FQR	0.0	0	100.0	1
	iAmpC	0.0	0	53.8	13
	NO	(45.6)	22	(76.6)	47
Enterobacter species in total	ALL	(55.2)		(74.4)	

BL—high-risk beta-lactamases (ESBL, AmpC, K1); iAmpC—inducible AmpC beta-lactamases; FQR—fluoroquinolone resistance; NO—no resistance.

2.2. Clinical Efficacy of Fosfomycin

The clinical effects were analyzed in 300 patients treated with fosfomycin trometamol for UTIs (Cohort 3). The basic demographic data of the patients are shown in Table 3. In total, 428 fosfomycin trometamol doses were prescribed, i.e., 1.43 doses on average for a patient, with a maximum of four doses per patient. Altogether, 66.0% ($n = 198$) of patients were administered a single dose and 34.0% ($n = 102$) of patients received multiple doses. Multiple-dose therapy was used mostly in patients with complicated (in 51.0% of these cases) or recurrent (in 43.7% of these cases) infections, but it was relatively rare in patients with uncomplicated infections (in 19.5% of these cases). In 50.0% of patients, bacterial cultivation was performed before fosfomycin treatment, while 50.0% of patients were treated empirically without the culture. The type of UTI was clearly specified in 234 cases. In 67.1% ($n = 157$) of patients, complicated/recurrent UTIs were diagnosed, while 32.9% of patients had an uncomplicated UTI (all females). Nearly 30% of patients ($n = 88$) did not come for a follow-up visit, and the therapeutic effect could not be evaluated.

Table 3. Basic demographic data of patients from Cohort 3 (patients evaluated for fosfomycin treatment efficacy). UTI—urinary tract infection.

Demographic Characteristics of Patients			
Variables	Parameters		%
Gender	Male	77	25.7
	Female	223	74.3
Age (years)	Average	51 years	Range 16–93 years
UTI type *	Uncomplicated	77	32.9
	Recurrent	110	47.0
	Complicated	47	20.1

* Only patients with available data.

The clinical effects of fosfomycin treatment in the individual groups are shown in Table 4. Among those, where the effects could be evaluated, fosfomycin had an immediate curative effect in 79.7% of cases ($n = 169$); however, in 20.1% of cases ($n = 43$), the drug had no positive effect. The highest fosfomycin immediate cure rate was observed in patients with infections caused by *Escherichia* species (69.8%) and *Enterococcus faecalis* (50.0%). In cases with no detectable antibiotic effect of fosfomycin, the bacterial culture (before antibiotic administration or control culture) was performed in 79.1% of patients. In one-third of these patients, susceptible bacteria were detected (*Escherichia* species or *Enterococcus faecalis*), while the culture was negative in 26.5% of cases ($n = 9$) and 14.7% ($n = 5$) had mixed culture; the remaining cases involved bacteria with no EUCAST susceptibility breakpoints of fosfomycin in the disc diffusion test (*Klebsiella pneumoniae*, *Pseudomonas aeruginosa*, *Streptococcus agalactiae*).

Table 4. Results of clinical efficacy evaluation of fosfomycin treatment, case distribution according to UTI type, and clinical follow-up after fosfomycin administration. Statistically significant differences (at $p < 0.05$) are shown in brackets.

UTI Type	Relapse (in %)				Total
	No Relapse/Fully Cured	No Effect	Relapse ≤2 M	Relapse 2–12 M	
Complicated	38.1	33.3	16.7	11.9	42
Recurrent	29.6	23.2	28.7	18.5	108
Uncomplicated	(77.8)	11.1	(5.6)	5.6	36

M—months.

The second evaluation criterion was the recurrence level after the administration of fosfomycin up to one year after drug use. Sufficient data could only be obtained from 186 patients, since 114 patients escaped the evidence of the Urology Clinic. The fact, the relatively high number of patients with uncomplicated UTIs that were not present for their follow-up visit may indicate that the antibiotic had a curable effect (according to standard procedures, in the case of successful treatment, no follow-up visit is needed). However, since there was no evidence for it, these patients were excluded from the analysis. From the included cases, 40.9% ($n = 76$) had no relapse of the same UTI, 21.5% ($n = 43$) had a relapse during the first two months after fosfomycin treatment, and 14.5% ($n = 27$) of patients had recurrence in the time period of 2–12 months after fosfomycin administration. From the patients with an early relapse, 57.5% were administered a single dose and 42.5% were administered multiple doses of the drug. In most cases, fosfomycin had no effect or the UTI showed early recurrence in patients with complicated UTIs (complicated UTIs created more than 90% of acute fosfomycin failure cases or cases with early recurrence). However, in patients with uncomplicated UTIs, cure failure or recurrence was very rare (5.6–11.1%). Thus, the statistical evaluation showed a much lower relapse rate in the group with uncomplicated UTIs in comparison to complicated or recurring UTIs for all three analyzed time periods, which was highly significant ($p = 0.00004$).

The dosage impact on immediate effect was not seen, as the same percentage of single-dose therapy (60.4% and 60.3%) was found in cases with no cure effect and with immediate cure effect.

3. Discussion

In this study, urine samples from patients experiencing urinary tract infections were analyzed with the aim to assess the efficacy of fosfomycin treatment and to identify whether the introduction of this drug into the treatment regime led to any increase in antimicrobial resistance to fosfomycin. Although many patients did not come for their follow-up visits, thereby decreasing the numbers available for analysis, the size of our cohort is comparable to the studies cited throughout this report and elsewhere [9]; therefore it represents, in our opinion, a valid set of data, which can be used for further treatment guidance.

Our study showed a relatively stable proportion of bacterial species isolated from the UTIs with a dominance of *E. coli*, *Enterococcus faecalis*, and *Klebsiella* species. These bacterial species represent the most prevalent isolates from urinary tract infections worldwide [10,11]. Previous studies showed that fosfomycin remains very effective for the treatment of urinary tract infections caused by various bacteria, including *E. coli* or enterococci, in which the susceptibility to the drug was reported around 90% [7,10,12,13]. This was fully confirmed by our data, where the overall susceptibility in both cohorts (pre- and post-fosfomycin introduction) was 96.5% for all *E. coli* isolates and 100.0% for *Enterococcus faecalis* (data not shown). While there is some evidence of similarly high susceptibility to fosfomycin in ESBL-producing bacteria [13], most studies showed significantly lower numbers (around 80%) than in non-beta-lactamase producers [7,10,14]. This overall trend was also reflected in the data presented here. For example, while the resistance level in non-ESBL isolates of *E. coli* was 3.0%, the resistance increased to 9.7% in ESBL-positive isolates.

According to a previously published meta-analysis, the risk of selecting resistant mutants during fosfomycin monotherapy was calculated at 3.4% [15]. This is likely why some countries, such as China, Spain, Turkey, and some regions of India, reported alarmingly increasing fosfomycin resistance levels associated with its increased application. Thus, the fosfomycin resistance levels of non-beta lactamase-producing *E. coli* reached as high as 15% in some of these countries [16]. On the contrary, in some other areas, including Japan and the majority of the European and American countries, fosfomycin resistance was maintained at low levels around 4.5% despite the increase in drug use [12,16,17]. Moreover, reports from Hungary showed inconsistent fosfomycin resistance levels of *Citrobacter*, *Enterobacter*, and *Serratia* isolates over five years of study, with an overall resistance level of 9.3% in outpatient and 13.8% in inpatient settings. The resistance level of Tribus *Proteae* members to fosfomycin from the same country was calculated to be 18.7% in inpatients and 30.3% in outpatients over 10 years of study [18,19]. A study from Israel conducted during a time period almost identical to that in our study showed a notable increase in overall fosfomycin resistance in Gram-negative bacteria from 20.7% in 2015 to 30.9% in 2016 [20]. Our data show low resistance levels in *Escherichia coli* isolates and high resistance levels in isolates of *Klebsiella* and *Enterobacter*. With the exception of *Enterobacter*, the resistance levels were, however, maintained over time with no demonstrated effect of increased fosfomycin use after its registration. The reason for this relatively stable susceptibility to fosfomycin in our country can be explained by the relatively infrequent prescription of this drug in the Czech Republic overall. In our system, fosfomycin is fully paid for by patients with no contribution from the health insurance system; as such, it is not usually the first drug of choice.

Fosfomycin was reported as a relatively effective drug for the treatment of UTIs. For example, one United States (US) study reported a microbiological cure rate of 59.0% [21] and a similar Chinese study showed an overall 15-day cure rate of 65.07%, with variability in accordance with gender, age, and infection type [22]. Our data show an overall seven-day clinical cure rate of 79.7%, which is slightly higher than the rates mentioned above. One potential explanation for the better results in our study may lie in the differences in the spectrum of bacteria isolated. Thus, in our cohort extended-spectrum beta-lactamase-producing bacteria represented only 14.0% of isolates, while, in the studies above, the numbers of multidrug-resistant isolates were higher. Our data also confirmed the correlation between the treatment efficacy and the type of UTI. Thus, a report from China showed the effectivity of fosfomycin treatment in 97.71% of uncomplicated and 62.69% of complicated UTIs [22], while our data show efficacies of 94.8% and 70.2%, respectively. A high percentage of our patients showed relapses of UTIs in our study. In total, 21.5% of patients treated with fosfomycin experienced a relapse of infection in the first two months after therapy. Fosfomycin therapy in the complicated UTIs was, according to our data, ineffective in 51.3% of cases (i.e., the drug has no effect, or there is early relapse of symptoms within two months). In the treatment of complicated UTIs or UTIs caused by multidrug-resistant microbes, many studies suggested multiple dose regimens of fosfomycin [1,21–26] with three-dose regimens being the most common. Patients in our cohorts were mostly treated with a single-dose regimen; however, about one-third of them received multiple doses. Our data support the approach to apply multiple doses of fosfomycin in complicated UTIs, because early relapses were much more frequent when single-dose regimens were used. The treatment assessment studies mostly showed multiple dose regimens within the range of 1.4 to 2.0 doses per patient in accordance with the NICE guidelines, with administration of single-dose treatments in female and double-dose regimens in male patients. In our study, the average regimen consisted of 1.4 doses per patient, and multiple-dose regimens were used more frequently in the male subgroup (in 48.7% of cases, compared to 29.0% in females), which is fully in accordance with other published data [9,21,27]. Some studies showed a significantly higher failure level in UTIs associated with *Klebsiella* infections than in those caused by *E. coli* [9,27]. Similarly, we found a higher failure rate in infections caused by *Klebsiella* isolates (35.7%) than *E. coli* (17.0%), but the highest treatment failure rate of 44.4% was present in UTIs associated with bacterial mixtures (combinations of *Kl. pneumoniae*, *E. coli*, *Proteus* spp., or *Enterococcus*).

The strength of the presented study is in the comparison of resistance levels in a naïve bacterial population (before oral fosfomycin use) with those in a bacterial population after the introduction and wide use of fosfomycin in treatment regimens. The other important aspect of the presented data lies in the evaluation of oral fosfomycin cure effectivity in urinary tract infections. Although our study had a limitation in the relatively low number of patients (in part due to the fact that many patients did not come for their follow-up visits), the size of our cohort is comparable to those cited in studies throughout this report and elsewhere (e.g., 24). The fact, that a relatively high number of patients with uncomplicated UTIs did not present for their follow-up visit may indicate that the antibiotic had a curable effect. According to standard procedures, in the case of a successful treatment, no follow-up visit is required; thus, the long-term curable effect of oral fosfomycin in uncomplicated urinary tract infections may, in fact, be even better. Nevertheless, since this could not be supported by any evidence, these patients were excluded from the analysis.

4. Materials and Methods

4.1. Patient Cohorts and Samples

Urine samples were obtained from patients treated at the Urology Clinic, University Hospital in Hradec Kralove, Czech Republic during the period 2013–2018. Samples were collected from patients with UTI signs including dysuria, flank pain, urinary frequency or urgency, leukocyturia and/or positive culture, and fever. Negative samples and all samples positive for the following microorganisms were excluded from the study: yeast, coagulase-negative staphylococci (with the exception of *Staphylococcus saprophyticus*), and other non-pathogenic bacteria (e.g., lactobacilli, corynebacteria). Moreover, all positive isolates without available fosfomycin susceptibility data were excluded.

The antimicrobial resistance of bacteria to fosfomycin prior to and following the drug's introduction into the UTI treatment guidelines was evaluated in samples from two cohorts of patients. Cohort 1 (before fosfomycin registration) consisted of samples collected in the period 2013–2014 and contained a total of 594 bacterial isolates. Cohort 2 (post fosfomycin introduction) consisted of 2935 bacterial isolates obtained from patients treated at the Urology Clinic in the years 2015–2018. The evaluation of fosfomycin treatment efficacy was performed in 300 patients (Cohort 3) treated at the Urology Clinic in the period 2015–2018 for UTIs. Of these patients, 25.7% ($n = 77$) had uncomplicated UTIs (defined as acute cystitis in women or acute cystitis in young men), 22.0% had undefined UTIs, and 52.3% ($n = 157$) had complicated UTIs (defined as recurrent UTIs, UTIs after urinary tract surgery, UTIs in men with benign prostate hyperplasia or carcinoma, or UTIs associated with lithiasis). Data from the electronic records of patients and microbiological test results were used for the assessment of clinical outcome. The patient data were strictly anonymized; thus, according to the Ethics Committee of the University Hospital, no patient consent was needed.

4.2. Susceptibility Evaluation

Standard Mueller–Hinton agar (Trios, Czech Republic) and a disc diffusion test with a 200 μg fosfomycin disc with the 50 μg of G-6-P (glucose-6-phosphate) supplement were used according to the EUCAST and CLSI guidelines. For the susceptibility evaluation of *Enterobacteriales*, the EUCAST guideline was applied (EUCAST Clinical breakpoint tables v. 09, valid from 2019-01-01). *Escherichia coli* isolates were considered susceptible to fosfomycin in the case of zone diameters ≥ 24 mm. Similar criteria were adopted to show the resistance levels in two other Gram-negative bacteria (*Klebsiella* species and *Enterobacter* species) for illustration, as used in some previous publications [10,14]. For other bacteria (*E. faecalis*), the CLSI susceptibility criteria (M100 S29, valid from 2019-01-01) were used. The following susceptibility criteria for *E. faecalis* were used: zone diameters ≥16 mm indicated susceptible isolates and zone diameters ≤ 12 mm indicated resistant ones.

4.3. Clinical Efficacy Evaluation

The clinical effects of the applied treatment were evaluated by urologists according to the criteria described below. The classification of UTIs was adopted from EAU Urological Infection Guidelines 2020 with three groups presented: uncomplicated, complicated, and recurrent (classification available on EAU website: https://uroweb.org/guideline/urological-infections/#3). The first assessment was the drug's acute effect, meaning the curative effect in the first seven days after drug administration; cases were classified as cured (the symptoms of UTI disappeared and/or negative culture result in control sample), no effect or acute failure (without any positive effect; the UTI symptoms were present despite the treatment), or not assessed (no data available, patients did not come for follow-up). The second criterion was the recurrence of the same clinical unit in the first year after drug administration with a focus on the first two months, which would indicate a relapse and treatment failure. All these data were correlated with the culture results, dose regime, and type of UTI.

4.4. Statistics

Statistical evaluation was performed using Pearson's chi-squared test with a significance level of $p = 0.05$. In the case of low numbers for the chi-squared test, the modified Fisher's exact test was used. The statistical evaluations were performed using the NCSS 11 Statistical Software (2016) (NCSS, LLC. Kaysville, UT, USA, ncss.com/software/ncss).

5. Conclusions

Our data confirmed the high susceptibility of Escherichia coli and Enterococcus faecalis to fosfomycin. The results did not show any increase of resistance levels after the registration and introduction of this drug to UTIs treatment regimes. The oral fosfomycin showed a high treatment efficacy in uncomplicated urinary tract infections. However, in complicated or recurrent infections the treatment led to a relatively high recurrence index.

Author Contributions: Conceptualization, M.F.; methodology, M.B. and M.F.; validation, M.F.; formal analysis, M.F.; investigation, M.B. and M.F.; resources M.B.; data curation and statistical analysis, E.C.; writing—original draft preparation, M.F.; writing—review and editing, P.B.; supervision, P.B. and M.F.; funding acquisition, P.B. All authors read and agreed to the published version of the manuscript.

Funding: This research was funded supported by the Ministry of Health of the Czech Republic DRO plan (UHHK, 00179906) and by the long-term organization development plan by the Ministry of Defense of the Czech Republic.

Conflicts of Interest: The authors declare no conflicts of interest. The funders had no role in the design of the study; in the collection, analyses, or interpretation of data; in the writing of the manuscript, or in the decision to publish the results.

References

1. Frimondt-Møller, N. Fosfomycin. In *Kucers' the Use of Antibiotics*, 6th ed.; Grayson, L.M., Ed.; CRC Press: Boca Raton, FL, USA, 2010.
2. Bader, M.S.; Loeb, M.; Brooks, A.A. An update on the management of urinary tract infections in the era of antimicrobial resistance. *Postgrad. Med.* **2017**, *129*, 242–258. [CrossRef] [PubMed]
3. Grabe, M.; Bartoletti, R.; Bjerklund Johansen, T.E.; Cek, M.; Koves, B.; Naber, K.; Pickard, R.S.; Tenke, P.; Wagenlehner, F.; Wullt, B. Guidelines on Urological Infections. Available online: https://uroweb.org/wp-content/uploads/18-Urological-Infections_LR.pdf (accessed on 12 April 2016).
4. Oteo, J.; Bautista, V.; Lara, N.; Cuevas, O.; Arroyo, M.; Fernandez, S.; Lazaro, E.; de Abajo, F.J.; Campos, J.; Spanish, E.-E.-N.S.G. Parallel increase in community use of fosfomycin and resistance to fosfomycin in extended-spectrum beta-lactamase (ESBL)-producing Escherichia coli. *J. Antimicrob. Chemother.* **2010**, *65*, 2459–2463. [CrossRef] [PubMed]
5. Sastry, S.; Doi, Y. Fosfomycin: Resurgence of an old companion. *J. Infect. Chemother.* **2016**, *22*, 273–280. [CrossRef] [PubMed]
6. Stefaniuk, E.; Suchocka, U.; Bosacka, K.; Hryniewicz, W. Etiology and antibiotic susceptibility of bacterial pathogens responsible for community-acquired urinary tract infections in Poland. *Eur. J. Clin. Microbiol. Infect. Dis.* **2016**, *35*, 1363–1369. [CrossRef]
7. Fajfr, M.; Louda, M.; Paterova, P.; Ryskova, L.; Pacovsky, J.; Kosina, J.; Zemlickova, H.; Brodak, M. The susceptibility to fosfomycin of Gram-negative bacteria isolates from urinary tract infection in the Czech Republic: Data from a unicentric study. *BMC Urol.* **2017**, *17*, 33. [CrossRef]
8. Liu, H.Y.; Lin, H.C.; Lin, Y.C.; Yu, S.H.; Wu, W.H.; Lee, Y.J. Antimicrobial susceptibilities of urinary extended-spectrum beta-lactamase-producing Escherichia coli and Klebsiella pneumoniae to fosfomycin and nitrofurantoin in a teaching hospital in Taiwan. *J. Microbiol. Immunol. Infect.* **2011**, *44*, 364–368. [CrossRef]
9. Matthews, P.C.; Barrett, L.K.; Warren, S.; Stoesser, N.; Snelling, M.; Scarborough, M.; Jones, N. Oral fosfomycin for treatment of urinary tract infection: A retrospective cohort study. *BMC Infect. Dis.* **2016**, *16*, 556. [CrossRef]
10. Demir, T.; Buyukguclu, T. Evaluation of the in vitro activity of fosfomycin trometamine against Gram-negative bacterial strains recovered from community- and hospital-acquired urinary tract infections in Turkey. *Int. J. Infect. Dis.* **2013**, *17*, e966–e970. [CrossRef]

11. Sobel, J.D.; Kaye, D. Urinary tract infection. In *Mandell, Douglas and Bennett's Principle and Practice of Infectious Diseases*, 7th ed.; Mandell, G., Bennett, J., Dolin, R., Eds.; Churchill Livingstone: Philadelphia, PA, USA, 2010.
12. Falagas, M.E.; Kastoris, A.C.; Kapaskelis, A.M.; Karageorgopoulos, D.E. Fosfomycin for the treatment of multidrug-resistant, including extended-spectrum beta-lactamase producing, Enterobacteriaceae infections: A systematic review. *Lancet. Infect. Dis.* **2010**, *10*, 43–50. [CrossRef]
13. Maraki, S.; Samonis, G.; Rafailidis, P.I.; Vouloumanou, E.K.; Mavromanolakis, E.; Falagas, M.E. Susceptibility of urinary tract bacteria to fosfomycin. *Antimicrob. Agents. Chemother.* **2009**, *53*, 4508–4510. [CrossRef]
14. Diez-Aguilar, M.; Canton, R. New microbiological aspects of fosfomycin. *Rev. Esp. Quimioter.* **2019**, *32*, 8–18. [PubMed]
15. Grabein, B.; Graninger, W.; Rodriguez Bano, J.; Dinh, A.; Liesenfeld, D.B. Intravenous fosfomycin-back to the future. Systematic review and meta-analysis of the clinical literature. *Clin. Microbiol. Infect.* **2017**, *23*, 363–372. [CrossRef] [PubMed]
16. Aghamali, M.; Sedighi, M.; Zahedi Bialvaei, A.; Mohammadzadeh, N.; Abbasian, S.; Ghafouri, Z.; Kouhsari, E. Fosfomycin: Mechanisms and the increasing prevalence of resistance. *J. Med. Microbiol.* **2019**, *68*, 11–25. [CrossRef] [PubMed]
17. Aris, P.; Boroumand, M.A.; Rahbar, M.; Douraghi, M. The Activity of Fosfomycin Against Extended-Spectrum Beta-Lactamase-Producing Isolates of Enterobacteriaceae Recovered from Urinary Tract Infections: A Single-Center Study Over a Period of 12 Years. *Microb. Drug. Resist.* **2018**, *24*, 607–612. [CrossRef] [PubMed]
18. Gajdacs, M.; Urban, E. Comparative Epidemiology and Resistance Trends of Proteae in Urinary Tract Infections of Inpatients and Outpatients: A 10-Year Retrospective Study. *Antibiotics* **2019**, *8*, 91. [CrossRef] [PubMed]
19. Gajdacs, M.; Urban, E. Resistance Trends and Epidemiology of Citrobacter-Enterobacter-Serratia in Urinary Tract Infections of Inpatients and Outpatients (RECESUTI): A 10-Year Survey. *Medicina (Kaunas)* **2019**, *55*, 285. [CrossRef]
20. Peretz, A.; Naamneh, B.; Tkhawkho, L.; Nitzan, O. High Rates of Fosfomycin Resistance in Gram-Negative Urinary Isolates from Israel. *Microb. Drug. Resist.* **2019**, *25*, 408–412. [CrossRef]
21. Neuner, E.A.; Sekeres, J.; Hall, G.S.; van Duin, D. Experience with fosfomycin for treatment of urinary tract infections due to multidrug-resistant organisms. *Antimicrob. Agents. Chemother.* **2012**, *56*, 5744–5748. [CrossRef]
22. Qiao, L.D.; Zheng, B.; Chen, S.; Yang, Y.; Zhang, K.; Guo, H.F.; Yang, B.; Niu, Y.J.; Wang, Y.; Shi, B.K.; et al. Evaluation of three-dose fosfomycin tromethamine in the treatment of patients with urinary tract infections: An uncontrolled, open-label, multicentre study. *BMJ Open* **2013**, *3*, e004157. [CrossRef]
23. Gupta, V.; Rani, H.; Singla, N.; Kaistha, N.; Chander, J. Determination of Extended-Spectrum beta-Lactamases and AmpC Production in Uropathogenic Isolates of Escherichia coli and Susceptibility to Fosfomycin. *J. Lab. Physicians.* **2013**, *5*, 90–93. [CrossRef]
24. Hagiya, H.; Ninagawa, M.; Hasegawa, K.; Terasaka, T.; Kimura, K.; Waseda, K.; Hanayama, Y.; Sendo, T.; Otsuka, F. Fosfomycin for the treatment of prostate infection. *Intern. Med.* **2014**, *53*, 2643–2646. [CrossRef] [PubMed]
25. Kaase, M.; Szabados, F.; Anders, A.; Gatermann, S.G. Fosfomycin susceptibility in carbapenem-resistant Enterobacteriaceae from Germany. *J. Clin. Microbiol.* **2014**, *52*, 1893–1897. [CrossRef] [PubMed]
26. Perdigao-Neto, L.V.; Oliveira, M.S.; Rizek, C.F.; Carrilho, C.M.; Costa, S.F.; Levin, A.S. Susceptibility of multiresistant gram-negative bacteria to fosfomycin and performance of different susceptibility testing methods. *Antimicrob. Agents. Chemother.* **2014**, *58*, 1763–1767. [CrossRef] [PubMed]
27. Giancola, S.E.; Mahoney, M.V.; Hogan, M.D.; Raux, B.R.; McCoy, C.; Hirsch, E.B. Assessment of Fosfomycin for Complicated or Multidrug-Resistant Urinary Tract Infections: Patient Characteristics and Outcomes. *Chemotherapy* **2017**, *62*, 100–104. [CrossRef]

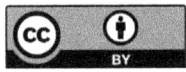

© 2020 by the authors. Licensee MDPI, Basel, Switzerland. This article is an open access article distributed under the terms and conditions of the Creative Commons Attribution (CC BY) license (http://creativecommons.org/licenses/by/4.0/).

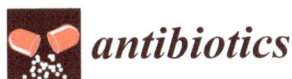

Review

Transitioning of *Helicobacter pylori* Therapy from Trial and Error to Antimicrobial Stewardship

David Y. Graham

Department of Medicine, Michael E. DeBakey VA Medical Center and Baylor College of Medicine, RM 3A-318B (111D), 2002 Holcombe Boulevard, Houston, TX 77030, USA; dgraham@bcm.edu;
Tel.: +713-795-0232; Fax: +713-795-4471

Received: 15 September 2020; Accepted: 1 October 2020; Published: 3 October 2020

Abstract: Helicobacter pylori is the only major infection for which antimicrobial therapy is not designed using the principles of antimicrobial stewardship. Traditionally, antimicrobial therapy is a susceptibility-based therapy, achieves high cure rates, and includes surveillance programs to regularly provide updated data regarding resistance, outcomes, and treatment guidelines. Current *H. pylori* therapies identified by trial-and-error, and treatment recommendations and guidelines are based on comparisons among regimens that rarely take into account the prevalence or effect of resistance. The majority of patients currently treated achieve suboptimal results. A paradigm shift is required to abandon current approaches and embrace antimicrobial stewardship, and therefore reliably achieve high cure rates; develop, propagate, and update best practice guidelines; and provide surveillance of local or regional susceptibility/resistance patterns. These also require timely updates to clinicians regarding the current status of resistance, antimicrobial effectiveness, and ways to prevent antimicrobial misuse to extend the useful life of currently available antibiotics. Here, we discuss the differences among current approaches to *H. pylori* therapy and antimicrobial stewardship and identify what is required to achieve the transition. Conceptually, the differences are significant, and the transition will likely need to be both abrupt and complete. Recommendations for therapy during the transition period are given.

Keywords: *Helicobacter pylori*; antimicrobial stewardship; therapy; antibiotics; metronidazole; clarithromycin; fluoroquinolones; amoxicillin; proton pump inhibitors; ethical trials

1. Introduction

The widespread misuse of antibiotics has resulted in increasing antimicrobial resistance which threatens the continued usefulness of currently available antimicrobials. The consequences of critical antibiotics becoming clinically ineffective have resulted in strong pressure to utilize the principles of antimicrobial stewardship for selecting and managing therapy for infectious diseases [1,2]. Management of *Helicobacter pylori* infections has long been within the purview of *Gastroenterology* which has been slow to accept the paradigm shift needed to change the approach to therapy from one utilizing trial-and-error to one based on the principles of antimicrobial stewardship. *H. pylori* was officially recognized as an infectious disease in 2015 [3], and those involved in studying *H. pylori* therapy are only now gradually beginning to accept that *H. pylori* therapy should no longer be exempt from the guidelines and practices governing treatment of other infectious diseases (i.e., the principles of antimicrobial stewardship).

2. Antimicrobial Stewardship in Traditional Infectious Disease Therapy

The principles of antimicrobial stewardship codified and extended thinking and practices involved in the development and implementation of methods to simultaneously improve antimicrobial therapy, prevent antimicrobial misuse, and reliably achieve high cure rates, while minimizing the risk of developing resistance in order to prolong the useful life of antibiotics. Until now, the approach to *H. pylori* therapy has not routinely involved elements critical to antimicrobial stewardship, such as optimization of the therapy in terms of drugs, dosing, or duration of therapy. As a result, current therapies have subsequently failed to reliably achieve high cure rates without prescribing unnecessary antimicrobials or prolonging therapy beyond the experimentally identified optimal duration. Stewardship elements that are also lacking include the development, propagation, and regular updating of best practice guidelines, as well as susceptibility/resistance surveillance to update clinicians of the current status of resistance and antimicrobial effectiveness, and the availability and potential role of new antimicrobials.

Fundamentally, a successful antimicrobial therapy is a susceptibility-based therapy, as success is predicated on the target organism being susceptible to the antimicrobial agents utilized. Antimicrobial therapies are also optimized so as to reliably achieve excellent results (i.e., high cure rates such as >95%) (Table 1) [4]. Comparisons among therapies are infrequent and, when done, compare proven highly effective regimens using noninferiority methodology [5–7]. As we discuss below, *H. pylori* therapy is most often prescribed empirically and most often fails to reliably achieve high cure rates [8]. Comparisons of empiric therapies are the rule and they focus on which is the better of the two regimens with seemingly little regard to the actual, often poor, cure rates achieved. In addition, consensus and guideline recommendations regarding *H. pylori* therapy rarely involve the principles of antimicrobial stewardship and are based on principles used for other gastrointestinal diseases, such as irritable bowel syndrome, which fail to reflect the marked differences and realities of antimicrobial therapy.

Table 1. Definitions of terms to describe outcome of therapy.

Term	Definition
Successful	Excellent or good results
Excellent results	Reliably achieve 95% or greater cure rates in adherent patients with susceptible infections
Good results	Reliably achieve 90% or greater cure rates in adherent patients with susceptible infections
Optimum duration	Days of therapy required to reliably achieve good to excellent results
Doses and frequency of administration	Those that will reliably achieve good to excellent results

From [4], with permission.

3. Original Development of *H. pylori* Antimicrobial Therapies

Soon after the discovery of *H. pylori*, it was shown that, in vitro, the organism was susceptible to a wide variety of commonly used antimicrobials. However, the infection proved to be difficult to cure using those antimicrobials, and it also proved impossible to reliably achieve high cure rates [9] (reviewed in [10]). This prompted a period of trial-and-error during which clinical trials were done with a wide variety of antimicrobials (reviewed in [10]). Eventually Tom Borody in Australia discovered an effective three-drug regimen consisting of bismuth, metronidazole, and tetracycline called bismuth triple therapy regimen [11].

H. pylori therapy was initially focused on treatment of peptic ulcer disease which was extremely common and one of the major gastrointestinal causes of morbidity, surgery, and medical costs. The basic approach was to treat the ulcer with a histamine-2 receptor antagonist (H2RA) and the infection with bismuth triple therapy [12]. It was soon recognized that the presence of metronidazole resistance greatly reduced the effectiveness of bismuth triple therapy, but that this could be partially or completely overcome by adding a proton pump inhibitor (PPI) and increasing both the dosage of metronidazole and the duration of therapy (e.g., to 14 days) (reviewed in [13]). This modified regimen is called bismuth quadruple therapy.

Bismuth triple therapy was commercially marketed in 1996 and while widely used with a PPI, the commercialization of bismuth quadruple therapy, in 2006, was delayed until after the patent regarding the addition of a PPI expired.

4. Development of *H. pylori* Therapies with Different Antibiotics

One of the initial attempts to produce an *H. pylori* therapy was with the macrolide, erythromycin. Erythromycin was able to suppress the infection but was unable to cure the infection [14]. Thus, macrolides were considered to be ineffective in vivo, until the introduction of clarithromycin which, when combined with a PPI or H2RA to increase gastric pH, proved effective. The initial dual therapy combination of clarithromycin and a PPI ultimately failed because of emergence of clarithromycin resistance during therapy [15–17]. However, with the addition of amoxicillin, it proved both well tolerated and effective [17]. This three-drug regime is called clarithromycin triple therapy or, alternatively, standard triple therapy. The effectiveness of clarithromycin triple therapy subsequently resulted in the development of additional triple therapies consisting of PPI and amoxicillin plus metronidazole, a fluoroquinolone, or rifabutin.

The original bismuth quadruple therapy was also modified by replacing the metronidazole with amoxicillin or furazolidone. Other recent successful iterations include bismuth and a PPI plus tetracycline and amoxicillin or metronidazole and amoxicillin (reviewed in [13,18,19]). The most recent advance has been with a dual therapy consisting of omeprazole plus amoxicillin. This was originally introduced in 1989 but proved unable to reliably achieve high cure rates and, until recently, was generally considered to be a failure [20–22] (reviewed in [19]). However, the introduction of potassium competitive acid blockers (P-CABs), such as vonoprazan, have reinvigorated interest in dual therapies (see below) [23].

5. The Effect of Gastroenterology Rather Than Infectious Disease Being Responsible for Development of *H. pylori* Therapies

Within a few years of discovery, the diagnosis and management of *H. pylori* had primarily become the responsibility of gastroenterology. Gastroenterologists found little need, or desire, to incorporate susceptibility testing as a key element required for choosing, defining, optimizing, and evaluating the results of *H. pylori* therapies. Instead, they adopted the trial-and-error approach which focused on comparison of therapies. This approach has remained the standard despite evidence that overall cure rates were often both poor and declining.

The gastroenterologist's approach to the development of *H. pylori* therapies was most likely based on the long experience with common gastroenterology diseases, such as constipation or irritable bowel syndrome. Most diseases in gastroenterology are characterized as follows: (a) the cause is largely unknown, (b) there is a large placebo response to therapy, and (c) the success of most therapies is low requiring a comparator which is often a placebo. The fact that the etiologies were unknown required a focus on the results rather than an explanation for a poor response. This contrasts with infectious disease where the cause of a poor response is discoverable. These differences resulted in two different approaches, one that focused on outcome as a comparison (the what school) and the other that focused on the actual outcome (i.e., cure rate) (the why school). In gastroenterology, the "what school" has dominated planning, analysis, and reporting of clinical trials which can be best characterized as comparisons of arbitrary regimens focusing on the difference, despite the fact that often none of the arms achieved a high cure rate. This approach was abetted by medical journals which expected, even demanded, comparative trials. Eventually, thousands of patients were enrolled in *H. pylori* treatment trials of which many, if not most, achieved poor cure rates in at least one treatment arm. The fact that at least one arm in a trial achieved a poor result was, however, often not a result of chance. The published study design confirmed that based on prior experience, the authors reliably predicted which regime would produce the unacceptably low cure rate. By definition, informed consent requires this information to be shared with the subjects, but it was withheld [24,25]. Informed consent also requires informing patients about any new information arising during the trial and allowing them to reconsider. This also was not done. These issues with informed consent have continued to plague *H. pylori* comparative trials up to the present.

The development of sequential therapy, probably, best illustrates the differences between gastroenterology and the traditional development of therapy for an infectious disease. Sequential therapy is a regimen in which a dual therapy with a PPI and amoxicillin are given for five days, followed by five days with the PPI, clarithromycin, and metronidazole. It was developed in Italy and was prompted by increasing treatment failures with triple therapy. By 2001, it had been conclusively shown (e.g., studies involving more than 53,000 patients) that, because of increased clarithromycin resistance, clarithromycin triple therapy was no longer able to reliably achieve high cure rates [26,27]. Clarithromycin triple therapy was used as the straw man in multiple studies in which more than 1800 patients participated. The investigators were able to show that, in the mid-2000s, in one region of Italy, sequential therapy yielded higher cure rates than clarithromycin triple therapy [28]. The fact that prior trials in the same population had already proven that one regime was inferior, was also withheld from the consent of subjects in subsequent trials. Despite many iterations of the same trials, sequential therapy was neither optimized nor explored for its weaknesses. When sequential therapy was tested in different geographic areas with different resistance patterns (e.g., resistance to clarithromycin and metronidazole vs. increased resistance to clarithromycin but low resistance to metronidazole) sequential therapy proved ineffective and was abandoned [28,29].

The traditional infectious disease approach focuses on attainment of a prespecified cure rate (e.g., $\geq 95\%$) (i.e., the why school) using susceptibility-based therapy and would never have been included in the empiric comparisons described above. Attempts to optimize sequential therapy would have discovered that (a) the duration of therapy of 14 days provided a higher cure rate, (b) that sequential therapy was only effective in the presence of isolated clarithromycin resistance, and (c) that all those with clarithromycin resistance received the clarithromycin with no benefits. As noted previously, comparisons of highly effective susceptibility-based therapies are rare and, when preformed, are generally limited to head-to-head comparisons of proven, highly reliable, optimized regimens using noninferiority methods with both regimens expected to achieve high cure rates [7]. Typically, in science, observation (the what) is typically followed by experiments to understand the phenomenon (the why) (i.e., they are complimentary). *H. pylori* therapy has generally stopped with the what.

6. Meta-Analysis and *H. pylori* Therapy

Although meta-analysis has become the holy grail for analysis of studies in gastroenterology, it was often used inappropriately for assessing *H. pylori* therapy. The main problem has been that the comparisons involved were often fatally flawed. For example, if one compared 14-day sequential therapy with 14-day clarithromycin triple therapies in treatment of adherent patients with susceptible infections, one would expect both to have very similar high cure rates. Different patterns of resistance would be an obvious important difference (e.g., to clarithromycin and to metronidazole which is only present in one of the therapies), whereas relative potency of the PPI used is not (i.e., 40 mg of pantoprazole = 9 mg of omeprazole, whereas 40 mg of esomeprazole = 64 mg omeprazole [30,31]. If the populations did not differ in relation to resistance patterns or PPI relative potency, one would expect both to yield high cure rates. Failure to do so would signify the presence of important differences between the two populations such that they could not be compared as the results would be nongeneralizable and produce flawed conclusions. When meta-analyses compare trials where the data for each population is population specific and not generalizable, they are best described as Shmeta analyses [4,30]. Generalizability is one of the key requirements for valid and ethical research (Table 2) [32].

Table 2. Guidelines to implement antimicrobial stewardship for treatment of *H. pylori* infections.

- Therapies must be optimized to reliably achieve high cure rates.
- Optimization should include the effects of resistance to the different components. Preferably, optimization should be confirmed in different regions.
- Surveillance programs should be instituted. At a minimum, this should include tests of cure and, preferably, with susceptibility testing available for treatment failures.
- Treatment of *H. pylori* should be integrated with ongoing or planned prescription and treatment monitoring utilized for other bacterial infections.
- Data from sites where culture and susceptibility testing and/or molecular testing are done locally should be published and kept up to date.
- Susceptibility testing should be reimbursed as for other bacterial pathogens and the results data should be submitted to local and central repositories responsible for monitoring resistance among bacterial pathogens.
- To avoid unethical studies, studies should adhere to the guidelines of the Infectious Diseases Society of America regarding conduct of superiority and organism-specific clinical trials of antibacterial agents for the treatment of infections caused by drug-resistant bacterial pathogens.

Adapted from [32].

Another example of misuse of meta-analyses has been when it was used to provide guidance regarding therapy. For example, the 2017 American College of Gastroenterology guideline used a meta-analysis to show that bismuth quadruple therapy should replace triple therapy. They provided "an updated meta-analysis, which included 12 randomized controlled trials (RCTs) with 2753 patients; the intention-to-treat (ITT) eradication rate was 77.6% with bismuth quadruple therapy vs. 68.9% with clarithromycin triple therapy" [33]. However, because both regimens achieved clinically unacceptably low cure rates, the appropriate conclusion, based on the results presented, would be that neither should be used as an empiric therapy (at least in the regions where the studies were done).

Although *H. pylori* gastritis is an infectious disease of known cause for which reliably high cure rates are possible and there is no placebo response, the current status is that consensus statements and guidelines have been ineffective, and most patients continue to receive largely poor effective therapy [8,34].

7. The Role of Pharmaceutical Companies in Developing *H. pylori* Therapy

Pharma became involved with *H. pylori* when PPIs were new drugs and peptic ulcer was the major disease for which antisecretory drugs were used. H2RA's were proven effective for treatment of peptic ulcers and omeprazole was having a difficult time becoming accepted. *H. pylori* represented an opportunity as it was a new problem without a simple and effective therapy. PPIs also appeared to possibly have a role to play in therapy and, in order to promote omeprazole, AstraZeneca sponsored a series of consensus conferences regarding *H. pylori* (including Maastricht I) [35,36]. This proved to be a win-win for AstraZeneca, as well as for spreading interest and knowledge regarding *H. pylori*. It also helped solidify *H. pylori* as a gastroenterology disease. Other pharmaceutical companies' subsequent involvement primarily was to promote their anti-*H. pylori* therapies. The most recent example has been designed to promote the bismuth quadruple therapy, Pylera®, in Europe. Pharma's goals included ensuring that their regimens, plus their suggested duration of therapy, were included in lectures, consensus conferences, and guidelines. Most regimens are now off-patent which has reduced, but not eliminated, pharmaceutal company influence on the knowledge and recommendations disseminated.

8. The Role of the U.S. Food and Drug Administration

The original approvals of *H. pylori* therapies by the U.S. Food and Drug Administration (FDA) were obtained during the period when high cure rates could not be reliably achieved (Figure 1) [37–40]. Although it is a common misconception, FDA approval does not carry with it any implication that the regimen has been optimized in terms of doses or duration of therapy or that it will reliably achieve high cure rates. For example, the cure rates reported in the studies used to obtain approval of clarithromycin triple therapies ranged from 79% to 86%. The cure rates with clarithromycin triple therapies were the following: 77% with omeprazole (for 10 days), lansoprazole (for 10 and 14 days), rabeprazole (for 7 days); 78% with rabeprazole (for 10 days); and 83% with esomeprazole (for 10 days) [17,41–43] (Figure 1) [37–40]. The pivotal study with pantoprazole was not submitted for FDA approval, likely because the per protocol cure rates were relatively low (70% for the clarithromycin and 76% for the metronidazole seven-day triple therapy) [37]. Of interest, whenever two durations of therapy were examined (e.g., 7 and 10 days or 10 and 14 days), the shorter duration was always selected for the marketed version.

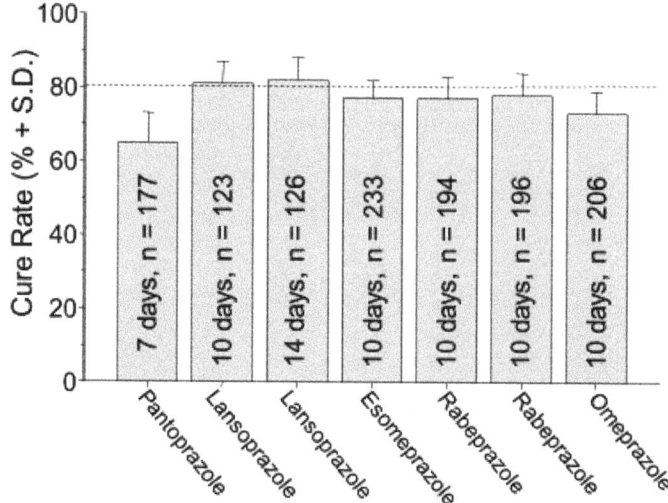

Figure 1. Intention to treat cure rates and standard deviations reported from the clinical trials published for studies designed to obtain FDA approval for triple therapy with PPI, clarithromycin, and amoxicillin, in the United States. From [4] with permission.

The original bismuth triple therapy (Helidac®) was approved using small studies that had been completed independently of the pharmaceutical company [44]. It was marketed for 14 days and could be used directly or with an H2RA. The more recent version as a three-in-one combination product (Pylera®) was studied and subsequently marketed for 10 days to offer a commercial advantage over the traditional product [45]. No comparisons were, or have been, done to address what is the optimum duration of therapy in the presence of metronidazole resistance (see below). The optimum duration must be defined experimentally rather than by marketing efforts of Pharma.

9. Basis for the General Recommendation for a Treatment Duration of 14 Days

H. pylori is one of those organisms, like *Mycobacterium tuberculosis*, that can enter a dormant state (persister state) in which its metabolism slows as does the need for replication. This process allows the organism to survive despite the presence of antibiotics [46–48]. As noted above, although therapy would appear to have eliminated the infection, early experiments found that, *H. pylori* was only suppressed and would rapidly reappear. Reappearance either denoted emergence of resistance or, if the organism remained susceptible to the antibiotics used, the duration of therapy was inadequate. The traditional response to recurrence without resistance is to lengthen the duration of therapy. With tuberculosis, this may require many months of therapy, with *H. pylori* 14 days appears to be sufficient. With *H. pylori*, this phenomenon is most often seen with amoxicillin-containing therapies. Because *H.*

pylori only replicates within a narrow pH range (near pH 7), strategies to enhance killing would be to maintain an intragastric pH of greater than six, increasing the duration of therapy, or both [46,49,50].

10. Optimization: Duration of Therapy

The principles of antimicrobial stewardship require that therapies be optimized to achieve the highest cure rates while taking into consideration safety and cost-effectiveness. Because of the general observation regarding amoxicillin-containing regimens that 14-day therapy is generally superior to shorter durations, it has been recommended that the initial trial should be for 14 days and, only if the 14-day therapy proves highly effective, should one consider testing shorter durations [24]. The effectiveness of PPI plus amoxicillin-containing triple therapies is duration dependent. For example, when these triple therapies are given to patients with susceptible infections, the cure rate is typically between 88 and 92% with a 7-day regimen, 90–94% with a 10-day regimen, and 94–98% with a 14-day regimen [51,52]. PPI, amoxicillin, fluoroquinolone triple therapy is an excellent example of a marked delay in recognizing that it was possible to achieve high cure rates with this regimen. A possible bias by clinical investigators toward shorter durations resulted in a large number of studies and meta-analyses with PPI, amoxicillin, fluoroquinolone triple therapy [53] before it was recognized that cure rates ≥95% were obtainable with 14-day therapy [54].

With many regimens, particularly with amoxicillin-containing triple therapies, one can predict the population cure rate based on the prevalence of resistance or vice versa. For example, since amoxicillin resistance is currently very rare, it can generally be ignored. In contrast, clarithromycin resistance is all-or-none and clarithromycin is functionally removed from the regimen making the cure rate dependent on the remaining amoxicillin PPI dual therapy [55]. The cure rate for any population can be estimated as follows: (cure rate with susceptible infections x the proportion with susceptible infections) + (cure rate with resistant infections x the proportion with clarithromycin resistance). An alternate approach would be to use an *H. pylori* treatment nomogram (Figure 2) [55]. The nomogram has the advantage of allowing one to easily visualize the effect of the relation of prevalence of resistance on cure rates with different durations of therapy.

Although 14-day therapy may prove to be optimal, clinicians may still be obliged to use a shorter, government-approved duration which may be less effective. Clinicians may also be confused by the recommendations from consensus conferences which, until recently, recommended 7-day triple therapy or, in other instances, recommended a range of durations such as 7 to 14 days. Optimal duration can never be expressed as a range. In addition, consensus recommendations often fail to include the caveats needed to understand when any specific duration would be recommended. The reasons for this lack of clarity are unclear. Possibilities include not wishing to appear opposed to what is approved locally, or bias related to one or more conference sponsors.

Bismuth quadruple therapy does not contain amoxicillin and the antimicrobials used are relatively acid insensitive, such that the lessons learned with amoxicillin-containing therapies may not apply. As noted above, early studies showed that, with metronidazole susceptible infections, a duration of 4 to 7 days was sufficient to achieve cure rates of >95% [56–59]. However, consensus conferences have almost exclusively recommended 14-day bismuth quadruple therapy [60–63]. This recommendation was based on the fact that, in many areas, metronidazole resistance is common and increasing, and susceptibility testing is rare. Thus, as a general rule, unless proven otherwise, resistance should be considered to be present which requires one to lengthen the duration of therapy and increase the dosage of metronidazole [13]. In areas where metronidazole resistance is rare or, when metronidazole susceptibility has been confirmed, durations shorter than 14 days are effective and 7-day therapy is generally recommended.

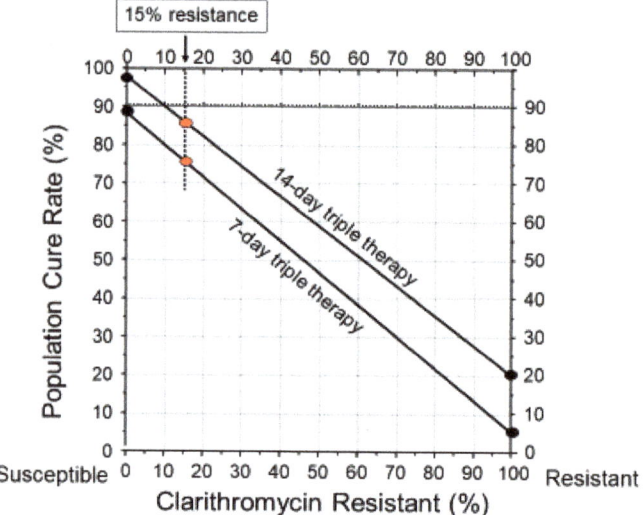

Figure 2. *Helicobacter pylori* treatment nomogram illustrating the duration-related difference in cure rate with 7- and 14-day clarithromycin triple therapy and the effect of clarithromycin resistance on the outcome. As shown, 15% clarithromycin resistance results in a decline in the population cure rate to approximately 85% with 14-day therapy and to approximately 75% with 7-day therapy. It also shows the lack of utility of consensus conference recommendations to use 15% resistance as a yes-no guide to therapy.

The approval of Pylera® in Europe resulted in an effort to shorten the recommended duration to 10 days to coincide with the approved and marketed duration. In the USA, the duration issue was not a problem, as Pylera® was offered in bottles of capsules which allowed the physician to prescribe, and the pharmacist to dispense, whatever the physician decided was the best duration of therapy for the individual patient. At the same time that tetracycline became very difficult to obtain, the company changed the packaging of Pylera® from bottles to a 10-day dose pack. This requires purchasing two packs to achieve a 14-day therapy for treatment of patients with metronidazole resistant infections, which represents a problem in the USA because the average retail price of Pylera® is $1110/10-day dose pack.

The optimum duration of bismuth quadruple therapy remains unknown, largely untested, and is impossible to prove without head-to-head comparisons in populations where the pattern of resistance is known. Another problem related to doing comparisons is that whether a strain is considered resistant or susceptible to metronidazole may depend in part on the test used. It is unclear why Etest may overestimate metronidazole resistance as compared with results obtained with agar dilution [64,65]. Etest is widely used because it is easier to perform. Because of Etest's tendency to overestimate the prevalence of metronidazole resistant infections, it has been our practice to always confirm metronidazole resistant results by agar dilution which correlates better with clinical outcome. Efficacy studies relying on Etest to determine metronidazole resistance are more likely to overestimate the therapies' efficacy in the presence of resistant strains. There are a number of studies ostensibly done to test whether 10-day bismuth quadruple therapy is highly effective. These have been studied in populations with an unknown, but generally low, prevalence of metronidazole resistance [66]. Such studies often achieve cure rates between 88% and 92% which appear suboptimal [8,66,67]. Studies are needed that are designed using the principles of antimicrobial stewardship and all treatment components, including the antisecretory activity of the PPI chosen, antimicrobial dosages, frequency of administration, administration in relation to meals, and the duration of therapy. The question "What is the optimal duration for bismuth quadruple therapy with susceptible infections, with resistant infections, and for populations where the resistant pattern is unknown?" remains unanswered. It is likely that, for susceptible infections, 10 and 14 days are too long and, for resistant infections, both may be too short.

11. Poly-Antimicrobial Therapies

The discovery of *H. pylori* and the search for effective treatment coincided with the problem of increasing global antimicrobial resistance. The worldwide increase in macrolide resistance resulted in a precipitous decline in *H. pylori* cure rates with clarithromycin-containing therapies. One response was to modify the current empiric regimens by increasing the number of antimicrobials used (i.e., if two antimicrobials were no longer effective, why not add a third or a fourth?) (reviewed in [30]). This led to the use of a variety of empirically administered regimens containing combinations of a PPI, amoxicillin, clarithromycin, and metronidazole named sequential, concomitant, hybrid, and reverse hybrid therapies. As noted above, 10-day sequential therapy consists of a five-day course of a PPI plus amoxicillin followed by five-day course of a PPI, clarithromycin, and metronidazole. Although the 14-day therapy was more effective, the longer duration has not been widely used, as overall, the regimen has been considered to be obsolete [52].

The alternative was to give all four drugs concomitantly as a concomitant therapy, and proceeded or followed by a dual PPI-amoxicillin therapy (as a hybrid or reverse hybrid therapies). Concomitant therapy is representative of the group. It is functionally equivalent to giving both metronidazole and clarithromycin triple therapies simultaneously [68,69], with success being dependent on the infection being susceptible to amoxicillin and clarithromycin or to metronidazole. Treatment failure requires resistance to both metronidazole and clarithromycin. Although effective, the potential for these three antimicrobial-containing therapies to contribute to the global problem of antimicrobial misuse was not considered. The problem is that all subjects receive at least one antimicrobial not required to cure the infection and whose only function is to potentially contribute to the global antimicrobial resistance (Table 3) [4,69].

Table 3. Hypothetical scenario of number of unnecessary antibiotics given in relation to antibiotic susceptibility patterns.

Sensitivity Pattern of *H. pylori* to Clarithromycin and Metronidazole		Prevalence of Pattern	Successful Treatment of *H. pylori*	Number of Ineffective Drugs Used	Number of Unnecessary Drugs Used
Clarithromyin: Susceptible 80%; Resistant 20%	Metronidazole: Susceptible 60%; Resistant 40%				
Susceptible	Susceptible	48%	Yes	0	1
Susceptible	Resistant	32%	Yes	1	1
Resistant	Susceptible	12%	Yes	1	1
Resistant	Resistant	8%	No	2	2

Legend: Table showing the number of ineffective or unnecessary antibiotics used by a population of patients similar to those seen in Texas with the *H. pylori* resistance pattern of 20% resistant to clarithromycin, 40% resistant to metronidazole (8% dual resistance) which receives concomitant therapy with a PPI, amoxicillin, clarithromycin, and metronidazole. From [69] with permission.

The quantity of unnecessary antibiotic misuse with these therapies is not trivial. For example, successful therapy with 14-day concomitant therapy containing 1 gm of metronidazole and clarithromycin would produce 14,000 kg of unneeded antibiotic per 1 million successful treatments and 28,000 kg per 1 million treatment failures. Empiric concomitant therapy was recommended by the Maastricht V, Toronto, and American College of Gastroenterology guidelines [33,61,62], but not by the Houston consensus which considered concomitant therapy to be obsolete [60]. The tendency to add antimicrobials has continued with new sequential therapies and even therapies containing four antimicrobials [30,70].

12. Requirements and Impediments for Transition of *H. pylori* Therapy to the Principles of Antimicrobial Stewardship

Although susceptibility testing for human pathogens is available in most hospitals and clinics worldwide, local susceptibility testing for *H. pylori* is almost universally unavailable. In the United States, culture and susceptibility testing for *H. pylori* is currently available from the Mayo Clinic laboratory and a few other major commercial laboratories. However, the details of how to obtain this service remain the responsibility of the individual physician or endoscopy unit. Molecular susceptibility testing of biopsies or stool specimens is also available commercially from a few sources (e.g., American Molecular Laboratories, http://amlaboratories.com/clinical-lab-menu/amhpr-h-pylori-antibiotic-resistance-panel). Consensus statements have typically recommended susceptibility testing only for patients with at least two treatment failures. The reasons why susceptibility testing is lacking are many and include lack of demand, difficulties with reimbursement, lack of a tradition of susceptibility-based therapy to treat *H. pylori*, and lack of surveillance programs to provide local or regional resistance patterns and to guide therapy. This may change in the USA as the Centers for Medicare and Medicaid Services (CMS) has recently published a regulation requiring all hospitals participating in its programs to establish antimicrobial stewardship programs [71]. They require the appointment of a physician and a pharmacist to be responsible for developing plans and procedures to ensure appropriate therapy. Their requirements also include providing susceptibility testing, treatment guides, as well as monitoring of therapy and prescriptions which are included in the U.S. Centers for Disease Control (CDC) guidelines [72]. These include creation and promotion of susceptibility-based treatments, tracking of antibiotic dispensing, and setting targets for improvement (i.e., monitoring and reporting). It is not yet clear whether *H. pylori* infections are included in the mandate.

The current *H. pylori* treatment guidelines have proven to be ineffective, as they have failed to provide recommendations to reliably yield high cure rates and for creation and promotion of susceptibility-based treatments, tracking of antibiotic dispensing, as well as setting targets for improvement [34]. The prevalent A vs. B comparison mentality has been concerned with differences in (a) actual results, (b) rather than whether either achieved acceptable cure rates, or (c) for understanding the reason for the differences (i.e., the data required to reliably achieve high cure rates). As noted above, most meta-analyses have involved studies whose results are only relevant to the individual study included and are not generalizable or useful for any other population [30].

Consensus conferences and guidelines have often failed to provide clinically useful guidance regarding therapy. For example, as noted above, by 2001 empiric clarithromycin triple therapy was proven to no longer achieve clinically acceptable cure rates in most areas. Rather than state outright that clarithromycin should no longer be used empirically, the 2006 Maastricht III conference suggested using a cutoff of 15–20% resistance above which clarithromycin should not be used empirically [73]. They noted, "Clarithromycin resistance is increasing. It is the main risk factor for treatment failure. Treatment should achieve an eradication rate of >80%. The threshold of clarithromycin resistance at which this antibiotic should not be used, or a clarithromycin susceptibility test should be performed is 15–20%." The cut-off was further refined to >15% in the 2012 Maastricht IV confirmed in the 2017 Maastricht V consensus [61,74]. In retrospect, these guidelines were both impractical and toothless as they were impossible to implement because the required susceptibility data was unavailable. Subsequent analyses of worldwide *H. pylori* resistance have confirmed that resistance exceeded 15% for clarithromycin, metronidazole, and levofloxacin in all WHO regions [75].

The more recent Houston consensus recommended that clarithromycin, metronidazole, and levofloxacin should not be used empirically unless proven to be reliably highly effective locally [60]. Post treatment test-of-cure is currently the only method that most clinicians can use to indirectly assess susceptibility/resistance patterns. With few exceptions, routine testing for cure has been recommended for decades. As a surveillance tool, the results, if heeded, provide information whether a regimen does, or does not, reliably achieve high cure rates. In theory, this information would be collected, shared, and used to indicate whether a regimen should be replaced or modified. Overall, it appears that while this simple measure may be used to assist in the management of individual patients it has been ineffective as a surveillance tool [8,33]

13. Adoption of the Principles of Antimicrobial Stewardship

While the goal is straightforward, accomplishing adoption of antimicrobial stewardship will not be easy as it requires a major paradigm shift (Table 4) [32].

Table 4. American Society of Infectious Diseases criteria for ethical active-controlled superiority studies of antibacterial agents.

1.	The control (i.e., the comparator drug) is active against most, or all, of the bacterial strains likely to be encountered in the study;
2.	All available drugs that could be used as comparators for the study are inadequately active against the strains likely to be encountered, such that there is no alternative effective therapy possible; or
3.	The infection under study is almost universally non-fatal, such that rescue therapy can be instituted rapidly enough to preclude serious sequelae upon recognition that the strain causing the infection is resistant to the comparator drug (e.g., uncomplicated urinary tract infection). The susceptibility of etiologic bacteria is almost never known at the time an infected patient is enrolled in a clinical trial that evaluates initial antimicrobial treatment. Therefore, the comparator drugs chosen for study in antibacterial clinical trials are selected because they are anticipated to be effective against all, or almost all, strains likely to be encountered during conduct of the study.

Adapted from reference [32].

One of the first steps is to develop treatment guidelines based on the principles of antimicrobial stewardship. All recommendations not based on antimicrobial stewardship should be replaced by ones proven to reliably produce high local cure rates. To date, none of the currently used or recommended treatment regimens have been optimized nor do they consider local resistance patterns. In addition to providing new treatment guidelines, surveillance of treatment outcomes must routinely be monitored to assure continuing effectiveness. Clinical trials should focus on achieving high cure rates (e.g., >95%). "Good enough" is not good enough. Comparative trials should be restricted to comparisons of proven highly effective therapies that utilize noninferiority methodology. Studies using a regimen known to have an inferior cure rate as a comparator without truly informed consent are unethical and should not be done and, if done, should not be published [25,32] (Table 2; Table 4). No regimen should be used empirically unless it has been proven to reliably achieve high cure rates in the target population. Surveillance programs should be implemented to provide early warning if the effectiveness of currently recommended therapies declines, so that new therapies and guidelines can be implemented. Until susceptibility testing becomes widespread, surveillance should consist of routine tests-of-cure and the results should be reported in order to alert clinicians when a regimen no longer should be prescribed empirically. Current ongoing local and regional antimicrobial surveillance programs should include *H. pylori*. Large effective consortia, such as the European Registry on *Helicobacter pylori* Management, should be repurposed from simply collecting treatment results to providing surveillance, susceptibility testing, and up-to-date treatment recommendations. Clearly, we still have a long way to go and many things to do to adopt antimicrobial stewardship for *H. pylori* therapy.

14. Proposal Regarding How to Improve Empiric Therapies While Introducing Antimicrobial Stewardship

Fundamentally, the goal is to reliably achieve high cure rates in routine clinical practice (Table 5). The principles are as follows: First, to use only regimens proven to achieve high cure rates locally; second, to provide real-time information about whether the goal is achieved by routinely monitoring and reporting outcomes based on test-of-cure data; third, to abandon or modify therapies that fail to reliably achieve the desired high cure rates.

Table 5. Reliable achievement of high cure rates with empiric therapies in clinical practice.

Principle 1 Only regimens proven to reliably achieve high cure rates.
Principle 2 Routinely monitor and report outcomes using test-of-cure result to provide real-time information about whether the goals are being met.
Principle 3 Abandon or modify the therapies that fail to reliably achieve the desired high cure rates.

Clinically, cure is defined using a noninvasive test such as a negative urea breath test at least four weeks after ending therapy or a negative stool antigen test preferably at least six weeks post therapy. Defining what is the minimal high cure rate is complicated by the fact that these noninvasive tests are only approximately 95% sensitive and specific. This limitation is overcome in clinical trials by requiring two positive or negative tests using different methodology (e.g., histology and UBT). This is not practical in daily practice and the cure rate that best approximates ≥95% needs to be identified experimentally. As noted above, the sensitivity and specificity of the noninvasive tests currently used to determine cure are at best 95%. Currently, only one test, typically the UBT, is used and it is practically impossible to reliably confirm that ≥95% have been cured. As such, we propose the cut-off of ≥93% until the testing required to define cure allows a more precise estimate. For population-based clinical results, the cure rate should be based on modified intention-to-treat results that include only those who have test-of-cure data. Obtaining a test-of-cure should be vigorously attempted on all patients irrespective of the duration of therapy (e.g., even for one day), as well as those on lost to follow-up for weeks or even months.

All locally or regionally approved therapies should be proven to reliably achieve high cure rates. These recommendations should include the following: (a) antibiotic doses and frequency of administration; (b) PPI minimum dosage should be 60 mg omeprazole equivalent (e.g., 60 mg omeprazole, 60 mg lansoprazole, 40 mg esomeprazole or rabeprazole, or vonoprazan 20 mg); (c) twice daily for 14 days; and (d) the duration should be 14 days unless the regimen has been formally optimized to use a different duration (Table 6).

Table 6. Elements of empiric regimens used while the principles of antimicrobial stewardship are being introduced.

• Antibiotic doses and frequency of administration should be identified experimentally.
• The duration should be 14 days, unless the regimen has been formally optimized to use a different duration.
• PPI minimum dosage should be 60 mg omeprazole or equivalent (e.g., 60 mg omeprazole, 60 mg lansoprazole, 40 mg esomeprazole or rabeprazole), or 20 mg vonoprazan given twice daily.

Therapies that contain unneeded antibiotics should not be prescribed (e.g., those with three antibiotics, such as concomitant or sequential therapies, or vonoprazan triple therapies) [76]. The test-of-cure result should also be used as part of ongoing surveillance. Ideally, the results should be reported to a central site so that data from an area/region can be pooled and shared.

Regimens that fail to achieve the prespecified endpoint in a prespecified percentage (e.g., 10%) should be removed from the list of approved empiric therapies, although they may remain on the list of approved susceptibility-based therapies.

Although all the approved therapies are expected to achieve high cure rates (i.e., they have been quasi-optimized), each should be formally optimized, as they most likely canfurther improved. Optimization of therapies should be one of the first goals in the introduction of antimicrobial stewardship. As noted above, any modification of an approved therapy should first be confirmed as reliably highly effective using pilot studies without a comparator that also include susceptibility testing. A head-to-head comparison using noninferiority methodology should only be considered after a new or modified regimen has been proven to achieve a high cure rate.

Funding: This research received no external funding.

Conflicts of Interest: Graham is a consultant for RedHill Biopharma and Phathom Pharmaceuticals regarding novel *H. pylori* therapies and has received research support for culture of *Helicobacter pylori* and is the PI of an international study on the use of anti-mycobacterial therapy for Crohn's disease.

Support: Graham is supported in part by the Office of Research and Development Medical Research Service Department of Veterans Affairs, Washington DC and Public Health Service grants DK56338 which funds the Texas Medical Center Digestive Diseases Center. The contents are solely the responsibility of the author and do not necessarily represent the official views of the VA or NIH.

References

1. Hulscher, M.E.J.L.; Prins, J.M. Antibiotic stewardship: Does it work in hospital practice? A review of the evidence base. *Clin. Microbiol. Infect.* **2017**, *23*, 799–805. [CrossRef] [PubMed]
2. Charani, E.; Holmes, A. Antibiotic Stewardship-Twenty Years in the Making. *Antibiotics* **2019**, *8*, 7. [CrossRef] [PubMed]
3. Sugano, K.; Tack, J.; Kuipers, E.J.; Graham, D.Y.; El-Omar, E.M.; Miura, S.; Haruma, K.; Asaka, M.; Uemura, N.; Malfertheiner, P. Kyoto global consensus report on Helicobacter pylori gastritis. *Gut* **2015**, *64*, 1353–1367. [CrossRef] [PubMed]
4. Graham, D.Y.; Dore, M.P. Helicobacter pylori therapy: A paradigm shift. *Expert. Rev. Anti Infect. Ther.* **2016**, *14*, 577–585. [CrossRef] [PubMed]
5. Geisler, W.M.; Uniyal, A.; Lee, J.Y.; Lensing, S.Y.; Johnson, S.; Perry, R.C.; Kadrnka, C.M.; Kerndt, P.R. Azithromycin versus Doxycycline for Urogenital Chlamydia trachomatis Infection. *N. Engl. J. Med.* **2015**, *373*, 2512–2521. [CrossRef] [PubMed]
6. Ghanem, K.G.; Erbelding, E.J.; Cheng, W.W.; Rompalo, A.M. Doxycycline compared with benzathine penicillin for the treatment of early syphilis. *Clin. Infect. Dis.* **2006**, *42*, e45–e49. [CrossRef]
7. Riedner, G.; Rusizoka, M.; Todd, J.; Maboko, L.; Hoelscher, M.; Mmbando, D.; Samky, E.; Lyamuya, E.; Mabey, D.; Grosskurth, H.; et al. Single-dose azithromycin versus penicillin G benzathine for the treatment of early syphilis. *N. Engl. J. Med.* **2005**, *353*, 1236–1244. [CrossRef]
8. Olga, P.; Nyssen, O.P.; Bordin, D.; Tepes, B.; Pérez-Aisa, A.; Vaira, D. European Registry on *Helicobacter pylori* management (Hp-EuReg): Patterns and trends in first-line empirical eradication prescription and outcomes of 5 years and 21,533 patients. *Gut* **2020**, in press.
9. McNulty, C.A.; Dent, J.; Wise, R. Susceptibility of clinical isolates of Campylobacter pyloridis to 11 antimicrobial agents. *Antimicrob. Agents Chemother.* **1985**, *28*, 837–838. [CrossRef]
10. Borsch, G.M.; Graham, D.Y. Helicobacter pylori. In *Pharmacology of Peptic Ulcer Disease, Handbook of Experimental Pharmacology Volume 99*; Collen, M.J., Benjamin, S.B., Eds.; Springer: Berlin, Germany, 1991; pp. 107–148.
11. George, L.L.; Borody, T.J.; Andrews, P.; Devine, M.; Moore Jones, D.; Walton, M.; Brandl, S. Cure of duodenal ulcer after eradication of Helicobacter pylori. *Med. J. Aust.* **1990**, *153*, 145–149. [CrossRef]
12. Graham, D.Y.; Lew, G.M.; Klein, P.D.; Evans, D.G.; Evans, D.J., Jr.; Saeed, Z.A.; Malaty, H.M. Effect of treatment of Helicobacter pylori infection on the long- term recurrence of gastric or duodenal ulcer. A randomized, controlled study. *Ann. Intern. Med.* **1992**, *116*, 705–708. [CrossRef]
13. Graham, D.Y.; Lee, S.Y. How to effectively use bismuth quadruple therapy: The good, the bad, and the ugly. *Gastroenterol. Clin. N. Am.* **2015**, *44*, 537–563. [CrossRef] [PubMed]
14. McNulty, C.A.; Gearty, J.C.; Crump, B.; Davis, M.; Donovan, I.A.; Melikian, V.; Lister, D.M.; Wise, R. Campylobacter pyloridis and associated gastritis: Investigator blind, placebo controlled trial of bismuth salicylate and erythromycin ethylsuccinate. *Br. Med. J. (Clin. Res. Ed.)* **1986**, *293*, 645–649. [CrossRef] [PubMed]
15. Peterson, W.L.; Graham, D.Y.; Marshall, B.; Blaser, M.J.; Genta, R.M.; Klein, P.D.; Stratton, C.W.; Drnec, J.; Prokocimer, P.; Siepman, N. Clarithromycin as monotherapy for eradication of Helicobacter pylori: A randomized, double-blind trial. *Am. J. Gastroenterol.* **1993**, *88*, 1860–1864. [PubMed]
16. Al-Assi, M.T.; Genta, R.M.; Karttunen, T.J.; Graham, D.Y. Clarithromycin-amoxycillin therapy for Helicobacter pylori infection. *Aliment. Pharmacol. Ther.* **1994**, *8*, 453–456. [CrossRef]

17. Prevacid (Lansoprazole) Lable, FDA Full Prescribing Information [Online]. 2012. Available online: https://www.accessdata.fda.gov/drugsatfda_docs/label/2012/020406s078-021428s025lbl.pdf (accessed on 16 September 2020).
18. Graham, D.Y.; Dore, M.P.; Lu, H. Understanding treatment guidelines with bismuth and non-bismuth quadruple Helicobacter pylori eradication therapies. *Expert Rev. Anti Infect. Ther.* **2018**, *16*, 679–687. [CrossRef] [PubMed]
19. Dore, M.P.; Lu, H.; Graham, D.Y. Role of bismuth in improving Helicobacter pylori eradication with triple therapy. *Gut* **2016**, *65*, 870–878. [CrossRef]
20. Unge, P.; Gad, A.; Gnarpe, H.; Olsson, J. Does omeprazole improve antimicrobial therapy directed towards gastric Campylobacter pylori in patients with antral gastritis? A pilot study. *Scand. J. Gastroenterol. Suppl.* **1989**, *167*, 49–54. [CrossRef]
21. Yang, J.C.; Lin, C.J.; Wang, H.L.; Chen, J.D.; Kao, J.Y.; Shun, C.T.; Lu, C.W.; Lin, B.R.; Shieh, M.J.; Chang, M.C.; et al. High-dose dual therapy is superior to standard first-line or rescue therapy for Helicobacter pylori infection. *Clin. Gastroenterol. Hepatol.* **2015**, *13*, 895–905. [CrossRef]
22. Furuta, T.; Yamade, M.; Kagami, T.; Uotani, T.; Suzuki, T.; Higuchi, T.; Tani, S.; Hamaya, Y.; Iwaizumi, M.; Miyajima, H.; et al. Dual Therapy with Vonoprazan and Amoxicillin Is as Effective as Triple Therapy with Vonoprazan, Amoxicillin and Clarithromycin for Eradication of Helicobacter pylori. *Digestion* **2019**, 1–9. [CrossRef]
23. Graham, D.Y.; Dore, M.P. Update on the use of vonoprazan: A competitive acid blocker. *Gastroenterology* **2018**, *154*, 462–466. [CrossRef] [PubMed]
24. Graham, D.Y. Efficient identification and evaluation of effective Helicobacter pylori therapies. *Clin. Gastroenterol. Hepatol.* **2009**, *7*, 145–148. [CrossRef] [PubMed]
25. Graham, D.Y. Helicobacter pylori eradication therapy research: Ethical issues and description of results. *Clin. Gastroenterol. Hepatol.* **2010**, *8*, 1032–1036. [CrossRef]
26. Laheij, R.J.; Rossum, L.G.; Jansen, J.B.; Straatman, H.; Verbeek, A.L. Evaluation of treatment regimens to cure Helicobacter pylori infection- a meta-analysis. *Aliment. Pharmacol. Ther.* **1999**, *13*, 857–864. [CrossRef] [PubMed]
27. Janssen, M.J.; Van Oijen, A.H.; Verbeek, A.L.; Jansen, J.B.; de Boer, W.A. A systematic comparison of triple therapies for treatment of Helicobacter pylori infection with proton pump inhibitor/ranitidine bismuth citrate plus clarithromycin and either amoxicillin or a nitroimidazole. *Aliment. Pharmacol. Ther.* **2001**, *15*, 613–624. [CrossRef]
28. Zullo, A.; De, F.V.; Hassan, C.; Morini, S.; Vaira, D. The sequential therapy regimen for Helicobacter pylori eradication: A pooled-data analysis. *Gut* **2007**, *56*, 1353–1357. [CrossRef]
29. Gatta, L.; Vakil, N.; Vaira, D.; Scarpignato, C. Global eradication rates for Helicobacter pylori infection: Systematic review and meta-analysis of sequential therapy. *BMJ* **2013**, *347*, f4587. [CrossRef]
30. Graham, D.Y. Illusions regarding Helicobacter pylori clinical trials and treatment guidelines. *Gut* **2017**, *66*, 2043–2046. [CrossRef]
31. Graham, D.Y.; Tansel, A. Interchangeable use of proton pump inhibitors based on relative potency. *Clin. Gastroenterol. Hepatol.* **2018**, *6*, 800–808. [CrossRef]
32. Infectious Diseases Society of America (IDSA). White paper: Recommendations on the conduct of superiority and organism-specific clinical trials of antibacterial agents for the treatment of infections caused by drug-resistant bacterial pathogens. *Clin. Infect. Dis.* **2012**, *55*, 1031–1046. [CrossRef]
33. Chey, W.D.; Leontiadis, G.I.; Howden, C.W.; Moss, S.F. ACG Clinical Guideline: Treatment of Helicobacter pylori Infection. *Am. J. Gastroenterol.* **2017**, *112*, 212–239. [CrossRef] [PubMed]
34. Graham, D.Y.; El-Serag, H.B. The European registry on Helicobacter pylori management shows that Gastroenterology has largely failed in its efforts to guide practitioners. *Gut* **2020**, in press. [CrossRef] [PubMed]
35. European Helicobacter Pylori Study Group. Current European concepts in the management of Helicobacter pylori infection. The Maastricht Consensus Report. *Gut* **1997**, *41*, 8–13. [CrossRef] [PubMed]
36. Lam, S.K.; Talley, N.J. Report of the 1997 Asia Pacific Consensus Conference on the management of Helicobacter pylori infection. *J. Gastroenterol. Hepatol.* **1998**, *13*, 1–12. [CrossRef] [PubMed]
37. Bochenek, W.J.; Peters, S.; Fraga, P.D.; Wang, W.; Mack, M.E.; Osato, M.S.; El Zimaity, H.M.; Davis, K.D.; Graham, D.Y. Eradication of Helicobacter pylori by 7-Day Triple-Therapy Regimens Combining Pantoprazole

with Clarithromycin, Metronidazole, or Amoxicillin in Patients with Peptic Ulcer Disease: Results of Two Double-Blind, Randomized Studies. *Helicobacter* **2003**, *8*, 626–642. [CrossRef]
38. Fennerty, M.B.; Kovacs, T.O.; Krause, R.; Haber, M.; Weissfeld, A.; Siepman, N.; Rose, P. A comparison of 10 and 14 days of lansoprazole triple therapy for eradication of Helicobacter pylori. *Arch. Intern. Med.* **1998**, *158*, 1651–1656. [CrossRef]
39. Vakil, N.; Lanza, F.; Schwartz, H.; Barth, J. Seven-day therapy for Helicobacter pylori in the United States. *Aliment. Pharmacol. Ther.* **2004**, *20*, 99–107. [CrossRef]
40. Laine, L.; Frantz, J.E.; Baker, A.; Neil, G.A. A United States multicentre trial of dual and proton pump inhibitor-based triple therapies for Helicobacter pylori. *Aliment. Pharmacol. Ther.* **1997**, *11*, 913–917. [CrossRef]
41. Prilosec (Omeprazole) Label, FDA Full Prescribing Information [Online]. 1909. Available online: https://www.accessdata.fda.gov/drugsatfda_docs/label/2012/019810s096lbl.pdf (accessed on 16 September 2020).
42. Aciphex (Rabeprazole Sodium) Label, FDA Full Prescribing Information [Online]. 2014. Available online: https://www.accessdata.fda.gov/drugsatfda_docs/label/2014/020973s035204736s005lbl.pdf (accessed on 16 September 2020).
43. Nexium (Esomprazole Magnesium) Label, FDA Full Prescribing Information [Online]. 2014. Available online: https://www.accessdata.fda.gov/drugsatfda_docs/label/2014/022101s014021957s017021153s050lbl.pdf (accessed on 16 September 2020).
44. Helicac. FDA Full Prescribing Information 2008. Available online: https://www.accessdata.fda.gov/drugsatfda_docs/label/2008/050719s013lbl.pdf (accessed on 16 September 2020).
45. Pylera. FDA Full Prescribing Information 2017. Available online: https://www.accessdata.fda.gov/drugsatfda_docs/label/2017/050786s016lbl.pdf (accessed on 16 September 2020).
46. Graham, D.Y.; Shiotani, A. New concepts of resistance in the treatment of Helicobacter pylori infections. *Nat. Clin. Pract. Gastroenterol. Hepatol.* **2008**, *5*, 321–331. [CrossRef]
47. Keren, I.; Kaldalu, N.; Spoering, A.; Wang, Y.; Lewis, K. Persister cells and tolerance to antimicrobials. *FEMS Microbiol. Lett.* **2004**, *230*, 13–18. [CrossRef]
48. Lewis, K. Persister cells, dormancy and infectious disease. *Nat. Rev. Microbiol.* **2007**, *5*, 48–56. [CrossRef] [PubMed]
49. Scott, D.; Weeks, D.; Melchers, K.; Sachs, G. The life and death of Helicobacter pylori. *Gut* **1998**, *43* (Suppl. S1), S56–S60. [CrossRef] [PubMed]
50. Sachs, G.; Weeks, D.L.; Melchers, K.; Scott, D.R. The gastric Biology of Helicobactor pylori. *Annu. Rev. Physiol.* **2003**, *65*, 349–369. [CrossRef] [PubMed]
51. Graham, D.Y.; Lee, Y.C.; Wu, M.S. Rational Helicobacter pylori therapy: Evidence-based medicine rather than medicine-based evidence. *Clin. Gastroenterol. Hepatol.* **2014**, *12*, 177–186. [CrossRef] [PubMed]
52. Liou, J.M.; Chen, C.C.; Chen, M.J.; Chen, C.C.; Chang, C.Y.; Fang, Y.J.; Lee, J.Y.; Hsu, S.J.; Luo, J.C.; Chang, W.H.; et al. Sequential versus triple therapy for the first-line treatment of Helicobacter pylori: A multicentre, open-label, randomised trial. *Lancet* **2013**, *381*, 205–213. [CrossRef]
53. Saad, R.J.; Schoenfeld, P.; Kim, H.M.; Chey, W.D. Levofloxacin-based triple therapy versus bismuth-based quadruple therapy for persistent Helicobacter pylori infection: A meta-analysis. *Am. J. Gastroenterol.* **2006**, *101*, 488–496. [CrossRef]
54. Miehlke, S.; Krasz, S.; Schneider-Brachert, W.; Kuhlisch, E.; Berning, M.; Madisch, A.; Laass, M.W.; Neumeyer, M.; Jebens, C.; Zekorn, C.; et al. Randomized trial on 14 versus 7 days of esomeprazole, moxifloxacin, and amoxicillin for second-line or rescue treatment of Helicobacter pylori Iinfection. *Helicobacter* **2011**, *16*, 420–426. [CrossRef]
55. Graham, D.Y. Hp-normogram (normo-graham) for assessing the outcome of H. pylori therapy: Effect of resistance, duration, and CYP2C19 genotype. *Helicobacter* **2015**, *21*, 85–90. [CrossRef]
56. de Boer, W.A.; Driessen, W.M.; Potters, V.P.; Tytgat, G.N. Randomized study comparing 1 with 2 weeks of quadruple therapy for eradicating Helicobacter pylori. *Am. J. Gastroenterol.* **1994**, *89*, 1993–1997.

57. de Boer, W.A.; Driessen, W.M.; Tytgat, G.N. Only four days of quadruple therapy can effectively cure Helicobacter pylori infection. *Aliment. Pharmacol. Ther.* **1995**, *9*, 633–638. [CrossRef]
58. de Boer, W.A.; van Etten, R.J.; Schade, R.W.; Ouwehand, M.E.; Schneeberger, P.M.; Tytgat, G.N. 4-day lansoprazole quadruple therapy: A highly effective cure for Helicobacter pylori infection. *Am. J. Gastroenterol.* **1996**, *91*, 1778–1782. [PubMed]
59. de Boer, W.A.; van Etten, R.J.; Lai, J.Y.; Schneeberger, P.M.; van de Wouw, B.A.; Driessen, W.M. Effectiveness of quadruple therapy using lansoprazole, instead of omeprazole, in curing Helicobacter pylori infection. *Helicobacter* **1996**, *1*, 145–150. [CrossRef] [PubMed]
60. El-Serag, H.B.; Kao, J.Y.; Kanwal, F.; Gilger, M.; LoVecchio, F.; Moss, S.F.; Crowe, S.; Elfant, A.; Haas, T.; Hapke, R.J.; et al. Houston Consensus Conference on testing for Helicobacter pylori infection in the United States. *Clin. Gastroenterol. Hepatol.* **2018**, *16*, 992–1002. [CrossRef]
61. Malfertheiner, P.; Megraud, F.; O'Morain, C.A.; Gisbert, J.P.; Kuipers, E.J.; Axon, A.T.; Bazzoli, F.; Gasbarrini, A.; Atherton, J.; Graham, D.Y.; et al. Management of Helicobacter pylori infection-the Maastricht V/Florence Consensus Report. *Gut* **2017**, *66*, 6–30. [CrossRef] [PubMed]
62. Fallone, C.A.; Chiba, N.; van Zanten, S.V.; Fischbach, L.; Gisbert, J.P.; Hunt, R.H.; Jones, N.L.; Render, C.; Leontiadis, G.I.; Moayyedi, P.; et al. The Toronto Consensus for the Treatment of Helicobacter pylori Infection in Adults. *Gastroenterology* **2016**, *151*, 51–69. [CrossRef] [PubMed]
63. Howden, C.W.; Hunt, R.H. Guidelines for the management of Helicobacter pylori infection. Ad Hoc Committee on Practice Parameters of the American College of Gastroenterology. *Am. J. Gastroenterol.* **1998**, *93*, 2330–2338. [CrossRef] [PubMed]
64. Osato, M.S.; Graham, D.Y. Etest for metronidazole susceptibility in H. pylori: Use of the wrong standard may have led to the wrong conclusion. *Am. J. Gastroenterol.* **2004**, *99*, 769. [CrossRef] [PubMed]
65. Osato, M.S.; Reddy, R.; Reddy, S.G.; Penland, R.L.; Graham, D.Y. Comparison of the Etest and the NCCLS-approved agar dilution method to detect metronidazole and clarithromycin resistant Helicobacter pylori. *Int. J. Antimicrob. Agents* **2001**, *17*, 39–44. [CrossRef]
66. Nyssen, O.P.; McNicholl, A.G.; Gisbert, J.P. Meta-analysis of three-in-one single capsule bismuth-containing quadruple therapy for the eradication of Helicobacter pylori. *Helicobacter* **2019**, *24*, e12570. [CrossRef] [PubMed]
67. Nyssen, O.P.; Perez-Aisa, A.; Rodrigo, L.; Castro, M.; Mata, R.P.; Ortuno, J.; Barrio, J.; Huguet, J.M.; Modollel, I.; Alcaide, N.; et al. Bismuth quadruple regimen with tetracycline or doxycycline versus three-in-one single capsule as third-line rescue therapy for Helicobacter pylori infection: Spanish data of the European Helicobacter pylori Registry (Hp-EuReg). *Helicobacter* **2020**, e12722. [CrossRef]
68. Shiotani, A.; Lu, H.; Dore, M.P.; Graham, D.Y. Treating Helicobacter pylori effectively while minimizing misuse of antibiotics. *Cleve. Clin. J. Med.* **2017**, *84*, 310–318. [CrossRef] [PubMed]
69. Dang, B.N.; Graham, D.Y. Helicobacter pylori infection and antibiotic resistance: A WHO high priority? *Nat. Rev. Gastroenterol. Hepatol.* **2017**, *7*, 383–384. [CrossRef] [PubMed]
70. Riahizadeh, S.; Malekzadeh, R.; Agah, S.; Zendehdel, N.; Sotoudehmanesh, R.; Ebrahimi-Dariani, N.; Pourshams, A.; Vahedi, H.; Mikaeli, J.; Khatibian, M.; et al. Sequential metronidazole-furazolidone or clarithromycin-furazolidone compared to clarithromycin-based quadruple regimens for the eradication of Helicobacter pylori in peptic ulcer disease: A double-blind randomized controlled trial. *Helicobacter* **2010**, *15*, 497–504. [CrossRef] [PubMed]
71. A Rule by the Centers for Medicare & Medicaid Services Federal Register [Online]. 2019. Available online: https://federalregister.gov/d/2019-20736 (accessed on 15 July 2020).
72. Core Elements of Antibiotic Stewardship. Centers for Disease Control and Prevention [Online] 2019. Available online: https://www.cdc.gov/antibiotic-use/core-elements/resource-limited.html (accessed on 15 July 2020).
73. Malfertheiner, P.; Megraud, F.; O'Morain, C.; Bazzoli, F.; El-Omar, E.; Graham, D.; Hunt, R.; Rokkas, T.; Vakil, N.; Kuipers, E.J. Current concepts in the management of Helicobacter pylori infection: The Maastricht III Consensus Report. *Gut* **2007**, *56*, 772–781. [CrossRef] [PubMed]
74. Malfertheiner, P.; Megraud, F.; O'Morain, C.A.; Atherton, J.; Axon, A.T.; Bazzoli, F.; Gensini, G.F.; Gisbert, J.P.; Graham, D.Y.; Rokkas, T.; et al. Management of Helicobacter pylori infection–the Maastricht IV/ Florence Consensus Report. *Gut* **2012**, *61*, 646–664. [CrossRef]

75. Savoldi, A.; Carrara, E.; Graham, D.Y.; Conti, M.; Tacconelli, E. Prevalence of Antibiotic Resistance in Helicobacter pylori: A Systematic Review and Meta-analysis in World Health Organization Regions. *Gastroenterology* **2018**, *155*, 1372–1382. [CrossRef]
76. Graham, D.Y.; Lu, H.; Shiotani, A. Vonoprazan-containing H, pylori triple therapy contributes to increasing global antimicrobial resistance. *J. Gastroenterol. Hepatol.* **2020**, in press.

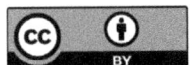

© 2020 by the author. Licensee MDPI, Basel, Switzerland. This article is an open access article distributed under the terms and conditions of the Creative Commons Attribution (CC BY) license (http://creativecommons.org/licenses/by/4.0/).

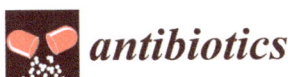

Review

Update on Acute Bone and Joint Infections in Paediatrics: A Narrative Review on the Most Recent Evidence-Based Recommendations and Appropriate Antinfective Therapy

Giovanni Autore, Luca Bernardi and Susanna Esposito *

Pediatric Clinic, Pietro Barilla Children's Hospital, Department of Medicine and Surgery, University of Parma, 43126 Parma, Italy; giovanniautore@gmail.com (G.A.); bernardi.luca91@gmail.com (L.B.)
* Correspondence: susanna.esposito@unimi.it; Tel.: +39-0521-903524

Received: 7 July 2020; Accepted: 4 August 2020; Published: 6 August 2020

Abstract: Acute bone and joint infections (BJIs) in children may clinically occur as osteomyelitis (OM) or septic arthritis (SA). In clinical practice, one-third of cases present a combination of both conditions. BJIs are usually caused by the haematogenous dissemination of septic emboli carried to the terminal blood vessels of bone and joints from distant infectious processes during transient bacteraemia. Early diagnosis is the cornerstone for the successful management of BJI, but it is still a challenge for paediatricians, particularly due to its nonspecific clinical presentation and to the poor specificity of the laboratory and imaging first-line tests that are available in emergency departments. Moreover, microbiological diagnosis is often difficult to achieve with common blood cultures, and further investigations require invasive procedures. The aim of this narrative review is to provide the most recent evidence-based recommendations on appropriate antinfective therapy in BJI in children. We conducted a review of recent literature by examining the MEDLINE (Medical Literature Analysis and Retrieval System Online) database using the search engines PubMed and Google Scholar. The keywords used were "osteomyelitis", OR "bone infection", OR "septic arthritis", AND "p(a)ediatric" OR "children". When BJI diagnosis is clinically suspected or radiologically confirmed, empiric antibiotic therapy should be started as soon as possible. The choice of empiric antimicrobial therapy is based on the most likely causative pathogens according to patient age, immunisation status, underlying disease, and other clinical and epidemiological considerations, including the local prevalence of virulent pathogens, antibiotic bioavailability and bone penetration. Empiric antibiotic treatment consists of a short intravenous cycle based on anti-staphylococcal penicillin or a cephalosporin in children aged over 3 months with the addition of gentamicin in infants aged under 3 months. An oral regimen may be an option depending on the bioavailability of antibiotic chosen and clinical and laboratory data. Strict clinical and laboratory follow-up should be scheduled for the following 3–5 weeks. Further studies on the optimal therapeutic approach are needed in order to understand the best first-line regimen, the utility of biomarkers for the definition of therapy duration and treatment of complications.

Keywords: antibiotic; bone infection; joint infection; osteomyelitis; pediatric infectious disease; septic arthritis

1. Introduction

Acute bone and joint infections (BJIs) in children may clinically occur as osteomyelitis (OM) or septic arthritis (SA). BJIs generally present clinically within 2 weeks of disease onset [1]. In clinical practice, one-third of cases present a combination of both conditions, and this combination may occur in as many as 75% of cases in newborns [2]. BJIs are usually caused by the haematogenous dissemination of septic emboli carried to the terminal blood vessels of bone and joints from distant infectious processes during transient bacteraemia. Less common infection routes are direct inoculation due to open fractures or invasive procedures and extension from contiguous infections, such as cellulitis and sinusitis. BJI can be classified as acute, subacute and chronic according to its duration: <2 weeks, <3 months and >3 months from onset, respectively. Chronic infections are relatively rare conditions in paediatric patients, could be caused by the establishment of biofilm, and different surgical approaches must be considered [3].

The mean annual incidence of BJI in high-income countries is approximately 8 per 100,000 children [4,5]. Despite the high variability between different reports, an increasing trend has been observed over the last few decades, probably due to increased diagnostic effectiveness. Gafur et al. observed that the annualised per capita incidence of OM increased 2.8-fold in the same paediatric hospital within two decades [4]. Children aged ≤ 5 years showed a higher prevalence, accounting for half of all cases [6]. Although uncommon, BJI in children should not be underestimated because local and systemic complications may result in life-threatening conditions and severe disabilities. If not promptly diagnosed and treated, the infection may extend to soft tissues, causing pyomyositis (especially in young infants) and sepsis [7]. Local progression may result in subperiosteal or intraosseous abscesses, pathological fractures, and abnormal bone growth due to the involvement of the epiphysis [8–10]. Venous thrombosis and septic embolism may also occur, more commonly in children aged >8 years [11,12].

Early diagnosis is the cornerstone for the successful management of BJI, but it is still a challenge for paediatricians, particularly due to its nonspecific clinical presentation and to the poor specificity of the laboratory and imaging first-line tests that are available in emergency departments. Moreover, microbiological diagnosis is often difficult to achieve with common blood cultures, and further investigations require invasive procedures. The indications and effectiveness of available diagnostic tools are still debated. In addition, the resistance pattern of aetiological agents and poor bone penetration of antibiotics represent a challenge for an appropriate therapeutic approach. Therefore, the aim of this narrative review is to provide the most recent evidence-based recommendations on appropriate antinfective therapy in BJI in children.

2. Aetiology and Pathogenesis

BJI commonly occurs in primarily healthy children without clear predisposing conditions. However, a higher prevalence is described in patients affected by immunodeficiencies and haemoglobinopathies, particularly sickle cell disease (SCD) and chronic granulomatous disease (CGD) [13,14]. Previous experimental studies on animal models have suggested that minor trauma may increase the susceptibility of bone and joint tissues to bacterial seeding [15]. More recent clinical studies question this association because children affected by BJIs show the same rate of previous minor trauma observed in the general paediatric population [16].

More than 80% of the cases of OM occur in the metaphysis of long tubular bones, and the most common localisations are the femur and tibia, followed by the pelvis and calcaneus among nontubular bones [17,18]. A nationwide survey conducted in the USA revealed that osteomyelitis in the pelvis, upper arm, hand and forearm was associated with a higher risk of septic arthritis and bacteraemia or septicaemia [19]. The knee and hip are the most commonly involved joints, accounting for more than half of SA cases [18]. In a large multicentre study recently conducted in Spain, the involvement of the hip in children affected by combined osteomyelitis and septic arthritis was the main negative prognostic factor associated with a higher risk of complications and sequelae [20].

The choice of proper empiric treatment is the main issue in the management of paediatric BJI. First-line antibiotics should cover the most likely aetiologies according to the patient's age and local prevalence of community-acquired and nosocomial pathogens. In addition, they should have an appropriate bone penetration. According to the largest studies in recent literature, methicillin-sensitive

Staphylococcus aureus (MSSA) may still be considered the most common pathogen in Europe, with a prevalence ranging from 30% to 63% of confirmed cases [5]. However, the emerging role of *Kingella kingae* has been confirmed by several studies reporting its isolation in up to 53% of all cases [5]. In addition, *Streptococcus pneumoniae* and Group A β-haemolytic *Streptococcus pyogenes* (GABHS) maintain a relevant role in patients aged ≥ 6 months. On the other hand, the prevalence of *Haemophilus influenzae* type b has drastically decreased in the post-vaccination era, accounting for less than 1% of cases [21].

The aetiology, however, largely depends on the patient's age (Table 1). A recent multicentre study conducted in France on 71 patients aged under 3 months reported that *Streptococcus agalactiae* is the main community-acquired pathogen accounting for 45% of these cases, followed by *S. aureus* (22% of all cases) which was the most frequent microorganism in infants aged over 2 months, and *Escherichia coli* (18%) [22]. These findings were confirmed by Juchler et al. in infants aged 0–6 months, reporting *S. aureus*, *S. agalactiae*, and *E. coli* as the most frequently isolated pathogens, accounting for 31%, 15%, and 8% of these cases, respectively [23]. In this age group, both studies observed that *Klebsiella pneumoniae* and *Candida albicans* are particularly frequent nosocomial pathogens, and they each account for 7% of cases [22]. Among children aged between 6 months and 5 years, *K. kingae* is the most frequent cause of osteoarticular infections, accounting for half of these cases [23]. Less frequent pathogens in this age group are *S. pneumoniae* and GABHS, which were isolated in 29% and 7% of cases, respectively [23]. In the post-vaccination era, *S. pneumoniae* still represents a causative agent of septic arthritis, accounting for over 4% of all cases [4,17]. The detection of *K. kingae* requires specific PCR assays. *K. kingae* seems to be very specific for the age group under 5 years. In fact, a large review of 566 osteoarticular infections caused by this pathogen reported that 80% of these cases occurred in children aged under 4 years [24]. Moreover, Ferroni et al. observed a higher prevalence of *K. kingae* among children affected by SA than OM [25]. A prospective case-control study revealed that oropharyngeal carriage of *K. kingae* is strongly associated with haematogenous BJI in children aged under 4 years. Using a specific polymerase chain reaction (PCR) assay, the authors identified the microorganism in the oropharynx of 71% of previously confirmed cases of osteoarticular infections and only in 6% of age-matched healthy controls, reporting an odds ratio of approximately 38.3 (95% CI, 18.5–79.1) [26].

Table 1. Most common pathogens causing bone and joint infection in children and recommended first-line intravenous (IV) empiric treatment of different age groups.

Age Group	Pathogen	Empiric First-Line IV Treatment
<6 months	Staphylococcus aureus Streptococcus agalactiae (<2 months) Escherichia coli Klebsiella pneumoniae, Candida albicans (nosocomial infections)	First/second generation cephalosporin or anti-staphylococcal penicillin + gentamicin (if age <3 months)
6–48 months	Kingella kingae Staphylococcus aureus Group A β-haemolytic Streptococcus pyogenes Streptococcus pneumoniae	First/second-generation cephalosporin Clindamycin (if local MRSA prevalence >10%)
>5 years	Staphylococcus aureus Kingella kingae Group A β-haemolytic Streptococcus pyogenes	First/second-generation cephalosporin or anti-staphylococcal penicillin Clindamycin (if local MRSA prevalence >10%)

MRSA, methicillin-resistant *S. aureus*.

BJIs in children aged over 5 years are most frequently caused by *S. aureus*, which accounts for up to 61% of these cases [23]. *K. kingae* is isolated in less than 13% of cases in this age group, followed by GABHS [20,23]. Once considered mainly nosocomial, the prevalence of particularly virulent strains of community-acquired *S. aureus* (CA-SA) is increasing, causing severe forms of BJI. Approximately 70–90% of confirmed cases caused by CA-SA involve methicillin-sensitive strains (MSSA), but there has been an increase in cases of BJI from community-acquired methicillin-resistant

S. aureus (CA-MRSA) [27,28]. Studying the regional prevalence of CA-MRSA is mandatory because, according to the recent guidelines published by the European Society for Paediatric Infectious Diseases (ESPID), a local prevalence over 10% should induce clinicians to choose a different empiric treatment from conventional first-line drugs. Another virulence factor causing severe forms of staphylococcal infections with issues of management is Panton–Valentine leukocidin (PVL). PVL is a bicomponent, pore-forming toxin produced by some strains of S. aureus (PVL-SA) that kills leukocytes. A multicentre European study conducted in 7 countries reported that PVL-SA reached an incidence up to 18%, and PVL was produced more frequently by MSSA strains in Europe, whereas it was more common among MRSA strains in the United States [29]. In the same study, MRSA isolates represented 6% of all cases caused by CA-SA [29]. Nationwide studies conducted in Spain and the UK observed rates of CA-MRSA ranging from 2.5% to 3% of all community-acquired staphylococcal infections, while PVL-SA has been isolated in 10% of these cases in Italy [20,30]. CA-MRSA seems to be less prevalent in European populations than in the USA, where its prevalence reached 30% in some regions within the last two decades [31].

3. Clinical Presentation

Onset symptoms of BJI are usually nonspecific in children. Children with osteomyelitis usually present acutely with fever and constitutional symptoms, such as irritability and decreased activity. Once the infection progresses, focal symptoms and signs of bone inflammation may occur. According to a large systematic review conducted over a population of 12,000 children with BJI, the most common onset features included localised pain (81%); focal warmth, swelling and point tenderness (70%), fever (62%) and limitation of function (50%) [17]. Clinical suspicion may be difficult in newborns and toddlers because they often lack focal findings and may continue to feed well. Although osteomyelitis is rare in this age group, it should be considered for the differential diagnosis in infants with skin infections, urinary tract anomalies, prematurity, and neonatal sepsis. Mediamolle et al. reported that 94% of infants aged under 3 months showed pain, and 87% of them had functional limitations, but only 52% were febrile [22]. BJI should also be suspected in older children presenting with fever without a source, bacteraemia, and abnormal radiological findings in the evaluation of trauma. A recent history of infections is uncommon, and this makes it difficult to identify the initial source of haematogenous dissemination. Ferroni et al. were able to tentatively identify the portal of entry in only 55% of cases, of which 55% were upper respiratory tract infections; 15%, skin trauma; 11%, gastro-enteritis; 8%, varicella; and 2%, congenital infections [25].

Special populations of children at higher risk of BJI may present with atypical features. Patients with haemoglobinopathy (i.e., sickle cell disease) may present multifocal infections that are difficult to distinguish from vaso-occlusive crisis [13]. Children with chronic granulomatous disease may have BJIs caused by uncommon bacterial or fungal pathogens that usually remain asymptomatic even in advanced stages [14].

When OM is suspected, the differential diagnosis should include traumatic fracture, cellulitis or pyomyositis, rheumatic fever, thrombophlebitis, leukaemia, tumours, sickle cell infarction, tuberculosis, scurvy, and other bone inflammatory processes such as hypophosphatasia and chronic recurrent multifocal osteomyelitis (CRMO). Sepsis should also be ruled out in neonates. Moreover, some clinical signs of SA may also occur in cases of transient synovitis, viral arthritis, reactive arthritis, juvenile idiopathic arthritis, Henoch–Schoenlein purpura, and Perthes disease.

4. Diagnosis

4.1. Blood Examination

Initial blood tests for children with suspected BJI include the complete blood count (CBC), erythrocyte sedimentation rate (ESR), and level of C-reactive protein (CRP) [32]. Elevated ESR and CRP show a high sensitivity at disease onset but a low specificity. Dartnell et al. observed that CRP was elevated in 81% of patients at the time of presentation, with a peak on the second day from onset; instead, ESR peaked 3–5 days after onset [17]. The same study showed that the WBC count was elevated in only 36% of children at the time of diagnosis [17]. However, the CBC is helpful in the differential diagnosis of children with bone pain (e.g., leukaemia). A prospective study of 265 children with osteomyelitis and septic arthritis reported a mean CRP value of approximately 87 mg/L and a mean ESR value of approximately 51 mm/h at the time of presentation [33]. The combination of elevated CRP and ESR showed the best sensitivity to suspect BJI in children [33]. Several studies observed that CRP and ESR are higher and remain abnormal for a longer period in patients with MRSA infection [34]. In addition, MRSA is associated with greater elevations in CRP, ESR and WBC levels [18]. At this time, the role of procalcitonin is unclear, and its effectiveness compared to CRP is debated [32]. Blood culture should always be obtained at the same time as initial blood tests, as well as in afebrile patients, if the clinical suspicion of BJI is well-founded [32].

4.2. Imaging

The initial imaging study should be the radiograph of the suspected area in order to exclude other causes of pain [32]. However, radiographs are usually normal at the beginning of BJIs, and other advanced techniques are often required. Exceptions may be presented by newborns, who more commonly show abnormal radiographs at the onset [35].

The main X-ray features that suggest a BJI are periosteal reaction, periosteal elevation (suggesting a periosteal abscess), lytic lesions or sclerosis, and narrowing of the intervertebral disc space. At the onset, these alterations are often undetectable, and the timing of radiographic changes depends on the involved bones and the age of the patient. In long bones, cortical thickening and periosteal reaction/elevation are shown only 10 to 21 days after the onset of symptoms (7 to 10 days in newborns) [36]. Lytic sclerosis usually occurs only after more than a month. Due to the indolent course of the discitis that delays the onset of symptoms, X-ray signs of this category of BJI are often evident at the time of presentation [37].

Indications for additional imaging studies are confirmation of the diagnosis in clinically suspected BJI with normal radiographs, further evaluation of detected lesion and its extension (i.e., the involvement of epiphysis and adjacent soft tissues), surgical planning, and guidance for percutaneous procedures.

Magnetic resonance imaging (MRI) can be considered the gold standard imaging method for the diagnosis of BJI and to evaluate the involvement of surrounding soft tissues or joints [32]. The sensitivity and specificity of this technique range from 80% to 100% and from 50% to 100%, respectively [17]. The variability observed between the reported specificity rates may also depend on radiologist-specific experience. The use of intravenous gadolinium is not routinely required, but it is useful to detect intramedullary or muscular abscesses or necrosis, although it should be avoided in patients with renal insufficiency due to the risk of nephrogenic systemic fibrosis [38,39].

MRI can highlight multiple alterations that suggest the diagnosis of BJI. Areas of active inflammation show a decreased signal in T1-weighted images and an increased signal in T2-weighted images [40]. Fat-suppression sequences, including short-tau inversion recovery (STIR), decrease the signal from fat and are more sensitive for the detection of bone marrow oedema. In discitis, MRI easily detects the reduction of disc space, the increased T2-weighted signal in the adjacent vertebral endplates, and bone oedema in the vertebral body [38].

MRI is superior to other imaging methods, particularly to identify early infections affecting the bone marrow before the involvement of the cortical bone, to detect pelvic OM and discitis that are usually undetected by X-rays, to evaluate the involvement of the growth plates, joint structures, and soft tissues (e.g., pyomyositis, muscular abscesses) and to exclude deep venous thrombosis associated with BJI [41–43]. Furthermore, MRI is usually required in presurgical planning and surgical follow-up when drainage is indicated. MRI is also preferred because it prevents children from exposure to ionising radiation.

The main disadvantages of MRI are the longer scan time than CT and the need for sedation in young children. Furthermore, MRI is not always easily available, and it is more expensive. Because of its high sensitivity, the diagnosis of BJI is unlikely if the MRI is negative [44]. False-positive results can occur in patients with primary infections in adjacent soft tissues.

Regarding other imaging methods, computerised tomography (CT) scans are not generally recommended because they are less sensitive than MRI and expose children to ionising radiation. It should be considered in diagnosis only when MRI is not feasible [32]. However, CT scans may play a role when there is important bone destruction on radiographs to assess the extent of bone damage for a surgical approach [41]. It should also be useful in chronic OM when inflammation is too weak to be detected by MRI. In these cases, a CT scan can be performed without sedation and takes less time than MRI. BJI can be detected by the evidence of increased bone marrow density, new periosteal bone formation with periosteal purulence and irregular erosion of bone surfaces.

Bone scintigraphy is used to identify multifocal OM or when localised signs of bone involvement are too poor. It may be more accessible than MRI, and sedation is required less frequently. Technetium radionuclide scanning (^{99m}Tc) has high sensitivity but lower specificity compared to MRI; furthermore, scintigraphy has proven to be scarcely sensitive (53%) for OM caused by MRSA [44,45]. ^{99m}Tc scanning is triphasic, consisting of the flow phase (2 to 5 s after injection), blood pool phase (5 to 10 min after injection), and delayed phase (2 to 4 h after injection). BJI causes focal absorption in the third phase, and signal intensity is related to the level of osteoblastic activity. Localisation of a lesion near a growth plate can complicate the interpretation. Using ^{99m}Tc-methylene diphosphonate (^{99m}Tc-MDP), early evidence of infection can be detected 24 h after onset. Hsu et al. observed that specificity may increase with Gallium scanning and In-labelled leukocytes, although these techniques are more complex and add higher radiation exposure [46]. The disadvantages of scintigraphy are the lack of information on the size of pus collections that could be drained (i.e., in cases of intramedullary abscess), exposure to ionising radiation, and false-negative results that may occur if the blood flow to the periosteum is interrupted (i.e., in cases of subperiosteal abscess) [44].

Ultrasonography (US) is not useful for the diagnosis of BJI. With US, it is possible to identify the fluid collections in soft tissues associated with bone infections, and US can be a support for percutaneous diagnostic and therapeutic drainage [47]. Table 2 summarises indications and features of imaging methods in bone and joint infection in pediatric age.

Table 2. Indications and features of imaging methods in bone and joint infection in pediatric age.

Imaging	Indications	Features
Plain radiographs	Baseline in the emergency department Excluding other conditions in the differential diagnosis	Sensitivity: <20% Specificity: 80–100% Only late signs of infections are usually detected. A normal radiograph at onset does not exclude osteomyelitis.
MRI	Confirming the diagnosis and evaluating the extension of the infection to joints and soft tissues Monitoring disease progression Surgical planning	Sensitivity: 80–100% Specificity: 70–100% Gold-standard imaging test to confirm the diagnosis Less useful in multifocal or poorly localised infections
Scintigraphy	Poorly localised or multifocal disease	Sensitivity: 53–100% Specificity: 50–100% More useful in multifocal infections Does not evaluate the extent of purulent collections
CT	When MRI is not available or is contraindicated Surgical planning	Sensitivity: <70% Specificity: <50%
US	Evaluation and monitoring of purulent collections in joints and muscles	Sensitivity: <55% Specificity: <45%

MRI, magnetic resonance imaging; CT, computed tomography; US, ultrasonography.

4.3. Microbiological Diagnosis

With the increasing prevalence of antibiotic-resistant microorganisms and emerging pathogens, it is important to collect as many microbiological specimens as possible, and different microbiological tests are often required (Table 3). A microbiological diagnosis is achieved in barely more than half of all cases. In their systematic review, Dartnell et al. reported that microbiological diagnosis is achieved in approximately 50% of all cases of BJI [17]. In the context of a paediatric emergency department, Akinkugbe et al. reported microbiological isolation in only 38% of their cases [30]. On the other hand, a significantly higher success rate, approximately 70%, was reported in a population of patients aged under 3 months [22]. Calvo et al. also observed that the rate of microbiological diagnosis reached 61% in the combined form of OM and SA [20].

Table 3. Indications for microbiological tests.

Test	Indications
Blood culture	In every patient at initial evaluation if BJI is clinically suspected even without fever To be repeated at fever peaks if the previous blood culture is negative
Arthrocentesis (synovial fluid culture)	Easily accessible joints: in every patient at initial evaluation if SA is clinically suspected Proximal joints: in complicated/nonresponsive cases
Bone biopsy	In complicated/nonresponsive cases if a bone abscess occurs Always when orthopaedic surgery is indicated

Blood culture has the lowest sensitivity, but it is also the most accessible technique. Reported rates of positive blood cultures are highly variable in the literature. McNeil et al. estimated a general sensitivity of approximately 46%, and other studies observed even lower rates for SA [20,48]. Juchler et al. observed that sensitivity may be increased by performing PCR assays on negative cultures; in this way, the authors reported an increase of +4.5% [23]. However, according to the ESPID guidelines, blood culture should always be analysed in cases where there is clinical suspicion (including afebrile patients); the culture should be performed at the same time as the initial laboratory evaluations and should be repeated at fever peaks [32].

When joint involvement is clinically suspected, synovial fluid can be obtained for microbiological analysis. For easily accessible joints (e.g., knee), arthrocentesis may be performed under conscious sedation in the emergency room. Less accessible joints, such as the ankle and hip, need an interventional radiologist. The sensitivity of synovial fluid culture is higher than that observed for blood culture and can be higher than 50% [48]. Arthrocentesis should always be performed when the involvement of accessible joints is clinically evident, and it should also be considered in complicated or nonresponsive cases affecting proximal joints. In order to increase the diagnostic yield of joint aspirate, synovial fluid can be inoculated in blood culture vials.

Bone samples can be obtained with a minimally invasive percutaneous needle biopsy, especially when subperiosteal abscesses occur, or with surgical biopsy in the operating room. The reported sensitivity rates for these invasive techniques may reach 82%, but they expose patients to higher risks [48]. Bone biopsy should be performed in complicated cases with negative blood culture that do not respond to empiric treatment, but it may also be considered when a bone abscess is easily accessible [32]. In fact, for most uncomplicated BJIs, invasive biopsy does not affect the clinical outcomes [49,50]. Nevertheless, surgical biopsy should be performed in every patient who undergoes surgical treatment. In their large prospective study, Ferroni et al. performed arthrocentesis for every SA and bone biopsy only when a subperiosteal abscess occurred; in this way, the authors reported high rates of microbiological isolation, reaching 40% for synovial fluid and 87% for bone samples [25].

Nucleic acid amplification methods, such as conventional and real-time polymerase chain reaction (PCR), improved the detection of pathogens even after the administration of antibiotics. Synovial fluid PCR may remain diagnostic up to 6 days after the first antibiotic dose, and similar results have been observed for bone samples [51]. Specific PCR analysis may also be the only way to identify *K. kingae* and its isolation can be enhancement by inoculation of samples in blood culture vials [51,52].

5. Antinfective Treatment

Empiric antinfective treatment should be started as soon as BJI is clinically suspected. The choice of empiric antimicrobial therapy is based on the most likely causative pathogens according to patient age, immunisation status, underlying disease, and other clinical and epidemiological considerations, including the local prevalence of MRSA. In addition, antibiotic bioavailability and bone penetration should be considered [53]. Then, management is guided by the results of the antibiograms obtained from the microbiological investigations performed before starting antimicrobial therapy [36].

In neonates younger than two months, empirical treatment should be oxacillin or cefazolin and gentamicin to cover *S. agalactiae* and other gram-negative organisms that are common causes of BJI in this age group [22,54,55]. In children aged 3 months and over, anti-staphylococcal penicillin or a cephalosporin such as cefazolin or cefuroxime should be used to target MSSA, *S. pneumoniae*, GABHS and *K. kingae* [32]. Among the anti-staphylococcal penicillins, the use of flucloxacillin should be preferred because it is well tolerated and shows high bone penetration, even if it is difficult to use for the type of formulation.

In areas with a local prevalence of MRSA higher than 10%, the administration of empirical therapies active against these pathogens is indicated [32,49]. In these cases, the first-choice drugs are clindamycin, vancomycin or linezolid [32,56]. Peltola et al. suggested the empirical use of clindamycin in areas where the prevalence of MRSA is over 10%, and the clindamycin resistance rate is under 10% or vancomycin if the prevalence of MRSA is over 10% and the clindamycin resistance rate is over 10%, with linezolid as the second-line choice [49]. Dalbavancin, even as a single dose, appeared effective in children with BJI due to MRSA [57,58]. Compared to other available antibiotics that are active against MRSA, the advantages of dalbavancin include a lower potential for drug interactions and the possibility of fewer required doses due to a longer half-life [59]. Another second-line drug after the failure of previous antibiotics may be daptomycin [60,61]. In complicated severe cases, when the involvement of PVL SA is suspected, antibiotic therapy should aim to inhibit toxin production. In these cases, inhibitors of protein synthesis, such as clindamycin, linezolid, and rifampicin, are the first choice [62,63]. Among less common pathogens, *Salmonella* spp. is a frequent cause of BJI in developing countries and in patients with sickle cell anaemia, and it should be treated with a third-generation cephalosporin or fluoroquinolone [5]. Candida spp. is mainly isolated in spondylodiscitis and requires prolonged antifungal treatment and surgical debridement [5].

The total duration of antibiotic treatment is widely debated in the literature. Classically, BJIs are treated with long courses of intravenous therapy and prolonged hospitalisation, with OM usually treated for 3–6 weeks and SA for 2–4 weeks. Peltola et al. have shown that even 10 days of treatment is sufficient for SA [64]. Moreover, a recent paper from France has shown that 15 days of treatment is sufficient in most of the cases [65]. Another prospective French study on 70 cases reported no failures of treatment with an intravenous regimen prolonged up to 8 days [25]. A retrospective study was conducted in Spain on 607 children with a mean duration of intravenous therapy of 12.9 days and reported good outcomes [20]. A multicentre randomised trial was conducted in Finland on 252 children randomly assigned to two therapeutic groups. The treatment involved a common short cycle of 2–4 days of intravenous antibiotics for both groups, followed by oral therapy with clindamycin or a high-dose first-generation cephalosporin for 20 days in the first group or 30 days in the second group. The authors observed no significant differences between the two groups, suggesting the effectiveness of shorter treatment regimens [66]. However, a limitation of this study was the absence of cases due to MRSA or PVL-SA. When spondylodiscitis occurs, it is still recommended to carry out intravenous therapy for 1–3 weeks [66]. A similar observational study conducted in the United States showed excellent outcomes with an early transition to oral antibiotics within 4 days; the researchers reported no significant difference in the treatment failure rate compared to that with longer intravenous regimens [67]. Only in case of patients with infection due to PVL-SA prolonged antimicrobial treatment and multiple surgical procedures are recommended since these infections are often complicated with abscesses and venous thrombosis [64].

The timing for switching from an intravenous to an oral regimen is still debated. Clinical criteria are apyrexia, compliance with oral therapy, pain reduction, and both general and local clinical improvement. Clinical conditions should be in accordance with the reduction in inflammatory markers such as CRP, ESR, and WBC count. Different cut-offs have been proposed for the evaluation of laboratory markers. Some authors prefer to wait until the complete normalisation of CRP before switching the antibiotic regimen [68]. Faust et al. considered acceptable a CRP value under 20 mg/L or at least a decrease of 2/3 of its maximum peak [36]. The ESPID guidelines recommend switching to oral therapy only when the patient presents an improvement in clinical conditions without fever for at least 24 h and a decrease of 30–50% from the CRP maximum peak is observed. However, the guidelines suggested prolonging the intravenous regimen if drug-resistant or more virulent pathogens are isolated [35].

In most observational studies and randomised clinical trials, oral therapy consists of high-dose cephalosporin or clindamycin [59,69–71]. Trials conducted by Peltola et al. showed a failure rate under 1% at follow-up [64]. Trimethoprim/sulfamethoxazole (TMP/SMX) has been successfully used in oral treatment of BJI in children [72–74]. The duration of oral therapy in uncomplicated BJIs is frequently approximately 3–4 weeks with rigorous monitoring of inflammatory markers and drug tolerability [32]. In this way, therapy can be continued at home, allowing patient discharge and subsequent outpatient follow-up.

6. Conclusions

The clinical presentation of BJI in children may be nonspecific and paucisymptomatic, especially in newborns and immunocompromised patients. Indirect functional signs of OM or SA should be carefully evaluated. All children with negative or inconclusive initial radiographic examination should undergo further highly sensitive imaging studies, such as MRI or bone scintigraphy. MRI is the gold-standard imaging method. It should always be performed in a diagnostic dilemma when the initial radiograph is negative. Contrast enhancement is not routinely required.

Empiric antibiotic therapy should be started as soon as possible. The choice of empiric antimicrobial therapy is based on the most likely causative pathogens according to patient age, immunisation status, underlying disease, and other clinical and epidemiological considerations, including the local prevalence of virulent pathogens, antibiotic bioavailability and bone penetration.

Despite the high success rate reported with empirical therapies, aetiological diagnosis is highly recommended. Blood culture should be obtained in every patient (even if he/she is afebrile) at the initial evaluation and repeated at the fever peak. Synovial fluid samples should also be obtained in the case of SA if antibiotics have already been administered. Bioptic samples are not routinely required in uncomplicated BJI. Instead, minimally invasive percutaneous bone biopsy and surgical biopsy should be considered in complicated infections and when surgery is indicated.

Multidisciplinary management is necessary to achieve an early diagnosis. Paediatricians should consult an experienced radiologist (or an interventional radiologist if percutaneous procedures are indicated) and an orthopaedic surgeon. Microbiological laboratories should also be directly consulted if the involvement of pathogens that are difficult to isolate is suspected (e.g., *K. kingae*).

Empiric antibiotic treatment consists of a short intravenous cycle based on anti-staphylococcal penicillin or a cephalosporin in children aged over 3 months with the addition of gentamicin in infants aged under 3 months. An oral regimen may be an option depending on the bioavailability of the antibiotic chosen and clinical and laboratory data. Further studies on the optimal therapeutic approach are needed in order to understand the best first-line regimen, the utility of biomarkers for the definition of therapy duration and treatment of complications.

7. Methods

We conducted a review of recent literature by examining the MEDLINE (Medical Literature Analysis and Retrieval System Online) database using the search engines PubMed and Google Scholar. The keywords used were "osteomyelitis", OR "bone infection", OR "septic arthritis", AND "p(a)ediatric" OR "children". We included clinical trials, observational studies, reviews and meta-analyses on acute haematogenous osteomyelitis and septic arthritis in children. The exclusion criteria were patients older than 18 years, non-acute or non-haematogenous infections, case series with fewer than 20 patients, articles published before 2005, and non-English language articles.

Author Contributions: G.A. and L.B. co-wrote the manuscript; S.E. supervised the project and made substantial scientific contributions. All authors have read and agreed to the published version of the manuscript.

Funding: This research received no external funding.

Conflicts of Interest: The authors declare no conflict of interest.

References

1. Islam, G.; Tomlinson, J.; Darton, T.; Townsend, R. Bone and Joint Infections. Available online: http://www.surgeryjournal.co.uk (accessed on 28 July 2020).
2. Perlman, M.H.; Patzakis, M.J.; Kumar, P.J.; Holtom, P. The incidence of joint involvement with adjacent osteomyelitis in pediatric patients. *J. Pediatr. Orthop.* **2000**, *20*, 40–43. [CrossRef] [PubMed]
3. Rousset, M.; Walle, M.; Cambou, L.; Mansour, M.; Samba, A.; Pereira, B.; Ghanem, I.; Canavese, F. Chronic infection and infected non-union of the long bones in paediatric patients: Preliminary results of bone versus beta-tricalcium phosphate grafting after induced membrane formation. *Int. Orthop.* **2018**, *42*, 385–393. [CrossRef] [PubMed]
4. Gafur, O.A.; Copley, L.A.; Hollmig, S.T.; Browne, R.H.; Thornton, L.A.; Crawford, S.E. The impact of the current epidemiology of pediatric musculoskeletal infection on evaluation and treatment guidelines. *J. Pediatr. Orthop.* **2008**, *28*, 777–785. [CrossRef] [PubMed]
5. Castellazzi, L.; Mantero, M.; Esposito, S. Update on the Management of Pediatric Acute Osteomyelitis and Septic Arthritis. *Int. J. Mol. Sci.* **2016**, *17*, 855. [CrossRef] [PubMed]
6. Gutierrez, K. Bone and joint infections in children. *Pediatr. Clin. N. Am.* **2005**, *52*, 779–794. [CrossRef] [PubMed]
7. Pannaraj, P.S.; Hulten, K.G.; Gonzalez, B.E.; Mason, E.O., Jr.; Kaplan, S.L. Infective pyomyositis and myositis in children in the era of community-acquired, methicillin-resistant Staphylococcus aureus infection. *Clin. Infect. Dis.* **2006**, *43*, 953–960. [CrossRef]
8. Belthur, M.V.; Birchansky, S.B.; Verdugo, A.A.; Mason, E.O., Jr.; Hulten, K.G.; Kaplan, S.L.; Smith, E.O.; Phillips, W.A.; Weinberg, J. Pathologic fractures in children with acute Staphylococcus aureus osteomyelitis. *J. Bone Jt. Surg. Am.* **2012**, *9*, 34–42. [CrossRef]
9. Peters, W.; Irving, J.; Letts, M. Long-term effects of neonatal bone and joint infection on adjacent growth plates. *J. Pediatr. Orthop.* **1992**, *12*, 806–810. [CrossRef]
10. El-Sayed, A.M.M. Treatment of early septic arthritis of the hip in children: Comparison of results of open arthrotomy versus arthroscopic drainage. *J. Child. Orthop.* **2008**, *2*, 229–237. [CrossRef]
11. Mantadakis, E.; Plessa, E.; Vouloumanou, E.K.; Michailidis, L.; Chatzimichael, A.; Falagas, M.E. Deep venous thrombosis in children with musculoskeletal infections:the clinical evidence. *Int. J. Infect. Dis.* **2012**, *16*, e236–e243. [CrossRef]
12. Gonzalez, B.E.; Teruya, J.; Mahoney, D.H., Jr.; Hulten, K.G.; Edwards, R.; Lamberth, L.B.; Hammerman, W.A.; Mason, E.O., Jr.; Kaplan, S.L. Venous thrombosis associated withstaphylococcal osteomyelitis in children. *Pediatrics* **2006**, *117*, 1673–1679. [CrossRef] [PubMed]
13. Fontalis, A.; Hughes, K.; Nguyen, M.P.; Williamson, M.; Yeo, A.; Lui, D.; Gelfer, Y. The challenge of differentiating vaso-occlusive crises from osteomyelitis in children with sickle cell disease and bone pain: A 15-year retrospective review. *J. Child. Orthop.* **2019**, *13*, 33–39. [CrossRef] [PubMed]
14. Bennett, N.; Maglione, P.J.; Wright, B.L.; Zerbe, C. Infectious Complications in Patients with Chronic Granulomatous Disease. *J. Pediatr. Infect. Dis. Soc.* **2018**, *7*, S12–S17. [CrossRef] [PubMed]

15. Morrissy, R.T.; Haynes, D.W. Acute hematogenous osteomyelitis: A model with trauma as an etiology. *J. Pediatr. Orthop.* **1989**, *9*, 447–456. [CrossRef] [PubMed]
16. Pääkkönen, M.; Kallio, M.J.; Lankinen, P.; Peltola, H.; Kallio, P.E. Preceding trauma in childhood hematogenous bone and joint infections. *J. Pediatr. Orthop. B* **2014**, *23*, 196–199. [CrossRef]
17. Dartnell, J.; Ramachandran, M.; Katchburian, M. Haematogenous acute and subacute paediatric osteomyelitis: A systematic review of the literature. *J. Bone Jt. Surg Br.* **2012**, *94*, 584. [CrossRef]
18. Peltola, H.; Pääkkönen, M. Acute osteomyelitis in children. *N. Engl. J. Med.* **2014**, *370*, 352–360. [CrossRef]
19. Okubo, Y.; Nochioka, K.; Testa, M. Nationwide survey of pediatric acute osteomyelitis in the USA. *J. Pediatr. Orthop. B* **2017**, *26*, 501–506. [CrossRef]
20. Calvo, C.; Núñez, E.; Camacho, M.; Clemente, D.; Fernández-Cooke, E.; Alcobendas, R.; Mayol, L.; Soler-Palacin, P.; Oscoz, M.; Saavedra-Lozano, J. Epidemiology and Management of Acute, Uncomplicated Septic Arthritis and Osteomyelitis: Spanish Multicenter Study. *Pediatr. Infect. Dis. J.* **2016**, *35*, 1288–1293. [CrossRef]
21. Howard, A.W.; Viskontas, D.; Sabbagh, C. Reduction in osteomyelitis and septic arthritis related to Haemophilus influenzae type B vaccination. *J. Pediatr. Orthop.* **1999**, *19*, 705–709. [CrossRef]
22. Mediamolle, N.; Mallet, C.; Aupiais, C.; Doit, C.; Ntika, S.; Vialle, R.; Grimprel, E.; Pejin, Z.; Bonacorsi, S.; Lorrot, M. Bone and joint infections in infants under three months of age. *Acta Paediatr.* **2019**, *108*, 933–939. [CrossRef] [PubMed]
23. Juchler, C.; Spyropoulou, V.; Wagner, N.; Merlini, L.; Dhouib, A.; Manzano, S.; Tabard-Fougère, A.; Samara, E.; Ceroni, D. The Contemporary Bacteriologic Epidemiology of Osteoarticular Infections in Children in Switzerland. *J. Pediatr.* **2018**, *194*, 190–196. [CrossRef] [PubMed]
24. Al-Qwbani, M.; Jiang, N.; Yu, B. Kingella kingae-Associated Pediatric Osteoarticular Infections: An Overview of 566 Reported Cases. *Clin. Pediatr. (Phila)* **2016**, *55*, 1328–1337. [CrossRef] [PubMed]
25. Ferroni, A.; Al Khoury, H.; Dana, C.; Quesne, G.; Berche, P.; Glorion, C.; Péjin, Z. Prospective survey of acute osteoarticular infections in a French paediatric orthopedic surgery unit. *Clin. Microbiol. Infect.* **2013**, *19*, 822–828. [CrossRef]
26. Gravel, J.; Ceroni, D.; Lacroix, L.; Renaud, C.; Grimard, G.; Samara, E.; Cherkaoui, A.; Renzi, G.; Schrenzel, J.; Manzano, S. Association between oropharyngeal carriage of Kingella kingae and osteoarticular infection in young children: A case-control study. *CMAJ* **2017**, *189*, E1107–E1111. [CrossRef]
27. Godley, D.R. Managing musculoskeletal infections in children in the era of increasing bacterial resistance. *JAAPA* **2015**, *28*, 24–29. [CrossRef]
28. Ratnayake, K.; Davis, A.J.; Brown, L.; Young, T.P. Pediatric acute osteomyelitis in the postvaccine, methicillin-resistant Staphylococcus aureus era. *Am. J. Emerg. Med.* **2015**, *33*, 1420–1424. [CrossRef]
29. Gijón, M.; Bellusci, M.; Petraitiene, B.; Noguera-Julian, A.; Zilinskaite, V.; Sanchez Moreno, P.; Saavedra-Lozano, J.; Glikman, D.; Daskalaki, M.; Kaiser-Labusch, P.; et al. Factors associated with severity in invasive community-acquired Staphylococcus aureus infections in children: A prospective European multicentre study. *Clin. Microbiol. Infect.* **2016**, *22*, e1–e6. [CrossRef]
30. Akinkugbe, O.; Stewart, C.; McKenna, C. Presentation and Investigation of Pediatric Bone and Joint Infections in the Pediatric Emergency Department. *Pediatr. Emerg. Care* **2019**, *35*, 700–704. [CrossRef]
31. Saavedra-Lozano, J.; Mejías, A.; Ahmad, N.; Peromingo, E.; Ardura, M.I.; Guillen, S.; Syed, A.; Cavuoti, D.; Ramilo, O. Changing trends in acute osteomyelitis in children: Impact of methicillin-resistant Staphylococcus aureus infections. *J. Pediatr. Orthop.* **2008**, *28*, 569–575. [CrossRef]
32. Saavedra-Lozano, J.; Falup-Pecurariu, O.; Faust, S.N.; Girshick, H.; Hartwig, N.; Kaplan, S.; Lorrot, M.; Mantadakis, E.; Peltola, H.; Rojo, P.; et al. Bone and Joint Infections. *Pediatr. Infect. Dis. J.* **2017**, *36*, 788. [CrossRef] [PubMed]
33. Pääkkönen, M.; Kallio, M.J.; Kallio, P.E.; Peltola, H. Sensitivity of erythrocyte sedimentation rate and C-reactive protein in childhood bone and joint infections. *Clin. Orthop. Relat. Res.* **2010**, *468*, 861. [CrossRef] [PubMed]
34. Hawkshead, J.J., 3rd; Patel, N.B.; Steele, R.W.; Heinrich, S.D. Comparative severity of pediatric osteomyelitis attributable to methicillin-resistant versus methicillin sensitive Staphylococcus aureus. *J. Pediatr. Orthop.* **2009**, *29*, 85. [CrossRef]
35. Wong, M.; Isaacs, D.; Howman-Giles, R.; Uren, R. Clinical and diagnostic features of osteomyelitis occurring in the first three months of life. *Pediatr. Infect. Dis. J.* **1995**, *14*, 1047. [CrossRef]

36. Faust, S.N.; Clark, J.; Pallett, A.; Clarke, N.M. Managing bone and joint infection in children. *Arch. Dis. Child.* **2012**, *97*, 545–553. [CrossRef]
37. Fernandez, M.; Carrol, C.L.; Baker, C.J. Discitis and vertebral osteomyelitis in children: An 18-year review. *Pediatrics* **2000**, *105*, 1299. [CrossRef]
38. Averill, L.W.; Hernandez, A.; Gonzalez, L.; Peña, A.H.; Jaramillo, D. Diagnosis of osteomyelitis in children: Utility of fat-suppressed contrast-enhanced MRI. *AJR Am. J. Roentgenol.* **2009**, *192*, 1232–1238. [CrossRef]
39. Kan, J.H.; Young, R.S.; Yu, C.; Hernanz-Schulman, M. Clinical impact of gadolinium in the MRI diagnosis of musculoskeletal infection in children. *Pediatr. Radiol.* **2010**, *40*, 1197–1205. [CrossRef]
40. Guillerman, R.P. Osteomyelitis and beyond. *Pediatr. Radiol.* **2013**, *43*, S193. [CrossRef] [PubMed]
41. Saigal, G.; Azouz, E.M.; Abdenour, G. Imaging of osteomyelitis with special reference to children. *Semin. Musculoskelet Radiol.* **2004**, *8*, 255. [CrossRef]
42. Connolly, L.P.; Connolly, S.A.; Drubach, L.A.; Jaramillo, D.; Treves, S.T. Acute hematogenous osteomyelitis of children: Assessment of skeletal scintigraphy-based diagnosis in the era of MRI. *J. Nucl. Med.* **2002**, *43*, 1310. [PubMed]
43. Poyhia, T.; Azouz, E.M. MR imaging evaluation of subacute and chronic bone abscesses in children. *Pediatr. Radiol* **2000**, *30*, 763. [PubMed]
44. Browne, L.P.; Mason, E.O.; Kaplan, S.L.; Cassady, C.I.; Krishnamurthy, R.; Guillerman, R.P. Optimal imaging strategy for community-acquired Staphylococcus aureus musculoskeletal infections in children. *Pediatr. Radiol.* **2008**, *38*, 841–847. [CrossRef]
45. Blickman, J.G.; van Die, C.E.; de Rooy, J.W. Current imaging concepts in pediatric osteomyelitis. *Eur. Radiol.* **2004**, *14*, 55–64. [CrossRef]
46. Hsu, W.; Hearty, T.M. Radionuclide imaging in the diagnosis and management of orthopaedic disease. *J. Am. Acad. Orthop. Surg.* **2012**, *20*, 151–159. [CrossRef] [PubMed]
47. Jaramillo, D.; Dormans, J.P.; Delgado, J.; Laor, T.; St Geme, J.W. Hematogenous Osteomyelitis in Infants and Children: Imaging A Chang. Disease. *Radiology* **2017**, *283*, 629. [CrossRef]
48. McNeil, J.C.; Forbes, A.R.; Vallejo, J.G.; Flores, A.R.; Hultén, K.G.; Mason, E.O.; Kaplan, S.L. Role of Operative or Interventional Radiology-Guided Cultures for Osteomyelitis. *Pediatrics* **2016**, *137*, e20154616. [CrossRef]
49. Pääkkönen, M.; Peltola, H. Bone and joint infections. *Pediatr. Clin. N. Am.* **2013**, *60*, 425–436. [CrossRef]
50. Dodwell, E.R. Osteomyelitis and septic arthritis in children: Current concepts. *Curr. Opin. Pediatr.* **2013**, *25*, 58–63. [CrossRef]
51. Yagupsky, P. Use of blood culture vials and nucleic acid amplification for the diagnosis of pediatric septic arthritis. *Clin. Infect. Dis.* **2008**, *46*, 1631–1632. [CrossRef]
52. Bidet, P.; Collin, E.; Basmaci, R.; Courroux, C.; Prisse, V.; Dufour, V.; Bingen, E.; Grimprel, E.; Bonacorsi, S. Investigation of an outbreak of osteoarticular infections caused by Kingella kingae in a childcare center using molecular techniques. *Pediatr. Infect. Dis. J.* **2013**, *32*, 558–560. [CrossRef] [PubMed]
53. Chiappini, E.; Camposampiero, C.; Lazzeri, S.; Indolfi, G.; De Martino, M.; Galli, L. Epidemiology and Management of Acute Haematogenous Osteomyelitis in a Tertiary Paediatric Center. *Int. J. Environ. Res. Public Health* **2017**, *14*, 477. [CrossRef] [PubMed]
54. Harik, N.S.; Smeltzer, M.S. Management of acute hematogenous osteomyelitis in children. *Expert Rev. Antinfect. Ther.* **2010**, *8*, 175–181. [CrossRef] [PubMed]
55. Thabit, A.K.; Fatani, D.F.; Bamakhrama, M.S.; Barnawi, O.A.; Basudan, L.O.; Alhejaili, S.F. Antibiotic penetration into bone and joints: An updated review. *Int. J. Infect. Dis.* **2019**, *81*, 128–136. [CrossRef]
56. Howard-Jones, A.R.; Isaacs, D. Systematic review of duration and choise of systemic antibiotic therapy for acute haematogenous bacterial osteomyelitis in children. *J. Pediatr. Child. Health* **2013**, *49*, 760–768. [CrossRef]
57. Wunsch, S.; Krause, R.; Valentin, T.; Prattes, J.; Janata, O.; Lenger, A.; Bellmann-Weiler, R.; Weiss, G.; Zollner-Schwetz, I. Multicenter clinical experience of real life Dalbavancin use in gram-positive infections. *Int. J. Infect. Dis.* **2019**, *81*, 210–214. [CrossRef]
58. Bradley, J.S.; Puttagunta, S.; Rubino, C.M.; Blumer, J.L.; Dunne, M.; Sullivan, J.E. Pharmacokinetics, Safety and Tolerability of Single Dose Dalbavancin in Children 12–17 Years of Age. *Pediatr. Infect. Dis. J.* **2015**, *34*, 748–752. [CrossRef]
59. Esposito, S.; Bianchini, S. Dalbavancin for the treatment of paediatric infectious diseases. *Eur. J. Clin. Microbiol. Infect. Dis.* **2016**, *35*, 1895–1901. [CrossRef]

60. DeRonde, K.J.; Girotto, J.E.; Nicolau, D.P. Management of Pediatric Acute Hematogenous Osteomyelitis, Part II: A Focus on Methicillin-Resistant Staphylococcus aureus, Current and Emerging Therapies. *Pharmacotherapy* **2018**, *38*, 1021–1037. [CrossRef]
61. McNeil, J.C.; Kaplan, S.L.; Vallejo, J.G. The Influence of the Route of Antibiotic Administration, Methicillin Susceptibility, Vancomycin Duration and Serum Trough Concentration on Outcomes of Pediatric Staphylococcus aureus Bacteremic Osteoarticular Infection. *Pediatr. Infect. Dis. J.* **2017**, *36*, 572–577. [CrossRef]
62. Diep, B.A.; Afasizheva, A.; Le, H.N.; Kajikawa, O.; Matute-Bello, G.; Tkaczyk, C.; Sellman, B.; Badiou, C.; Lina, G.; Chambers, H.F. Effects of linezolid on suppressing in vivo production of staphylococcal toxins and improving survival outcomes in a rabbit model of methicillin-resistant Staphylococcus aureus necrotizing pneumonia. *J. Infect. Dis.* **2013**, *208*, 75–82. [CrossRef] [PubMed]
63. Rojo, P.; Barrios, M.; Palacios, A.; Gomez, C.; Chaves, F. Community-associated Staphylococcus aureus infections in children. *Expert Rev. Anti. Infect. Ther.* **2010**, *8*, 541–554. [CrossRef]
64. Peltola, H.; Pääkkönen, M.; Kallio, P.; Kallio, M.J.; Osteomyelitis-Septic Arthritis Study Group. Short-versus long-term antimicrobial treatment for acute hematogenous osteomyelitis of childhood: Prospective, randomized trial on 131 culture-positive cases. *Pediatr. Infect. Dis. J.* **2010**, *29*, 1123–1128. [CrossRef] [PubMed]
65. Filleron, A.; Laurens, M.E.; Marin, G.; Marchandin, H.; Prodhomme, O.; Alkar, F.; Godreuil, S.; Nagot, N.; Cottalorda, J.; L'Kaissi, M.; et al. Short-course Antibiotic Treatment of Bone and Joint Infections in Children: A Retrospective Study at Montpellier University Hospital From 2009 to 2013. *J. Antimicrob. Chemother.* **2019**, *74*, 3579–3587. [CrossRef]
66. Fucs, P.M.; Meves, R.; Yamada, H.H. Spinal infections in children: A review. *Int. Orthop.* **2012**, *36*, 387–395. [CrossRef] [PubMed]
67. Islam, S.; Biary, N.; Wrotniak, B. Favorable Outcomes With Early Transition to Oral Antibiotics for Pediatric Osteoarticular Infections. *Clin. Pediatr. (Phila)* **2019**, *58*, 696–699. [CrossRef]
68. Street, M.; Puna, R.; Huang, M.; Crawford, H. Pediatric Acute Hematogenous Osteomyelitis. *J. Pediatr. Orthop.* **2015**, *35*, 634–639. [CrossRef]
69. Chiappini, E.; Krzysztofiak, A.; Bozzola, E.; Gabiano, C.; Esposito, S.; Lo Vecchio, A.; Govoni, M.R.; Vallongo, C.; Dodi, I.; Castagnola, E.; et al. Risk factors associated with complications/sequelae of acute and subacute haematogenous osteomyelitis: An Italian multicenter study. *Expert Rev. Anti. Infect. Ther.* **2018**, *16*, 351–358. [CrossRef]
70. Keren, R.; Shah, S.S.; Srivastava, R.; Rangel, S.; Bendel-Stenzel, M.; Harik, N.; Hartley, J.; Lopez, M.; Seguias, L.; Tieder, J.; et al. Pediatric research in inpatient settings network. Comparative effectiveness of intravenous vs. oral antibiotics for postdischarge treatment of acute osteomyelitis in children. *JAMA Pediatr.* **2015**, *169*, 120–128. [CrossRef]
71. Sánchez-Moreno, P.; Ardanuy-Pizarro, A.V.; Navarro, L.; Melón, M.; Falcón-Neyra, M.D.; Camacho-Lovillo, M. Acute osteoarticular infections in children in a tertiary hospital: Our experience across 5 years. *Ann. Rheum. Dis.* **2015**, *74*, 1233. [CrossRef]
72. Chiappini, E.; Serrano, E.; Galli, L.; Villani, A.; Krzysztofiak, A. Italian Paediatric Collaborative Osteomyelitis Study Group. Practical Issues in Early Switching from Intravenous to Oral Antibiotic Therapy in Children with Uncomplicated Acute Hematogenous Osteomyelitis: Results from an Italian Survey. *Int. J. Environ. Res. Public Health* **2019**, *16*, 3557. [CrossRef] [PubMed]
73. Al-Hasan, M.N.; Rac, H. Transition from intravenous to oral antimicrobial therapy in patients with uncomplicated and complicated bloodstream infections. *Clin. Microbiol. Infect.* **2020**, *26*, 299–306. [CrossRef] [PubMed]
74. Deconinck, L.; Dinh, A.; Nich, C.; Tritz, T.; Matt, M.; Senard, O.; Bessis, S.; Bauer, T.; Rottman, M.; Salomon, J.; et al. Efficacy of cotrimoxazole (Sulfamethoxazole-Trimethoprim) as a salvage therapy for the treatment of bone and joint infections (BJIs). *PLoS ONE* **2019**, *14*, e0224106. [CrossRef] [PubMed]

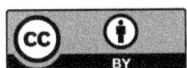

© 2020 by the authors. Licensee MDPI, Basel, Switzerland. This article is an open access article distributed under the terms and conditions of the Creative Commons Attribution (CC BY) license (http://creativecommons.org/licenses/by/4.0/).

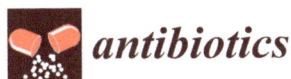

Article

Opportunities and Challenges for Improving Anti-Microbial Stewardship in Low- and Middle-Income Countries; Lessons Learnt from the Maternal Sepsis Intervention in Western Uganda

Louise Ackers [1,*], Gavin Ackers-Johnson [1], Maaike Seekles [1], Joe Odur [2] and Samuel Opio [3]

1. School of Health and Society, University of Salford, Salford M66PU, UK; g.ackersjohnson@edu.salford.uk (G.A.-J.); m.l.seekles1@salford.ac.uk (M.S.)
2. Knowledge For Change, Bradford BD232HX, UK; joeodur@gmail.com
3. Pharmaceutical Society of Uganda, Kampala 920102, Uganda; opixam25@gmail.com
* Correspondence: h.l.ackers@salford.ac.uk; Tel.: +44 7977 409985

Received: 29 April 2020; Accepted: 4 June 2020; Published: 9 June 2020

Abstract: This paper presents findings from an action-research intervention designed to identify ways of improving antimicrobial stewardship in a Ugandan Regional Referral Hospital. Building on an existing health partnership and extensive action-research on maternal health, it focused on maternal sepsis. Sepsis is one of the main causes of maternal mortality in Uganda and surgical site infection, a major contributing factor. Post-natal wards also consume the largest volume of antibiotics. The findings from the Maternal Sepsis Intervention demonstrate the potential for remarkable changes in health worker behaviour through multi-disciplinary engagement. Nurses and midwives create the connective tissue linking pharmacy, laboratory scientists and junior doctors to support an evidence-based response to prescribing. These multi-disciplinary 'huddles' form a necessary, but insufficient, grounding for active clinical pharmacy. The impact on antimicrobial stewardship and maternal mortality and morbidity is ultimately limited by very poor and inconsistent access to antibiotics and supplies. Insufficient and predictable stock-outs undermine behaviour change frustrating health workers' ability to exercise their knowledge and skill for the benefit of their patients. This escalates healthcare costs and contributes to anti-microbial resistance.

Keywords: antimicrobial stewardship; pharmacy; sepsis; wound management; culture and sensitivity testing; resistance patterns; low-and middle-income countries; Uganda

1. Introduction

A recent review of research on antibiotic stewardship [1] found limited evidence of effective and feasible stewardship interventions in low- and middle-income countries (LMICs) and, where examples of effective interventions were identified, emphasised the essential need for contextualised. This paper reports on a recent, highly contextualized, facility-level intervention in a Regional Referral Hospital (RRH) in Uganda, known as the Maternal Sepsis Intervention (MSI). Funding for this action-research intervention came from the Commonwealth Partnerships for Antimicrobial Stewardship (CwPAMS) [2]. The funding body stipulated a focus on antimicrobial use (stewardship) and a project completion within 15 months with a budget of £60,000. The intervention was necessarily aligned with the Ugandan National Action Plan on Anti-Microbial Resistance or 'NAP' [3]. The NAP was launched in 2018 in an attempt to 'slow down and contain' [3] (p. 3) anti-microbial resistance (AMR). It sets out five Strategic Objectives focused on Awareness-Raising; Infection Prevention; Optimal Access and Use of Antimicrobials; Surveillance and Research.

The CwPAMS objectives resonate most directly with Strategic Objective 3 of the NAP with a primary emphasis on Antimicrobial Stewardship (AMS). The NAP describes the use of antimicrobial agents as 'the major modifiable driver of AMR'. According to the Plan, achieving optimal antimicrobial use 'will require strengthening technical and regulatory frameworks, ensuring availability of appropriate medicines and changing behaviour amongst prescribers, dispensers and consumers' [3] (p. 14).

This articulation of the funding body's objectives with the NAP on AMR framed the design of the MSI. Building on strong pre-existing relationships especially in the field of maternal and new-born health, the project partners decided to focus the intervention on the Post-Natal and Gynaecology (PNG) ward in a RRH in Western Uganda. Fort Portal Regional Referral Hospital (FPRRH) has the second highest maternal mortality rate in the country. The most recent Ministry of Health report indicates a maternal mortality rate of 632/100,000 almost double the reported national average [4]. Sepsis competes with haemorrhage as the leading causes of maternal mortality [4–6] and Reinhart et al. [7] describe sepsis as a 'Global Health Priority'.

Surgical site infection (SSI) following caesarean section contributes significantly to maternal mortality and morbidity [8] and to antimicrobial consumption. As a component of hospital acquired infection, it is also largely preventable. The decision to focus on the PNG ward reflected the opportunity to assess the potential for preventive intervention through improved infection prevention control (IPC) to reduce post-caesarean section SSIs. This focus also enabled us to address stewardship practices on a ward associated with the highest levels of antibiotic consumption in the hospital.

The intervention built on the long-established Kabarole Health Partnership which involves a UK and Ugandan registered NGO (Knowledge For Change (K4C)) as the key operational partner together with the University of Salford; Kabarole Health District, FPRRH and the Pharmaceutical society of Uganda. The Health Partnership model has been actively developed through the Tropical Health and Education Trust (THET) as a more democratic and grounded approach to foreign engagement in global health.

Substantial pre-existing research conducted in partnership with Knowledge For Change (K4C) has established the principle of co-presence to the achievement of effective knowledge mobilisation and behaviour change in health partnerships [9]. In practice, the mechanism involves the deployment of UK professionals working alongside Ugandan staff employed by K4C and local health workers in what can best be described as 'knowledge mobilisation clusters.' Long term continuity of engagement is the hallmark of K4C's approach. Understanding the contextual dynamics of AMS is critical to behaviour change at individual and organisational levels. Capturing the effectiveness of this approach – based on continuous and active co-working—requires a longitudinal ethnographic methodology with in-built reflexivity.

The MSI is reported in full in Ackers et al. [10]. This paper focuses on the mechanism that has supported the emergence of clinical pharmacy at FPRRH, and could form the basis of highly effective AMS. The development of this 'mechanism' has taken place over the past year. It has evolved in an iterative fashion as part of a continuous, exploratory, journey supported by on-going ethnographic co-researching. This type of approach does not lend itself to a linear, before-and-after, hypothesis testing structure. The paper instead charts the evolution of the MSI and the data collected along the way. As data presents new theories, this then creates new opportunities for data collection.

The intervention team started with a focus on SSI wounds, which led to an initial emphasis on wound care. Nurses and midwives are the custodians of wounds in Ugandan public facilities. The quality of wound care was found to be grossly inadequate at project inception; wound dressing was infrequent, and health workers were avoiding this task. Improvements in wound care led by nurses and midwives created the opportunity for swabbing and laboratory testing. Active engagement between nurses, midwives and laboratory scientists then created the evidence base, stimulating the opportunity for highly effective and impactful clinical pharmacy and multi-disciplinary team working. The first part of the paper tracks this process. Ultimately the effectiveness of this team in achieving optimal AMS is limited by access to antibiotics and IPC supplies. The second part of the paper presents data evidencing the dynamics of supply chain failures in the Ugandan public health system.

2. Methods

The approach can best be described as a multi-method ethnography, commencing with observational work on the ground. Observational work was undertaken on a co-researching basis with a lead role played by Ugandan staff employed through K4C, supported by repeated and extended site visits by the Principal Investigator and virtual co-presence over a 15-month period. The team were joined by the Ugandan lead and attended Hospital IPC meetings on two occasions. Observations, complemented by on-going WhatsApp and Skype conversations were recorded in notebooks, minutes, reports and emails, and entered into NVIVO for storage and analysis.

This observational research generated theory inductively which, in turn, stimulated the search for other sources of data. Although we had anticipated accessing facility data on antibiotic consumption we could not have known or understood the complexity of this process and the challenges of even defining consumption in a public hospital setting prior to the start of the project. In such situations and given the essentially inductive quality of ethnographic research, where context is 'everything' [11], a simple a priori (deductive) hypothesis setting is inappropriate. In that respect, a process of conceptualisation, theory generation and data collection took place simultaneously. Every attempt to record or collate data stimulated intense on-going discussions about the recording processes and the nuances of its interpretation. In most cases it led us to new lines of enquiry (theories) and approaches to data collection. Much of the data, as is normal in this context, was not collated and had to be manually and painstakingly searched for from casefiles or record books. The very poor quality of documentation in patient files and subsequent records management is a critical dimension of context with implications for AMR [8]. Data collection became a process of exploration, involving forms of local capacity-building along the way on methods of organising and storing hospital records and entering them into excel spreadsheets. In this context (as in many others), much of the facility-based data could not be interpreted at face value as facts; but rather, as artefacts reflecting their (social) construction.

Facility data has been collected from a wide range of sources. Firstly, data on drug orders and supplies from National Medical Stores (NMS), was obtained through an on-line national pharmacy data base, known as the Rx system, the use of which was functionalised through the project. This was supplemented by data from paper-based records (the Dispensing Log) of supplies distributed from the central hospital stores to the wards over a 4-month period, from December 2019 to April 2020. Further, the Infectious Diseases Institute (IDI) supported hospital laboratory have proved key partners both in the intervention itself, with laboratory results providing a critical stimulus to multi-disciplinary team working, but also in generating research data. This commenced prior to the project as part of Ackers-Johnson's microbiology doctorate [12] and has continued throughout, generating valuable data on resistance patterns. The laboratory provided data on test results of samples taken from the PNG ward in 2019. This complemented a data set generated from 142 cases of suspected sepsis between January 2019 and February 2020 that were identified through a manual search of paper-based patient records.

In January 2020, a phase of qualitative interviewing took place to capture perceptions of the impact and effectiveness of the intervention. Twenty-five interviews were conducted with all cadres involved in the MSI, including 50% of the nurses, midwives, intern doctors, laboratory technicians and pharmacists working on the PNG ward, two hospital managers and three UK volunteers. The interviews were transcribed and thematically analysed using NVivo 12. Ethical approval for the work was gained from the University of Salford, Makerere University and the Ugandan National Council of science and technology (HS249ES).

3. Results and Discussion

The MSI built on on-going under-pinning research including three PhD studies. One of these (Ackers-Johnson) involved active co-researching on emerging AMR patterns with microbiologists in the hospital laboratory. The team was aware that the laboratory was struggling to obtain adequate samples from the hospital wards for testing and that maternal sepsis was one of several priorities for their research.

In common with all projects funded by THET, the CwPAMS funding stream identified a knowledge transfer mechanism based on the harnessing of UK (National Health Service) health worker expertise as the basis for behaviour change interventions. The role and contribution of professional volunteer engagement has been researched extensively by the authors, with an emphasis both on the impacts on LMICs [9,13] and, in a study financed by Health Education England, the benefits to the NHS [13]. Our approach to the MSI was informed by this research and resulted in the decision to deploy professional volunteers in co-working, mentoring roles for the duration of the intervention. The aim was to have continual presence on the ground with UK volunteers working alongside locally recruited staff (through K4C) and health workers in the hospital. One of the volunteers recruited was a member of the Ugandan diaspora working in the NHS. This volunteer knew the region, spoke the local language and specialised in wound care and SSIs. The importance of creating the conditions for serendipitous opportunities to influence action-research interventions has been reported elsewhere [14–16].

3.1. The Maternal Sepsis Intervention and Wound Management as the Focus for Change

The MSI proposal made no specific reference to wound care; wounds were something to be swabbed in order to test resistance patterns, and we had not anticipated the value of wound care to AMR work and patient outcomes. The early decision to focus on post c-section wounds turned out to be pivotal; it encouraged a very grounded approach focusing on multi-disciplinary team working at the patient's bedside. The lack of effective wound care was found to be contributing to extended patient stays and inappropriate use of antibiotics. More immediately, the ward had become associated with the stench of infection; nurses and midwives were reluctant to spend time with patients with badly infected wounds. They considered the work to be unpleasant and, in the absence of hand washing and protective clothing, staff feared the risk to their own health. The initial engagement in wound cleaning and dressing by the K4C midwives, the UK volunteers and a pioneering local midwife stimulated an holistic investment in IPC measures. This very quickly delivered major and very tangible results: Critically, it created a safer and more comfortable environment for wound swabbing. Working closely with our hospital laboratory colleagues, the project began to see a transformation of practice from a situation where no wounds were being swabbed (or other samples taken) to one where wounds were being dressed (and seen) twice daily; all patients with suspected infections were being identified, having samples taken and sent to the laboratory for culture and sensitivity testing. Table 1 presents the results of data collected from case files of all suspected sepsis cases in the 12 months commencing 1st January 2019. They show the lack of swabbing and culture and sensitivity testing on the wards prior to project commencement. The implementation aspect of the project began to impact in July, after a short initial transition period with few cases swabbed. After 22nd July 2019, nearly all suspected sepsis cases have been identified and samples sent to the laboratory for testing.

Laboratory results from these tests were present in the files of 67 of the 74 (90.5%) patients who had had a swab taken. For four patients, the results had gone missing from the file; for two patients the test was not completed because the IDI hospital laboratory was closed over Christmas and New Year and one patient's lab test was not completed because the patient had discharged herself against medical advice. Although this emphasises the importance of improving record-keeping, this level of documentation represents a remarkable achievement in the context.

Table 1. Volume and Proportion of Suspected Sepsis Cases Sent for Laboratory Testing.

Time Frame	Suspected Sepsis Cases	Culture and Sensitivity Tests Performed	% Tested
1st January 2019–8th July 2019	50	0	0%
9th July 2019–21st July 2019	16	3	19%
22nd July 2019–31st January 2020	76	74 (2 had missing data)	95%

The impact of the focus on wound care and culture and sensitivity testing is explained by a local midwife. She had taken a particular interest in the use of sugar in wound care prior to the project (in Sudan) and had previously worked alongside K4C staff and British nursing students on the labour ward, so relationships were strong. She describes the impact the project has had on her personally and on the ward and patients. She notes that, prior to the project, empirical prescribing of antibiotics lacked the desired effectiveness, and this lack of effectiveness was compounded by prolonged prescribing of the same antibiotics. Importantly, she also specifically recognises the role that clinical pharmacists are now playing:

> You came in at a critical time [and] brought new skills. Before there was no culture and sensitivity testing. Some of us knew about it but had never used it—even the doctors. When you came in it is me who benefitted most; I was carrying a very heavy burden and you helped me. You came as a combined team. We have not lost any women from sepsis since the project started and Dorothy (a Ugandan midwife employed by K4C) came. I had worked with her on labour ward with your students. Even the laboratory has started to respond—the burden was lifted, and everyone started getting involved.

> We did use culture and sensitivity tests in Mulago (National Referral Hospital) but with not much emphasis and sometimes you have your interests on other things and we left it to the doctors. Here much of the things are now done by nurses/midwives—like doing culture and sensitivity tests. We knew culture and sensitivity would get results. Now I try to do the septic patients first. Before we noticed some were not getting better and we did not pay much attention to how this woman has been on this treatment for so long and you just gave her more antibiotics. [. . .] now [the pharmacist] comes on the ward daily and looks around and helps us as sometimes the intern doctors are busy and lack supervision. Before we used the same medicines—same—same—we just gave what was prescribed.

In addition to describing the importance that swabbing and testing has made to progress, the midwife alludes to a major change in team-working and task-shifting with midwives and nurses now playing a very central role in these processes. This has been critical to the effectiveness of the MSI. Midwives and nurses are barely mentioned in the NAP. In the Ugandan context their active engagement and empowerment is absolutely essential to AMS, not least because they are most often the only cadres continually present on the ground. The presence of senior doctors is at best sporadic with rotating and largely unsupervised intern doctors providing most medical input [10,17,18]. This evidence adds weight to Brink et al.'s proposal for new nurse-led models of AMS in Africa [19].

The following section examines how the presence of laboratory results has created the opportunity for improved antimicrobial stewardship through clinical pharmacy engagement.

3.2. AMS Performance Indicators: The Engagement of Clinical Pharmacy at FPRRH

One of the key AMS performance indicators identified by the pharmacy team at FPRRH is the 'Review of Pharmacotherapy' by pharmacists. In practice we are concerned here with the extent to which pharmacists are directly engaged in multi-disciplinary decision-making following the receipt of laboratory test results showing resistance patterns. The data collated from patient notes showed that pharmacists reviewed the pharmacotherapy in 91.8% of cases where test results showed a bacterial growth.

We must not underestimate the impact of the introduction and embedding of culture and sensitivity testing to the team-building process. Test results trigger team-based activity; they engage all staff irrespective of cadres. Having the laboratory results provides a focus for interests to coalesce around; they stimulate team discussion and active pharmacy engagement and create the environment for genuinely patient-centred care. Having the evidence-base for rational prescribing undermines entrenched disciplinary hierarchies. It was clear from the discussion in a hospital-wide Infection Prevent Control (IPC) Committee that the tension between doctors and pharmacists persists in other areas of the hospital and had been evident, on occasion, on the PNG ward:

Sometimes you find a pharmacist has changed a prescription and then on the ward round the doctor changes it back to a drug the patient is resistant to. (Midwife)

A pharmacy intern responded to this comment:

I think it should be teamwork here and respect for each other. If we advise and then the prescription is changed the clinicians come and undermine that decision without listening to the pharmacist. We can see that post-natal is taking the lead in consulting with pharmacy, but other units are relying on empirical usage designed for health centres and not for hospitals. If you are rigid on the usage you will not use the pharmacists/laboratory's advice.

Evidence of a transformational increase in direct clinical pharmacy engagement on the wards is supported by qualitative findings. One midwife refers to the impact of laboratory results on these hierarchies:

Sometimes there can be ego—that the doctor or pharmacist thinks, 'I am the overall boss so I can't be directed on what to do', but with the data that goes down.

Every respondent identified the improvement in teamwork and identified this as the source of change on the wards:

We are now working hand-in-hand with the pharmacists, the laboratory and the doctors—in-charge nurse.

An intern doctor also describes how useful he has found the expertise of the pharmacy team:

It's changed a lot now; the senior pharmacist comes regularly, and you may find there are 2 microorganisms sensitive to different antibiotics. Now I don't have the time to walk to the pharmacy and those people have studied medicines. I have textbook knowledge; if someone has a UTI (Urinary tract infection) I give x. I did study this but as time goes on you get used to giving certain medicines quite often and you are not so equipped to understand how one medicine interacts with another one or if a patient has TB or is HIV positive or how to combine drugs—so a pharmacist being available on the ward has really brought in great improvement.

A midwife shows her appreciation of the teamworking environment that has developed. She refers to the presence of pharmacy on the ward and the lengths the pharmacists have gone to, to try to secure appropriate antibiotics:

It has greatly improved because right now we have pharmacists who come on a daily basis or if not, every day we can't go 3 days without seeing one who can guide us on the mothers and which drugs to take. They interact with the doctors; if you don't interact there is that collision. Right now, there is no tension. They say, 'what if we do this' and there is a discussion. We never used to have any pharmacists coming on the wards, so it was majorly the doctors dealing with the prescriptions. We have managed to reduce the irrational use of antibiotics.

The use of language in this response by the midwife illustrates the growing status of midwives and nurses in the multi-disciplinary teams and their ability to talk confidently about 'rational' prescribing; a concept they would not have been aware of prior to the MSI. It also illustrates the 'boundary spanning' role nurses and midwives are playing on the wards mediating professional hierarchies and tensions. Pharmacists were also very aware of their role in mediating these boundaries, and take care not to 'clash' with doctors:

> *[Pharmacy] don't see all the cases. We try to pick cases where we feel pharmacists can have an input and that way, we don't clash so much with the doctors. We work within our mandates so there are no clashes. Intern doctors are also using this as a chance to learn about AMR.*

The MSI has achieved optimal pharmacy engagement (in an RRH context) on the PNG ward. The impact of laboratory testing has played an important role in empowering pharmacy. This is evident in the new policy, initiated by pharmacy with strong support from the laboratory, of only permitting use of high-end antibiotics when laboratory test results are available. A midwife respondent makes the point that there is a limited role for pharmacy on the ward in the absence of laboratory results:

> *Pharmacy will tell you there is no point in them coming unless there are cultures. Clinicians are not allowed to change antibiotics now without cultures.*

Discussions have taken place in the hospital's IPC committee to extend this policy to all wards, illustrating the wider impact of the MSI on the hospital as a whole. The laboratory respondent welcomes this achievement, which also represents the growing recognition of the pharmacy presence in the hospital:

> *The policy of only prescribing high end antibiotics to patients who have had culture and sensitivity testing has really worked; these antibiotics are being guarded jealously now. In fact, (the pharmacy team) are very strict on that. I really feel this could work on other wards. It is only working on post-natal ward at present because they have laboratory reports.*

3.3. Creating the Evidence Base and Momentum for a Hospital Antibiogram

Another important aspect of this wider impact can be seen in the role that the MSI has played in creating the evidence base for a hospital antibiogram. An antibiogram is a collection of data, based on laboratory testing of the pathogens in a specific facility that summarises patterns of resistance to different antimicrobial agents (or antibiotics). Although international and national trends in resistance patterns can be identified, regional and facility-specific patterns enable even closer targeting of antibiotics.

Whilst we have seen the benefits of culture and sensitivity testing in terms of trying to identify the optimal antibiotic for individual patients; in cases of suspected sepsis, health workers cannot wait for the test results, but must immediately start the patient on an antibiotic, whilst awaiting the testing process. This is known as 'empirical prescribing'. In FPRRH (as in many other facilities), the prescribing decision, usually made by a junior doctor, will be based on their usual practice, perhaps with reference to the formulary—and is very much tempered by their perception of what is available in stores. Where a hospital antibiogram exists, this initial empirical prescribing can be informed by local evidence and has a much higher chance of success. The presence of an antibiogram with associated awareness raising and sensitisation amongst all staff, and especially medical interns, would have major impacts on empirical prescribing across the hospital. Prior to the MSI, FPRRH did not have the volume of laboratory results to create the necessary evidence base for a hospital antibiogram. A member of the pharmacy team describes how this has changed:

> *If you go to maternity, you will notice a very big change. The ward sends the biggest volume of swabs now to the laboratory because those people [midwives] are aware.*

The laboratory scientist confirms this:

> *On the basis of the increased swabbing we hope to be in a position to have an antibiogram. This will be very informative—the sample size is now very adequate, but we want to enter this information into a comprehensive database which has different parameters—length of stay–age–sex–ward–so that when you are doing the analysis it is very comprehensive. The antibiogram will be good for the clinicians to guide prescribing—it will be good for the patients.*

The results presented above demonstrate the ability to make considerable progress in AMS at a RRH.

3.4. Access to Antibiotics in FPRRH: Supply Dynamics

Ultimately, the model that has evolved on PNG ward has the potential to significantly reduce infection, improve prescribing practice, reduce antibiotic consumption and overcome some of the effects of AMR on patient outcomes. The major challenge facing the MSI model is access to the right antibiotics and antimicrobials at the right time. The laboratory scientist is clear about this:

> Antibiotic stock-outs remain a serious constraint; in many cases patients can only be given the right antibiotics if they pay and many of them can't pay. We have to be very clear, antibiotic stock-outs are a key factor fueling AMR. If we look at the scenario where we have investigations done and antibiotics are available, and the outcomes are good, but we have done the investigations and the antibiotics are out of stock we won't have a good outcome.

There is a bigger concern here too; if supplies are not available and the ward staff are unable to respond effectively to laboratory results this can be predicted to have a major impact on staff motivation and the behaviour change gains. Problems of access critically restrict pharmacy's ability to engage in rational prescribing; prescribing the drug most likely to work according to laboratory results. This in turn leads to over-consumption of poorly performing antibiotics and poor patient outcomes. The following section describes the supply chain system at FPRRH and presents data on consumption. Critical problems include:

1. The hospital may only order against a budget prescribed by the Ministry of Finance and held by NMS.
2. The hospital can only order antibiotics from a prescribed catalogue which excludes many of the antibiotics indicated as necessary from laboratory results and present on the 'Essential Medicines and Health Supplies List for Uganda' [20].
3. There are major and unpredictable discrepancies in what is ordered and what is delivered ('Order Fill Rates').
4. As a result of the above, most IPC supplies and antibiotics run out half-way through the bi-monthly supply cycle (Stock-Outs).

3.5. The Impact of the MSI Project on the 2020/2021 Procurement Plan

In Uganda, the funds for procurement of drugs and supplies in the public sector are highly centralised and inadequate. NMS procures and distributes supplies to health facilities based on a centrally allocated Annual Supplies Budget. Each hospital is required to produce an Annual Procurement Plan. Once agreed, this Plan is fixed and cannot be varied over the year reducing the opportunity for flexibility and responsiveness to the hospital laboratory results and any changes indicated by a future antibiogram. This budget is held by NMS. With the exception of private wards, it is not possible for a RRH to source supplies from elsewhere. NMS deliveries take place bi-monthly.

During the annual procurement process, the hospital may only order those items authorised by the 'Essential Medicines and Health Supplies List for Uganda'. However, not all essential drugs feature in the NMS catalogue. A hospital pharmacist describes the situation as follows:

> As much as we may desire a certain antibiotic, we can't plan for it if it is not present in the catalogue. A case in point is Amikacin and Moxifloxacin.

Out of the nine antibiotics tested against *Acinetobacter* samples in the laboratory, only two—doxycycline and amikacin—showed greater levels of susceptibility than resistance (for details of these test results, see Supplement 1). Given the much higher success rate of amikacin, it is paramount that the antibiotic can be obtained for cases of severe *Acinetobacter* infections where other avenues have failed.

Within the constraints described above, the MSI has influenced procurement planning for 2020/21. Figure 1 evidences significant changes in antibiotic ordering and consumption arising directly from the intervention, where antibiotics in red denote project-related increases and those in blue denote decreases.

	Unit	Price	2019/2020 Plan	Past Av. Consumpt.	2020/2021 Plan	Bi-monthly Cost
Amoxicillin 250g capsules	1000	54,100	101	134	90	4869000
Ampicillin/cloxacillin capsules	100	14,400	30	42	50	720000
Metronidazole tablets	1000	17,100	50	70	70	1197000
Chloramphenicol 250mg tabs	1000	100,200	0	0	5	501,000
Ciprofloxacin 50mg tablet	100	10,500	70	118	70	735000
Ceftriaxone 1g vials	1	1,700	6000	6000	5000	8500000
Cloxacillin 500mg inj	50	33,000	0	2	1	33000
Ampicillin/cloxaciline 250mg inj	100	71,700	2	5	2	143400
Meropenem 500mg inj	1	16,000	0	92	150	2400000
Gentamycin 80mg inj	100	32,800	40	0	0	0
Ciprofloxacin IV 200mg	50	33,000	100	217	150	195000
Metronidazole 500mg infus	1	800	7000	5833	7000	5600000
Cefotaxime inj	1	13,400	1	767	0	0
Penicillin Benzathene 2.4MU amp	10	11,400	5	4	5	57,000
Chloramphenicol 1g inj.	50	80,200	0	0	5	401,000

Figure 1. Extract from the 2020/2021 Procurement Plan (with bi-monthly figures) focusing on key Antibiotics used on PNG Wards. In this table, the column 'unit' shows the number of doses per unit as sold. 'Price' is the price per unit in Ugandan Shillings (1 USD = 3780 UGX, May 2020). The column '2019/2020 plan' shows the number of units ordered for delivery every other month in 2019, with 'past av consumption' detailing the average bi-monthly consumption of the past year. The column '2020/2021' details the set number of units ordered every other month for this year, with the corresponding bi-monthly cost reported in the final column.

The pharmacy team involved in procurement planning pointed out the severe budgetary constraints they faced when attempting to order new antibiotics in response to laboratory results. In practice, this meant making difficult 'trade-offs', especially when the new antibiotics are so much more expensive than those they were able to reduce. The reduction in supply of amoxicillin for example is explained as follows:

> We realised that the majority of patients using amoxicillin were mothers discharged after giving birth. They are usually given amoxicillin as prophylaxis to prevent infection. Some were being given for a longer duration than necessary. As pharmacy staff, we intervened so that the duration of treatment would be reflective of the nature of risk. This led to a reduction in use. We had to increase certain antibiotics or include new antibiotics as well. Due to budget constraints, it was agreed during the planning stage that we cut on the quantity of Amoxicillin to free up some budget to cater for other needed antibiotics.

The laboratory results indicated very high levels of resistance to both amoxicillin and ampicillin, both of which are derived from penicillin (Supplement 1). Based on these assumptions, ampicillin and amoxicillin will have minimal effects on the three primary bacterial causes of infection.

Significant changes in planned use of Meropenem can also be directly attributed to the MSI. The pharmacist explains that consumption of this drug over the past year has been reliant entirely on donated supplies (it was not ordered in 2019):

> [The increased order] can be supported by evidence generated by the laboratory. Due to the increased culture and sensitivity reporting, we noticed that there was improved sensitivity to meropenem. This ensured that we were able to convince members involved in planning to include it on the 2020/2021 plan. We were able to get some donations last year and that's why it shows that we consumed it. What's more, we wrote to NMS to allow us procure it, even though it's not in the current plan.

This action, of communicating directly with NMS on procurement, represents one example of a scenario where the pharmacy team have attempted to advocate as a result of the MSI. The impact of this procurement may be to the benefit of other hospitals if NMS are influenced to place it on their catalogue in future.

The decision to increase orders of Meropenem required the team to make stark choices, which led to the reduction in orders of cefotaxime:

> *Just like Meropenem, this particular consignment of Cefotaxime (used in 2019) was a donation. It wasn't in the procurement plan. While working on the 2020/2021 plan, we had to prioritise between Cefotaxime and Meropenem. We had to go with Meropenem. We did factor in the cost and resistance profile per the lab reports.*

Cefotaxime has shown high levels of resistance in the laboratory tests (Supplement 1). The marked rise in procurement of Ciprofloxacin is also directly attributable to the MSI, although the pharmacy team were concerned about the volume needed:

> *What we require is actually a lot more. Again, [the increase] can be explained by the results of culture and sensitivity. There seems to be less resistance to ciprofloxacin.*

The pharmacist sums up the impact that the project has had on procurement planning and the constraints the team had to work with:

> *We had to reduce the quantity of Ceftriaxone by a significant margin. This again was supported by laboratory data which showed a lot of resistance to ceftriaxone. Some of the monies freed up were used to plan for chloramphenicol and meropenem, drugs which are showing less resistance as per lab reports. There is no significant increase in this current budget and the incoming budget for drugs and medical sundries. It's therefore painstaking to reallocate priorities in terms of drugs while maintaining the same budget. Our [MSI] efforts to encourage and support Culture and Sensitivity testing and sharing this with the procurement planning team lead us to include some much-needed antibiotics (Meropenem and Chloramphenicol) on next year's plan and reduce the procurement of antibiotics with a lot of resistance (Ceftriaxone).*

Figure 1 also provides an indication of the cost implications of the changes in antibiotic procurement as a result of the MSI. Most of the increases in procurement involve more expensive antibiotics. The procurement plan reflects the negotiations the pharmacy team have engaged in, to balance the need for rational prescribing against the cost implications of buying more expensive antibiotics. Unfortunately, the constraints of the NMS budget-line are not the end of the story.

3.6. Discrepancies between Order and Supply (Order Fill Rates)

In practice, not all that is ordered by the hospital from NMS is supplied. The 'Order Fill Rate' gauges the delivery performance of total number of items ordered against the total number of items delivered. As clearly seen in Table 2, NMS supplies about 75% of orders. More specific discrepancies may also arise. Unusually, NMS failed to deliver Ceftriaxone in September 2019, for example.

Table 2. The Order Fill Rate at Fort Portal Regional Referral Hospital (FPRRH) (2019/2020).

Financial Year Cycle	Total Items Ordered	Total Items Delivered	Fill Rate
CYCLE 1 (July–August 2019)	307	236	77%
CYCLE 2 (September–October 2019)	306	232	76%
CYCLE 3 (November–December 2019)	309	226	73%

Source: Rx on-line medicines management system (National Medical Stores (NMS) do not provide data on fill rates for specific medications)

3.7. Key Challenges to Sustained Behaviour Change: The impact of Stock-Outs on AMS

Stock-outs (the exhaustion of supplies) are a feature of Ugandan public health facilities at all levels, and are a major factor contributing to sepsis deaths in maternal and new-born health [21]. Inevitably, the bi-monthly deliveries tend to be exhausted quite rapidly and often by the end of the first month, when 'stock-outs' become a major feature of life and cause of morbidity and mortality at FPRRH. A pharmacist describes the situation as follows:

> For example, when we get 6000 vials of Ceftriaxone, we consume all of it in maybe 4 weeks, then we stay without for another 3–4 weeks. And the following cycle, we get the same quantity. Therefore [consumption data] are merely an average of what is not enough.

Stock-outs are caused by a combination of misuse and overall shortfalls. The pharmacists noted that the project had improved antibiotic use on the wards:

> When these antibiotics are received [from NMS] they tend to run out quickly. Again, this is attributed to the small budget and probably misuse/irrational prescribing. However [MSI's] endeavour to link the ward, pharmacy and the Lab has to a great extent solved the issue of irrational antibiotic prescribing.

By way of illustration this shortfall, on 18th February 2020 the PNG ward contacted K4C to request support in the purchase of gauze. Without this, they would not be able to continue with the wound dressing established on the ward. This would have resulted in increased infection and sepsis (and antibiotic consumption). We were aware during the project visit in January 2020 that the hospital had also run out of disinfectants, iodine and spinal needles (amongst many other things). In such circumstances the only option is for staff to ask patients to pay for the necessary items, and if they are unable to pay then operations will not happen, and major delays occur in treatment. On 19th February 2020 we established that 13 key items for use on the PNG ward were out of stock and had been for over a month:

1. Ceftriaxone injection;
2. Intravenous metronidazole;
3. Intravenous Normal Saline;
4. Intravenous Ringers Lactate;
5. Intravenous Ciprofloxacin;
6. Meropenem 1 g injection;
7. Gentamicin 80 mg injection;
8. JIK (Sodium hypochlorite) solution;
9. Alcohol hand rub;
10. Chlorhexidine Gluconate;
11. Cotton Wool 1 kg (hospital quality);
12. Gauze (Hospital quality);
13. Povidone Iodine;

The next supplies were expected on 25th February.

3.8. Antibiotic Consumption Patterns at Ward Level in FPRRH

When supplies arrive at FPRRH from NMS, they are located at the Main Stores. At this point, supply data is recorded electronically in the on-line ordering system (Rx). The process of distributing supplies within the hospital is, unfortunately, not covered by this electronic system. Instead, the in-patient pharmacy (located a short distance from the Stores) orders from the Stores. Individual wards then visit the in-patient pharmacy to requisition supplies, and this is recorded manually on forms and in a records ledger book (the HMIS Dispensing Log). Figure 2 presents data on the distribution of oral antibiotics between the main hospital wards in January and February 2020. As can be seen, the level of antibiotic consumption on the PNG wards as a proportion of overall consumption is high and indicates the importance of this to overall AMS. The data presented in this figure illustrates three important trends, which were also seen in the use of intravenous antibiotics:

- The dominance of Amoxicillin and Metronidazole in antibiotic consumption.
- The significant contribution that PNG ward makes to overall antibiotic consumption.

- The profound impact of stock-outs on access to antibiotics with a reduction in oral antibiotic use in February, showing a reduction in consumption to between 25% and 30% compared to the January figures.

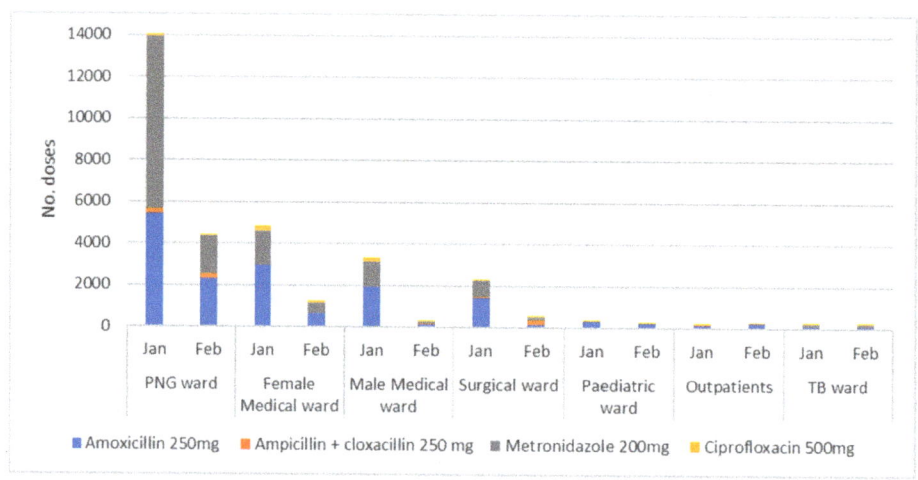

Figure 2. Supply of Oral Antibiotics to All Wards in January and February 2020.

Figures 3 and 4 present data collected from the in-patient pharmacy on key antibiotics used in the PNG wards only. NMS deliveries were made on 13th December 2019 and 24th February 2020. The dispensing patterns show stark evidence of stock-outs.

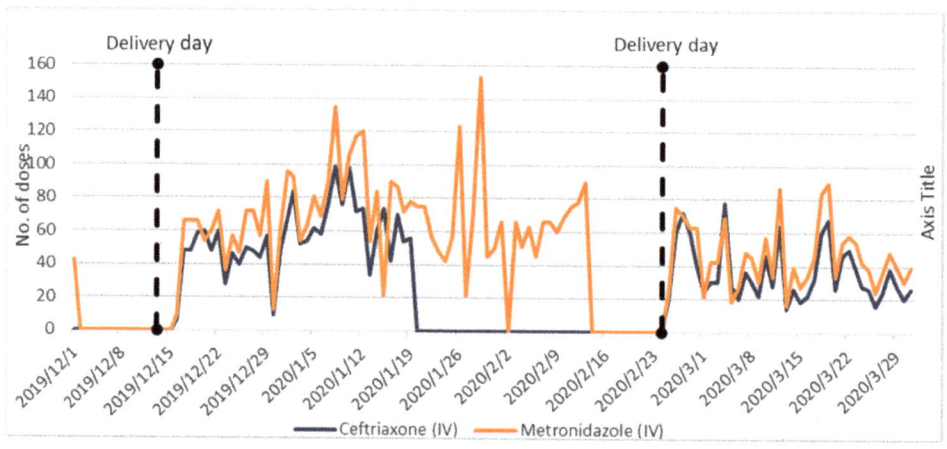

Figure 3. Dispensing of IV Ceftriaxone and Metronidazole from In-Patient Pharmacy to Post-Natal and Gynaecology (PNG) Wards (1/12/2019–29/03/2020).

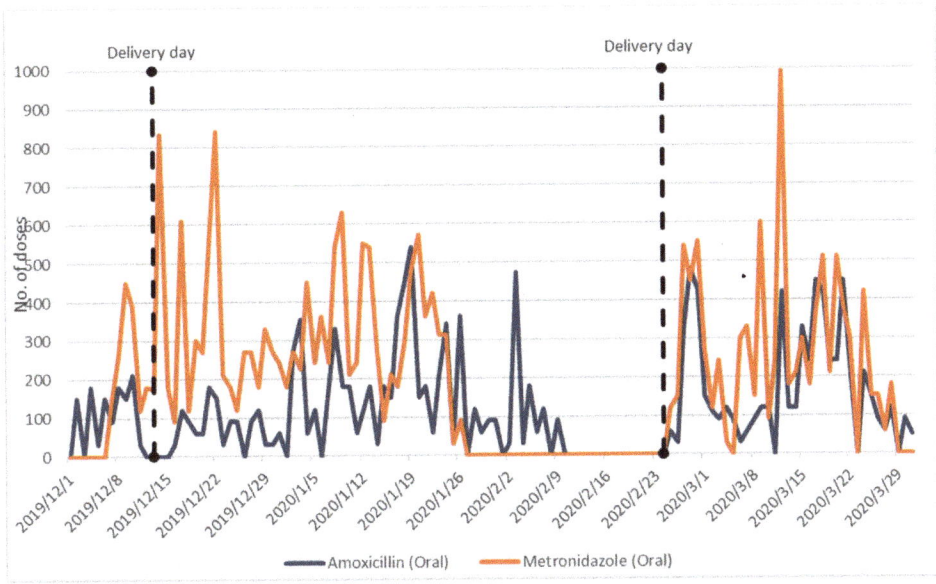

Figure 4. Dispensing of Oral Amoxicillin and Metronidazole from In-Patient Pharmacy to PNG Wards (1/12/2019–29/03/2020).

The higher consumption of metronidazole can be attributed to the high dosing regimen (three times daily), plus its empirical indication as a broad-spectrum therapy for prophylaxis against anaerobes. IV Ceftriaxone (dosed once daily) is also being used empirically and for prophylaxis, especially in surgical cases. Dispensing of IV metronidazole showed evidence of stock-outs but for shorter periods than Ceftriaxone. In the period between 15th and 23rd February, neither IV Metronidazole or IV Ceftriaxone was available to the PNG wards. Similar falls can be seen at Christmas and New Year.

Dispensing patterns for oral metronidazole show higher utilisation and longer periods of stock-outs than oral amoxicillin, with an extended stock-out from 26th January to 23rd February coinciding exactly with the stock out of IV Metronidazole.

3.9. Interpreting In-Patient Pharmacy Data—A Note

We discussed some of the challenges of collating and interpreting facility consumption data (above). The emphasis in instruments such as the WHO's Practical Toolkit for AMS programmes in health-care facilities in low- and middle-income countries [22], which prescribe 'outcome measures' aligned to Western consumption indicators (such as Defined Daily Dose and Direct Observed Therapy) fail to capture the reality of many LMIC contexts. Hantrais' work on comparative methods [23] discusses the idea of 'conceptual equivalence', arguing that 'concepts cannot be separated from contexts' [23] (p. 73). Operationalising the concept of direct observed therapy presents insurmountable challenges in Ugandan RRHs. Hospital pharmacists were very aware of these limitations:

> *We cannot measure performance by zeroing on antibiotic [consumption] only.*

Collecting and analysing the data on antibiotic 'consumption' patterns at FPPRH has emphasised the dangers of empiricist approaches to data analysis and presentation, and the importance of interrogating data rigorously. In most cases, data presents a myriad of questions and very few obvious and immediate answers. This is especially the case when attempting to collate data from public health facilities in Uganda and many other LMICs. Collecting data has been a continuous process of trial and error, merging with the underlying ethnographic journey. As described, in the case of in-patient pharmacy, the data is not yet managed electronically via the Rx system. Rather, individual wards come to a window in the in-patient pharmacy with paper forms requesting supplies for that day. The pharmacy then maintains a hand-written record of dispensing in a records book and this data is compiled into forms for the Ministry of Health. In the first instance, we believed that all wards behaved in this manner, but the initial data suggested otherwise. The TB ward, for example, appeared to collect very few drugs. We found that most of the drugs used on the TB ward are in fact provided by a donor and follow a different track. These drugs pass through the main stores and are directly requisitioned by the TB ward. As such, they do not pass through in-patient pharmacy and neither are they recorded as received from NMS on the Rx system, leaving a gap in overall supply and consumption data.

Our observational work on the wards, supplemented by qualitative interviews and many emails led us to question the relationship between this 'consumption' data and overall consumption patterns. We know, for example, that since laboratory results have been available, many women are getting higher-end antibiotics and that this is contributing to shortened stays and improved patient outcomes [10]. However, the supplies of these drugs were not visible in the data. It seems that the pharmacists have played a critical role in supporting access to these antibiotics through a combination of 'borrowing' from other hospital supplies. The following excerpt explains this process:

> There is a TB focal person who handles all TB related logistics, including the ordering of TB drugs. These drugs are stored in main stores. Rx only focuses on drugs from NMS. In most cases, we don't have the changed antibiotics in stock or in our procurement plan or we have limited quantities. Take Amikacin for example. We usually borrow from the TB program and give to the patients. The same applies to Moxifloxacin. These medicines are not available in the inpatient pharmacy. In fact, one time you had to use K4C money to purchase Amikacin. Because at times we have septic patients who are only responsive to these drugs, we 'beg'/borrow from the TB drugs. Apparently, this has caused audit queries.

This 'borrowing' behaviour clearly saves women's lives; it also compromises the pharmacists under pressure to assist, but potentially contravening donor conditionalities. We can anticipate similar situations in relation to anti-retroviral therapies (for HIV patients) and also, in the case of FPRRH given its proximity to Congo, some (necessary) stockpiling in the event of Ebola spread.

Other apparent 'discrepancies' in the data, including very sporadic and low use of antibiotics in the neo-natal intensive care unit (NICU) and the paediatric ward uncovered other variances in practice, which are undocumented and apparently do not comply with the published protocol. This was explained by one respondent as follows:

> The paediatric ward gets injectable drugs (directly) from main stores, including antibiotics, but oral antibiotics and other oral drugs from in-patient pharmacy.

When drugs are prescribed but not in-stock, patients are asked to buy them privately. Current recording systems cannot capture the consumption of privately purchased drugs. These examples underline the need to exercise caution when interpreting data on antibiotic consumption. The team is currently completing a more in-depth SSI follow-up on patients which will capture some of these processes.

4. Summary and Conclusions

Dyar's paper [24] reviews the use of the term 'antimicrobial stewardship' and concludes that there has been an overemphasis on conceptualisations focused on 'individual prescriptions', and insufficient emphasis on the societal implications of antimicrobial use. Furthermore, and of particular relevance to the MSI project, there has been insufficient translation of the concepts of 'responsible use' into context and time-specific actions. The authors conclude that AMS is not so much a concept, as it is a tool to assess whether organisations are identifying actions to improve responsible use in the specific context within which they are functioning. This idea fits very well with the action-research approach used in our intervention, and the results arising from that.

Sadly, the changes described above are essential to achieving 'responsible use' in a Ugandan RRH; but they are not sufficient. They create the opportunity for active pharmacy engagement in multi-disciplinary decision-making. This achievement could have a major impact on AMS at the hospital, as these wards consume by far the largest volume of antibiotics at the hospital. The cost-effectiveness of this intervention underlines the sustainability potential and the immediate opportunity for scale-up across the hospital as a whole, but also to other public health facilities in Uganda and beyond. Cox et al. make the important point that, 'delayed or no access to antibiotics kills more people than antibiotic resistant bacteria. . . . AMS is not only about reducing inappropriate use, but also assuring access to effective treatment' [1] (p. 813).

The findings evidence significant and impactful behaviour change on the PNG wards, with genuine multi-disciplinary team-working contributing to changes in prescribing behaviour and AMS. Wound care and laboratory testing lie at the heart of these changes centre staging nurses, midwives and laboratory scientists in AMS processes. The results of the microbiology testing then provide a platform for genuine multi-disciplinarity and, specifically, the first opportunity for clinical pharmacy engagement. This is true both at the level of rational (evidence-based) prescribing for individual patients and in improving the evidence base behind empirical prescribing (through an understanding on patterns of AMR). If access to a full range of antibiotics were available, this platform of behaviour change would transform antimicrobial use patterns, reduce the overuse and inappropriate use of antimicrobials and improve patient outcomes and deliver significant cost-benefits.

The second part of the paper has elaborated the complexity and opacity of the supply chain system in a RRH setting in Uganda. In the absence of effective supplies not only will these cost-savings elude facilities, but the patients involved will fail to thrive, and the motivation of health workers to apply the skills and knowledge they have demonstrated will inevitably decline. The paper has explained, in detail, the complex dynamics of supply chain management in a Ugandan public hospital. Understanding and piecing together these processes has required painstaking ethnographic research to unpick major errors in record-keeping and interpret the trends observed. In the first instance, the very centralised system creates huge dependency on the functionality of NMS and the adequacy of Ministry budgets. Centralisation may be seen as necessary in systems so damaged by corruption but where this undermines flexibility and responsiveness and generates extended and predictable stock-outs, the systems put in place to improve AMS will, inevitably, fail.

The MSI has demonstrated the potential for change and the efficiencies associated with this. We hope that publication of this evidence will stimulate discussion at national level amongst all key stakeholders, and generate a momentum for change. The COVID-19 pandemic has thrown a light on supply-chain effectiveness and the impact of weak supply chains on global and national inequalities. Although the poorest in societies will suffer disproportionately, the tentacles of AMR, as with all global pandemics will reverberate across the globe.

At a local level, after years of ongoing engagement, the Kabarole Health Partnership has recently signed a Public-Private-Partnership (PPP) agreement, which was triggered by the current project. The PPP will generate a more sustainable and integrated mechanism for supply-chain augmentation with an emphasis on IPC and antimicrobials. This will enable foreign organisations to cooperate on a co-decision and co-funding basis, guided by the hospital's Medicine Therapeutic Committee, and supported by a not for profit supplier, Joint Medical Stores. The objective will be to move away from dependency-generating donations to a more integrated approach with the agility to respond to local needs.

Supplementary Materials: The following are available online at http://www.mdpi.com/2079-6382/9/6/315/s1, File 1: Antimicrobial Resistance patterns at FPRRH. Figure 1: Extract from the 2020/2021 Procurement Plan (with bi-monthly figures) focusing on key Antibiotics used on Post Natal and Gynae Wards, Figure 2: Supply of Oral Antibiotics to All Wards in January and February 2020, Figure 3: Dispensing of IV Ceftriaxone and Metronidazole from In-Patient Pharmacy to PNG Wards (1/12/2019–29/03/2020), Figure 4: Dispensing of Oral Amoxicillin and Metronidazole from In-Patient Pharmacy to PNG Wards (1/12/2019–29/03/2020).

Author Contributions: L.A. was the Principal Investigator for the MSI and was involved in project conceptualisation; funding acquisition, research design; data collection, analysis and original draft application. G.A.-J. was involved in project design, data collection, formal analysis and draft preparation. M.S. was involved in investigation, formal analysis and writing–original draft preparation. J.O. was involved in investigation and writing–original draft preparation. S.O. was co-applicant and funding acquisition and review and editing. All authors have read and agreed to the published version of the manuscript.

Funding: This research was funded by the Commonwealth Partnership for Antimicrobial Stewardship (CwPAMS) Project Reference AMSB03.

Acknowledgments: The authors would like to acknowledge the support of Richard Walwema and Daniel Kibombo (Infectious Disease Institute); Louis Muhindo (Hospital Administrator); the nursing and midwifery team on Post Natal and Gynae ward; Alan Muwaza and Simon Sseguya (Hospital Pharmacists); the K4C team and Beatrice Waddingham, Project Manager at the Tropical Health and Education Trust.

Conflicts of Interest: The authors declare no conflict of interest. The funders had no role in the design of the study; in the collection, analyses, or interpretation of data; in the writing of the manuscript, or in the decision to publish the results.

References

1. Cox, J.A.; Vlieghe, E.; Mendelson, M.; Wertheim, H.; Ndegwa, L.; Villegas, M.V.; Gould, I.; Levy Hara, G. Antibiotic stewardship in low- and middle-income countries: The same but different? *Clin. Microbiol. Infect.* **2017**, *23*, 812–818. [CrossRef] [PubMed]
2. THET. Commonwealth Partnerships for Antimicrobial Stewardship Scheme. Available online: https://www.thet.org/our-work/grants/cwpams/ (accessed on 24 April 2020).
3. Government of Uganda. Antimicrobial Resistance National Action Plan. 2018. Available online: https://cddep.org/wp-content/uploads/2018/12/GoU_AMR-NAP.pdf (accessed on 20 May 2020).
4. Ministry of Health, Uganda. The National Annual Maternal and Perinatal Death Surveillance and Response (MPDSR) Report FY 2018/2019. 2019. Available online: http://library.health.go.ug/publications/maternal-health/maternal-and-perinatal-death-surveillance-and-response-guidelines (accessed on 10 May 2020).
5. Ngonzi, J.; Tornes, Y.F.; Mukasa, P.K.; Salongo, W.; Kabakyenga, J.; Sezalio, M.; Wouters, K.; Jacqueym, Y.; Van Geertruyden, J.P. Puerperal sepsis, the leading cause of maternal deaths at a tertiary university teaching hospital in Uganda. *BMC Pregnancy Childbirth* **2016**, *16*, 207. [CrossRef] [PubMed]
6. Mutyaba, S.T.; Mmiro, F.A. Maternal morbidity during labor in mulago hospital. *Int. J. Gynaecol. Obstet.* **2001**, *75*, 79–80. [CrossRef]
7. Reinhart, K.; Daniels, R.; Kissoon, N.; Machado, F.R.; Schachter, R.D.; Finfer, S. Recognizing sepsis as a global health priority—A WHO resolution. *N. Engl. J. Med.* **2017**, *377*, 414–417. [CrossRef] [PubMed]
8. Allegranzi, B.; Bagheri Nejad, S.; Combescure, C.; Graafmans, W.; Attar, H.; Donaldson, L.; Pittet, D. Burden of endemic health-care-associated infection in developing countries: Systematic review and meta-analysis. *Lancet* **2011**, *377*, 228–241. [CrossRef]
9. Ackers, H.L.; Ackers-Johnson, J. *Mobile Professional Voluntarism and International Development: Killing Me Softly?* Palgrave Macmillan: New York, NY, USA, 2016. [CrossRef]
10. Ackers, L. Containing Anti-Microbial Resistance in Low- and Middle-Income Countries. In *Ethnographic Insights on Intervention Opportunities in Public Hospital Contexts*, 1st ed.; Palgrave Macmillan: New York, NY, USA, in press.
11. Bate, P. Perspectives on Context: Context Is Everything. 2014. Available online: https://www.health.org.uk/publications/perspectives-on-context (accessed on 30 April 2020).
12. Ackers-Johnson, G. Comparing the Antimicrobial Diversity of Staphylococcus Aureus Strains Isolated from Clinical Cases of Infection and Those Found as a Commensal Organism in Fort Portal, Uganda and Salford, United Kingdom; and Further Investigating the Potential Mechanisms. Unpublished Ph.D. Thesis, University of Salford, Greater Manchester, UK, July 2020.
13. Ackers, H.L.; Ackers-Johnson, J.; Chatwin, J.; Tyler, N. *Healthcare, Frugal Innovation, and Professional Voluntarism: A Cost-Benefit Analysis*; Palgrave Macmillan: New York, NY, USA, 2017. [CrossRef]
14. Alvinius, A.; Starrin, B.; Larsson, G. Reflexive serendipity. grounded theory and serendipity in disaster management and military research. *QSR* **2016**, *12*, 28–42.
15. Martínez, F. The serendipity of anthropological practice the process of discovery as an anthropological problematic. *Anthropol. J. Eur. Cult.* **2018**, *27*, 1–6. [CrossRef]

16. Rivoal, I.; Salazar, N.B. Contemporary ethnographic practice and the value of serendipity. *Soc. Anthropol.* **2013**, *21*, 178–185. [CrossRef]
17. Ackers, L.; Ioannou, E.; Ackers-Johnson, J. The impact of delays on maternal and neonatal outcomes in Ugandan public health facilities: The role of absenteeism. *Health Policy Plan* **2016**, *31*, 1152–1161. [CrossRef] [PubMed]
18. Tweheyo, R.; Reed, C.; Campbell, S.; Davies, L.; Daker-White, G. "I have no love for such people, because they leave us to suffer": A qualitative study of health workers' responses and institutional adaptations to absenteeism in rural Uganda. *BMJ Glob. Health* **2019**, *4*, e001376. [CrossRef] [PubMed]
19. Brink, A.J.; van den Bergh, D.; Mendelson, M.; Richards, G.A. Passing the baton to pharmacists and nurses: New models of antibiotic stewardship for South Africa? *S. Afr. Med. J.* **2016**, *106*, 947–948. [CrossRef] [PubMed]
20. Ministry of Health. Essential Medicines and Health Supplies List 2016—Ministry of Health | Government of Uganda. Available online: https://www.health.go.ug/cause/essential-medicines-and-health-supplies-list-2016/ (accessed on 28 April 2020).
21. Bua, J.; Mukanga, D.; Lwanga, M.; Nabiwemba, E. Risk factors and practices contributing to newborn sepsis in a rural district of eastern uganda, august 2013: A cross sectional study. *BMC Res. Notes* **2015**, *8*, 350.
22. World Health Organization. Antimicrobial Stewardship Programme in Health-Care Facilities in Low and Middle-Income Countries: A WHO Practical Toolkit. 2019. Available online: https://apps.who.int/iris/bitstream/handle/10665/329404/9789241515481-eng.pdf (accessed on 30 May 2020).
23. Hantrais, L. *International Comparative Research: Theory, Methods and Practice*; Red Globe Press: London, UK, 2008.
24. Dyar, O.J.; Huttner, B.; Schouten, J.; Pulcini, C. What is antimicrobial stewardship? *Clin. Microbiol. Infect.* **2017**, *23*, 793–798. [CrossRef] [PubMed]

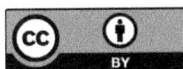

© 2020 by the authors. Licensee MDPI, Basel, Switzerland. This article is an open access article distributed under the terms and conditions of the Creative Commons Attribution (CC BY) license (http://creativecommons.org/licenses/by/4.0/).

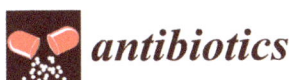

Article

Developing a Sustainable Antimicrobial Stewardship (AMS) Programme in Ghana: Replicating the Scottish Triad Model of Information, Education and Quality Improvement

Jacqueline Sneddon [1,*], Daniel Afriyie [2], Israel Sefah [3], Alison Cockburn [4], Frances Kerr [5,6], Lucie Byrne-Davis [7] and Elaine Cameron [7,8]

1. Scottish Antimicrobial Prescribing Group, Healthcare Improvement Scotland, Delta House, 50 West Nile Street, Glasgow G1 2NP, UK
2. Pharmacy Department, Ghana Police Hospital, Accra PO Box CT104, Ghana; dspdan77@yahoo.com
3. Department of Pharmacy, Keta Municipal Hospital, Keta-Dzelukope P.O. Box WT82, Ghana; isefah1980@gmail.com
4. NHS Lothian, Western General Hospital, Crewe Road South, Edinburgh EH4-2XU, UK; Alison.Cockburn@nhslothian.scot.nhs.uk
5. NHS Education for Scotland, Glasgow G3 8BW, UK; Frances.Kerr@nes.scot.nhs.uk
6. NHS Lanarkshire, Airdrie ML6 0JS, UK
7. School of Medical Sciences, The University of Manchester, Manchester M13 9PL, UK; lucie.byrne-davis@manchester.ac.uk (L.B.-D.); elaine.cameron@stir.ac.uk (E.C.)
8. Division of Psychology, University of Stirling, Stirling FK9 4LA, UK
* Correspondence: jacqueline.sneddon@nhs.net

Received: 24 August 2020; Accepted: 22 September 2020; Published: 23 September 2020

Abstract: (1) Background: Our aim was to develop robust and reliable systems for antimicrobial stewardship (AMS) in Keta Municipal Hospital and Ghana Police Hospital. Objectives were to build capacity through training staff in each hospital, establish AMS teams, collect data on antibiotic use and support local quality improvement initiatives. (2) Methods: The Scottish team visited Ghana hospitals on three occasions and the Ghanaian partners paid one visit to Scotland. Regular virtual meetings and email communication were used between visits to review progress and agree on actions. (3) Results: Multi-professional AMS teams established and met monthly with formal minutes and action plans; point prevalence surveys (PPS) carried out and data collected informed a training session; 60 staff participated in training delivered by the Scottish team and Ghanaian team cascaded training to over 100 staff; evaluation of training impact demonstrated significant positive change in knowledge of antimicrobial resistance (AMR) and appropriate antibiotic use as well as improved participant attitudes and behaviours towards AMR, their role in AMS, and confidence in using the Ghana Standard Treatment Guidelines and antimicrobial app. (4) Conclusions: Key objectives were achieved and a sustainable model for AMS established in both hospitals.

Keywords: antimicrobial stewardship; training; antibiotics use; behavior change

1. Introduction

The Scottish Antimicrobial Prescribing Group (SAPG) has established a comprehensive and robust national antimicrobial stewardship (AMS) programme coordinated by a national group working with regional antimicrobial multi-professional teams [1]. The national group is chaired by an Infection Specialist (Infectious Diseases Consultant or Microbiology Consultant) but the lead for the programme is an Antimicrobial Pharmacist. The regional AMS teams, in common with those in the rest of the UK and other European countries, are generally led by an Infection Specialist but the majority of their stewardship interventions are delivered by Antimicrobial Pharmacists and increasingly supported by specialist nurses. Close multi-professional working has been critical to the success of the Scottish AMS programme. This has been successful in changing prescribing practice, providing rich data on antimicrobial use and resistance, providing education for health and social care staff across all settings and applying quality improvement methodology at scale to tackle areas of poor practice [2]. The approach in Scotland is aligned with and informed by the United Kingdom (UK) Antimicrobial Resistance (AMR) National Action Plan [3] and supports the ambitions for stewardship within Europe [4] and those of the World Health Organisation (WHO) [5] as one of several important actions for tackling AMR.

The model for SAPG was adopted from the Swedish Strategic Programme Against Antibiotic Resistance (Strama) programme [6] following visits by key personnel. The Scottish triad approach utilises Information, Education and Quality Improvement as the three key elements required for effective stewardship. The SAPG model has informed approaches in several other countries including Wales [7], Kenya [8], South Africa [9] and Brazil [10].

In 2019 the SAPG secured a global volunteering grant from the Fleming Fund's Commonwealth Partnerships for Antimicrobial Stewardship (CwPAMS) [11] to work with two hospitals in Ghana. This was the first such grant that required partnership leads to be pharmacists, reflecting their major role in delivery of AMS. The Ghanaian Ministry of Health had developed national Standard Treatment Guidelines (STG) for the management of common infections and had a 5-year National Action Plan (NAP) for AMR (2017–2021) [12]. The NAP covers improving knowledge of AMR, establishing surveillance of antimicrobial consumption, optimising antimicrobial use, establishment of a functional antimicrobial stewardship (AMS) team in all health facilities in Ghana and supporting sustainable investment in AMR reduction. The implementation of the NAP included, among others, the establishment of a functional AMS team in all health facilities in Ghana, which was lacking [12]. At the time of this study few hospitals in Ghana had progressed with establishing an AMS team or programme. The two hospitals involved in this partnership were keen to progress AMS, management support had been agreed and AMS team members identified.

The SAPG team (antimicrobial pharmacists, antimicrobial nurses, Infectious Disease Consultants and researchers from the University of Strathclyde) created a partnership with lead pharmacists in Ghana Police Hospital (GPH), Accra, and Keta Municipal Hospital (KMH), Volta Region, to support the development of antimicrobial stewardship. These lead pharmacists were supported by medical and nursing managers within their hospitals to provide leadership for a multi-professional AMS team. The project was also supported by health psychologists from The Change Exchange, who provided behavioural science strategies in assessing and changing influences on AMS behaviours [13].

The aim of the project was to develop and implement robust and reliable systems (accountability) and processes (practical tools) for antimicrobial stewardship in GPH and KMH by April 2020. This was to include establishing a local AMS team for each hospital, building capacity through provision of training sessions for a total of up to 25 professionals (medical, pharmacy, nursing and laboratory staff) in each hospital to deliver a local stewardship programme and a supported point prevalence survey (PPS) across each hospital to provide baseline surveillance data on antibiotic use to inform improvements. A simplified behaviour change wheel approach was taken to supplement the SAPG model. In this approach, behaviours are specified, the influences on behaviour are studied and these influences targeted in the intervention [14]. The SAPG triad approach to stewardship (Information, Education and Quality Improvement) was applied with behaviour change concepts incorporated throughout with the aim of developing a robust and crucially sustainable antimicrobial stewardship programme in each hospital.

2. Results

2.1. Hospital AMS Teams

In advance of the initial visit by the SAPG team the Ghanaian lead pharmacists with their hospital management team each convened a local multi-professional antimicrobial stewardship team to support the project and to ensure long term sustainability in antimicrobial stewardship. A standardised assessment of current stewardship was undertaken in both hospital using a tool developed by the Commonwealth Pharmacy Association (CPA). This identified gaps and informed discussions with the SAPG team during the initial visit. The local AMS teams (specialist doctors, pharmacists and nurses) established regular meetings and acted as champions to promote and engage all professional staff in antimicrobial stewardship. These teams also supported the lead pharmacists on all three elements of the project.

2.2. Information

For the initial PPS in May 2019 data were collected from prescription charts and patient notes by the Scotland/Ghana teams from all wards on a single day in each hospital utilising paper-based Global Point Prevalence Survey [15] methodology. Prescriptions were compared for compliance with available STG prior to data entry into the online Global PPS system. The overall prevalence of antibiotic use was 65.0% in GPH and 82.0% in KMH. Prevalence rates ranged from 46.7% to 100.0%, depending on the clinical specialty and patient population (Table 1). Penicillins and other beta-lactam antibiotics were the most prescribed antibiotics in both hospitals, with amoxicillin/clavulanic acid being the most commonly prescribed antibiotic.

Table 1. Prevalence of antibiotic use in Ghana hospitals compared with Africa data from Global PPS.

Prevalence of Antibiotic Use	Adult Total	Paediatric Total
Ghana Police Hospital % ($n = 59$)	57.1 (49)	76.9 (10)
Keta Municipal Hospital % ($n = 101$)	55.6 (90)	100.0 (11)
Africa (Global PPS) % (70 hospitals)	64.2	79.4

Some differences were observed in the quality indicators between the two hospitals (Table 2) however in both hospitals there was good documentation of the indication for antibiotic treatment compared with the benchmark level for African hospitals in the Global PPS. For some indications, guideline compliance could not be assessed especially for antibiotic use for surgical procedures as they were not included in the STG. Where a guideline was available, compliance with the choice of agent was ≥50% in both hospitals for both medical and surgical patients.

Table 2. Quality indicators for antibiotic use in Ghana hospitals compared with Africa data from Global PPS.

Quality Indicator	Ghana Police Hospital % ($n = 59$)		Keta Municipal Hospital % ($n = 101$)		Africa Global PPS in 70 Hospitals	
	Medical	Surgical	Medical	Surgical	Medical	Surgical
Indication for antibiotic use recorded	100 (41)	85 (17)	88 (66)	84.5 (11)	60.8 (1839)	57.6 (1230)
Guidelines missing	46.3 (19)	70 (14)	1.3 (1)	46.2 (6)	24.1 (729)	43.9 (938)
Guideline compliant	62.5 (10)	66.7 (4)	55.4 (31)	50 (2)	55.9 (670)	61.2 (370)
Stop/review date in notes	92.7 (38)	95 (19)	98.7 (74)	100 (13)	29.1 (880)	32.4 (693)

No treatment was observed to be based on microbiology data in GPH and were only used for one patient in KMH on the day of survey. Duration of surgical prophylaxis was typically more than one day (GPH 69.0%, KMH 77.0%) with no single dose prophylaxis in either hospital.

Data collection for a follow up PPS was carried out in February 2020 by the Ghanaian teams and results were discussed with the SAPG team. Online data entry and reporting was paused due to the COVID-19 pandemic and will be completed in due course.

2.3. Education

2.3.1. Engagement

A total of 60 staff participated in a one day training session held across two days, delivered twice in each hospital by the SAPG team. Nurses made up the majority of participants (22, 36.7%) followed by medical doctors (10, 16.7%) and pharmacists (10, 16.7%). Laboratory scientists, hospital managers, midwives and a public health practitioner made up the remaining 30%.

Feedback forms on the SAPG training were completed by 48 of the 60 participants. Responses were positive with 39 participants rating the session as very good and 9 participants as good.

2.3.2. Knowledge Evaluation

For the knowledge quiz in GPH the participant mean scores were: pre-training 9.2 (SD2.2, range 5–13) and post-training 11.1 (SD1.8) (range 8–13), and in KMH the mean scores were: pre-training 9.4 (SD1.8, range 5–13) and post-training 10.9 (SD1.4) (range 8–13). The mean difference between pre and post-training participant scores in GPH was 1.88 (95% CI 0.753 to 3.008) ($p = 0.00002$) and in KMH the mean difference between the scores was 1.57 (95% CI 0.93 to 2.21) ($p = 0.00001$).

In GPH, training was cascaded by the local AMS team to a total of 25 staff across one session. A total of 18 participants completed the knowledge quiz before a session and 8 participants fully completed it post-training. The mean pre-training score was 8.5/13 (range 6–12) and the mean post-training score was 9.3/13 (range 8–11). During the final visit by the SAPG team, 2 of the original training participants completed a further knowledge quiz (4 months after the training session), scoring 10 and 13 points and total of 8 staff (additional 6 people trained by GPH team) completed the knowledge quiz and scored a mean of 10/13 (range 8–13).

In KMH, training was cascaded by the local AMS team to a total of 144 staff over two training sessions. During the final visit by the SAPG team, 2 of the original training participants completed a further knowledge quiz, scoring 9 and 13 points and a total of 12 staff (who completed SAPG or KMH team training) completed the knowledge quiz and scored a mean of 10.5/13 (range 6–13).

2.3.3. Attitudes and Behaviours Evaluation

Participants from both hospitals demonstrated improved attitudes and behaviours around use of antibiotics after the training session as shown in Tables 3 and 4. Attitudes and behaviours were similar across professional groups based on comments from the training sessions.

Sustained change in attitudes and behaviours were assessed during the final visit with the following findings: in GPH, staff agreed or strongly agreed with all but two of them having positive stewardship behaviours. Areas where some staff did not agree were the ease of adhering to guidelines and the need for peer support for adherence to guidelines. In KMH, a larger number of staff did not agree with these attitudes towards the guidelines and more staff said they could not access the guidelines.

Table 3. Pre and post education responses to survey questions by staff at GPH (Ghana Police Hospital).

Statement		Strongly Disagree	Disagree	Neither Agree nor Disagree	Agree	Strongly Agree	Don't Know
Antimicrobial resistance (AMR) is a serious problem	Pre				4	15	
	Post	1			4	14	
I am worried that antibiotics will soon become ineffective	Pre	1	1	1	7	8	1
	Post	1			4	13	1
I am worried patients will develop antibiotic resistant infections	Pre	1		1	7	10	
	Post	2			6	11	
Following national or local antibiotic prescribing guidelines will help to prevent the development of AMR	Pre			2	8	9	
	Post	1			5	13	
It is part of my professional role to reduce the risks of AMR	Pre	1			5	13	
	Post				5	13	1
I am able to access the GSTG easily	Pre	1			6	12	
	Post			6	6	6	1
I find it easy to adhere to GSTG whenever I prescribe or administer antimicrobials	Pre	1			9	9	
	Post		1	5	8	4	1
My peers support adherence to GSTG when prescribing or administering antimicrobials	Pre	1		2	10	5	1
	Post			7	11		
I feel confident about questioning a colleague about an antibiotic prescription not in line with the GSTG	Pre	1		4	11	3	
	Post		2	4	11	1	1
I plan to adhere to GSTG whenever I prescribe or administer an antibiotic	Pre	1			10	7	1
	Post			1	10	7	1

GSTG—Ghana Standard Treatment Guidelines.

Table 4. Pre and post education responses to survey questions by staff at KMH (Keta Municipal Hospital).

Statement		Strongly Disagree	Disagree	Neither Agree nor Disagree	Agree	Strongly Agree	Don't Know
Antimicrobial resistance (AMR) is a serious problem	Pre	2			4	21	1
	Post					28	
I am worried that antibiotics will soon become ineffective	Pre	1	1		11	14	1
	Post		1		1	26	
I am worried patients will develop antibiotic resistant infections	Pre	2	1		13	12	
	Post				4	23	1
Following national or local antibiotic prescribing guidelines will help to prevent the development of AMR	Pre	2	1	1	10	14	
	Post				3	25	
It is part of my professional role to reduce the risks of AMR	Pre	2			10	15	1
	Post				1	27	
I am able to access the GSTG easily	Pre	3	6	4	12	2	1
	Post		3	1	10	14	
I find it easy to adhere to GSTG whenever I prescribe or administer antimicrobials	Pre	1	2	10	14	1	
	Post		1	4	7	16	
My peers support adherence to GSTG when prescribing or administering antimicrobials	Pre		6	14	6	2	
	Post		2	5	13	8	
I feel confident about questioning a colleague about an antibiotic prescription not in line with the GSTG	Pre	2	4	11	9	2	
	Post	1		1	9	17	
I plan to adhere to GSTG whenever I prescribe or administer an antibiotic	Pre	2		3	16	7	
	Post			1	2	25	

GSTG—Ghana Standard Treatment Guidelines.

2.4. Quality Improvement

In both hospitals access to guidelines and gaps in local guidance were identified by AMS teams as a key target for improvement. Local guidelines in poster format were developed in collaboration with clinical teams for display in wards and departments to ensure staff were aware of which antibiotics should be used for common infections seen among inpatients. Colour laminated copies of these posters were provided by the SAPG team during the final visit.

In GPH, the AMS team agreed a local action plan with a focus on introducing interns (doctors, pharmacists, nurses) to AMS and developing local guidelines for antibiotic prescribing for wound management, as well as obstetric pre- and post-delivery (Figure S2). Other actions included addressing the need for surveillance and analysis of laboratory antimicrobial data for common infections such as urinary tract infections, initiating routine collection and analysis of antimicrobial prescribing at the outpatient department. All findings were to be shared periodically at clinical meetings and with the drug and therapeutic committee, as well as publishing findings as appropriate.

In KMH the AMS team agreed a local action plan that focused on: rollout of AMS education to all staff; improving the adherence to the local treatment guideline on empirical management of pneumonia for ambulatory patients; and increasing patient awareness (Figure S3). Their long term goal was to create and locally adapt antibiotic policies for KMH. Progress has already been made towards these goals with over 144 staff trained in antimicrobial stewardship locally, patient education initiated in some pharmacy led clinics and an ongoing Quality Improvement project in the out patients department which to date has increased compliance with policy and reduced amoxicillin/clavulanic acid prescribing.

3. Discussion

Immense progress has been made with the establishment of a robust and sustainable stewardship in GPH and KMH as a result of this project. Through the expert team from SAPG and The Change Exchange providing practical support and guidance, the Ghanaian lead pharmacists have been able to lead their local AMS teams to gain experience and knowledge of the requirements for a successful AMS programme. Building successful relationships has been key to the success of the project and having a single profession, pharmacists, as leaders has been helpful to demonstrate behaviours and capabilities amongst peers [16]. This will support long-term engagement beyond the project to provide continued advice and guidance as the Ghana AMS programmes mature, as well as potentially supporting the spread of AMS to other hospitals in Ghana. Using a multi-professional approach along with behavior change techniques has also been crucial as stewardship needs to be owned by clinical teams and practiced by all staff to be reliable and sustainable [17].

Regarding the Information element of the project, we demonstrated that the PPS assessment was feasible in both hospitals and can be achieved with limited resources and minimal training of a multi-disciplinary team. Now that staff are familiar with the process, further repeats of PPS will take less time and we are hopeful that eventually direct electronic data collection may be possible to reduce data entry time. The use of repeated PPS is a well-recognised method for measuring both the quantity and quality of antibiotic prescribing where electronic medicine management systems are not available [14]. This will allow progress with improvement work to be tracked and smaller bespoke PPS can also be used to investigate prescribing practice in specific clinical areas or of specific antibiotics.

Our approach to the Education element of the project involved developing training collaboratively to ensure the content met the needs of local clinicians. Delivery of the education by a multi-professional team was successful in imparting knowledge, skills and positive behaviours to support improved use of antibiotics. Key behaviours identified by the psychologists during the first visit around supporting access to guidelines and responsibilities of all staff groups for querying prescriptions that do not follow the guidelines featured in the role play scenarios, giving staff a chance to practice promoted behaviours in a non-threatening way. Participants rated the training highly and the use of lectures and interactive sessions supported good engagement and involvement of everyone in discussion of the issues. The 'train the trainer' approach has been successful in building local capacity for provision of ongoing training in both hospitals and potentially beyond to other hospitals in these regions of Ghana. This was demonstrated by the capacity of the local team to train more staff as means of cascading the knowledge of the principles of AMS to untrained staff. The training materials used for the project have been made available via the Commonwealth Pharmacist Association (CPA) website and can be used by others to support similar work. Key learning from the one day sessions was that participants would prefer lectures and interactive sessions to be interspersed rather than have all the lectures at the start. This would also help educators and participants to relax and get to know each other to make the most of the sessions.

The Quality Improvement element of the project was tailored to each hospital's priorities and ambitions based on the action plans agreed by the AMS teams. Both hospitals identified a need for improved access to guidelines so that staff without a smartphone to access the MicroGuide STG app could easily find the information required when prescribing or administering antibiotics. Locally designed posters proved a useful format and the SAPG team were able to produce a quantity of these for each hospital to support compliance with the guidelines across all wards and departments.

In GPH, the AMS team with obstetrics and gynaecology (OBG) and the surgical unit have developed their antibiotic guidelines for pre- and post-delivery and wound management, respectively. Furthermore, the guidelines for common infections seen at the OBG were developed with guidance from the STG. Currently, routine microbial antibiotic sensitivity data from the laboratory, as well as prescribing of antibiotics audits by the pharmacy department, are being done.

In KMH, weekly prescription analysis of compliance to empirical management of pneumonia of ambulatory patients by pharmacists showed an increasing change in behaviour towards the use of first line antibiotics, and work is ongoing.

Limitations of this project included the limited time spent in Ghana by the SAPG team and by the Ghana team in Scotland. With a large team of 10 experts from SAPG (5 for each hospital) and a limited budget, an intensive schedule was necessary to ensure all three elements of the work were delivered in each hospital. Reliance on email communication and some Skype/WhatsApp calls for discussion of the project was not ideal but in the current climate of virtual meetings and global collaboration that may be the way forward. Time for staff to work as volunteers on the project was also at times difficult to manage as all were full time employees with busy work schedules. A further limitation for the training element is potential bias in data collection as a clear protocol for mandatory participant completion of knowledge and behaviour surveys was not employed.

In the current context of the COVID-19 pandemic, future financial support for exchange visits to support development of AMS in low and middle income countries is unlikely and innovative virtual solutions will be a more feasible approach. There may also be merit in supporting the train the trainer approach employed in this study to spread local expertise for AMS to other Ghana hospitals.

4. Materials and Methods

4.1. Study Design

The study design was developed in late 2018 and detailed plans were progressed during March and April 2019 following the grant award. Implementation of the three elements of AMS was facilitated by exchange visits during a 9-month period from May 2019 to February 2020. There were three visits by the Scottish team and The Change Exchange to Ghana to support AMS implementation and one visit by the Ghanaian partners to Scotland to observe how AMS has been embedded at local and national level. Regular virtual meetings and email communication were used between visits to review progress, plan training sessions and agree actions. The study did not require ethics approval.

At the initial visit in May 2019 a small multi-professional group from SAPG visited both hospitals and supported data collection on antibiotic use for a baseline PPS using the Global PPS system. At this visit, in both hospitals, the health psychologists interviewed a variety of staff whose behaviours would impact on the use of antimicrobials. This included prescribers and dispensers. These discussions probed the behaviours that would support prescribers and dispensers to improve AMS and the barriers and facilitators to those behaviours.

On the second visit in September 2019, two separate multi-professional groups worked with Ghanaian Partners to provide 2 × 1-day 'train the trainer' education in each hospital following a training plan (Figure S1) informed by findings from the initial visit. Interactive training activities were developed using behaviour change principles, including a fun Antibiotic Guardian session where trainees pledged their commitment to AMS actions; an activity identifying barriers to changing practice and problem-solving potential solutions; generating action plans to initiate and maintain changes; role playing potentially difficult conversations with prescribers, patients and families; and practicing using the CwPAMS MicroGuide app to access antimicrobial guidelines. Local pharmacist-led antimicrobial teams agreed an action plan and a Quality Improvement (QI) project.

Local Ghana teams cascaded training to other staff and conducted a second PPS between October 2019 and February 2020.

On the 3rd visit by the SAPG team in February 2020, laminated guideline posters for each hospital were provided to increase access for all staff and progress with local action plans was discussed with the AMS teams to agree next steps. Health psychologists and nurses from the visiting team interviewed a range of healthcare staff at both hospitals to identify changes in AMS behaviours since the trainings and ongoing barriers.

4.2. Practical Delivery of the Project

The Global Point Prevalence Survey system [15] was used to collect, submit and generate reports on antibiotic use in each hospital.

Training sessions utilised Microsoft PowerPoint presentations and both plenary and small group workshop discussions. Some elements of the training were filmed using a smartphone camera as a record of AMS pledges made by staff. Staff who attended the training session received a signed certificate of participation. Training was evaluated to assess the change in knowledge and behaviours of participants before and after the session using paper forms. Participants were also asked to complete a paper-based feedback form about their perception of the training session. Participants were not asked for formal consent to use information they provided in the evaluation and feedback forms but consent was presumed from their participation in the training session.

Each facility was encouraged to identify a QI project to address the shortfalls identified in key quality indicators identified by the PPS.

5. Conclusions

Key objectives were achieved and a sustainable model for AMS was established in both hospitals. Support for spread of AMS at national level was discussed through partnership meetings with academics in the Medical and Pharmacy Schools, the Ministry of Health AMR lead and Pharmaceutical Society staff with commitment to ongoing collaboration. Overall, members of the SAPG team and the Ghanaian lead pharmacists learned much about each other's professional practice and countries' cultures which will remain important memories for all.

Supplementary Materials: The following are available online at http://www.mdpi.com/2079-6382/9/10/636/s1, Figure S1: Antimicrobial stewardship training plan—Ghana 2019, Figure S2: Ghana Police Hospital AMS Action Plan—2019/2020, Figure S3: Updated Action Plan Keta Hospital (February 2020).

Author Contributions: Conceptualization, J.S., D.A. and I.S.; methodology, J.S., A.C., F.K.; writing—original draft preparation, J.S.; writing—review and editing, D.A., I.S., A.C., F.K., L.B.-D., E.C.; funding acquisition, J.S., D.A., I.S. All authors have read and agreed to the published version of the manuscript.

Funding: This research was funded via a grant from the Commonwealth Partnerships on Antimicrobial Stewardship (CwPAMS) supported by Tropical Health and Education Trust (THET) and Commonwealth Pharmacists Association (CPA) using Official Development Assistance (ODA) funding, through the Department of Health and Social Care's Fleming Fund. The views expressed in this publication are those of the author(s) and not necessarily those of the NHS, the Fleming Fund, the Department of Health and Social Care, THET or CPA. UK partners involved were volunteers supported by their NHS host organisations.

Acknowledgments: We thank the members of the Healthcare Improvement Scotland and Ghana hospitals partnership for supporting development and delivery of the training sessions, and staff at Keta Municipal Hospital and Ghana Police Hospital for engaging with the sessions. Thanks to Jo Hart and Joanna Goldethorpe from the Change Exchange for their contributions to the project. Special thanks to Marion Pirie, SAPG Project Officer, for administrative support, organising all travel and budget management and to Lesley Cooper, SAPG Health Service Researcher, for help with literature evaluation and analysis of data.

Conflicts of Interest: The authors declare no conflict of interest. The funders had no role in the design of the study; in the collection, analyses, or interpretation of data; in the writing of the manuscript, or in the decision to publish the results.

References

1. The Scottish Antimicrobial Prescribing Group. Available online: https://www.sapg.scot/ (accessed on 22 July 2020).
2. Colligan, C.; Sneddon, J.; Bayne, G.; Malcolm, W.; Walker, G.; Nathwani, D. On behalf of the Scottish Antimicrobial Prescribing Group, Six years of a national antimicrobial stewardship programme in Scotland: Where are we now? *Antimicrob. Resist. Infect. Control* **2015**, *4*, 28. [CrossRef] [PubMed]
3. UK 5-Year Action Plan for Antimicrobial Resistance 2019 to 2024. Available online: https://www.gov.uk/government/publications/uk-5-year-action-plan-for-antimicrobial-resistance-2019-to-2024 (accessed on 22 July 2020).
4. European Centre for Disease Prevention and Control: Antimicrobial Stewardship. Available online: https://www.ecdc.europa.eu/en/publications-data/directory-guidance-prevention-and-control/prudent-use-antibiotics/antimicrobial (accessed on 22 July 2020).
5. World Health Organisation. Available online: https://www.who.int/health-topics/antimicrobial-resistance (accessed on 22 July 2020).
6. Mölstad, S.; Cars, O.; Struwe, J. Strama—A Swedish working model for containment of antibiotic resistance. *Euro Surveill.* **2008**, *13*, 19041. [CrossRef] [PubMed]
7. Public Health Wales. Available online: https://phw.nhs.wales/services-and-teams/harp/antimicrobial-resistance-and-prescribing-surveillance-and-reports/ (accessed on 29 July 2020).
8. Okoth, C.; Opanga, S.; Okalebo, F.; Oluka, M.; Baker Kurdi, A.; Godman, B. Point prevalence survey of antibiotic use and resistance at a referral hospital in Kenya: Findings and implications. *Hosp. Pract.* **2018**, *46*, 128–136. [CrossRef]
9. Brink, A.J.; Messina, A.P.; Feldman, C.; Richards, G.A.; Becker, P.J.; Goff, D.A.; Bauer, K.A.; Nathwani, D.; van der Bergh, D.; on behalf of the Netcare Antimicrobial Stewardship Study Alliance. Antimicrobial stewardship across 47 South African hospitals: An implementation study. *Lancet Infect Dis.* **2016**, *16*, 1017–1025. [CrossRef]
10. Piastrelli, F.S.R.; Sapienza, G.; Borges, K.; Rodrigues, F.; Borba, C.; Fernandez, J.G.; Lima, C. Results of a Successful Implementation of a Antimicrobial Stewardship Program in a Public Hospital in São Paulo, Brazil. *Open Forum Infect Dis.* **2018**, *26*, S504. [CrossRef]
11. Commonwealth Pharmacists Association. Commonwealth Partnerships for Antimicrobial Stewardship. Available online: https://commonwealthpharmacy.org/commonwealth-partnerships-for-antimicrobial-stewardship/ (accessed on 22 July 2020).
12. Ghana Ministry of Health, Ministry of Food and Agriculture, Ministry of Environment, Science, Technology and Innovation, Ministry of Fisheries and Aquaculture Development. Ghana National Action Plan for Antimicrobial Use and Resistance. 2017–2021. Available online: http://www.moh.gov.gh/wp-content/uploads/2018/04/NAP_FINAL_PDF_A4_19.03.2018-SIGNED-1.pdf (accessed on 22 July 2020).
13. Manchester Implementation Science Collaboration Collaboration. The Change Exchange. Available online: https://www.mcrimpsci.org/the-change-exchange/ (accessed on 22 July 2020).
14. Michie, S.; Atkins, L.; West, R. *The Behaviour Change Wheel: A Guide to Designing Interventions*; Silverback: London, UK, 2014.
15. Global Point Prevalence Survey. Available online: https://www.global-pps.com/ (accessed on 23 July 2020).
16. Gilchrist, M.; Wade, P.; Ashiru-Oredope, D.; Howard, P.; Sneddon, J.; Whitney, L.; Wickens, H. Antimicrobial stewardship from policy to practice: Experiences from UK antimicrobial pharmacists. *Infect Dis.* **2015**, *4*, 51–64. [CrossRef] [PubMed]
17. Currie, K.; Laidlaw, R.; Ness, V.; Gozdzielewska, L.; Malcom, W.; Sneddon, J.; Seaton, R.A.; Flowers, P. Mechanisms affecting the implementation of a national antimicrobial stewardship programme; multi-professional perspectives explained using normalisation process theory. *Antimicrob. Resist Infect Control* **2020**, *9*, 99. [CrossRef] [PubMed]

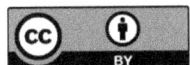 © 2020 by the authors. Licensee MDPI, Basel, Switzerland. This article is an open access article distributed under the terms and conditions of the Creative Commons Attribution (CC BY) license (http://creativecommons.org/licenses/by/4.0/).

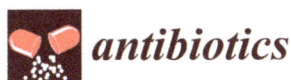

Review

Knowledge, Attitudes and Perceptions of Medical Students on Antimicrobial Stewardship

Panagiotis Efthymiou, Despoina Gkentzi * and Gabriel Dimitriou

Department of Paediatrics, Patras Medical School, University of Patras, 26504 Rio Achaia, Greece; panosefth@upatras.gr (P.E.); gdim@upatras.gr (G.D.)
* Correspondence: gkentzid@upatras.gr

Received: 14 October 2020; Accepted: 16 November 2020; Published: 17 November 2020

Abstract: Antimicrobial Resistance (AMR) is an ongoing threat to modern medicine throughout the world. The World Health Organisation has emphasized the importance of adequate and effective training of medical students in wise prescribing of antibiotics Furthermore, Antimicrobial Stewardship (AMS) has been recognized as a rapidly growing field in medicine that sets a goal of rational use of antibiotics in terms of dosing, duration of therapy and route of administration. We undertook the current review to systematically summarize and present the published data on the knowledge, attitudes and perceptions of medical students on AMS. We reviewed all studies published in English from 2007 to 2020. We found that although medical students recognize the problem of AMR, they lack basic knowledge regarding AMR. Incorporating novel and effective training methods on all aspects of AMS and AMR in the Medical Curricula worldwide is of paramount importance.

Keywords: knowledge; attitudes; medical students; antimicrobial; stewardship; prescribing; antibiotics

1. Introduction

Antimicrobial Resistance (AMR) is an ongoing threat to modern medicine throughout the world with a negative effect on patient treatment outcome. Pathogens are developing mechanisms of resistance, making it difficult to treat common infectious diseases like pneumonia, tuberculosis and foodborne diseases [1–4]. Antibiotic prescribing is determined by various factors, including the socio-cultural and socio-economic factors of each country and the beliefs of patients and professionals regarding antibiotic use [5,6]. In many developing countries, there is shortage of appropriate diagnostic tools, resulting in the unnecessary administration of antibiotics [7,8]. It has also been observed that the insufficient regulatory policies of each country can cause an increase in over-the-counter antibiotics [9]. The World Health Organisation (WHO) has clearly emphasized the importance of adequate and effective training of medical students in the wise prescribing of antibiotics [10]. In 2015, the WHO endorsed the Global Action Plan on Antimicrobial Resistance, which highlights the importance of training all healthcare professionals regarding AMS [11]. It is vital that healthcare students are aware of the challenges posed by AMR, and that there are investments in training them on topics relevant to responsible antibiotic use in their chosen specialties [11].

Thus, future medical professionals have to be prepared appropriately in order to face the challenges of antimicrobial use in everyday clinical practice [12]. Nowadays, medical education incorporates thorough knowledge of infectious diseases and diagnosis, as well as antibiotic utilization and pathogen resistance mechanisms. All the above-mentioned fields of knowledge are highly required for medical students [13]. Furthermore, Antimicrobial Stewardship (AMS) has been recognized as a rapidly growing field in medicine that sets a goal of rational use of antibiotics in terms of dosing, duration of therapy and route of administration [13–15].

Taking into consideration the importance of medical education on AMS and AMR, we undertook the current review to systematically summarize and present the published data on knowledge, attitudes and perceptions of medical students on AMS.

2. Results

In the present review, we included 25 studies. Fifteen of them were focused exclusively on medical students (Table 1), whereas ten were conducted on healthcare professional students with the inclusion of medical students amongst them (Table 2). All studies included final year medical students, three of them also included prefinal students, and three studies included medical students from all years of medical school. We found studies from all over the world in countries of Europe, America, Africa, Asia and Oceania. As for the studies focusing exclusively on medical students, five were conducted in Asia [16–20], three in Africa [21–23], one in Oceania [24], five in Europe [10,25–28] and finally one study in the USA [11]. All studies used questionnaires as research tools so they could collect data regarding the knowledge, attitudes, and perceptions of medical students about AMS. More precisely, questionnaires included questions on self-perceived preparedness to prescribe antibiotics and the importance of AMS. Knowledge regarding antibiotics was, in most cases, tested by clinical scenarios or general questions. The oldest study was conducted in 2012 and the latest in 2020. We also included 10 multidisciplinary studies (Table 2) that incorporated medical, pharmacy, dental, veterinary students, medical interns and physicians [29–38].

Table 1. Studies assessing knowledge, attitudes and perceptions of medical students regarding Antimicrobial Stewardship (AMS).

Country/Study Years	Type of Study	Number of Participants	Main Findings/Outcomes	Reference
France (2012)	Cross-sectional	54 medical students (prefinal and final year)	Medical students feel more confident diagnosing infections than treating them. Four in five wanted more education on antimicrobial use. Almost all of them (96%) found unnecessary prescription unethical. The majority think that AMR is a national problem.	Dyar et al. [27]
USA (2012)	Cross-sectional	317, 4th year medical students at University of Miami, John Hopkins University and the University of Washington	The majority perceive that antimicrobial use is very important and would like more education on it. Around half of them answered correctly in knowledge-related questions depending on their educational sources. Those who completed an elective in infectious diseases felt more confident, however, this had no significant connection with better knowledge scores.	Abbo et al. [12]
Europe (2012)	Multi-centre, cross-sectional study	338 final year medical students from 7 European universities	Students wanted more education on antibiotic prescribing. Most of the students incorrectly believed that MRSA bacteraemia had increased in their country the last decade. They overestimated the burden caused by resistant bacteria compared to lung cancer.	Dyar et al. [10]
China (2015)	Multi-centre, cross-sectional	611, 4th year medical students from 5 teaching university hospitals of Central China	Medical students wish for more training on antimicrobial use through AMS programs and clinical rotations. No significant difference in knowledge between students who used textbooks and smartphones as teaching material.	Yang et al. [16]
France, Sweden (2015)	Multi-centre, cross-sectional	2085 medical students in France and 302 students in Sweden (all in final year)	Preparedness for antimicrobial use was higher in Sweden than in France. Students in France perceive that they need further education on antibiotic use. Swedish students had more working experience at the hospital than French students.	Dyar et al. [28]
Europe, 29 countries (2015)	Multi-centre, Cross-sectional	7328 final year medical students from 179 medical schools	Medical students tend to be more confident in diagnosis of infections than choosing an accurate therapeutic plan. Over a third of the students wanted more education on antimicrobial use. Northern countries show a higher amount of confidence. Clinical cases and small-group teaching sessions are preferred by students.	Dyar et al. [25]
China (2015)	Multi-centre, Cross-sectional	1819 medical students in 6 Universities (all grades of medical school)	The majority of students self-medicated their own illnesses and had a stock of antibiotics, in most cases without medical prescription. One in seven used antibiotics for common cold and asked their doctors for antibiotics.	Hu et al. [17]

Table 1. Cont.

Country/Study Years	Type of Study	Number of Participants	Main Findings/Outcomes	Reference
Australia (2015)	Multi-centre, cross-sectional	163 final-year medical students from 8 universities in Australia	54% of medical students were 'confident' in their knowledge of infectious disease, while 70% were confident in Cardiology. They believe hands on clinical practise more helpful than lectures. Most of them were aware of AMR.	Weier et al. [24]
Thailand (2016)	Multi-centre, cross-sectional	455 final year medical students in 3 medical schools	Almost all of the participants perceive that prescribing board-spectrum antibiotics increases AMR. Half of them answered correct questions related to antibiotic use. Students evaluate bedside teaching as the most effective learning method for appropriate usage of antibiotics.	Chuenchom et al. [20]
South Africa (2017)	Multi-centre, cross-sectional	289 final year medical students in 3 medical schools	The majority assert that antibiotics are overused and that AMR is a major problem in South Africa. Only a third of the participants feel confident in prescribing antibiotics, which is related to use og guidelines and contact with infectious diseases specialists. Medical students who followed prescribing guidelines had a better score in the knowledge section of the questionnaire.	Wasserman et al. [22]
Nigeria (2018)	Cross-sectional	184 medical students (prefinal, final year) at Ebonyi State University, Nigeria	The vast majority wanted more training on antibiotic usage and resistance. Almost half of them had practical training on antibiotic use. Around 2/3 had adequate knowledge on antibiotic use and resistance. However, a high level of false antibiotic management was reported.	Oketo-Alex et al. [21]
Egypt (2018)	Multi-centre, Cross-sectional	963 medical students (all years) from 25 medical schools of Egypt	Almost all students had sufficient knowledge and attitudes towards AMR. Around 40% believed that antibiotics can treat the common cold. Nearly half of them would stop antibiotics when starting to feel well.	Assar et al. [23]
Spain (2019)	Multi-centre, cross-sectional	441 final year medical students from 21 Spanish medical schools	Medical students feel more confident diagnosing than treating infectious diseases. They want additional education regarding antibiotic usage.	Sánchez-Fabra et al. [26]
Japan (2019–2020)	Cross-sectional	661 undergraduate medical students at Okayama University Medical School (1st to 6th year)	90% of medical students knew the mechanism of action of antibiotics. 30% of all medical students believed that antibiotics could treat viral infections, while 46.4% considered antibiotics as treatment for the common cold. AMR plan awareness was poor (6.5%).	Hagiya et al. [18]
India (2020)	Cross-sectional	197 medical students (93 prefinal year and 104 final year) of a teaching institute in Southern Indian city	Insufficient knowledge of medical students about AMR and AMS. However, they recognize that appropriate use of antibiotics is essential, as well as training on AMS.	Meher et al. [19]

Table 2. Studies assessing knowledge, attitudes and perceptions of medical students as well as other healthcare professional students regarding AMS.

Country/Study Years	Type of Study	Number of Participants	Main Findings/Outcomes	Reference
India (2015)	Multidisciplinary, cross-sectional	120 medical and 48 dental students	98% of medical students had positive attitude and knowledge towards AMS.	Sharma et al. [34]
India (2017)	Multidisciplinary, cross-sectional	198 medical students, 89 dental students, 89 nursing students, 80 pharmacy students	A great amount of healthcare students tend to use antibiotics over the counter. 25% of medical students reported self-medication. 33% of medical students did not finish the course of antibiotics.	Virmani et al. [30]
UK (2018)	Multidisciplinary, multicentre, cross-sectional	255 students, 165 pharmacy students, 71 veterinary students, 12 medical students, 11 dental students, 3 physicians, 2 nurses	95% of the students believe that AMR will be a major issue in their future clinical practice. One out of five students felt confident about their knowledge about antimicrobial use	Dyar et al. [31]
Croatia (2018)	Multidisciplinary, cross-sectional	115 medical students 46 pharmacy students	90.7% of students believed that antibiotics are overused. No difference in average knowledge score between medical and pharmacy students.	Rusic et al. [32]
USA (2018)	Single-centre, cross-sectional	103 participants (31 medical students, 57 medical residents, 12 attending physicians)	85% of the responders believed that it would be beneficial for medical staff to be trained further and 75% agreed on the need for AMS education. Medical students had the lowest mean of correct answers compared to medical interns and physicians	Beatthy et al. [36]
USA (2019)	Single-centre, cross-sectional	50 medical students, 30 medical residents, 6 nurse practitioners	Lack of communication among senior and junior practitioners was observed regarding decision of antimicrobial treatment.	Smoke et al. [29]
Pakistan (2019)	Multidisciplinary, cross-sectional	247 prefinal and final year medical students, 203 prefinal and final year pharmacy students	79% of the participants believed that AMS is an important issue in their hospital. Knowledge of antimicrobial use and resistance was higher in pharmacy students than medical students. More pharmacy students would like further training regarding AMS compared to medical students.	Saleem et al. [37]
United Arab Emirates (2019)	Multidisciplinary, cross-sectional	Medical students, pharmacy students, veterinary students, dental students, engineering, technology and law students	Knowledge, attitude and perception score was better among medical students (58%) than in other groups of students (52%). High rates of antibiotic self-medication (38,2%).	Jairoun et al. [38]
Iran (2020)	Multicentre, cross-sectional	126 responders including infectious diseases practitioners, surgeons, medical interns, medical students, general practitioners, microbiology lab technicians and PhD students.	88.1% of participants agreed on establishment of local guidelines. 94.4% claimed that training regarding proper antibiotic use can bring positive effects on reducing AMR.	Firouzabadi et al. [35]
Rwanda (2020)	Multidisciplinary, cross-sectional	115 medical students, 41 dental students.	83% did not have knowledge of AMS. 23% did not agree that excessive antibiotic use can lead to AMR. 50% claimed that antibiotics can be used for pain and inflammation.	Nisabwe et al. [33]

A study in a Japan University in Japan showed that 92.6% of their medical students had sufficient knowledge of the mechanism of actions of antibiotics. However, 30% of the respondents worryingly answered that antibiotics could be used to treat viral infections and around half of them believed that they could be administered for the common cold. We should point out that wrong answers were significantly lower among final year medical students compared to the first-year students. Lastly, only 6.5% of the students were aware of the AMR plan that was promoted by the Japanese government [18].

In 2015, a survey in eight universities from Australia showed that 70% of medical students felt more confident regarding their knowledge in cardiology compared to infectious diseases, where 54% were confident of their knowledge. As for clinical knowledge, students scored better in cardiovascular disease questions (64%) contrary to antibiotic prescribing questions (45%). In addition, nearly all students were aware of guidelines referring to antimicrobial prescribing. A negative aspect of this study was the small number of participants, which may not give an accurate perception of the country's undergraduate students [24].

Our research revealed two studies from China, a country with the second largest antibiotic consumption in the world and high rates of dispensable use of antibiotics. The majority (92%) of medical students from Central China agree that misuse of antibiotic treatment increases AMR, where 67% found their training useful in antimicrobial management. Once again, the percentage of correct answers in a broad spectrum of questions around the treatment of different infections was low, with the total correct percentage being 34% [16]. Another study from China showed that 27% of medical students reported self-medication with antibiotics. Additionally, 64% of the respondents reported that they were stocking antibiotics for personal use, whilst 97% have bought antibiotics without medical prescription in the past [17].

The studies that we found from Europe were conducted under the European Society of Clinical Microbiology and Infectious Diseases Study Group of Antimicrobial Policies (ESGAP/ESCMID). In 2012, seven European medical schools competed an online survey which reported that medical students felt more confident about infection diagnosis in comparison to treatment, e.g., administration route, duration, necessity of antimicrobial use. A high percentage of them (83%) believed that incidence of methicillin-resistant *Staphylococcus aureus* (MRSA) bacteraemias has increased in their country, which was not true. Moreover, medical students overestimated possible death rate resulting from resistant bacteria compared to lung cancer. Nearly all medical students (98%) believed that AMR would be a major issue in the foreseeable future [10]. In another study, we have more detailed results from France, where 64% of the respondents were aware of the implementation of antibiotic guidelines in their hospital and 62% have used them in practice. Furthermore, 94% believed that AMR is a national problem. It should be noted at this point that this study was limited due to the small number of participants [27]. A Spanish study showed that 40.4% of medical students claimed that they would prescribe an antibiotic without consulting guidelines. On the other hand, only 24.3% believed they had adequate training regarding rational use of antibiotics [26]. In 2015, 29 European countries participated in an online survey of ESGAP to assess the preparedness of medical students using antibiotics in a judicious way. Countries that incorporate guidelines in clinical practice, like the United Kingdom, reported a higher rate of preparedness. This conclusion can also be related to quality of education on the use of antibiotics. Hence, there was some variability between different European countries [25]. For example, a study comparing France and Sweden showed that French medical students were less likely to feel prepared compared to the Swedish students and they suggest a need for more focused education in the field. A hypothesis that originated from this study claims that this concept may come from the fact that Swedish medical students tend to have more clinical exposure to the approach of antibiotic management [28]. In general, 37.3% of medical students requested more education on this subject. This is one of the greatest studies considering the preparedness of medical students on a topic [25].

Another study from India revealed that medical students have insufficient knowledge about AMR and AMS (39.7% of prefinal and 54.8 of final year medical students answered correct). Most of the students knew that viral infections cannot be treated with antibiotics. However, many of them had did not know how to treat and prevent MRSA infections effectively and could not recall the acronym *Enterococcus faecium*, *Staphylococcus aureus*, *Klebsiella pneumoniae*, *Acinetobacter baumannii*, *Pseudomonas aeruginosa*, and *Enterobacter* species (ESKAPE) pathogens [19]. Additionally, a study from a medical school in Nigeria showed that 64.7% of the students had a good understanding of antibiotic resistance and use, although a mere 39% of them would treat common cold with antibiotics. Furthermore, only 8.2% of the students took medical consultation before taking antibiotics [21]. In a multi-centre, cross-sectional study in Egypt, 43% of the respondents considered that skipping doses of antibiotic treatment does not affect AMR, which is a common misconception. Around 40% of the students would use antimicrobials for a sore throat. Furthermore, students in final years performed better in the knowledge section of the questionnaire [23].

On a survey taking place in the USA in 2012, 90% of medical students from 3 universities (University of Miami, John Hopkins University, University of Washington) reported that they would like more education on antibiotics. More specifically, mean correct knowledge score was 51% which has been significantly affected by study sources that students used as learning methods. For instance, medical students scored high on questions regarding the use of antibiotics and management of community-acquired pneumonia. In contrast, they scored low in urinary tract infections and in questions for recognition of Clostridium difficile infection. Students who referred to physicians, pharmacists and those who used guidelines had better scores. Except from that only 15% of the students had followed a rotation in Infectious Disease department during their studies [12]. In addition, in a study from three medical schools in Thailand, 90% of students affirmed that the misuse of antibiotics is a major problem in their hospital and their country. The majority (98%) believed that they were capable of prescribing antibiotics, while 71.4% would feel stressed when prescribing. Over 10% of medical students reported that they have never been taught the principles of prudent use of antibiotics and AMR [20].

Last but not least, a study including three medical Schools in Africa showed that one out of three medical students did not feel confident enough on antibiotic prescribing [22]. On the other hand, students claimed that antibiotic overuse (63%) and resistance (61%) is an essential problem in their hospital, while 92% believed that antibiotics are overused and that the AMR is a crucial issue in the South African region. They also had the perception that hand hygiene is not a large contributing factor to AMR [22].

3. Discussion

In the current review, our main goal was to reveal if and how medical students were taught the basic principles of AMS. Nowadays, we are living in an era of excessive and often irrational usage of antibiotics in some settings, resulting in a significant increase in AMR. As this is an intercontinental issue, several studies conducted around the world give us valuable data for the preparation of future medical professionals. Our research has shown noteworthy findings regarding the knowledge, attitudes and perception of medical students.

3.1. Knowledge

It is clearly shown that medical students today lack adequate basic and clinical knowledge on the principal concepts of infectious diseases. In all parts of the world, medical students score relatively low in the relevant knowledge questionnaires as well as in the included clinical scenarios, making it clear that there is a room for improvement in medical education in both developed and developing countries [12,20,23,33]. Notwithstanding that medical students know that inappropriate use of antibiotics increases bacterial resistance, there are some common misperceptions [22]. For example, many of them claim that antibiotics can be used for treating viral infections and common flu [23,33]. It is widely known that those practices can increase inappropriate antimicrobial usage, resulting in high rates of AMR. In contrast to the above, diagnosis seems to be an easier task for medical students [10].

These knowledge gaps can occur due to the ineffective curriculums of each Medical School, which do not thoroughly cover the fundamentals of antibiotic usage, management, and duration of treatment, although the situation varies among different countries [39]. However, students who were in their final years of their studies in Medicine or had completed a clinical rotation in the Infectious Diseases Department of their hospital scored better in the knowledge section [16,18,33]. On the other hand, students who followed guidelines and reliable sources for learning tend to have more structured knowledge [34]. This finding implicates the importance of guidelines in undergraduate medical education in the early stage of the curricula. In any case, in all studies, medical students would appreciate more education in both basic science as well as clinical grounds so that they feel better prepared in their future tasks of everyday clinical practice [10,12,16,18,19,22,31,35,36,39]. It is of interest to note that, overall, following the WHO Global Action Plan on Antimicrobial Resistance [11], medical education about AMS might be essentially different in individual countries. Although we observed a trend of better knowledge in the field from 2015 onwards, we cannot accurately assess this difference as we have no country-specific data on educational changes and their potential impact. In addition, none of the included studies were designed to address this particular question, ideally comparing knowledge and attitudes on AMR with the same research tool and in the same setting before and after the WHO Global Action Plan on AMR.

3.2. Attitudes and Perceptions

Medical students do believe that rational use of antimicrobials is an essential aspect of their career to avoid the spread of AMR among pathogens [10,12,19,20,31]. These findings indicate that medical students and tomorrow's doctors have a positive moral attitude towards this issue. They also believe that antibiotics should not be sold and administered without a medical prescription [17,19]. The recognition of AMR's severity is the major factor that will guide and assist professionals in searching for efficacious ways of fighting mild as well as more severe infectious diseases. Although most students assess that antimicrobial overuse and resistance are worldwide issues, they tend to underestimate that this problem also exists in their hospital environment [12,16,40]. Such behaviors can lead to improper prescribing. Another interesting point is that a large percentage of medical students lack confidence and preparedness referred to antibiotic prescription [20,34,35]. This can correlate with each country's AMR status, where students in countries with low resistance rates tend to feel more prepared, possibly because they are less exposed to severe infectious clinical challenges [36]. On the other hand, evidence exists that overconfidence in the field had a negative impact on antibiotic prescription [22,35].

3.3. Limitations of the Study

To the best of our knowledge, this is the first review that summarizes the relevant studies worldwide on AMS and medical students. However, our review has some limitations regarding data evaluation. First of all, medical students in the reviewed studies were questioned around different aspects of AMS, making it difficult to proceed to an equal assessment of the results. In addition to that, no international validated questionnaire exists in the field, which would obviously make the results of the studies more comparable and could be used for future studies. Moreover, different antibiotic policies and guidelines are in place in each country, and hence different behaviors and attitudes can be described. We should also take into consideration that learning and training resources do vary around the globe due to social and economic conditions. This can obviously have an impact on medical education strategies on AMS. Finally, depending on countries, the status of AMR is different, which may be related to medical education, but we do not have the data to proceed to such a comparison between countries.

3.4. Implications for Future Approach

With all above-mentioned issues, we understand the need to enhance medical education towards AMS. The majority of students worldwide consider traditional lectures and passive learning tools ineffective methods or an unsuccessful way of promoting knowledge on antibiotics and AMS [11,21,36,41]. Therefore, a more practical approach such as discussion of clinical scenarios and presence in clinical practice (e.g., clinical placements, clinical rotations [12,16,38]) seems to have a positive effect on knowledge of and attitude toward antibiotic usage and administration [20,35]. In addition, a more detailed teaching of basic microbiology knowledge could reinforce medical students with important information, which is necessary for a better understanding of antibiotics [42]. Another useful intervention would be cooperation between medical universities in order to exchange educational approaches, and also between medical schools and faculties like pharmacy schools (e.g., interprofessional workshops and simulations between medical and pharmacy students), so they can learn more about the uses and specific features of antibiotics, by introducing principles and the importance of AMR [43–45]. As far as time organization is concerned, curricula studies have shown that early introduction of AMR teaching as well as repetitive and enriched training upon antibiotic resistance, diagnosis, management, prescribing and communication skills would lead to a more comprehensive understanding of the challenges and complexities of infectious diseases [43,46–48]. Moreover, e-learning and online education about AMS is a desirable and effective method according to medical professionals and students [41,49], although a European survey questions the successfulness of this means [35,50]. Furthermore, a study based on a seminar for medical students included real patients and their advocates. Post this seminar, students believed that hearing patients' stories is an effective way of learning more about AMR and the importance of stewardship [51]. There should also be a change regarding the learning tools and resources which medical students study during their years of medical school. Of note, students who follow the updated guidelines [52] and those who referred to medical and pharmacy specialists tended to have a more completed and updated knowledge on AMS [12]. Another helpful implication would be to encourage medical students to get involved in undergraduate research to acquire new academic skills and be aware of both AMR and AMS [53]. However, there is need for further future assessment of current medical training methods so we can make clear assumptions about their effectiveness [54].

4. Materials and Methods

We reviewed all studies published in English from 2007 to 2020. The studies were included if they contained original results or had exceptional content with particular emphasis on studies Knowledge, Attitude, Perceptions (KAP) studies.

The initial search was conducted in the PUBMED and Scopus databases and the last search was performed on 1 September 2020. The following key words and their combinations were used for the search: antimicrobial stewardship*, medical students*, knowledge*, attitudes*, perceptions*. Duplicate publications were identified and removed.

We identified 160 potentially relevant articles through database searches. Of these, there were 48 duplicates and 70 were excluded on the basis of title and abstract screening. We also excluded studies that investigated training methods for promoting AMS. Hence, only studies with quantitative results regarding the knowledge and attitudes of medical students regarding AMS were included. We focused on medical students and no other health-related undergraduate students (e.g., pharmacy or dental students). Studies on the knowledge and attitudes of other healthcare professionals or students (i.e., non-medical students) are listed as Supplementary Materials (Table S1). Moreover, protocols and editorials were excluded. Figure 1 describes the details of the methodology and excluded studies.

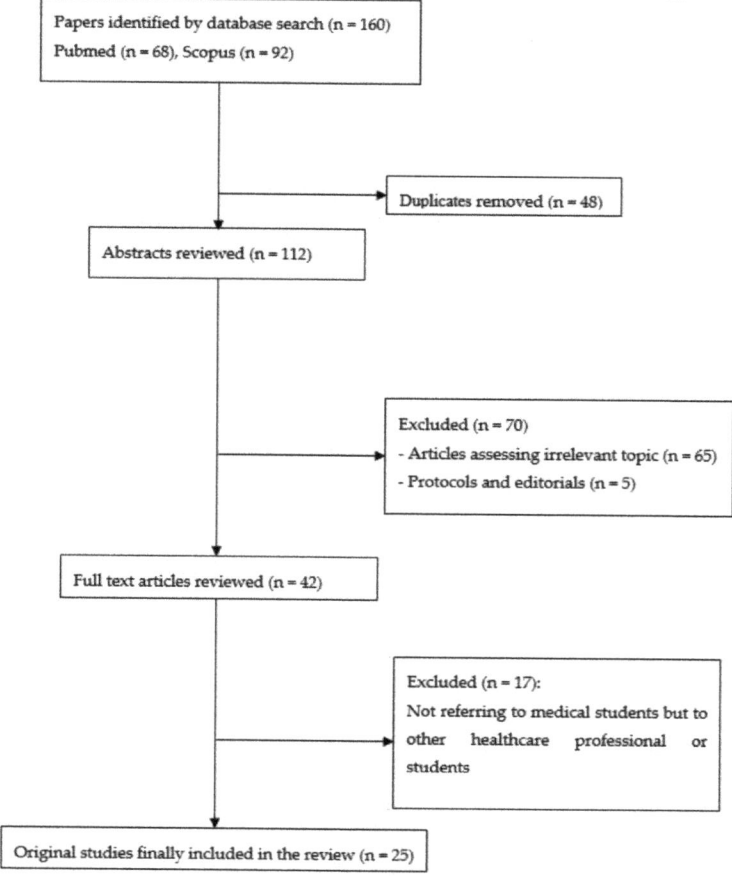

Figure 1. Flowchart of methodology and included studies.

5. Conclusions

Education on AMS is an emerging fundamental value for medicine around the world due to rapidly increasing AMR. Today's medical professionals will hand over the baton to medical students and hope for a greater improvement in AMR and antibiotic usage. Although medical students recognize the imminent issue of excessive resistance, they also lack basic knowledge regarding AMR. Consequently, at this time we should provide knowledge and confidence to medical students so that they will be able to face ongoing daily clinical challenges in the future. This could be achieved by incorporating novel and effective training methods on all aspects of AMS and AMR in the medical curricula worldwide.

Supplementary Materials: The following are available online at http://www.mdpi.com/2079-6382/9/11/821/s1, Table S1: Studies on knowledge and attitudes of other healthcare professionals and non-medical students.

Author Contributions: Conceptualization, D.G. and G.D.; methodology, D.G.; software, D.G., P.E.; validation, D.G., P.E. and G.D.; formal analysis, P.E. and D.G.; investigation, D.G. and P.E.; resources, D.G. and P.E.; data curation, D.G. and P.E.; writing—original draft preparation, P.E.; writing—review and editing, D.G. and G.D.; visualization, P.E., D.G., and G.D.; supervision, D.G. and G.D.; project administration, D.G. and G.D. All authors have read and agreed to the published version of the manuscript.

Funding: This research received no external funding.

Conflicts of Interest: The authors declare no conflict of interest.

References

1. Antibiotic Resistance. Available online: https://www.who.int/news-room/fact-sheets/detail/antibiotic-resistance (accessed on 26 September 2020).
2. Founou, R.C.; Founou, L.L.; Essack, S.Y. Clinical and economic impact of antibiotic resistance in developing countries: A systematic review and meta-analysis. *PLoS ONE* **2017**, *12*. [CrossRef]
3. Prestinaci, F.; Pezzotti, P.; Pantosi, A. Antimicrobial resistance: A global multifaceted phenomenon. *Pathog. Glob. Health* **2015**, *109*, 309–318. [CrossRef] [PubMed]
4. Cosgrove, S.E. The relationship between antimicrobial resistance and patient outcomes: Mortality, length of hospital stay, and health care costs. *Clin. Infect. Dis.* **2006**, *42*, 82–89. [CrossRef]
5. Moore, M.; McNulty, C. European Antibiotic Awareness Day 2012: TARGET antibiotics through guidance, education, and tools. *Br. J. Gen. Pract.* **2012**, *62*, 621–622. [CrossRef] [PubMed]
6. Aslam, B.; Arshad, M.I.; Khurshid, M.; Muzammil, S.; Rasool, M.H.; Nisar, M.A.; Alvi, R.F.; Aslam, M.A.; Qamar, M.U.; Salamat, M.K.F.; et al. Antibiotic resistance: A rundown of a global crisis. *Infect. Drug Resist.* **2018**, *11*, 1645–1658. [CrossRef]
7. Chaw, P.S.; Hoepner, J.; Mikolajczyk, R. The knowledge, attitude and practice of health practitioners towards antibiotic prescribing and resistance in developing countries-A systematic review. *J. Clin. Pharm. Ther.* **2018**, *43*, 606–613. [CrossRef] [PubMed]
8. Spellberg, B. The Maturing Antibiotic Mantra: "Shorter Is Still Better". *J. Hosp. Med.* **2018**, *13*, 361–362. [CrossRef] [PubMed]
9. Chokshi, A.; Sifri, Z.; Horng, H. Global Contributors to Antibiotic Resistance. *J. Glob. Infect. Dis.* **2019**, *11*, 36–42.
10. Dyar, O.J.; Pulcini, C.; Howard, P.; Nathwani, D. ESGAP (ESCMID Study Group for Antibiotic Policies). European medical students: A first multicentre study of knowledge, attitudes and perceptions of antibiotic prescribing and antibiotic resistance. *J. Antimicrob. Chemother.* **2014**, *69*, 842–846. [CrossRef]
11. World Health Organization. *Global Action Plan on Antimicrobial Resistance*; World Health Organization: Geneva, Switzerland, 2015.
12. Abbo, L.M.; Cosgrove, S.E.; Pottinger, P.S.; Sinkowitz-Cochran, R.; Srinivasan, A.; Webb, D.J.; Hooton, T.M. Medical students' perceptions and knowledge about antimicrobial stewardship: How are we educating our future prescribers? *Clin. Infect. Dis.* **2013**, *57*, 631–638. [CrossRef]
13. Mendelson, M.; Balasegaram, M.; Jinks, T.; Pulcini, C.; Sharland, M. Antibiotic resistance has a language problem. *Nat. News* **2017**, *545*, 23–25. [CrossRef] [PubMed]
14. Dellit, T.H.; Owens, R.C.; McGowan, J.E.; Weinstein, R.A.; Gerding, D.N.; Burke, J.P.; Huskins, W.C.; Paterson, D.L.; Fishman, N.O.; Carpenter, C.F.; et al. Infectious Diseases Society of America and the Society for Healthcare Epidemiology of America guidelines for developing an institutional program to enhance antimicrobial stewardship. *Clin. Infect. Dis.* **2007**, *44*, 159–177. [CrossRef] [PubMed]
15. Doron, S.; Davidson, L.E. Antimicrobial Stewardship. *Mayo. Clin. Proc.* **2011**, *86*, 1113–1123. [CrossRef] [PubMed]
16. Yang, K.; Wu, D.; Tan, F.; Shi, S.; Guo, X.; Min, Q.; Zhang, X.; Cheng, H. Attitudes and perceptions regarding antimicrobial use and resistance among medical students in Central China. *Springerplus* **2016**, *5*, 1779. [CrossRef] [PubMed]
17. Hu, Y.; Wang, X.; Tucker, J.D.; Little, P.; Moore, M.; Fukuda, K.; Zhou, X. Knowledge, Attitude, and Practice with Respect to Antibiotic Use among Chinese Medical Students: A Multicentre Cross-Sectional Study. *Int. J. Environ. Res. Public Health* **2018**, *15*, 1165. [CrossRef]
18. Hagiya, H.; Ino, H.; Tokumasu, K.; Ogawa, H.; Miyoshi, T.; Ochi, K.; Otsuka, F. Antibiotic literacy among Japanese medical students. *J. Infect. Chemother.* **2020**, *26*, 1107–1109. [CrossRef]
19. Meher, B.K.; Srinivasan, A.; Vighnesh, C.S.; Padhy, B.M.; Mohanty, R.R. Factors most influencing antibiotic stewardship program and comparison of prefinal- and final-year undergraduate medical students. *Perspect Clin. Res.* **2020**, *11*, 18–23. [CrossRef]
20. Chuenchom, N.; Thamlikitkul, V.; Chaiwarith, R.; Deoisares, P. Perception, Attitude, and Knowledge Regarding Antimicrobial Resistance, Appropriate Antimicrobial Use, and Infection Control Among Future Medical Practitioners: A Multicenter Study. *Infect. Control Hosp. Epidemiol.* **2016**, *37*, 603–605. [CrossRef]

21. Okedo-Alex, I.; Madubueze, U.C.; Umeokonkwo, C.D.; Oka, O.U.; Okeke, K.C. Knowledge of antibiotic use and resistance among students of a medical school in Nigeria. *Malawi Med. J.* **2019**, *31*, 133–137. [CrossRef]
22. Wasserman, S.; Potgieter, S.; Should, E.; Constant, D.; Stewart, A.; Mendelson, M.; Boyles, T.H. South African medical students' perceptions and knowledge about antibiotic resistance and appropriate prescribing: Are we providing adequate training to future prescribers? *S. Afr. Med. J.* **2017**, *107*, 405–410. [CrossRef]
23. Assar, A.; Abdelraoof, M.I.; Abdel-Maboud, M.; Shaker, K.H.; Menshawy, A.; Swelan, A.H.; Eid, M.; Khalid, R.; Mogahed, M.; Abushouk, A.I.; et al. Knowledge, attitudes, and practices of Egypt's future physicians towards antimicrobial resistance (KAP-AMR study): A multicenter cross-sectional study. *Environ. Sci. Pollut. Res. Int.* **2020**, *27*, 21292–21298. [CrossRef] [PubMed]
24. Weier, N.; Thursky, K.; Zaidi, S.T.R. Antimicrobial knowledge and confidence amongst final year medical students in Australia. *PLoS ONE* **2017**, *12*, e0182460. [CrossRef] [PubMed]
25. Dyar, O.J.; Nathwani, D.; Monnet, D.L.; Gyssens, I.C.; Stålsby Lundborg, C.; Pulcini, C.; ESGAP Student-PREPARE Working Group. Do medical students feel prepared to prescribe antibiotics responsibly? Results from a cross-sectional survey in 29 European countries. *J. Antimicrob. Chemother.* **2018**, *73*, 2236–2242. [CrossRef] [PubMed]
26. Sánchez-Fabra, D.; Dyar, O.J.; Del Pozo, J.L.; Amiguet, J.A.; Colmenero, J.D.; Fariñas, M.C.; López-Medrano, F.; Portilla, J.; Praena, J.; Torre-Cisneros, J.; et al. Perspective of Spanish medical students regarding undergraduate education in infectious diseases, bacterial resistance and antibiotic use. *Enferm. Infecc. Microbiol. Clin.* **2019**, *37*, 25–30. [CrossRef] [PubMed]
27. Dyar, O.J.; Howard, P.; Nathwani, D.; Pulcini, C.; ESGAP (the ESCMID [European Society of Clinical Microbiology, Infectious Diseases] Study Group for Antibiotic Policies). Knowledge, attitudes, and beliefs of French medical students about antibiotic prescribing and resistance. *Med. Mal. Infect.* **2013**, *43*, 423–430. [CrossRef]
28. Dyar, O.J.; Lund, M.; Lindsjö, C.; St ålsby Lundborg, C.; Pulcini, C.; French-Swedish Student-PREPARE ESGAP working group. Preparedness to prescribe antibiotics responsibly: A comparison between final year medical students in France and Sweden. *Eur. J. Clin. Microbiol. Infect. Dis.* **2019**, *38*, 711–717. [CrossRef]
29. Smoke, S.M.; Centrella, M.; Grigoriu, A.; Brust-Sisti, L. Antibiotic Decision-Making Among Medical Residents, Medical Students, and Nurse Practitioners: A Single-Center Survey. *J. Pharm. Pract.* **2019**, *32*, 372–374. [CrossRef]
30. Virmani, S.; Nandigam, M.; Kapoor, B.; Makhija, P. Antibiotic use among health science students in an Indian university: A cross sectional study. *Clin. Epidemiol. Glob. Health* **2017**, *5*, 176–179. [CrossRef]
31. Dyar, O.J.; Hills, H.; Seitz, L.T.; Perry, A.; Ashiru-Oredope, D. Assessing the Knowledge, Attitudes and Behaviors of Human and Animal Health Students towards Antibiotic Use and Resistance: A Pilot Cross-Sectional Study in the UK. *Antibiotics* **2018**, *7*. [CrossRef]
32. Rusic, D.; Bozic, J.; Vilovic, M.; Bukic, J.; Zivkovic, P.M.; Leskur, D.; Seselja Persin, A.; Tomic, S.; Modun, D. Attitudes and Knowledge Regarding Antimicrobial Use and Resistance Among Pharmacy and Medical Students at the University of Split, Croatia. *Microb. Drug Resist.* **2018**, *24*, 1521–1528. [CrossRef]
33. Nisabwe, L.; Brice, H.; Umuhire, M.C.; Gwira, O.; Harelimana, J.; Nzeyimana, Z.; Sebatunzi, O.R.; Rusingiza, E.K.; Hahirwa, I.; Muvunyi, C.M. Knowledge and attitudes towards antibiotic use and resistance among undergraduate healthcare students at University of Rwanda. *J. Pharm. Policy Pract.* **2020**, *13*. [CrossRef] [PubMed]
34. Sharma, K.; Jain, P.; Sharma, A. Knowledge, attitude and perception of medical and dental undergraduates about antimicrobial stewardship. *Indian J. Pharmacol.* **2015**, *47*, 676–679. [CrossRef] [PubMed]
35. Firouzabadi, D.; Mahmoudi, L. Knowledge, attitude, and practice of health care workers towards antibiotic resistance and antimicrobial stewardship programmes: A cross-sectional study. *J. Eval. Clin. Pract.* **2020**, *26*, 190–196. [CrossRef] [PubMed]
36. Beatthy, N.; August, J.; Saenz, J.A.; Nix, D.E.; Matthias, K.R.; Mohajer, M.A. Knowledge, attitude, and practices associated with the diagnosis and management of skin and soft-tissue infections among medical students, residents, and attending physicians. *Avicenna J. Med.* **2018**, *8*, 104–106. [CrossRef]
37. Saleem, Z.; Azmi Hassali, M.; Hashmi, F.; Azhar, F.; Mubarak, R.; Afzaal, A.; Munawar, U. Medical and pharmacy students' knowledge, attitude and perception concerning antimicrobial use and resistance in Pakistan. *Pharm Edu.* **2019**, *19*, 199–205.

38. Jairoun, A.; Hassan, N.; Ali, A.; Jairoun, O.; Shahwan, M.; Hassali, M. University students' knowledge, attitudes, and practice regarding antibiotic use and associated factors: A cross-sectional study in the United Arab Emirates. *Int. J. Gen. Med.* **2019**, 235–246. [CrossRef]
39. Pulcini, C.; Wencker, F.; Frimodt-Møller, N.; Kern, W.W.; Nathwani, D.; Rodríguez-Baño, J.; Simonsen, G.S.; Vlahović-Palčevski, V.; Gyssens, I.C.; ESGAP Curriculum Working Group. European survey on principles of prudent antibiotic prescribing teaching in undergraduate students. *Clin. Microbiol. Infect.* **2015**, *21*, 354–361. [CrossRef]
40. Brink, A.; Schoeman, J.; Muntingh, G. Undergraduate antibiotic stewardship training: Are we leaving our future prescribers 'flapping in the wind'? *S. Afr. Med. J.* **2017**, *107*, 357–358. [CrossRef]
41. Satterfield, J.; Miesner, A.R.; Percival, K.M. The role of education in antimicrobial stewardship. *J. Hosp. Infect.* **2020**, *105*, 130–141. [CrossRef]
42. O'Donnell, L.A.; Guarascio, A.J. The intersection of antimicrobial stewardship and microbiology: Educating the next generation of health care professionals. *FEMS Microbiol. Lett.* **2017**, *364*, fnw281. [CrossRef]
43. MacDougall, C.; Schwartz, B.S.; Kim, L.; Nanamori, M.; Shekarchian, S.; Chin-Hong, P.V. An interprofessional curriculum on antimicrobial stewardship improves knowledge and attitudes toward appropriate antimicrobial use and collaboration. *Open Forum Infect. Dis.* **2017**, *4*, ofw225. [CrossRef] [PubMed]
44. Nori, P.; Madaline, T.; Munjal, I.; Bhar, S.; Guo, Y.; Seo, S.K.; Porrovecchio, A.; Gancher, E.; Nosanchuk, E.; Pirofski, L.A.; et al. Developing Interactive Antimicrobial Stewardship and Infection Prevention Curricula for Diverse Learners: A Tailored Approach. *Open Forum Infect. Dis.* **2017**, *4*, ofx117. [CrossRef] [PubMed]
45. Frenk, J.; Chen, L.; Bhutta, Z.A.; Cohen, J.; Crisp, N.; Evans, T.; Fineberg, H.; Garcia, P.; Ke, Y.; Kelley, P.; et al. Health professionals for a new century: Transforming education to strengthen health systems in an interdependent world. *Lancet* **2017**, *376*, 1923–1958. [CrossRef]
46. Schwartz, B.S.; Armstrong, W.S.; Ohl, C.A.; Luther, V.P. Create Allies, IDSA Stewardship Commitments Should Prioritize Health Professions Learners. *Clin. Infect. Dis.* **2015**, *61*, 1626–1627. [CrossRef] [PubMed]
47. Ohl, C.A.; Luther, V.P. Health care provider education as a tool to enhance antibiotic stewardship practices. *Infect. Dis. Clin. North Am.* **2014**, *28*, 177–193. [CrossRef] [PubMed]
48. Shekarchian, S.; Schwartz, B.S.; Teherani, A.; Irby, D.; Chin-Hong, P.V. Is It Time for a Coordinated and Longitudinal Approach to Antibiotic Stewardship Education? *Clin. Infect. Dis.* **2016**, *63*, 848–849. [CrossRef]
49. Laks, M.; Guerra, C.M.; Miraglia, J.L.; Medeiros, E.A. Distance learning in antimicrobial stewardship: Innovation in medical education. *BMC Med. Educ.* **2019**, *19*, 191. [CrossRef]
50. Sikkens, J.J.; Caris, M.G.; Schutte, T.; Kramer, M.H.H.; Tichelaar, J.; van Agtmael, M.A. Improving antibiotic prescribing skills in medical students: The effect of e-learning after 6 months. *J. Antimicrob. Chemother.* **2018**, *73*, 2243–2246. [CrossRef]
51. Nori, P.; Cowman, K.; Jezek, A.; Nosanchuk, J.D.; Slosar-Cheah, M.; Sarwar, U.; Bartash, R.; Ostrowsky, B. Faces of Resistance: Using Real-World Patients and Their Advocates to Teach Medical Students About Antimicrobial Stewardship. *Open Forum Infect. Dis.* **2019**, *6*, ofz487. [CrossRef]
52. Southwick, F.; Katona, C.; Kauffman, C.; Monroe, S.; Pirofski, L.A.; del Rio, C.; Gallis, H.; Dismukes, W. Commentary: IDSA guidelines for improving the teaching of preclinical medical microbiology and infectious diseases. *Acad. Med.* **2010**, *85*, 19–22. [CrossRef]
53. Rawson, T.M.; Moore, L.S.P.; Gill, D.; Lupton, M.; Holmes, A.H. Promoting medical student engagement with antimicrobial stewardship through involvement in undergraduate research. *J. Infect.* **2017**, *74*, 200–202. [CrossRef] [PubMed]
54. Silverberg, S.L.; Zanella, V.E.; Countryman, D.; Lenton, E.; Friesen, F.; Law, M. A review of antimicrobial stewardship training in medical education. *Int. J. Med. Educ.* **2017**, *8*, 353–374. [CrossRef] [PubMed]

Publisher's Note: MDPI stays neutral with regard to jurisdictional claims in published maps and institutional affiliations.

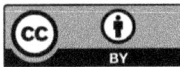

© 2020 by the authors. Licensee MDPI, Basel, Switzerland. This article is an open access article distributed under the terms and conditions of the Creative Commons Attribution (CC BY) license (http://creativecommons.org/licenses/by/4.0/).

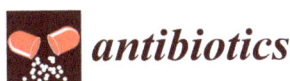 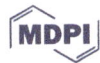

Article

Improving Access to Antimicrobial Prescribing Guidelines in 4 African Countries: Development and Pilot Implementation of an App and Cross-Sectional Assessment of Attitudes and Behaviour Survey of Healthcare Workers and Patients

Omotayo Olaoye [1], Chloe Tuck [1], Wei Ping Khor [1], Roisin McMenamin [1], Luke Hudson [2], Mike Northall [2], Edwin Panford-Quainoo [3], Derrick Mawuena Asima [4] and Diane Ashiru-Oredope [1,*]

1. Commonwealth Pharmacists Association, London E1W 1AW, UK; omotayo.olaoye@commonwealthpharmacy.org (O.O.); chloe.tuck@commonwealthpharmacy.org (C.T.); weiping.khor@commonwealthpharmacy.org (W.P.K.); R.Mcmenamin@uea.ac.uk (R.M.)
2. Horizon Strategic Partners, London EC3R 8HL, UK; luke@horizonsp.co.uk (L.H.); mike@horizonsp.co.uk (M.N.)
3. Liverpool School of Tropical Medicine, University of Liverpool, Liverpool L3 5QA, UK; 248964@lstmed.ac.uk
4. LEKMA Hospital, Teshie, Accra P.O. BOX MS 216, Ghana; mawuenaasima@gmail.com
* Correspondence: diane.ashiru-oredope@commonwealthpharmacy.org

Received: 4 August 2020; Accepted: 26 August 2020; Published: 29 August 2020

Abstract: Smartphone apps have proven to be an effective and acceptable resource for accessing information on antimicrobial prescribing. The purpose of the study is to highlight the development and implementation of a smartphone/mobile app (app) for antimicrobial prescribing guidelines (the Commonwealth Partnerships for Antimicrobial Stewardship—CwPAMS App) in Ghana, Tanzania, Uganda and Zambia and to evaluate patients' and healthcare providers' perspectives on the use of the App in one of the participating institutions. Two structured cross-sectional questionnaires containing Likert scale, multiple-choice, and open-ended questions were issued to patients and healthcare workers six months after the introduction of the app at one of the hospital sites. Metrics of the use of the app for a one-year period were also obtained. Download and use of the app peaked between September and November 2019 with pharmacists accounting for the profession that the most frequently accessed the app. More than half of the responding patients had a positive attitude to the use of the app by health professionals. Results also revealed that more than 80% of health care workers who had used the CwPAMS App were comfortable using a smartphone/mobile device on a ward round, considered the app very useful, and found it to improve their awareness of antimicrobial stewardship, including documentation of the indication and duration for antimicrobials on the drug chart. It also encouraged pharmacists and nurses to challenge inappropriate antimicrobial prescribing. Overall, our findings suggest that its use as a guide to antimicrobial prescribing sparked positive responses from patients and health professionals. Further studies will be useful in identifying the long-term consequences of the use of the CwPAMS App and scope to implement in other settings, in order to guide future innovations and wider use.

Keywords: CwPAMS App; smartphone apps; antimicrobial prescribing; pharmacy

1. Introduction

Antimicrobial stewardship programs in hospitals are focused on optimising antimicrobial prescribing to improve individual patient care, decrease healthcare costs and combat antimicrobial resistance [1]. The availability of accurate and up-to-date information is important to guide the right diagnosis and prescription of antimicrobials. Healthcare providers' attempts to access this information are influenced by previous training, availability of the information, ability to access and leverage technology [2]. There has been a recent rise in the use of smartphones generally across global population and it is predicted to be rising fastest in Africa. There has been increased development of smartphone apps designed for use in healthcare, including in the area of antimicrobial stewardship [3–7]. Current research in medicine has shown that the use of mobile phones and devices in medical settings is more popular and is increasingly being brought to the fore of international research [1]. For instance, recent studies have shown that 52% of smartphone users access medical information through their devices [8]. A study by Kamerow, Chief scientist and Associate editor for the British Medical Journal, revealed that there are approximately 100,000 health-oriented smartphone apps and, by the year 2015, over 500 million smartphone owners worldwide will use these apps [9]. The study also highlighted that, although designed for health professionals, around 15% of health apps are now marketed to patients to help them monitor, evaluate, and transmit medical data such as blood pressure and body weight among other health checks [9]. The author also stated that the use of these apps was higher amongst the younger population, females, and people who earned a higher income. Similarly, results from a longitudinal study of 206 medical doctors working at Hannover Medical School, Germany in the summer of 2012 and spring of 2014 also revealed a rapid increase in the use of mobile devices in medical settings during patient interaction and professional collaboration [10]. This significant increase was observed in both the frequency of use and the expansion of the areas of application of these devices. Smartphones have specific features that support their increasing use in healthcare delivery and behavioural interventions. They are highly portable, more convenient, cost-effective and interconnected compared to reference books and computers, thus promoting improved communication and the sharing of knowledge, data and resources among health professionals and as well as facilitating regular updates as new data becomes available [11–13]. Furthermore, the ability of smartphones to use internal sensors to deduce context including emotions, location and activity has greatly increased their relevance in the consistent monitoring and tracking of health-related behaviours and healthcare delivery [14–19]. In the early days of their use, there was a significant paucity of academic research on users' viewpoints and experiences with the use of these apps. The recent literature has provided positive feedback on the acceptability and workability of smartphone apps although it has also been recognized that this evolving technology may raise concerns regarding privacy and security [17,20]. In the past decade, there has been a rapid increase in the use of mobile phones in Africa [18]. There has also been a rapid integration of mobile health technologies and telecommunication into the healthcare system, especially in low and middle-income countries. In addition to this there has been an increased investment in mobile healthcare interventions including the use of these technologies for behavioural change communication [19]. With the increasing burden of communicable and non-communicable diseases in Africa, low-cost mobile health technology has the potential to make healthcare more accessible to disadvantaged communities [21]. For example, in Zambia and Ghana adverse event reporting apps were developed by medical regulatory authorities in 2019 [22]. The Zambia Medicines Regulatory Authority—ZAMRA also launched Adverse Drug Reaction Application (ADRA), a new mobile application for android phone users for reporting adverse medicines reactions in 2017 [23]. Furthermore, apps have been used to identify falsified and substandard medicines in Kenya [24]. These technologies also offer great solutions aimed at improving the speed, safety and quality of healthcare provision in resource-constrained settings by providing easy access to local and international guidelines and resources. The purpose of the study is to highlight the development and implementation of an app to support prudent antimicrobial prescribing and improved antimicrobial stewardship practice; as part of the Commonwealth Partnerships for Antimicrobial Stewardship (CwPAMS) programme in Ghana, Tanzania, Uganda and Zambia and to conduct a pilot study assessing patients and healthcare providers' perspectives on the use of the app in one of the hospitals in Ghana.

2. Results

2.1. App Metrics 1 Year from Launch (April 2019–May 2020)

The Commonwealth Partnerships for Antimicrobial Stewardship App was developed to improve antimicrobial prescribing and stewardship practices among health professionals in Ghana, Tanzania, Uganda and Zambia. The app provides, for the first time in the four countries, easy access to infection management resources to improve appropriate use of antimicrobials in line with national and international guidelines. Following the launch of the app in four countries, there were 530 downloads of the app and 2,795 guide opens within 12 months. Ghana had more page hits (50.3%) than Uganda (31%), Tanzania (13%), Zambia (1.9%) and others (3.8%) (Table 1). The most visited section of the app was the National Prescribing Guidelines, accounting for 66.1% of the total number of page hits while the section for Updates on antimicrobial resistance (AMR) (coming soon) was the least visited (0.7%). Pharmacists (51.1%) and nurses (20.4%) accounted for the highest number of registered users while pharmacists (64.1%) and medical doctors (20.3%) had the highest frequency of downloads and guide opens (Table 2).

Table 1. Frequency of monthly downloads, guide opens and page hits for Ghana, Tanzania, Uganda and Zambia.

Commonwealth Partnerships for Antimicrobial Stewardship (CwPAMS) App Metrics															
Months	2019									2020					Total (%)
	Apr	May	Jun	Jul	Aug	Sep	Oct	Nov	Dec	Jan	Feb	Mar	Apr	May	
Downloads (n)															
	35	12	20	75	21	67	66	124	27	28	27	9	9	40	100
Guide Opens (n)															
		36	26	354	237	453	375	457	147	141	130	127	122	155	100
National Guideline Page Hits by Country (n)															
Ghana		40	17	569	176	399	827	438	192	141	375	243	126	46	50.3
Tanzania		3	11	101	21	20	53	307	73	25	27	187	73	22	13
Uganda		21	81	196	223	663	322	368	64	101	96	10	13	45	31
Zambia		2	-	15	4	8	9	74	4	3	0	4	10	4	1.9
Nil		17	7	65	27	19	23	39	10	24	3	19	15	6	3.8
Individual Page Hits by App Sections (n)															
About the CwPAMS App		13	9	57	39	44	31	71	11	13	8	19	16	37	3.4
Userguide		3	4	58	31	38	29	58	17	17	8	9	22	15	2.9
National Prescribing Guidelines		83	116	946	451	1109	1234	1226	343	294	501	463	237	119	66.1
Access, Watch, Reserve (AWaRE)—WHO Essential Medicines List		132	17	140	212	184	54	202	45	39	18	40	49	42	11.0
Antimicrobial Stewardship (AMS) Tools		21	3	84	143	89	40	72	17	36	10	25	18	27	5.5
Training on AMS		26	4	105	105	66	46	51	7	33	10	20	10	4	4.5
Infection Prevention and Control		6	5	91	61	42	24	70	24	17	7	16	23	18	3.7
Antimicrobial Use Surveillance		11	2	44	43	39	15	26	8	14	4	11	16	3	2.2
Updates on Antimicrobial Resistance (AMR)—Coming Soon		4	1	8	7	7	9	11	0	11	1	0	8	0	0.7

Table 2. Frequency of registered users, downloads and guide opens by profession.

Profession	CwPAMS App Metrics (By Profession)		
	Registered Users	Downloads	Guide Opens
Dentistry	1	2	2
Physiotherapy	1	0	0
Clinical science	3	0	0
Healthcare management	6	2	1
Paramedic	6	1	1
Biomedical scientist	15	3	11
Physician Associate	15	1	12
Medicine	84	57	80
Nursing	103	29	36
Pharmacy	258	159	274
Other	13	2	3

2.2. Cross-Sectional Survey Studies

A cross-sectional attitude and behaviour survey was carried out on patients and healthcare professionals to determine their attitudes/views on the use of antimicrobial prescribing guidelines by health professionals. A total of 47 patients and 38 health professionals participated in the survey; response rates were 51% and 38%, respectively.

2.2.1. Demographics

Demographics presented in Table 3 shows that respondents comprise various age groups and educational qualifications and professions.

Table 3. Demographics of patients and healthcare professionals.

Patients							
Highest Level of Education Obtained							
Basic Primary Education		Secondary Education		Tertiary Education		No data provided	
4		23		19		1	
Age							
<18	18–25	26–35	36–45	46–55	56–67	68 above	Nil
1	25	7	1	3	5	3	2
Health Professionals							
Profession							
Doctor		Pharmacist		Nurse		Others	
4		6		18		10	

2.2.2. Patients

Patients' Responses to the Use of Smartphone Mobile Apps in Healthcare Delivery

Patients' views on the use of the app by health professionals obtained using a Likert scale of five options (Strongly agree, Agree, Neutral, Disagree and Strongly disagree) are presented in Table 4. More than 50% of patients had a positive attitude to the use of smartphone apps by health professionals and the fact that it increases the quality of healthcare offered by health professionals and quickens access to healthcare. Patients' greatest concern was that the use of smart phone mobile apps in healthcare delivery could be a distraction to healthcare provision. This was followed by concerns that their data may not be protected/secure and that mobile devices may not be technically reliable enough. Patients' least concern was that the health professional "may not be competent enough".

Table 4. Patients' responses to the use of smart phone mobile apps in healthcare delivery—5-point Likert scale from Strongly disagree (1) to Strongly agree (5) (n = 47).

Questions/Comments	Score (%)				
	1	2	3	4	5
What do you feel about the following?					
I am pleased with my doctor assessing a smart phone app while attending to me	21.3	36.2	23.4	6.4	12.8
Using smart phone apps will increase the quality of healthcare offered by my doctor	25.5	31.9	19.1	17.0	6.4
The use of smart phone apps quickens access to healthcare	17.0	40.4	25.5	12.8	4.3
The use of smart phone apps increases quality of healthcare delivery	14.9	36.2	36.2	6.4	6.4
Do you have any reservations/concerns with a doctor's use of a mobile app while attending to you? If yes, what are your concerns?					
The doctor may not be competent enough	4.3	17.0	8.5	10.6	12.8
It is a distraction to healthcare provision	4.3	25.5	12.8	10.6	2.1
My data may not be protected/secured	6.4	21.3	10.6	8.5	4.3
Mobile devices may not be technically reliable enough	6.4	21.3	10.6	17.0	0
The use of smart phones/mobile apps may be complicated when it comes to healthcare	4.3	17.0	12.8	17.0	2.1

Patients' Concerns with Their Health Professionals' Use of Smartphone Apps by Age and Education

The highest proportion of patients who had no concerns with their use of smartphone apps by health professionals were aged 26–35 (71.4%). This was followed by patients aged 68 and above (66.7%), 18–25 (64.0%), 56–67 (60.0%) and 46–55 (33.3%) in descending order. Patients aged 36–45 had concerns with health professionals' use of smartphone apps. Patients with the most concern with health professionals' use of smartphones were aged 46-55. With respect to patients' highest level of education, patients with tertiary education (63.2% had the least concern with health professionals' use of smartphone apps while patients with basic primary education (25%) had the most concern.

Patients' Preferences for Health Professionals' Use to Access Medicines Information

The highest proportion of patients wanted health professionals to use a computer or laptop (38.3%). This was followed by smartphone mobile apps (23.4%), reference books (6.4%) and tablets (6.4%) in descending order. A computer/laptop/reference book was preferred by 6.4% of patients while 2.1% preferred any of a smartphone, computer/laptop or tablet, a smartphone, computer/laptop or reference book, a smartphone or tablet, and a computer/laptop, reference book or tablet. Additionally, 10.6% of patients had no preference (n = 47).

2.2.3. Healthcare Workers

Use of the CwPAMS App and Other Sources of Information

Thirty-eight healthcare workers (HCWs) comprising of four doctors, eighteen nurses, six pharmacists and ten other healthcare workers participated in the survey. On a daily basis, mobile phones (28.9%) and printed posters (13.2%) were most predominantly used by the HCWs, while tablets and computers (7.9% each) were the least used devices (Table 5). Mobile phones were used more than once a day by 60.5% of healthcare workers. Percentages of healthcare workers who had never used a tablet, pocketbook, printed posters and computers were 47.4%, 28.9%, 26.3% and 21.0%, respectively. Healthcare workers' responses showed that many respondents had not consulted the CwPAMS App for antimicrobial prescribing information. The British National Formulary

(BNF)/National guidelines, a printed copy of standard treatment guidelines, senior colleagues and junior doctors were mostly consulted daily. In descending order, internet search engines, senior colleagues and pharmacists were consulted more than once a day. No additional source of information on antimicrobial prescribing was mentioned.

Table 5. Use of the Commonwealth Partnerships for Antimicrobial Stewardship (CwPAMS) App and other sources of information by healthcare workers (n = 38).

Device	Daily	More than once a day	Weekly	Monthly	Never	Nil
Frequency of Accessing Medical Information (%)						
Mobile phone	28.9	60.5	5.3	2.6	0	2.6
Tablet	7.9	13.2	5.3	0	47.4	26.3
Computer	7.9	10.5	5.3	26.3	21.0	28.9
Pocket book	10.5	2.6	13.2	10.5	28.9	34.2
Printed posters	13.2	15.8	7.9	13.2	26.3	23.7
Others	0	5.3	0	0	5.3	89.5
Frequency of Accessing Antimicrobial Prescribing Information (%)						
CwPAMS App	2.6	5.3	7.9	2.6	63.2	18.4
Printed copy of standard treatment guidelines	26.3	21.0	0	21.0	13.2	18.4
British National Formulary (BNF)/National guidelines	28.9	23.7	10.5	15.8	10.5	10.5
Microbiology/Infectious disease advice	13.2	10.5	15.8	7.9	31.6	21.0
Pharmacists	18.4	31.6	7.9	15.8	13.2	13.2
Senior colleagues	26.3	36.8	7.9	13.2	2.6	13.2
Other junior doctors	26.3	26.3	2.6	10.5	18.4	15.8
Internet search engines (e.g., Google)	18.4	50.0	13.2	2.6	2.6	13.2
Others	0	0	0	0	2.6	97.4

Use of the CwPAMS App and Other Sources of Information on Antimicrobial Prescribing by Profession

An assessment of the various sources of information on antimicrobial prescribing used by healthcare workers showed that the CwPAMS App was mostly used by nurses and other health workers. BNF and National guidelines were mostly used by doctors (100%) and pharmacists (66.7%) and least used by nurses (33.3%). Internet search engines were mostly used by pharmacists (100%) and least used by doctors (25%) (See Figure 1). Pharmacists were seen to refer to their senior colleagues for antibiotic information more than doctors, nurses and other health professionals. More doctors and other healthcare workers (midwives, dispensing technicians and medication counter assistants) sought information from pharmacists than nurses. Printed copies of the standard treatment guidelines were mostly used by pharmacists and least used by nurses.

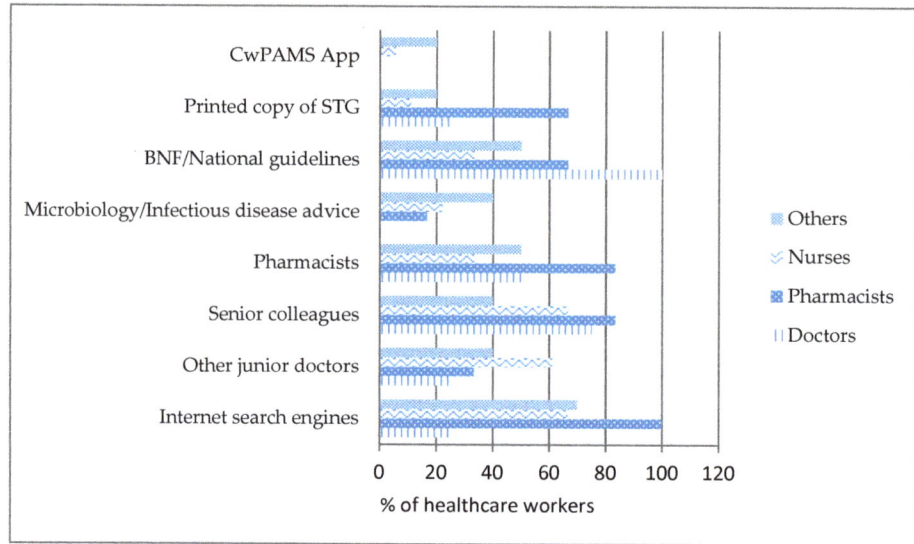

Figure 1. Use of the CwPAMS App and other sources of information on Antimicrobial prescribing by profession.

Assessment of Standard Treatment Guidelines and Drug Resistant Infections

All responding healthcare practitioners admitted being concerned about the emergence of drug resistant infections while 79.0% agreed or strongly agreed that these guidelines are easy to access. A total of 44.7% stated that they preferred their senior's preferences over standard treatment guidelines. Only 18.5% preferred to use non-standard treatment guidelines for antimicrobial prescribing while 13.2% felt the standard treatment guidelines did not apply to their patients (Table 6).

Table 6. Assessment of Standard treatment guidelines and drug resistant Infections on a 5-point Likert scale from Strongly Agree (1) to Strongly Disagree (5), median response category for each question marked in bold.

Questions/Comments	Score				
	1	2	3	4	5
Assessment of standard treatment guidelines and attitude to Antimicrobial Resistance (%) (n = 38)					
Standard antimicrobial treatment guidelines are easy to access	15.8	**63.2**	10.5	5.3	5.3
My seniors' preferences guide antimicrobial prescribing more than standard treatment guidelines	7.9	36.8	**26.4**	15.8	2.6
Standard antimicrobial treatment guidelines don't apply to my patients	7.9	5.3	13.2	**42.1**	26.4
I prefer to use non-standard treatment guidelines to guide my antimicrobial prescribing	5.3	13.2	7.9	**36.8**	28.9
I am concerned about the emergence of drug-resistant infections	**50**	44.7	0	0	0

Perception and Assessment of the CwPAMS Smartphone App

All healthcare workers who had used the App agreed that the app was very useful, relevant to their patient population and considered it the best way to access standard antimicrobial treatment guidelines. In addition, they all felt comfortable using a smartphone on a ward round, admitting that the app increased their awareness of antimicrobial stewardship and encouraged them to challenge inappropriate prescribing and to document the indication and duration for antimicrobials on the drug chart. Furthermore, participants found the country-specific standard treatment guidelines most useful. This was followed by the WHO Essential Medicines list section and the Antimicrobial Stewardship (AMS) resource section.

3. Discussion

3.1. CwPAMS App Metrics

Analysis of the CwPAMS App metrics revealed that the months with the highest downloads and page hits were September, October and November. The increase in September and October can be largely attributed to partnership project visits and antimicrobial stewardship interventions in all four countries. The spike in the month of November can most likely be linked to events during the World Antibiotic Awareness Week in all four countries as well as the app promotion by the Commonwealth Pharmacists Association during the World Antibiotic Awareness Week. Pharmacists accounted for the highest number of registered users and had more page hits and downloads than other health care professionals and workers. While this could mean that the app is more common among pharmacy teams, it calls for increased app promotion among doctors and other health professionals, who have also begun to use the app. The variations in the number of page hits and app downloads in each country can be explained by the number of partnerships in per country as Ghana and Uganda had the highest number of partnerships while Tanzania and Zambia had the lowest number of partnerships.

3.2. Cross-Sectional Survey

The use of smartphone mobile apps in healthcare delivery has gained acceptance over the years among patients and health professionals in sub-Saharan Africa and worldwide [19]. The CwPAMS App was developed by the Commonwealth Pharmacists Association to provide easy access to medicine management information for health professionals across Ghana, Tanzania, Uganda and Zambia. In addition to providing health professionals with relevant national and international guidelines, notable advantages of the app are its usability without internet access, a feature which suits low and middle-income countries, and its easy adaptability. Most recently, the app was updated to provide health care professionals across the commonwealth with links to relevant country-specific and international resources on COVID-19 from the World Health Organization (WHO), International Pharmaceutical Federation (FIP) and the Africa Centres for Disease Control and Prevention, among other relevant sources. The pilot study showed that more than 50% of patients were content with their health professional's use of smartphone apps while attending to them. Age and education level had an impact on the patient's acceptance of smartphone mobile technology as middle-aged patients had the least acceptance while the young and the most elderly had the greatest acceptance. Patients with tertiary education had the highest acceptance for these technologies while those with basic primary education had the least acceptance. These results correlate with a study carried out in 2014 on the acceptance and use of health technology by community-dwelling elders which revealed that income, education and age were found to significantly affect the acceptance of technology in healthcare. Patients with higher education and income used the internet at rates close to or exceeding the general population [25]. Another study also revealed that the acceptance of mobile phone technology among the older population was on the increase as they were found to constitute the fastest-growing group using the internet and computers [26]. Regarding patients' preferences, our survey reveals that more patients preferred their health professionals using a computer/laptop to access information over a smartphone or reference book. This can be explained by the fact that the patients' greatest concern was that smartphones could be a distraction to healthcare provision. This concern corroborates findings from a study by Wu et al. which revealed that on an average, physicians' smartphones received 21.9 emails and 6.4 telephone calls, sent out 6.9 emails and initiated 8.3 telephone calls within 24 h. The study also revealed that 55.6% of 439 perfusionists admitted that they had used a cellular phone for purposes other than healthcare delivery while performing their duties [27]. On the contrary, a cross-sectional survey of adult patients in metropolitan academic and private dermatological clinics carried out in 2015 revealed that most patients (69.7%) considered personal smartphones an acceptable reference tool to provide information in patient care [28]. To access medical information more than once a day, health care workers mostly use mobile phones (60.5%) and printed posters (15.8%). These sources were also the most predominantly used daily (28.9% and 13.2%), respectively. This supports previous studies which have highlighted an increase in the use of smartphone mobile apps by health professionals [3–5]. Healthcare workers were also found to mostly consult internet search engines (50%), senior colleagues (36.8%) and pharmacists (31.6%) to access antibiotic prescribing information more than once a day. This demonstrates the need to involve these groups in promoting the app as they have a significant influence on antibiotic prescribing behaviours and healthcare workers' decisions. Furthermore, healthcare professionals' responses to the use of the CwPAMS App was found to correspond with results obtained from a similar study by Panesar et al. involving 146 healthcare professionals. Both studies show that the health professionals found apps useful and relevant to their patient population. They also agreed that apps encouraged them to challenge inappropriate prescribing [6]. The concern displayed by healthcare workers for the emergence of drug-resistant infections and the use of the standard treatment guidelines as seen in Table 6 was highly impressive. Healthcare workers also found the country-specific section of the CwPAMS App most useful. This correlates with the app metrics from all four countries which revealed that the National prescribing guidelines had the highest number of page hits from May 2019 to May 2020. The study highlights the need for more healthcare workers, especially doctors, to use the CwPAMS App as app metrics and the pilot cross-sectional survey both reveal that more nurses and pharmacists than doctors had used the app. There is also the need for more focused implementation as well as app promotion at all partnership sites and among all health professionals, especially doctors who are prescribers. Furthermore, there may be a need for subsequent studies to be carried out within the hospital when a higher number of healthcare professionals have used the app, in order to have a broader perspective from patients and health professionals. It would also be important to incorporate regular reminders about the app into the implementation strategy. A recently published study by Lester et al. [29] highlighted that implementing a locally appropriate, pragmatic antibiotic guideline through an app, supported by a simple educational strategy of weekly 'reminders', led to a significant reduction in third generation cephalosporin usage as well as an increase in the proportion of 48-h antibiotic reviews.

3.3. Strengths and Limitations

The CwPAMS Microguide antimicrobial prescribing app is the first of its kind to combine country-specific and international guidelines and information on antimicrobial prescribing for Ghana, Tanzania, Uganda and Zambia. Hence, based on our knowledge, this study on the development, implementation and use of the app in these four countries is novel. One of the limitations is the low sample size for the surveys, which was due to the time constraint in carrying out the survey, limited time spent by patients at the waiting room of a single hospital site and health care workers' busy schedules. However, it is important to note that this section of the full study was intended to be a pilot in one setting and to provide initial descriptive findings. Extensive surveying across other sites would enable a test of significance and to confirm trends. In addition, the survey encompassed a wide range of health care workers, including doctors, pharmacists, nurses, midwives and other health care workers. Patients' who participated where across a broad range with respect to age and education, providing a wide perspective. The response rate was greater for patients than health professionals, most likely because patients were available to fill questionnaires whilst in waiting rooms compared to health professionals. The proportion of healthcare workers groups that responded to the survey were not comparable. This is due to more nurses and other health care workers being available in the hospital compared to doctors and pharmacists. Though not all healthcare workers had used the app, there was an 85.7% response rate from those who had used the app to questions on the use of the

App. Frequent updates and increased use of the app by health care workers highlight the need for further studies.

4. Materials and Methods

4.1. Development of the App

The CwPAMS App was developed by the Commonwealth Pharmacists Association using the MicroGuide platform (http://www.microguide.eu). The platform provides a cloud-based service that allows local pharmacists to develop, manage, update and publish clinical guidelines to various apps for any mobile operating system including iOS (Apple, Cupertino, CA, USA), Android (Google, Mountain View, CA, USA), Windows devices (Microsoft, Redmond, WA, USA) among other operating systems. It offers healthcare professionals offline access to clinical guidelines and content autonomously managed by pharmacy teams. It is also available online via https://viewer.microguide.global/CPA/CWPAMS. The CwPAMS App contains national and international guidelines listed into various sections including the WHO Essential Medicines List, surveillance tools, antimicrobial stewardship training, Infection Prevention and Control (IPC) resources, and country-specific Standard Treatment Guidelines. The App metrics and statistics were derived from routine data collection by Horizon Strategic Partners.

4.2. Study Site

The CwPAMS App was developed for use by 14 secondary care institutions that were part of the CwPAMS programme in four countries Ghana, Tanzania, Uganda and Zambia (S1–S3, Video S1). One of the hospitals in the partnership was used as the pilot study site. The hospital is a secondary health facility with a 100-bed capacity.

CwPAMS is a health partnership programme funded by the UK Department of Health and Social Care's Fleming Fund to tackle antimicrobial resistance (AMR) globally. CwPAMS will support partnerships between the UK NHS and institutions in Ghana, Tanzania, Uganda and Zambia to work together on AMS initiatives. This aims to enhance implementation of protocols and evidenced based decision making to support antimicrobial prescribing, as well as capacity for antimicrobial surveillance. Further information about CwPAMS is available via https://commonwealthpharmacy.org/commonwealth-partnerships-for-antimicrobial-stewardship/. CwPAMS is being run by the Commonwealth Pharmacists Association (CPA) and Tropical Health Education Trust (THET).

4.3. Study Design

The CwPAMS App metrics were obtained from data collected by the Horizon Strategic Partners. These assessed the frequency of page hits, guide opens and the number of registered users and downloads. The pilot study was a cross-sectional survey with patients and healthcare workers in one of the hospital sites, six months after the introduction of the App using questionnaires adapted from Panesar et al. [6]. Patients' questionnaires comprised of four sections with eight questions using a Likert scale and multiple-choice questions. The first section comprised of demographics including age, gender, highest education qualification and occupation. The second section assessed patients' attitudes to health professionals' use of smart phone mobile apps in healthcare delivery. The third section was designed to obtain patients' concerns about the use of these smart phone apps, while the last section requested patients' preferences for health professionals reference ranging from a smart phone mobile app to a tablet, computer/laptop and a reference book. The health care workers' questionnaires comprised of nine sections with 15 questions designed as a Likert scale and open-ended questions. The first section obtained healthcare workers' demographics including country, specialty, year of graduation, grade, type of institution and profession and role. The eight sections following comprised of health professionals' attitudes to the use of the CwPAMS App and current practices.

4.4. Sample Size Determination/Sample Size and Sampling Technique

A convenience sample size determination of maximum 100 each was used for the cross-sectional study.

4.5. Procedure for Data Collection

4.5.1. CwPAMS App metrics

App metrics for user engagement evaluating the number of registered users, downloads, guide opens and page hits for various sections of the App from April 2019 to May 2020 were obtained through the MicroGuide platform. (http://www.microguide.eu).

4.5.2. Pilot Cross-Sectional Survey

Health Professionals Survey: Questionnaires were distributed among healthcare workers comprising of doctors, pharmacists, nurses and other healthcare workers at various points of care in the hospital including consulting rooms, nurses' station, pharmacy sections and wards. A total of 100 questionnaires were distributed to health professionals with 38 returned questionnaires completed anonymously.

Patients Survey: Patients' questionnaires were distributed to patients in the waiting room within the consulting area. Patients' questionnaires comprised of demographic data and questions regarding attitude to the use of smartphone apps among health professionals over a one-week period. Patients' consent was sought for before administration of the questionnaires. A total of 93 questionnaires were distributed to patients based on patients available in hospital during the study period. All 47 questionnaires (S4: Questionnaires) were completed anonymously with no personally identifiable information documented.

4.5.3. Study Approval

Study was conducted under service improvement as part of the CwPAMS project therefore no ethical approval was required but the Ghana Health Service and the Ghana AMR Platform were made aware of the pilot project.

4.6. Procedure for Data Analysis

Microsoft Excel 2013 was used to analyse the data obtained from the pilot study using descriptive statistics.

5. Conclusions

Our study provides insight into the overall perception of the use of mobile apps as a means to improve antimicrobial stewardship, demonstrating general acceptance among patients and healthcare professionals. In general, the patients and healthcare workers surveyed had a positive attitude following the introduction of the CwPAMS App as a fundamental resource for accessing information on antimicrobial prescribing. Hence, increased and more comprehensive use of all sections of the App could contribute to improved antimicrobial stewardship practices among healthcare workers and increased acceptance of the use of smartphone apps among patients. App downloads and utilization were found to be highest during partnership visits and App promotion, highlighting the need for more focused implementation and promotion of the App among all health professionals, especially doctors. Further studies will be useful in evaluating the impact of the App on antimicrobial prescribing as well as guide future Antimicrobial Stewardship interventions.

Supplementary Materials: The following are available online at http://www.mdpi.com/2079-6382/9/9/555/s1: S1: Launch Communications presentation, S2: AMS App–Commonwealth Pharmacists Association (CPA) Press Release https://commonwealthpharmacy.org/ams-app-cpa-press-release/, Video S1: Commonwealth Partnerships for Antimicrobial Stewardship App https://www.youtube.com/watch?v=MJ7fa_aLgCI, S3: App Launch Posters, S4: Questionnaires Healthcare workers and patients.

Author Contributions: Conceptualization, C.T. and D.A.-O.; Data curation, O.O., C.T., W.P.K., R.M., L.H., E.P.-Q., D.M.A. and D.A.-O.; Formal analysis, O.O.; Funding acquisition, D.A.-O.; Methodology, O.O., C.T., W.P.K., R.M., E.P.-Q. and D.A.-O.; Project administration, O.O.; Resources, D.A.-O.; Supervision, D.A.-O.; Writing—original draft, O.O.; Writing—review and editing, C.T., W.P.K., L.H., M.N., E.P.-Q., D.M.A. and D.A.-O. All authors have read and agreed to the published version of the manuscript.

Funding: This project was funded as part of the Commonwealth Partnerships on Antimicrobial Stewardship (CwPAMS) supported by Tropical Health and Education Trust (THET) and Commonwealth Pharmacists Association (CPA) using Official Development Assistance (ODA) funding, through the Department of Health and Social Care's Fleming Fund. The views expressed in this publication are those of the author(s) and not necessarily those of the NHS, the Fleming Fund, the Department of Health and Social Care, THET or CPA.

Acknowledgments: Charlotte Ashton, Communications and External Engagement Manager THET for design of launch materials and Comms for CwPAMS App launch. Victoria Rutter, Sarah Cavanagh, (Commonwealth Pharmacists Association), Richard Skone-James, Beatrice Waddingham, William Townsend (THET) for CwPAMS contributions.

Conflicts of Interest: The funders had no role in the design of the study; in the collection, analyses, or interpretation of data; in the writing of the manuscript, or in the decision to publish the results. MK and LH work at Horizon Strategic Partners who own and manage the Microguide app.

References

1. MacDougall, C.; Polk, R.E. Antimicrobial stewardship programs in health care systems. *Clin. Microbiol. Rev.* 2005, *18*, 638–656. [CrossRef] [PubMed]
2. Smith, C.; van Velthoven, M.H.; Truong, N.D.; Nam, N.H.; Anh, V.P.; AL-Ahdal, T.M.A.; Hassan, O.G.; Kouz, B.; Huy, N.T.; Brewster, M.; et al. How primary healthcare workers obtain information during consultations to aid safe prescribing in low-income and lower middle-income countries: A systematic review. *BMJ Glob. Health* 2020, *5*, e002094. [CrossRef] [PubMed]
3. Johns Hopkins ABX Guide App. Available online: http://www.unboundmedicine.com/products/johns_hopkins_abx_guide (accessed on 24 August 2015).
4. Payne, K.F.; Weeks, L.; Dunning, P. A mixed methods pilot study to investigate the impact of a hospital-specific iPhone application (iTreat) within a British junior doctor cohort. *Health Inform. J.* 2014, *20*, 59–73. [CrossRef] [PubMed]
5. Horizon Strategic Partners. MicroGuide. Available online: http://www.microguide.eu/ (accessed on 27 August 2020).
6. Panesar, P.; Jones, A.; Aldous, A.; Kranzer, K.; Halpin, E.; Fifer, H.; Macrae, B.; Curtis, C.; Pollara, G. Attitudes and behaviours to antimicrobial prescribing following introduction of a smartphone App. *PLoS ONE* 2016, *11*, e0154202. [CrossRef] [PubMed]
7. Tran, K.; Morra, D.; Lo, V.; Quan, S.D.; Abrams, H.; Wu, R.C. Medical students and personal smartphones in the clinical environment: The impact on confidentiality of personal health information and professionalism. *J. Med. Internet Res.* 2014, *16*, e132. [CrossRef] [PubMed]
8. Fox, S.; Duggan, M. Pew Research Center. Mobile Health 2012. Available online: https://www.pewresearch.org/internet/2012/11/08/mobile-health-2012/ (accessed on 7 May 2014).
9. Kamerow, D. Regulating medical apps: Which ones and how much? *BMJ* 2013, *347*, f6009. [CrossRef] [PubMed]
10. Illiger, K.; von Jan, U.; Albrecht, U.V. Professional use of mobile devices at a university medical center. *Biomed. Tech.* 2014, *59*, S691.
11. Morris, M.E.; Aguilera, A. Mobile, social, and wearable computing and the evolution of psychological practice. *Prof. Psychol. Res. Pract.* 2012, *43*, 622–626. [CrossRef] [PubMed]
12. Patrick, K.; Griswold, W.G.; Raab, F.; Intille, S.S. Health and the mobile phone. *Am. J. Prev. Med.* 2008, *35*, 177–181. [CrossRef] [PubMed]
13. Preziosa, A.; Grassi, A.; Gaggioli, A.; Riva, G. Therapeutic applications of the mobile phone. *Br. J. Guid. Counc.* 2009, *37*, 313–325. [CrossRef]
14. Lane, N.; Mohammod, M.; Lin, M.; Yang, X.; Lu, H.; Ali, S.; Doryab, A.; Berke, E.; Choudhury, T.; Campbell, A.T. BeWell: A smartphone application to monitor, model and promote wellbeing. In Proceedings of the 5th International Conference on Pervasive Computing Technologies for Healthcare, Dublin, Ireland, 23–26 May 2011.

15. Mascolo, C.; Musolesi, M.; Rentfrow, P.J. Mobile sensing for mass-scale behavioural intervention. In Proceedings of the NSF Workshop on Pervasive Computing at Scale (PeCS), University of Washington, Seattle, WA, USA, 27–28 January 2011.
16. Rachuri, K.K.; Musolesi, M.; Mascolo, C.; Rentfrow, P.J.; Longworth, C.; Aucinas, A. EmotionSense: A mobile phones based adaptive platform for experimental social psychology research. In Proceedings of the 12th ACM International Conference on Ubiquitous Computing, Copenhagen, Danmark, 26–29 September 2010; pp. 281–290.
17. Yardley, L. The potential of Internet-delivered behaviour change interventions. *Eur. Health Psychol.* **2011**, *13*, 40–43.
18. Temitope, F. mHealth in Africa: Challenges and opportunities. *Perspect. Public Health* **2014**, *134*, 14.
19. Gurmana, T.A.; Rubin, S.E.; Roess, A.A. Effectiveness of mHealth behavior change communication interventions in developing countries: A systematic review of the literature. *J. Health Commun.* **2012**, *17*, 82–104. [CrossRef] [PubMed]
20. Buhi, E.R.; Trudnak, T.E.; Martinasek, M.P.; Oberne, A.B.; Fuhrmann, H.J.; McDermott, R.J. Mobile phone-based behavioural interventions for health: A systematic review. *Health Educ. J.* **2013**, *72*, 564–583. [CrossRef]
21. Julian, S.; Christina, S. The Economics of eHealth and mHealth. *J. Health Commun.* **2012**, *17*, 73–81.
22. Access and Delivery Partnership. Updates-FDA Launches Med Safety App to Improve Health Care Delivery in Ghana. Available online: https://www.adphealth.org/news/66/FDA-launches-Med-Safety-App-to-improve-health-care-delivery-in-Ghana.html (accessed on 20 August 2020).
23. Chan, A.H.Y.; Rutter, V.; Ashiru-Oredope, D.; Tuck, C.; Babar, Z.-U.-D. Together we unite: The role of the Commonwealth in achieving universal health coverage through pharmaceutical care amidst the COVID-19 pandemic. *J. Pharm. Policy Pract.* **2020**, *13*, 13. [CrossRef] [PubMed]
24. mPedigree. Recent News-Kenya's e-Health Department has begun Piloting a System to Curb Fake Goods. Available online: https://mpedigree.com/news/kenyas-e-health-department-has-begun-piloting-a-system-to-curb-fake-goods-2/ (accessed on 20 August 2020).
25. Smith, A. Pew Research Center. Older Adults and Technology Use. Available online: https://www.pewresearch.org/internet/2014/04/03/older-adults-and-technology-use/ (accessed on 3 April 2020).
26. Wagner, N.; Hassanein, K.; Head, M. Computer use by older adults: A multi-disciplinary review. *Comput. Hum. Behav.* **2010**, *26*, 870–882. [CrossRef]
27. Wu, R.; Rossos, P.; Quan, S.; Reeves, S.; Lo, V.; Wong, B.; Cheung, M.; Morra, D. An evaluation of the use of smartphones to communicate between clinicians: A mixed-methods study. *J. Med. Internet Res.* **2011**, *13*, e59. [CrossRef] [PubMed]
28. Hsieh, C.; Yun, D.; Bhatia, A.C.; Hsu, J.T.; Ruiz de Luzuriaga, A.M. Patient perception on the usage of smartphones for medical photography and for reference in dermatology. *Dermatol. Surg.* **2015**, *41*, 149–154. [CrossRef] [PubMed]
29. Lester, R.; Haigh, K.; Wood, A.; MacPherson, E.E.; Maheswaran, H.; Bogue, P.; Hanger, S.; Kalizang'oma, A.; Srirathan, V.; Kulapani, D.; et al. Sustained reduction in third-generation cephalosporin usage in adult inpatients following introduction of an antimicrobial stewardship program in a large urban hospital in Malawi. *Clin. Infect. Dis.* **2020**. [CrossRef] [PubMed]

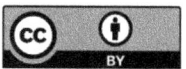

© 2020 by the authors. Licensee MDPI, Basel, Switzerland. This article is an open access article distributed under the terms and conditions of the Creative Commons Attribution (CC BY) license (http://creativecommons.org/licenses/by/4.0/).

MDPI
St. Alban-Anlage 66
4052 Basel
Switzerland
Tel. +41 61 683 77 34
Fax +41 61 302 89 18
www.mdpi.com

Antibiotics Editorial Office
E-mail: antibiotics@mdpi.com
www.mdpi.com/journal/antibiotics

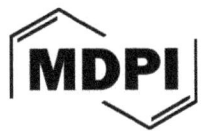

www.ingramcontent.com/pod-product-compliance
Lightning Source LLC
LaVergne TN
LVHW070239100526
838202LV00015B/2151